AF709741

The American Civil War Medical Series

Ira M. Rutkow, M.D., Dr.P.H.

1. John Ordronaux. *Hints on the Preservation of Health in Armies.* New York: 1861. BOUND WITH: Ordronaux. *Manual of Instructions for Military Surgeons.* New York: 1863.
2. Joseph Janvier Woodward. *The Hospital Steward's Manual.* Philadelphia: 1862.
3. Frank Hastings Hamilton. *A Practical Treatise on Fractures and Dislocations.* Philadelphia: 1860.
4. Francis Peyre Porcher. *Resources of the Southern Fields and Forests, Medical, Economical, and Agricultural.* Richmond: 1863.
5. William Alexander Hammond. *A Treatise on Hygiene.* Philadelphia: 1863.
6. Roberts Bartholow. *A Manual of Instructions for Enlisting and Discharging Soldiers.* Philadelphia: 1863.
7. Claude Bernard and Charles Huette. *Illustrated Manual of Operative Surgery and Surgical Anatomy.* Edited, with notes and additions . . . by William H. Van Buren and Charles E. Isaacs. New York: 1861.
8. Samuel Preston Moore. *Regulations of the C.S.A. Medical Department* IN: *Regulations for the Army of the Confederate States. Richmond:* 1862.
9. Charles Ravenscroft Greenleaf. *A Manual for the Medical Officers of the United States Army.* Philadelphia: 1864.
10. William Grace. *The Army Surgeon's Manual.* New York: 1864.
11. Joseph Janvier Woodward. *Outlines of the Chief Camp Diseases of the United States Armies.* Philadelphia: 1863.
12. *Confederate States Medical and Surgical Journal.* Richmond: January 1864 – February 1865.

A PRACTICAL TREATISE ON FRACTURES AND DISLOCATIONS

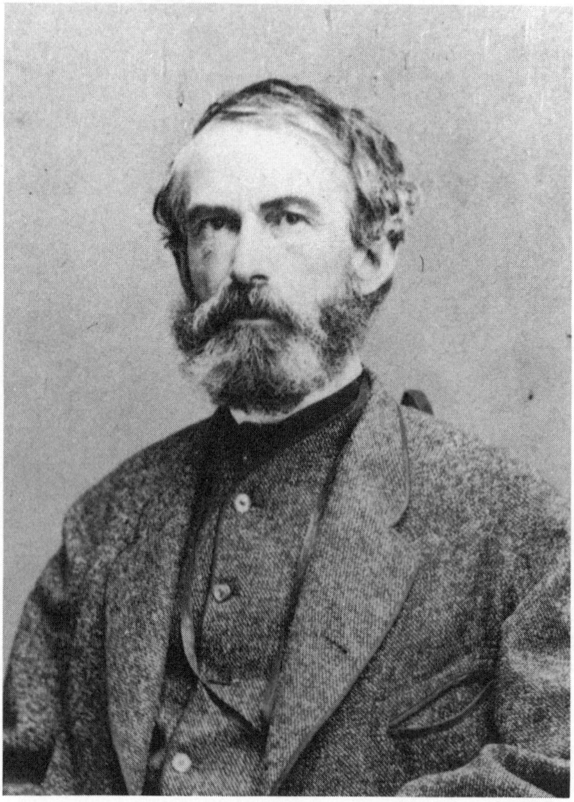

Frank Hastings Hamilton
1813–1886

National Library of Medicine

A PRACTICAL TREATISE ON FRACTURES AND DISLOCATIONS

by Frank Hastings Hamilton, M.D.

Reprinted with a Biographical Introduction
by Ira M. Rutkow, M.D., Dr.P.H.

Norman Publishing
San Francisco
1991

Copyright © 1991 by Norman Publishing

Published by Norman Publishing
720 Market Street
San Francisco, California 94102–2502

All rights reserved. No part of this publication may be reproduced, stored in a retrieval system, or transmitted, in any form or by any means, electronic, mechanical, photocopying, recording, or otherwise, without the prior written permission of the publishers, except in the case of brief quotations embodied in critical articles and reviews.

Library of Congress Cataloging-in-Publication Data

Hamilton, Frank Hastings, 1813–1886.
A practical treatise on fractures and dislocations / by Frank Hastings Hamilton ; reprinted with a biographical introduction by Ira. M. Rutkow.
p. cm. — (The American Civil War medical series ; 3)
Reprint. Originally published: Philadelphia ; Lea, 1860.
Includes index.
ISBN 0–930405–32–3 (alk. paper)
1. Fractures—Treatment. 2. Dislocations—Treatment. 3. United States—History—Civil War, 1861–1865—Medical care—Sources. 4. United States—History—Civil War, 1861-1865—Medical care—Sources. I. Title. II. Series.
[DNLM: 1. Dislocations—Treatment. 2. Dislocations—therapy. 3. Fractures —therapy. WEA H217p 1860a]
RD101.H22 1991
DNLM/DLC
for Library of Congress 90–14279
CIP

The American Civil War Medical Series, No. 3

This book was reproduced from the original edition loaned from the Francis A. Countway Library of Medicine, Boston.

This book is printed on acid-free paper, and its binding materials have been chosen for strength and durability.

Manufactured in the United States of America.

Frank Hastings Hamilton

Frank Hastings Hamilton was born in Wilmington, Vermont, on September 10, 1813, the second son of Calvin and Lucinda Hamilton. His parents were farmers and also owned the local stagecoach line. For unknown reasons his family moved to Schenectady, New York, in 1816, and there Hamilton attended the Lancasterian School and the Schenectady Academy. He was an exceptional student and at age fourteen entered the sophomore class of Union College. Union was the first nondenominational college in the United States and was considered one of the foremost institutions of higher education in nineteenth-century America. Its liberal arts curriculum was quite comprehensive, and there Hamilton developed an interest in the classics that was later reflected in his work.

Hamilton graduated from Union in 1830 and registered as a private student of medicine with John Morgan, who was physician-surgeon to the state prison in Auburn, New York. During his three years of study with Morgan, Hamilton's greatest interest was anatomy. He was able to pursue this avocation through numerous dissections of recently deceased prisoners. As a consequence of this research, he painted life-size oils of nearly every part of the human body. During 1831 Hamilton attended a full course of lectures at the Western

College of Physicians and Surgeons at Fairfield, New York. Although he received a license to practice medicine in 1833 from the Cayuga County Medical Censors, he decided instead to obtain a formal medical degree from the University of Pennsylvania. He completed this work and graduated in 1835.

Immediately following his graduation, Hamilton was appointed demonstrator of anatomy in the medical college at Fairfield. He continued this through the end of 1838, and then was promoted to professor of surgery in January 1839. Hamilton's reputation grew and nineteen months later, in August 1840, he was given the chair of surgery in the medical college at Geneva, New York. Hamilton remained at this institution for eight years, although he interrupted his work at Geneva for seven months in 1843–44 for travel and study in Europe. This European trip supplied literary materials for an extended diary, which soon appeared in installments in the *Buffalo Medical Journal.*

In 1846 Hamilton accepted appointments as professor of surgery at Buffalo Medical College and surgeon to the Buffalo Charity Hospital. He held his joint professorships at both Geneva and Buffalo for two years, resigning from the former in 1848 to attend more fully to his rapidly growing practice in Buffalo.

In Buffalo Hamilton became friends with Austin Flint, Sr. (1812–1886), and James Platt White (1811–1881). Together they founded a medical department within the University of Buffalo and Hamilton was named professor of surgery and the first dean of the medical faculty. His career in Buffalo blossomed. He soon became politically active in the profession and was elected president of the New York State Medical Society in 1855.

Hamilton remained in Buffalo until 1860, when he joined Flint in a newly organized faculty at the Long Island College Hospital in Brooklyn as professor of the principles and practice of surgery and as surgeon-in-chief. In May 1861 he was appointed professor of military surgery at the College. This was the first professorship of its kind established in the United States. Its development was closely related to the outbreak of the Civil War and the need for greater expertise in the management of traumatic war injuries. At the same time, Hamilton joined a group of physicians who helped found the Bellevue Hospital Medical College, where he was subsequently named professor of military surgery and fractures and dislocations.

Just prior to the commencement of hostilities, Hamilton entered the U.S. Army as surgeon to the Thirty-First Volunteer Infantry of New York, also known as the Montezuma Battalion. He did this not only for its patriotic allure but also with an earnest desire to gain greater practical insight into military surgery. While with the Thirty-First Regiment of the Army of the Potomac he was in charge of a field hospital during the first Battle of Bull Run (July 21, 1861). He remained with the regiment until September 1861. In August 1861 an examination was given by the Army Medical Corps to find men who could participate in the establishment of a new corps of brigade surgeons not attached to regiments. Of the 130 applicants, Hamilton ranked second in the examination. He was soon appointed brigade surgeon and by the end of the year medical director of General Franklin's Sixth Corps. In May 1862 Hamilton was transfered to General Keyes's Fourth Corps. That same year he helped organize the army's Central Park General Hospital in New York. In July 1863 Hamilton was selected as medical inspector of the U.S. Army with a rank of lieutenant-colonel. He was immediately reassigned to the Army of the Cumberland under General Rosecrans. Hamilton continued in active service up to September 10, 1863, when he resigned his commission. While in the army he participated in a number of field campaigns and was captured twice: first by a party of Texas Rangers in Tennessee and later by a Confederate unit in Kentucky. He was well treated by the Confederates, who released him in both cases after a short period of internment.

With a return to civilian life Hamilton resigned his appointment at the Long Island College Hospital but continued his professorial duties at Bellevue. After the retirement of James Rushmore Wood (1813–1882) in 1868, Hamilton assumed his position as professor of the practice of surgery, with operations, and of clinical surgery in Bellevue Hospital Medical College. He held this post until his resignation in March 1875. Subsequently, he continued in his position as one of the surgeons to Bellevue Hospital and conducted weekly surgical clinics.

Hamilton's professional career was notable for an influential body of written work. His major texts include a *Monograph on Strabismus, with Cases* (1845), *A Practical Treatise on Fractures and Dislocations* (1860), *A Practical Treatise on Military Surgery* (1861), *A Treatise on Military Surgery and Hygiene* (1865), *The Principles and Practice of Surgery* (1872), and *Fracture of the Patella: A Study of One Hundred and Twenty-Seven Cases* (1880). He also edited the massive two-volume *Surgical Memoirs of the War of the Rebellion: Collected and Published by the United States Sanitary Commission* (1870–71). Among Hamilton's most important journal articles were those on deformities after fractures [*Transac-*

tions of the American Medical Association 8(1855):349–443], and the earliest description of a crossleg pedicle flap as a treatment for chronic ulcer (termed elkoplasty or anaplasty) [*New York Journal of Medicine*, n.s., 13(1854): 163–73]. He also authored a short pamphlet entitled *Fracture Tables* (1853), which is a statistical study intended to be utilized in legal cases where an authoritative source is needed. Hamilton wrote about medical ethics in *Health Aphorisms and an Essay on the Struggle for Life Against Civilization, Luxury, and Aestheticism* (1882), and *Conversations Between Drs. Warren and Putnam on the Subject of Medical Ethics: With an Account of the Medical Empiricisms of Europe and America* (1884). Among his other literary contributions is the translation from the French of Alphonse-Auguste Amussat's *On the Employment of Water in Surgery* (1851), and a biography, *The Life and Character of Theodoric Romeyn Beck, M.D.* (1856), who, like Hamilton, was also a graduate of Union College (1807).

Hamilton's *Practical Treatise on Fractures and Dislocations* was initially available in a cloth cover for $4.25. Further editions were published in 1863, 1866, 1871, 1875, 1880, 1884, and 1891. The latter was revised by Stephen Smith (1823–1922), a well-known New York surgeon. The work was also translated into French and German and brought Hamilton his greatest fame within the profession. This was due to its being the first complete book written in English on the treatment of fractures and dislocations. The work grew out of Hamilton's previously authored pamphlet, *Fracture Tables*. This work is a collection of data on the results of the treatment of fractures that was assembled in an effort to provide physicians with information to use in defending malpractice actions. Patients in the United States in the nineteenth century were quite litigious, and most of the cases involved the results of the treatment of fractures and dislocations.

Hamilton is remembered eponymically for Hamilton's pseudophlegmon (a trophic affection of the subcutaneous connective tissue, marked by a circumscribed swelling that may become indurated and red but never suppurates), and for Hamilton's test (a rod that touches both the acromion process and the outer condyle of the humerus in axillary dislocation of the shoulder).

Always active in organized medicine, Hamilton was president of the New York Pathological Society (1866), the New York Medico-Legal Society (1876), the American Academy of Medicine (1878), and the New York Society of Medical Jurisprudence (1885). From 1880 to 1884 he was vice-president of the New York Academy of Medicine. In 1869 the trustees of Union College conferred upon him the degree of Doctor of Laws.

Shortly after the assassination attempt on President James Garfield (1831–1881), Hamilton was consulted by Mrs. Garfield. Garfield suffered a lingering septic course secondary to an abdominal gunshot wound. Hamilton remained a constant and conspicuous figure during the ordeal, remaining in attendance until Garfield died in Long Branch, New Jersey. Hamilton's candor in later joining in the publication of a report that criticized the poor quality of medical care that the president received and the repercussions of this report have become part of American surgical lore.

Hamilton had discriminating social and literary tastes. He assembled a large medical library, which was detailed in a 36-page catalogue published shortly after his death. The collection was eventually purchased by John B. Hamilton (1847–1898), no relation to Frank

Hastings. Hamilton's unique assemblage of surgical specimens was bequeathed to the United States Army Medical Museum.

Hamilton was married twice. His first wife was Mary Virginia (Van Arsdale) McMurran, whom he married in October 1834. They had one son, Theodore B. Hamilton. Mary Hamilton died on April 8, 1838, following a short illness. In September 1840, Hamilton married Mary Gertrude Hart. He had three children by his second wife, who died in July 1885. Their oldest child was Frank Hastings, Jr. (1841–1869), who followed in his father's medical footsteps but died prematurely. Only two of his children were alive at the time of his death, his son Theodore and daughter Mary, wife of Daniel Davis, a lawyer in New York.

In December 1885 Hamilton suffered severe and repeated pulmonary hemorrhage due to tuberculosis. For the next year and a half his health continued to deteriorate, and he died in his New York City home on 32d Street on August 11, 1886. Interment was at the Sleepy Hollow Cemetery in Tarrytown, New York.

A

PRACTICAL TREATISE

ON

FRACTURES AND DISLOCATIONS.

BY

FRANK HASTINGS HAMILTON, M. D.,

PROFESSOR OF SURGERY IN THE UNIVERSITY OF BUFFALO;
SURGEON TO THE BUFFALO HOSPITAL OF THE SISTERS OF CHARITY;
CONSULTING SURGEON TO THE BUFFALO GENERAL HOSPITAL, AND TO THE BUFFALO CITY DISPENSARY.

ILLUSTRATED WITH

TWO HUNDRED AND EIGHTY-NINE WOOD-CUTS.

PHILADELPHIA:
BLANCHARD AND LEA.
1860.

Entered according to the Act of Congress, in the year 1860, by
BLANCHARD AND LEA,
in the Office of the Clerk of the District Court of the United States in and for the Eastern District of Pennsylvania.

PHILADELPHIA:
COLLINS, PRINTER.

TO

VALENTINE MOTT, M. D.,

IN RECOGNITION OF HIS JUSTLY DISTINGUISHED REPUTATION AS A SURGEON,

AND IN

TESTIMONY OF PERSONAL ESTEEM,

This Volume

IS RESPECTFULLY DEDICATED

BY

THE AUTHOR.

PREFACE.

THE English language does not at this moment contain a single complete treatise on Fractures and Dislocations. The two small volumes of Desault, and the one of Boyer, issued near the close of the last century, and translated into English early in this, may perhaps properly enough have been regarded as complete treatises at the time of their publication, but they certainly cannot be so considered now. The several chapters on "*Diseases and Injuries of the Bones*," contained in the *Leçons Orales* of Dupuytren, translated in 1846, and the *Treatise on Fractures in the Vicinity of Joints, and on Certain Forms of Accidental and Congenital Dislocations*, by Robert Smith, are invaluable monographs, but neither of them claims to be anything more than a collection of occasional and miscellaneous papers. The writings of Amesbury and of Lonsdale relate only to fractures. Even the justly celebrated quarto of Sir Astley Cooper is no more than what its title plainly declares it to be, *A Treatise on Dislocations and on Fractures of the Joints;* but since the announcement of the present volume, a translation of Malgaigne's great and crowning work on Fractures and Dislocations has been commenced by Dr. Packard, of Philadelphia, and the first volume has been placed in the hands of the American profession. Should the remaining volume be rendered into English, the gap in our literature will be measurably filled.

Under these circumstances I might scarcely have thought it worth while to continue my labors, already so near their completion, had it not seemed to me that Malgaigne, whose researches have been truly marvellous, had failed in some measure to give a just representation of the observations and improvements which have been made from time to time by my own countrymen.

The contributions of American surgeons to this department had to be sought chiefly in medical journals, many of which have long been discontinued, and most of which were inaccessible to the great French writer. Even to an American, the labor of exhumation from archives hitherto almost unexplored has not been small; and it is probable that many valuable papers have been overlooked; indeed it is impossible that it should be otherwise.

I am free to say, also, that I have been encouraged by a hope that my own personal experience, obtained during many years of public and private service, might be of some value to my contemporaries.

Very little space has been devoted to what is now only historical, except so far as was necessary to correct certain time-consecrated errors, or to confirm and illustrate the practice of the present day; but, by a pretty full report of characteristic examples, selected from more than one thousand cases already published by myself, by copious references to the examples recorded by others, and by a careful exclusion of whatever has not been confirmed by experience or established by dissection, I have endeavored to make this treatise useful both to the student and practical man, and a reliable exponent of the present state of our art upon those subjects of which it treats.

In order to render the description of the various forms of apparatus employed in the treatment of fractures more intelligible, and to avoid the necessity of lengthened explanations, a large number of illustrations have been introduced, more, perhaps, than might be thought necessary, especially as in several instances the apparel which is figured is not that which is recommended by the author. It is believed, however, that by a study of the principal forms of approved dressings, the reader will be better prepared for the exigencies of practice; and that by the simultaneous presentation of those which are not approved, he will be saved from a wasteful expenditure of his time, in the contrivance of useless apparatus. It is not in the discovery and multiplication of mechanical expedients that the surgeon of this day declares his superiority, so much as in the skilful and judicious employment of those which are already invented.

The author desires to acknowledge his indebtedness to very many of his professional brethren, throughout the United States, for the promptness with which they have responded from time to time to his inquiries, and for the generosity with which they have opened their pathological collections and placed valuable specimens at his disposal.

He wishes also to express his special obligations to Dr. J. R. Lothrop, of this city, who has kindly aided him in revising most of the proof sheets as they have been issued from the press.

FRANK H. HAMILTON.

BUFFALO, N. Y., December, 1859.

CONTENTS.

PART I.

FRACTURES.

CHAPTER I.

CHAPTER II.

CHAPTER III.

CHAPTER IV.

CHAPTER V.

CHAPTER VI.

CHAPTER VII.

CHAPTER VIII.

CHAPTER IX.

CHAPTER X.

CHAPTER XI.

CHAPTER XII.

CHAPTER XIII.

CHAPTER XIV.

CHAPTER XV.

CHAPTER XVI.

CHAPTER XVII.

CHAPTER XVIII.

CHAPTER XIX.

CHAPTER XX.

CHAPTER XXI.

CHAPTER XXII.

CHAPTER XXIII.

CHAPTER XXIV.

CHAPTER XXV.

CHAPTER XXVI.

CHAPTER XXVII.

CHAPTER XXVIII.

CHAPTER XXIX.

CHAPTER XXX.

CHAPTER XXXI.

CHAPTER XXXII.

CHAPTER XXXIII.

CHAPTER XXXIV.

CHAPTER XXXV.

PART II.

DISLOCATIONS.

CHAPTER I.

CHAPTER II.

CHAPTER III.

CHAPTER IV.

CHAPTER V.

CHAPTER VI.

CHAPTER VII.

CHAPTER VIII.

CHAPTER IX.

CHAPTER X.

CHAPTER XI.

CHAPTER XII.

CHAPTER XIII.

CHAPTER XIV.

CHAPTER XV.

CHAPTER XVI.

CHAPTER XVII.

CHAPTER XVIII.

CHAPTER XIX.

CHAPTER XX.

CHAPTER XXI.

CHAPTER XXII.

CHAPTER XXIII.

CHAPTER XXIV.

CHAPTER XXV.

CHAPTER XXVI.

LIST OF ILLUSTRATIONS.

FRACTURES.

DISLOCATIONS.

PART I.

FRACTURES.

FRACTURES.

CHAPTER I.

GENERAL DIVISION OF FRACTURES.

FRACTURES are divided into Complete and Incomplete, Simple, Comminuted, Compound, and Complicated.

A "Complete" fracture is one in which the line of division completely traverses the bone.

An "Incomplete" fracture implies only a partial separation of the bone.

A "Simple" fracture is one in which the bone is broken at only one point. The term has no reference to the question of complications, but in its technical meaning, as employed by both English and American surgeons, it has reference only to the number of fragments into which the bone is broken. So that we may, without a paradox, say of a fracture that it is both simple and complicated, or simple and compound. It would be more correct, perhaps, to substitute the word "single" for "simple," as has been done by Malgaigne and some other French writers, but I fear that to American surgeons the substitution would be rather a source of confusion than otherwise.

A "Comminuted" fracture, called by Malgaigne "multiple," is a fracture in which the bone is broken at more than one point, and in which, consequently, the bone is divided into more than two fragments. It also is used in a technical sense, and by no means implies minute division or comminution of the fragments.

A "Compound" fracture is technically one in which there exists also an external wound communicating with the bone at the point of fracture. It may be either partial or complete, simple or comminuted, or even complicated, while at the same time it is also compound.

"Complicated" fractures are such as present additional complications, or complications for which no other specific term has been invented. Thus the fracture may be complicated with the lesion of an important bloodvessel or nerve, or with great contusion or laceration of the soft parts, with a dislocation, or with fractures of other bones, or even with some constitutional fault.

Fractures are also divided into Transverse, Oblique, and Longitudinal, according as the direction of the line of separation is at a right angle with the axis of the bone at the point of fracture, or as it deviates more or less from this direction. But a fracture is called transverse when it does not traverse the bone precisely at a right angle; indeed, we usually apply this term whenever the obliquity is only moderate, not exceeding, perhaps, fifteen or twenty degrees, or when, in the examination of a limb, although we are unable to detect the precise line of the fracture, we ascertain that, without being impacted or serrated, the ends of the bones continue to rest upon each other, or being replaced, do not spontaneously become displaced.

Longitudinal fractures occur generally in connection with oblique or transverse fractures; as when the lower end of the femur is split vertically into the socket, and the shaft of the bone is traversed horizontally by a fracture which intercepts the vertical or longitudinal fracture. The fracture of a condyle or of any projection from the body of the bone is called longitudinal if the direction of the line of fracture is parallel, or nearly so, to the axis of the shaft.

Fig. 1.

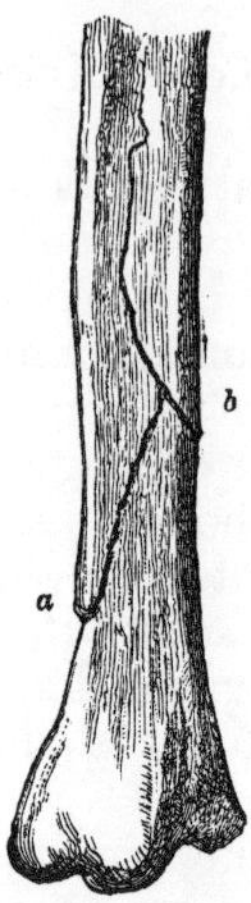

Longitudinal and oblique fracture.

Fig. 2.

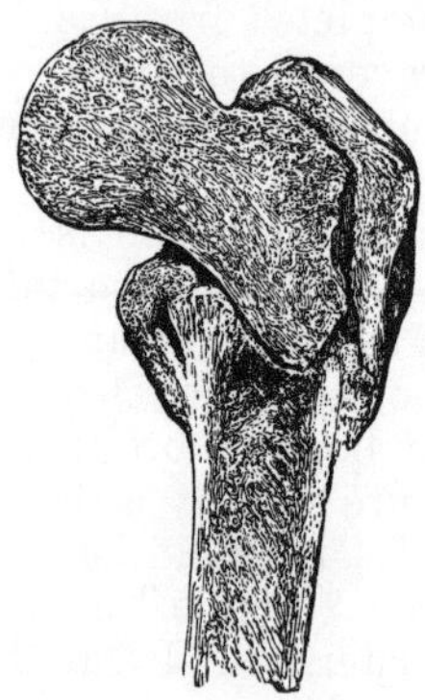

Impacted extra-capsular fracture of neck of femur.

A "Serrated" fracture is one in which the opposite surfaces denticulate, the elevations upon one fragment being reflected by corresponding depressions upon the other.

"Impacted" fractures are driven into each other, the lamellated structure of one fragment penetrating the cancellous structure of the other.

The French writers also occasionally speak of fractures *en rave*, or radish-like, and of fractures *en bec de flûte*, the latter being so called from a supposed resemblance to the mouth-piece of a clarionet; but we scarcely see the necessity of multiplying the divisions and encumbering our nomenclature by these fancied resemblances. For all useful purposes, the divisions above given are sufficient.

Epiphyseal separations we do not hesitate to class with fractures, and to submit them to the same rules of nomenclature.

CHAPTER II.

GENERAL ETIOLOGY OF FRACTURES.

THE causes of fractures may be considered as predisposing and exciting.

Predisposing Causes.—Partial fractures, with bending of the bones, are most frequent in infancy and childhood; but complete fractures occur most often during manhood; and if they are again less frequent in old age, it is because the exciting causes are less operative, since the fragility of the bones, as a general rule, increases with the age. It will be noticed, also, that somewhat in proportion as the bone is more brittle, its fracture will be more nearly transverse, so that very old persons have frequently what has been not inaptly termed the "pipe-stem fracture;" but we must except from this rule fractures occurring in children, which are also not unfrequently transverse, often denticulated or splintered, and but rarely oblique. In all of the intermediate periods of life, oblique fractures are by far the most common. Females are less liable to fractures than males, except in old age, when the law seems, in general, to be reversed. As to the season of the year, it has been generally observed by surgical writers, that fractures were more frequent in winter than in summer, and an explanation has been sought for in the greater rigidity of the muscles during the cold weather, and the greater liability to falls upon the ice and frozen ground. Some have affirmed that the bones themselves were more brittle; but aside from the improbability of this last explanation, it is really a matter of question whether fractures are actually any more frequent in the winter than in the summer. If, on the one hand, the rigidity of the muscles and falls upon slippery walks are active causes in the production of fractures in the one season, on the other hand, falls from buildings and accidents from a great variety of similar causes, are equally active agents in the other.

Mollities ossium, fragilitas ossium, rickets, cancer, tertiary lues, scrofula, gout, scurvy, mercurialization, and, in short, all of those diseases dependent upon vicious cachexiæ, more or less predispose to the occurrence of fractures. Inflammation of the periosteum, also, or of the bone itself, may predispose to fracture. It is said, moreover, that the bones of persons who have lain a long time in bed break easily.

Exciting Causes.—The exciting, determining, or immediate causes of fractures are of two kinds: mechanical violence and muscular action.

Of these two, mechanical or external violence is much the most frequent cause; and this violence may operate in two ways: by acting directly upon the bone at the point at which it separates, and then we say the fracture is "direct," or from "direct violence;" or by acting upon some point remote from the seat of fracture, and then we say the fracture is "indirect," or from a "counter stroke." When a person falls from a height, alighting upon his feet, and the leg or thigh is broken, the fracture is indirect; so also if the bone is broken by flexion or torsion. Even direct pressure upon one side of a long bone in a child may produce a partial fracture upon the opposite side, which is properly an indirect fracture; or a direct blow upon the trochanter major may occasion a counter fracture through the neck of the femur.

Fractures from muscular action occur most often in the patella, calcaneum, humerus, femur, tibia, and olecranon process of the ulna. These accidents imply generally some conditions of the bones themselves which predispose them to fracture; but I have seen one example of a fracture of the shaft of the femur in a large and perfectly healthy man, occasioned by a twist of the leg in rolling tenpins. I have also known the tibia and patella to break from natural muscular action in persons of uncommon vigor. Fractures sometimes occur in the violent contractions of the muscles during convulsions, and where no abnormal condition of the bones could be assumed to exist. Parker, of New York, relates a case of fracture of the humerus in a negro preacher, which occurred in the act of gesticulation; also, a fracture of the clavicle occasioned by striking a dog with a whip; in another case the humerus was broken in attempting to throw a peach; but the most singular case of all was a fracture of the humerus caused by an effort to extract a tooth.[1]

Nearly all of the cases of fractures occasioned by muscular contraction seen by me were transverse, or nearly so, indicating, perhaps, also, the existence of some unusual fragility; and most of these have been unattended with shortening, the ends of the bones not becoming completely displaced from each other. The example of fracture of the shaft of the femur just mentioned, was, however, an exception. The bone shortened to the extent of an inch or more, in consequence of overlapping, and in this position it has finally united.

Intra-uterine fractures are not yet fully explained, but it is probable that they, like extra-uterine fractures, may be ascribed sometimes to external violence, and at other times to simple muscular contraction, both perhaps acting upon bones already somewhat predisposed by a peculiar constitutional cachexy.

Lawrence Proudfoot, of New York, has related a case of compound fracture *in utero* occurring in the practice of Dr. Freeman, which was apparently caused by external violence. Mrs. F., æt. 38, always having enjoyed good health, during the sixth month of gestation, while attempting to pass through a very narrow passage, was severely pressed upon the abdomen, and immediately experienced a severe pain in that region, accompanied with nausea and faintness. The following day, uterine hemorrhage with pain, commenced; and these symptoms continued at intervals, in a form more or less severe, up to the period

[1] Parker, New York Journ. Med., July, 1852, p. 95.

of her delivery, which occurred at full time, and was perfectly natural. At birth, the right foot of the child, a female, was found to be much distorted, and in a condition of valgus with equinus, the outer side of the foot being laid against the side of the leg above the external malleolus. The tibia, also, of the same limb, near its middle, seemed to have been the seat of a compound fracture; the two ends of the bone having united at an angle slightly salient anteriorly, and the skin presenting over the point of fracture an old cicatrix. The soft tissues adjacent were considerably thickened. Seventeen months after birth, when the child was seen by Drs. Proudfoot, Van Buren, and Isaacs of New York, the foot, although much improved by the means employed by Dr. Freeman, was still considerably deformed in consequence of the contraction of the tendo-Achillis; on cutting which, the limb was found to be of the same length with the other.[1]

Dr. Aristide Rodrigue, of Hollidaysburg, Pa., has communicated a case of fracture with dislocation, which he ascribes to a similar cause. The woman, when about four months with child, fell on her left side, striking upon a board, and hurting herself severely. At the full period she was delivered of a well-grown male child. Its left humerus was found to be dislocated into the axilla, and both the radius and ulna of the same limb had been broken through their lower thirds, but were now united by bony callus at an angle of about 45°, and slightly overlapped. In all other respects the child was perfect. It does not appear that anything was done to the fracture, and the attempt to reduce the humerus was unsuccessful. Four years later Dr. R. saw the lad and found him strong and hearty, the dislocated humerus having grown nearly at the same rate with the opposite, but the forearm remained "short and deformed as at birth." The hand was of the same size as the hand of the sound limb.[2]

Devergie has given an account of a woman, who, when seven months with child, struck her abdomen against the corner of a table. Intense pain followed, lasting some time. She went her full period, however, and the child was then found to have a fracture of the left clavicle, the fragments being overlapped somewhat, and united in this position by a firm and large callus.[3] A woman also six months gone met with a similar accident, and at the full time she gave birth to a feeble child, having in one leg a separation of the shaft of the tibia from its lower epiphysis. The end of the shaft was necrosed and projected through a wound in the integument. This child died on the thirteenth day.[4]

Schubert reports the case of a female delivered before her term, of twins, one of whom was born with a fracture of the left thigh which had occurred *in utero;* the fractured bone had pierced the flesh, through which it projected more than an inch, and it was carious. The mother stated that about six weeks before the accouchement, during a movement of the fœtus, she had heard a noise like that

[1] Proudfoot, New York Journ. Med., Sept. 1846, p. 199.
[2] Rodrigue, Amer. Jour. Med. Sci., Jan. 1854, p. 272.
[3] Devergie, Rev. Méd., 1825.
[4] Malgaigne, from Archiv. Gén. de Méd., t. xvi. p. 288.

produced by breaking a stick, and from that moment she had felt pricking pains in her belly.[1] It is probable that in this instance the fracture was the result of a muscular action, although it is possible that it was occasioned by the thigh having become entangled between the legs of the twin.

In many other examples upon record, the explanation is plainly enough to be sought for in the abnormal condition of the bones. Monteggia saw in a newly born infant, twelve ununited fractures. Chaussier, who has published a memoir upon this subject, mentions two very extraordinary cases, in one of which the child presented forty-three fractures, and in the other, one hundred and twelve.[2] I myself was permitted to see, on the 29th of June, 1853, with Drs. Hawley and White, of this city, an infant only four days old, who was born at the full time, of a healthy mother, in whom nearly all of the long bones were separated and movable at their epiphyses, the motion being generally accompanied with a distinct crepitus. The bones were also much enlarged in their circumference; the bones of the forearm and the femur were greatly curved; the fontanelles unusually open, and the clavicles were entirely wanting. The child was of full size, but looked feeble. It died in a condition of marasmus six months after birth; at which time some degree of union had taken place at several of the points of separation, the limbs having been supported constantly with pasteboard splints and rollers.

I have also seen one example of complete separation of the tibia and fibula near the middle of the leg, which I was disposed to regard as defective development rather than as an instance of intra-uterine fracture; and a gentleman in Michigan has recently sent me an account of another, which I am inclined to think belongs to the same class of deformities, although he thought it might be a case of intra-uterine fracture.

Fractures occurring from violence inflicted upon the child by the accoucheur, or from contractions of the neck of the womb while the child is *in transitu*, are more common occurrences, and do not require a separate consideration. I shall mention several in connection with the various bones in which they have taken place; among which, one of the most interesting is that published by Dr. Jacob H. Vanderveer, of Long Branch, N. J. The mother came to bed on the 18th of January, 1847, after a labor of more than twelve hours. It was a foot presentation; the child weighed fourteen pounds, and was perfectly healthy, but one of the thighs had suffered a complete fracture, occasioned probably by the strong contractions of the cervix uteri. With careful splinting and bandaging, the bone was finally, but not without some difficulty, kept in position and made to unite, so that at the date of the report one would not discover that the bone had been broken, except by close inspection.[3]

[1] Amer. Jour. Med. Sci., May, 1828, p. 223; from Zeitsch. für Staatsarz von Henke, 7e. Erg. Heft., p. 311.

[2] Chaussier, Bullet. de la Faculté de Méd. de Paris, 1813, p. 301.

[3] Vanderveer, Amer. Journ. Med. Sci., May, 1847, p. 378.

CHAPTER III.

GENERAL SEMEIOLOGY AND DIAGNOSIS.

FRACTURES are liable to be confounded with contusions, and with various other local injuries, but most often with dislocations; and especially when the fracture has taken place near one of the articulations, is the differential diagnosis sometimes rendered exceedingly difficult. It is with particular reference, therefore, to the general points of distinction between fractures and dislocations, that I now propose to speak. The special signs or points of difference which belong to each individual case, will be considered in their proper places.

The most important general, or common signs of a fracture—and by "common" signs I mean those which are common to most fractures—are crepitus, mobility, and an inability on the part of the fragments to maintain their positions when reduced; indeed, in many cases, this constantly recurring displacement is due to the fact that the surgeon is unable to accomplish a complete reduction. While on the other hand, dislocations are almost as uniformly characterized by the absence of crepitus, by preternatural immobility, and by the fact that when reduced the bones do not usually require support to retain them in place, or indeed we may say, by the fact that they are generally reducible.

Let us study these phenomena a little more in detail.

Crepitus, occasioned by the chafing of the broken surfaces upon each other, when actually present, is almost positive evidence of the existence of a fracture. It is possible, however, to confound the chafing of engorged tendinous sheaths, or of inflamed joints upon which fibrinous effusions have occurred, or of emphysema even, for the true crepitus of a fracture; but to the experienced ear and well practised touch these sensations are seldom a source of error. The one is rough, crackling, or even clicking sometimes, while the other is more subdued, and imparts a more uniform sensation to the hand, and but rarely conveys an actual sound, unless the ear is directly applied or the stethoscope is employed. It is only when the crepitus is transmitted obscurely through a great mass of soft tissues, or sufficient time has elapsed for the ends of the fragments to become softened by inflammation, and partially covered with a plastic material, or when indeed a dislocation is actually coincident with the fracture, that the surgeon is left in doubt. Occasionally, also, the existence of caries or of necrosis, in connection with a dislocation, might lead to the supposition of a fracture; but the history of the case, aside from the remaining common signs, and the special symptoms hereafter to be enumerated, would prevent any possibility of error.

It must not be forgotten, moreover, that a fracture at one point may transmit the sensation of crepitus distinctly enough, but in such a direction, owing to the relations of other bones to the one broken, as to mislead the surgeon, and induce him to locate the fracture in the wrong bone. Several examples of this species of deception I shall hereafter have occasion to mention.

Valuable and important, as is crepitus in its relations to differential diagnosis, unfortunately it is not always present, and for reasons which must be plainly stated. First; we cannot, in a pretty large proportion of cases, bring the broken ends again into apposition. Whatever mere theorists may say to the contrary, and notwithstanding surgeons up to this time have rarely ventured to allude to this subject, the fact is so that we do not usually "set" broken bones. We do not, even at the first, bring them into complete apposition, unless it is as the exception. I speak of bones once completely displaced by overlapping, and these constitute the majority of examples which come under the surgeon's observation. Second; in transverse fractures of the patella, and in fractures of the olecranon and coronoid process of the ulna, of the coracoid and acromion process of the scapula, and in all similar detachments of processes and apophyses, the action of the muscles by displacing the fragments prevents crepitus from being readily produced. Third; in a few cases, such as certain fractures of the neck of the femur, of the neck and head of the humerus, &c., the broken ends are impacted, or so driven into each other as to forbid the production of motion and crepitus; or they may be simply denticulated, and the consequences, so far as crepitus is concerned, will be the same.

Finally, in very many incomplete fractures, crepitus does not exist, and even when it is present the sensation is feeble, or very much modified, sometimes resembling the chafing of lymph, and at other times giving only a faint and single click.

Preternatural mobility, less valuable as a means of diagnosis than crepitus, is nevertheless more constantly present, being never absent, in some degree, in all complete, non-impacted, and non-denticulated fractures; but its presence does not, like crepitus, render the existence of a fracture quite certain. Whenever the bony lesion takes place in the vicinity of a joint, it may be difficult or impossible to determine whether the mobility of the limb is due to motion in the joint or to motion at the supposed seat of fracture. While, on the other hand, the preternatural immobility so generally observed in dislocations, may give place to preternatural mobility, as when the ligaments and tendons surrounding the joint are extensively torn, or the system itself is laboring under the shock of the accident, or when from any other cause there exists great general prostration.

As to the third common sign mentioned, namely, that in the case of fractures the bones do not generally support themselves, but demand for this purpose the interposition of splints, bandages, and even of extending and counter-extending forces, its authority rests upon the same evidence as does the assertion already made that bones once separated entirely, cannot generally be "set," that is, placed again end to end in such a manner as to be made effectually to support each other. It rests upon the evidence of my own personal experience; to which I am permitted to add, also, the personal experience of Malgaigne, who, with a frankness which does him great credit, and which, I am sorry to say, has hitherto found few imitators, remarks: "Second. That overlapping is the most stubborn of all. Here I will add a disagreeable truth, which classical authors have kept too much out of sight, namely, that it is so stubborn that in an immense majority of cases the efforts of art are unable to overcome it."[1] And it must be observed further, that if we shall often find it possible to bring the broken surfaces sufficiently into contact to develop crepitus, they may still be unable to maintain themselves in this position, owing to the obliquity of the line of fracture.

The other common signs of fracture may be briefly stated. Pain at the seat of fracture; swelling; ecchymosis; deformity, produced by either an angular, transverse, or rotary displacement of the fragments, and which is much more often due to the direction and force of the impulse which occasioned the fracture than to the action of the muscles; separation of the fragments, as in fractures of the patella and olecranon process; and inability to move the limb, a phenomenon due in part to the breaking of the bony lever upon which the muscles acted, and in part to the intense pain caused by any such attempts. This latter symptom is, however, often entirely absent. It is not generally present in impacted fractures, in serrated and partial fractures, or in many other fractures in which the periosteum has not yet completely given way.

Velpeau was the first, I think, to call attention to the fact that patients with broken clavicles could very generally raise the arm above the shoulder and even to the head, and I have repeatedly verified the observation, notwithstanding the separation of the fragments has been complete, and the overlapping considerable. In fractures of the neck of the femur and of the tibia it is no uncommon thing for the patient to walk some distance after the receipt of the injury.

I cannot dismiss this subject without calling attention to the necessity of exercising care and gentleness as well as skill in the examination of broken limbs. Nothing, in my opinion, betrays a lack of judgment as well as of common humanity on the part of the surgeon, so much as a rude and reckless handling of a limb already pricked and goaded into spasms by the sharp points of a broken bone. It is not enough to say that such rough manipulation is generally unnecessary, it is positively mischievous, provoking the muscles to more violent contractions; increasing the displacement which already exists, and not unfrequently producing a complete separation of impacted, denticulated, transverse, or partial fractures, which can never afterwards be wholly remedied; augmenting the pain and inflammation, and not unfrequently, I have no doubt, determining the occurrence of suppuration, gangrene, and death.

In proceeding to establish the diagnosis in any case, the surgeon should sit down quietly and patiently by the sufferer, so as to inspire

[1] Malgaigne, Traité des Fractures et des Luxations, Paris ed., t. i. p. 102.

in him from the first a confidence that he is not to be hurt, at least unnecessarily. He ought then to inquire of him minutely as to all the circumstances immediately relating to the accident, in order that he may determine as nearly as possible its cause, which alone, to the experienced surgeon, often affords presumptive, if not conclusive evidence as to the nature and precise point of the injury. From this, he should proceed to examine the disabled limb; removing the clothes with the utmost care by cutting them away rather than by pulling; and, when completely exposed, he should notice with his eye its position, its contour, the points of abrasion, discoloration, or of swelling; and not until he has exhausted all these sources of information, ought the surgeon to resort to the harsher means of touch and manipulation. Nor will his sensations guide him to the point of fracture by any other method so accurately as when, the patient being composed and his muscles at rest, he moves his fingers lightly along the surface of the limb, pressing here and there a little more firmly, according as a trifling indentation or elevation may lead him to suspect this or that to be the point of fracture. If the skin is more than usually tender, a few drops of sweet oil or of fresh lard laid upon its surface, or even moistening the skin with tepid water, will render this examination less painful, whilst it will facilitate the diagnosis, by rendering the tactile sensation somewhat more acute.

The limb, in case of a supposed fracture of a long bone, may now be measured with a tape line, and compared with the opposite limb, having first marked with a soft pencil or with ink the several points from which the measurements are to be made.

Finally, if any doubt remains, the limb must be firmly but steadily held while the necessary manipulations are performed, for the purpose of ascertaining the existence of mobility and of crepitus. Mobility is most easily determined by giving to the limb a lateral motion, but in general, crepitus is most effectually developed by gentle rotation. If the place of fracture is already pretty well declared by the previous examinations, the surgeon should place one finger over the suspected point, during this manipulation, by which means the crepitus will be more certainly recognized.

I do not often find it necessary to resort to anæsthetics for the purpose of insuring quietude and annihilating pain in making these examinations, since it is seldom that the patient need to be much disturbed; but if the examination is not satisfactory, and the diagnosis is important, I do not hesitate to render the patient completely insensible, after which the questions in doubt may be more thoroughly investigated and perhaps definitively settled.

It is scarcely necessary to say that the earlier the examination is entered upon, the more readily will the diagnosis be made out; and if, unfortunately, some time has already elapsed before the patient is seen by the surgeon, and much swelling has taken place, the examination is still not to be omitted, and whatever doubts remain we must endeavor to remove by repeated examinations made from day to day until the subsidence of the tumefaction has brought the surfaces of the bone again within the reach of our observation.

CHAPTER IV.

REPAIR OF BROKEN BONES.

It is not my intention to enter very fully into a consideration of the process of repair in fractures, preferring to leave this subject where it more properly belongs, to the general treatises on surgical pathology. And especially am I disinclined to this topic, because of the discrepancy of opinion which has all along existed upon many of the points involved, and which differences still continue to exist, even among the best informed pathologists, and to the final settlement of which I confess I have not brought, except perhaps in relation to one single point, any new observations or labors.

I only propose to state very briefly a few practical, and I trust I may now say, pretty well established facts, such as the manner or position in which this reparative material, whenever it is employed, is applied to the broken bones, the length of time which is usually required for the completion of the process of repair, and the causes which may impede or prevent bony union.

If I think it necessary to say anything more upon this subject, it will be simply to announce my belief that the reparative material, consisting originally of a plastic lymph, is poured out from the vessels of the medullary membrane, the periosteum, the broken ends of the bone, and more or less from all of the lacerated tissues which are immediately adjacent to the seat of fracture; that after a period, longer or shorter, this lymph becomes organized, and begins to receive from the same sources particles of bony matter, through which the consolidation is finally effected; that the transition from the original plastic material to bone is almost constantly through the interposition of a fibrous tissue, rarely, unless in the case of children, through a cartilaginous tissue, and sometimes through both consentaneously or consecutively; that in a few fortunate examples bones unite directly or immediately, without the intervention of a reparative material, and finally, that granulations, or inflammatory exudations become transformed into bone, or perhaps we are only authorized to say that they immediately precede ossification, in certain cases of compound fractures, or of fractures in which the process of inflammation exceeds certain limits.

This last proposition, in reference to the agency of granulations in the production of callus, or their mutual pathological relations, is at the present more in debate than either of the others; but, with this exception, it will be seen that I have carefully avoided all of those points upon which the observations and opinions of pathologists are still greatly at variance.

Dupuytren, enlarging upon the doctrines taught by Galen, Duhamel, Camper, and Haller, declared that "nature never accomplishes the immediate union of a fracture save by the formation of two successive deposits of callus;" one of which is derived from the periosteum and from the adjacent tissues, and from the medulla; while the other, derived, perhaps, from the broken extremities of the bone itself, is found at a later period directly interposed between these surfaces. The material or callus derived from the tissues outside of the bone, and which Galen compared to a ferule, but which Mr. Paget calls "ensheathing," together with the material derived from the medulla, compared often to a plug, and by Mr. Paget named "interior" callus, is by Dupuytren spoken of as the "provisional," or temporary callus; by which the fragments are supported, and maintained in contact until the permanent callus is formed. This temporary splint is completed, or has arrived at the condition of bone in a spongy form at periods varying from twenty to sixty days; but it does not assume the character of compact bone until a period varying from fifty days to six months have elapsed; after which it is gradually removed by absorption. The second process, by which the ends of the bone are definitively or permanently united, commences when the provisional callus has arrived at the stage of spongy bone, and is not completed usually within less than eight, ten, or twelve months, "when," says Dupuytren, "it acquires a solidity greater than the original bone."

While it is certain that this eminent surgeon and most accurate observer has described faithfully the various phenomena which usually accompany the repair of bones in those animals which were the subjects of his experiments, and that his conclusions have a certain degree of application to the human species, it is equally certain that he erred in assuming that in man simple fractures always unite by this double process; yet, such is the power of authority, these doctrines were accepted from the first without hesitation or debate, and for nearly half a century they have occupied the minds of surgeons to the almost complete exclusion of every other theory. Mr. Stanley was among the first to question the solidity of the doctrines of Dupuytren, but it remained for Mr. Paget to fully expose their many fallacies; nor has Malgaigne, although not strictly a disciple of Paget, failed to detect certain of these errors.

I should also do injustice to myself were I not to mention that at the very moment when Mr. Paget was making his observations upon the specimens in "the large collection of fractures in the museum of the University College," I was myself employed in similar researches both among cabinet specimens and in the hospitals of this country and of Europe; and that the conclusions to which I had arrived were nearly identical with, although the inferences were far from being so complete in their detail, as those to which this distinguished pathologist was himself brought.[1] I do not, however, wish to make Mr. Paget responsible for any of the opinions upon this subject which I shall

[1] Paper on "Provisional Callus," by Frank H. Hamilton. Buffalo Medical Journal, Feb. 1853.

hereafter express, except so far as they may be found to agree with his own published views.[1]

I think it may now be fairly stated that the repair of bones by the double process described by Dupuytren, is, in man, only an exception to a very general rule; and that fractures unite by the following modes:—

First. Immediately, or in the same manner that the soft tissues sometimes unite, by the direct reunion of the broken surfaces, and without the interposition of any reparative material. This happens not unfrequently in the spongy bones, and in the extremities or spongy portions of the long bones, especially when one portion of bone is driven into another and becomes impacted; as in certain fractures of the neck of the humerus or of the femur.

Second. By interposition of a reparative material between the broken ends; as when the fragments remain in exact apposition, but immediate union fails. This is especially apt to occur in superficial bones, such as the tibia; or upon those sides of the bone which are most superficial. It is not an unusual circumstance to find the shaft of the tibia during the process of union presenting no exterior callus upon its anterior and inner surface, whilst the posterior and outer section of its circumference is covered with an abundant deposit. In other cases, however, of fractures of the shaft as well as of the epiphyses, the intermediate callus secures a prompt union, but no ensheathing callus is ever formed.

Third. Bones broken and not separated, unite occasionally by the process described by Dupuytren, namely, by the formation, first, of an ensheathing callus, whilst at the same moment the cylindrical cavity becomes closed by a spongy plug or a compact septum of bone; and second, by definitive callus deposited between the broken ends. It is probable that this happens generally in children, and it is a common mode of union in the ribs, which bones, during the whole progress of the case, are necessarily kept in motion. My cabinet furnishes many illustrations of ensheathing callus in ribs; and also a few in fractures of the tibia and fibula.

Fourth. Under similar circumstances, where no displacement exists, the fracture may unite by ensheathing and interior callus alone, no intermediate callus ever being formed between the broken ends; in which case it may be properly said that the bone itself has never united, and the ensheathing callus instead of being provisional is permanent or definitive. This was essentially the doctrine of Galen, Haller, and Duhamel before Dupuytren added his "fifth period," or the formation of definitive callus; and by these older surgeons it was held to be of universal application, except perhaps in the case of children. To this doctrine also Malgaigne has returned—at least to the question "Is there always a definitive callus, or complete union of the fragments?" he has made this laconic reply: "Galen admitted its occurrence, but only in young subjects; it has been obtained in animals, where there had been no displacement. I would willingly believe that such is

[1] Lectures on Surgical Pathology, by James Paget, Phila. ed., 1854, Chapter XI.

sometimes the case in human adults; but I must confess I have seen only the instance above cited, which might just as well be used to prove the compact ossification of the provisional callus." He accepts it, therefore, as not only an occasional mode of union, but as the most common mode; and in support of this extreme view he finds that the exterior callus, which Dupuytren called provisional or temporary, is actually permanent unless removed by the absorption consequent upon pressure.

To all of which we can only say that an examination of five or six specimens in our own cabinet, after having carefully divided them with a saw, has furnished only one illustration of union by ensheathing and interior callus alone. In each of the other specimens the union was completed by definitive or intermediate callus. We cannot, therefore, avoid the conclusion that Malgaigne has been deceived as to the relative frequency of these different modes of union, and that union without intermediate callus is exceptional.

Fifth. When bones are broken and overlap, they may unite by the interposition of a callus between the opposing surfaces, that is, by an

Fig. 3.

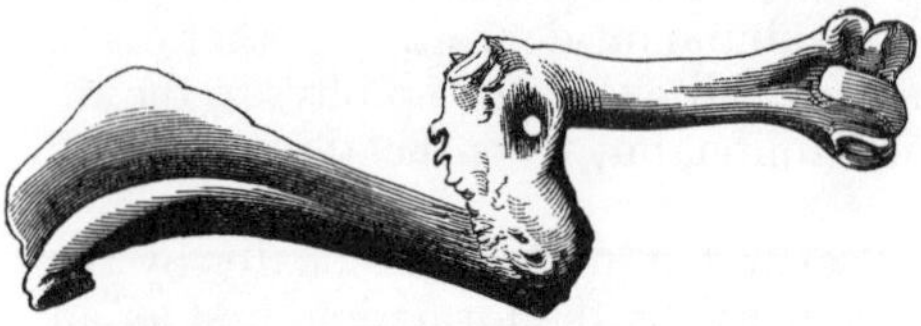

Fracture of the thigh of a turkey; united with the fragments widely separated. From a specimen in the author's cabinet.

Fig. 4.

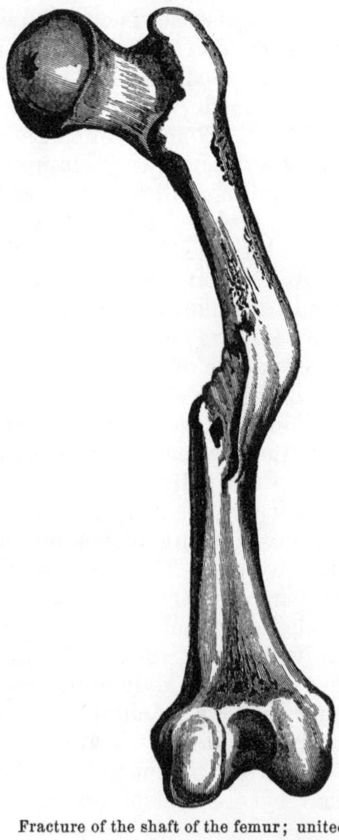

Fracture of the shaft of the femur; united with an oblique callus. From a specimen in the author's cabinet.

intermediate callus, but which will differ from that described as the second method, inasmuch as the new material will be deposited upon the sides of the fragments and not upon their extremities. The limb being kept perfectly at rest, and all other circumstances proving favorable, this union may take place without any excess or irregularity in the deposit. The surfaces will unite firmly where they are in actual contact, and smooth and well-formed buttresses will fill up all the spaces between the bones where they are not in actual contact sufficient generally to give the requisite strength to this new bond of union. This mode of union will be completed sometimes when the two ends of the bones are separated laterally an inch or more from each other. I have in my collection the bone of a turkey's thigh thus united by a transverse bony shaft, although separated more than one inch, and what is less common, I possess also a specimen of the human adult thigh in which an oblique shaft of solid callus has, after many months, and while no splints were employed, bound together firmly the two opposite extremities of the broken bone.

Sixth, the fragments being overlapped more or less, and suffering unusual disturbance, or the adjacent tissues having been much torn, or much blood being effused so that considerable inflammation is caused, the amount of callus will exceed what is necessary for the complete union of the bones; and this redundancy may be deposited around and upon the broken ends of the bones, or anywhere in their immediate vicinity, in layers, or in masses of irregular shape and size. Even the bones which are not broken, but which are near, as in the case of the fibula, after a fracture of the tibia, may become inflamed, or their coverings may inflame, and they may also contribute to the general mass of bony callus.

Compound fractures, or rather, we ought to say, fractures accompanied with granulations and suppuration, obey no uniform law of repair, so far as the manner and position of the deposit is concerned; but they come together finally with more or less irregular distributions of ossified matter, according to the varying circumstances of imperfect coaptation, mobility, &c., in which they may chance to be placed. Occasionally the amount of callus is less than occurs in simple fractures, and at other times the excess is very great.

In short, we conclude that fractures of adult human bones, whether placed end to end or overlapped, unite most naturally and most promptly either immediately or mediately, and in the same manner that soft tissues unite; that is to say, without the interposition of any reparative material, or through the medium of an intermediate, permanent callus; and that all deviations from these simple methods are accidental, or the result of disturbing influences.

That was, no doubt, a beautiful thought, which ascribed the formation of provisional callus to an intelligent efficient cause, which in this manner sought to support the fragments until a reunion of their divided ends was accomplished; nor would the beauty of the conception be marred by ascribing to it a more limited application, and invoking its interference only when the ordinary resources of nature had failed. We no longer hold that such intelligent interposition is necessary in the first instance, but that if demanded at all it is only for an exigency; and we have grave doubts whether nature ever allows any interference with her laws even in an exigency, unless by the substitution of a miracle. Provisional callus is just as much the necessary result of natural laws, as is definitive. It is formed because in that condition of the parts and of the general life its formation was inevitable. Whether useful for the purposes of repair or not, it will under certain circumstances exist. In the repair of certain fractures, provisional callus, it is conceded, seldom occurs. Thus it is with the cranium, the acromion, coracoid and olecranon processes, the patella, and with all those portions of bones which are immediately invested with a synovial capsule. Will it be affirmed that in the examples just named this callus is not formed because it is not required? To us it seems that nowhere could it prove more useful, since, with the single exception of the cranium, it is in these very cases that the obstacles to a reunion are the most serious. In fractures of the patella, olecranon, &c., the action of the muscles tends constantly and powerfully to displace the fragments, and gladly would the surgeon avail himself of the assistance of a temporary callus, but it is rarely present, at least in any useful degree. So also in fractures of the neck of the femur within the capsule, and in other similar cases, we cannot say that temporary callus would not be advantageous in facilitating the retention of the fragments, yet the "intelligent efficient agent" neglects to furnish it.

The only satisfactory reason which, as we think, can be assigned for the absence of callus in these cases, is found in the doctrines we now advocate; that is to say, it is usually absent because that amount of excitement and irritation is usually absent which alone determines its formation. In the case of the olecranon, patella, &c., the fragments being separated from each other by muscular action, so that no painful pinchings or chafings occur and their rough surfaces or sharp points being rather drawn away from than protruded into the flesh, no sufficient provocation exists for the production of inflammation and effusion. Hence the failure of provisional callus, but wherever the fracture occurs, and however moderate the action, definitive callus does not fail, still the broken surfaces of the patella and olecranon are softened, and smoothed, and covered over with a new matter, which, if contact could have been secured and preserved, would certainly have served to consolidate and repair the breach. The natural reparative process proceeds, but only the accidental process is omitted. This latter, however, is seen again even here, when from other and unusual causes a sur-excitement is established.

Temporary callus is not formed upon bones invested with synovial membranes, because here, too, as in the neck of the femur, there are not so many structures lacerated and irritated, and the supply of this effusion must be the less not only in proportion to the less intensity of the inflammation, but also to the less amount of structures implicated.

Possibly other and more satisfactory reasons may be assigned why provisional callus is not formed usually when the neck of the femur is broken within the capsule; but we certainly can never admit the common, and as here applied, the too palpably absurd explanation, that it is not wanted. It is wanted, and in no case so much as in the one now supposed.

Provisional callus has, therefore, no final purpose, but is the unavoidable result of certain abnormal conditions. It still occurs everywhere when against and in the vicinity of the bone there is the requisite lesion and action, and it will occur as certainly when there is no fracture at all, but only a caries, a necrosis, or a simple bony or periosteal inflammation; and whilst it is doubtless true that in fractures it sometimes renders valuable aid to the surgeon, it is equally true that it often proves a source of hindrance.

From these remarks I choose to except fractures occurring in children, in relation to which the observations are not yet sufficiently numerous to determine absolutely the laws of repair. If, however, I was to venture an opinion based upon a few examinations, I should say that in children we may accept with but little qualification the doctrine of Dupuytren as already explained.

Dupuytren, in determining the limits of his "third" period, or of that in which a provisional callus is formed of sufficient strength to support the fragments, has given what has been usually quoted as the natural period within which bones may be said to be united, that is, "from the twentieth or twenty-fifth day, to the thirtieth, fortieth, or sixtieth." But this depends so much upon the age of the patient, his general condition of health, the condition and position of the broken ends, as well as upon the bone itself, and the point at which it is broken, with many other circumstances, that it would be unsafe to establish any absolute laws in reference to this point.

In very early infancy, union is accomplished in half the time required in adult life, and it is generally thought to be still more retarded in advanced age, but Malgaigne has not found this latter observation confirmed by his own experience. Various constitutional causes, as we shall hereafter explain more fully, retard bony union. Motion, also, sometimes delays consolidation: fragments which are overlapped do not unite as speedily as those which are placed end to end, and other complications interfere in a similar manner, such as lesions of nerves, of bloodvessels, comminution of the bone, &c. It is affirmed, moreover, that in general the bones of the lower extremities, independently of their size, unite more slowly than the bones of the upper extremities.

For a more complete consideration of the causes which retard the union of bones, I beg to refer the reader to the chapter on "Delayed and Non-Union of Bones."

CHAPTER V.

GENERAL TREATMENT OF FRACTURES.

ALL that has been said in relation to the propriety of handling a broken limb gently when the surgeon is examining the position and character of the fracture, is equally applicable to the lifting and transporting of the patient to his bed, to the removal of the clothing, and to the general management of the limb before it is dressed. Rude or awkward manipulations, by which needless pain is inflicted, are not simply acts of wanton cruelty, but they are sources, and I think I may say frequent sources, of inflammation, suppuration, and gangrene. Here, as in all the subsequent handlings, everything should be done slowly, thoughtfully, and systematically. Yet it is difficult to state the precise manner in which the surgeon ought to proceed. Much will depend upon the circumstances of the case, something upon one's natural tact, and upon the amount of experience, but more, I think, upon natural kindness of heart, and social education. The man of refinement and sensibility will know instinctively how to proceed, and needs no instruction. They who lack these qualities can never learn, and it would be quite useless to undertake to teach them. I sincerely wish such men as these latter would find some more suitable employment than the practice of a humane art.

Nearly all fractures present three principal indications of treatment, namely, to restore the fragments to place as completely as possible, to maintain them in place, and to prevent or to control inflammation, spasms, and other accidents.

It ought to be regarded as a rule, liable only to rare exceptions, that broken bones should be restored to place, or to the position in which we hope to maintain them, as soon as possible after the occurrence of the accident. If the patient is seen within the first few hours, or before much swelling has taken place, we scarcely know the circumstance which would warrant an omission to adjust the fragments either end to end or side by side, as the one or the other might be found to be practicable. We have before sufficiently explained the general impossibility of again restoring to place, end to end, and fibre to fibre, fragments which have been made to override. We are therefore in no danger of being understood to say that bones should in all cases be immediately "set," in the popular sense of this term. They ought to be "set," no doubt, if this can be accomplished through the application of a prudent amount of force; but if they cannot be thus placed end to end, they may at least be laid in such a manner side by side as to restore, in some measure, the natural axis of the limb, and prevent the points of the bone from pressing unnecessarily into the flesh.

Experience has indeed furnished us with four or five very good reasons why broken bones should be reduced as soon as possible. When the injury is recent, the muscles offer less resistance; their resistance being increased after a time not only by the reaction which ensues upon the shock, but also by actual adhesion between their fibres; effusions distend both the muscles and the skin, and compel the limb to shorten; the constant goading of the flesh by the sharp points of the broken bones increases the muscular contractions; the patient will submit readily to manipulation and extension at first, but after the lapse of a few days, it is very seldom that he will permit the limb to be in any manner disturbed, even if he is assured that his refusal entails upon him a great deformity. If it is true that no callus or bony structure is deposited earlier than the seventh or tenth day, it is also true that the renewed attempt to adjust the bones at this period, by chafing and tearing again the tissues, reduces the fracture, in some degree, to the same condition in which it was at the first, and, consequently, the time which has elapsed, or, at least, a portion of it, may be regarded as lost.

We cannot, therefore, understand the argument by which Bromfield, South, and a few other surgeons have persuaded themselves that reduction should never be attempted before the third or fourth day; nor, indeed, do we fully appreciate the refinement which Malgaigne has given to this question in itself so simple. To affirm that we ought not to reduce the bones to their original positions during the period of intense inflammation, or of great swelling, or while the muscles are acting spasmodically, is only to affirm that we may not do what is impossible; and the attempt to do which, therefore, can only be mischievous; but to authorize their restoration to a better position, by such manipulation, extension, and lateral support as they may comfortably bear, is warrantable under any circumstances. The practice is not only defensible but imperative, and we do not think any really sound and practical surgeon ever intended to teach the contrary. We say still, if bones can be easily reduced, or the position

Fig. 5.

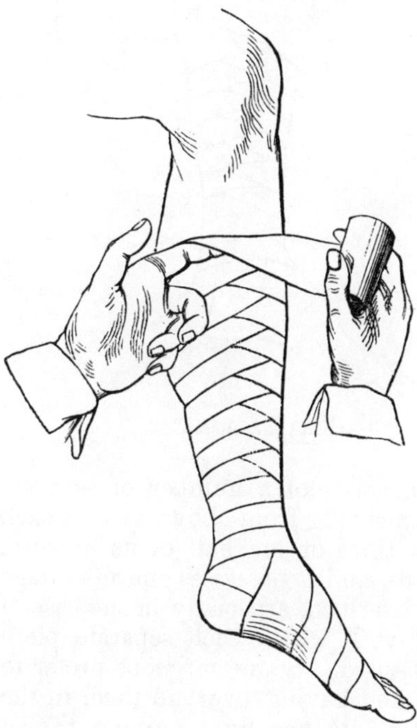

Application of the "roller" by circular and reversed turns.

Fig. 6.

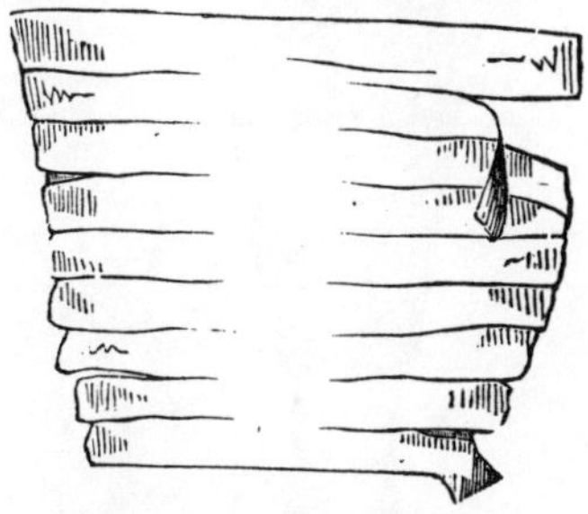

Many-tailed bandage.

of the fragments improved at any moment or under any circumstances, it ought to be done; and if we fail in accomplishing all that we wish to do in the first instance, we must remain incessantly watchful to seize the earliest opportunity which presents, to complete the adjustment. No doubt our efforts will prove fruitless very much in proportion to the amount of swelling, inflammation, or muscular spasm which exists, and also in proportion to the time which has elapsed, but this will not excuse us for omitting to do all which the circumstances permit.

It has been the practice of most surgeons, for a long period, to cover the broken limb with some form of a bandage or roller before applying the lateral splints.

Of these primary dressings there are two principal varieties: first; the "roller," or simple bandage, applied to the limb in circular and reversed turns; and, second; the "many-tailed bandage," consisting of a piece of muslin, or other cloth, torn down from each side into a suitable number of strips, leaving the centre, which is to be applied to the back of the limb, entire.

Fig. 7.

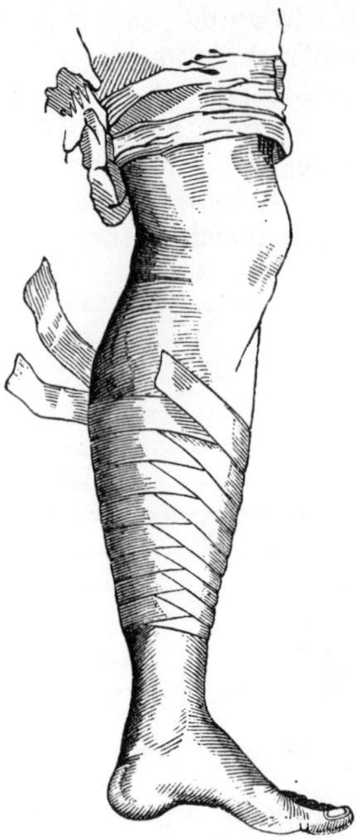

Application of the many-tailed bandage.

Fig. 8.

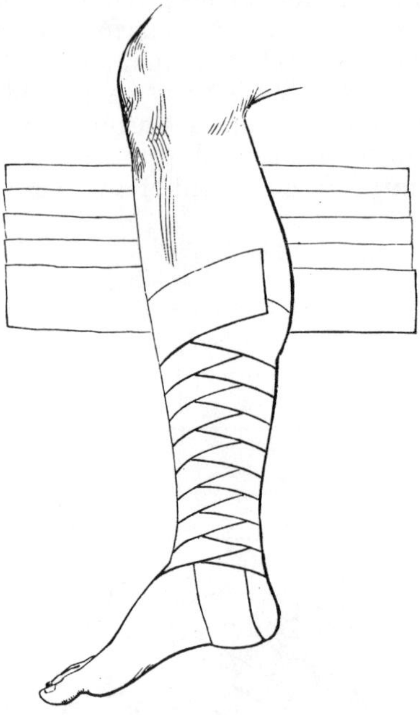

Bandage of Scultetus.

A modification of this bandage consists of a number of separate strips, so laid upon one another, commencing from above, as that each strip shall overlap the other by one-third or one-half of its breadth. This is called the bandage of Scultetus, and it possesses one advantage over the many-tailed bandage just described, especially in the case of compound fractures, in the facility with which each separate piece may be removed and another substituted. Some surgeons prefer to form the bandage of separate strips, and having overlaid them in the manner directed, to unite them again into one by running a thread through the whole mass along the centre.

Whichever of these several varieties of strips are employed, the mode of applying them is the same. They are folded alternately around the limb, being made to overlap and cross upon each other in front, and only the last strip or two is fastened with a pin.

The object proposed in the use of the roller or of the many-tailed bandage is twofold: first, to compress and support the muscles, by which their tendency to contraction is in some measure controlled; and second, to protect the limb against the direct pressure of the side splints.

A moment's consideration will convince us that the first of these objects is in most cases fully attained by the lateral splints themselves, and by the bandages by which they are retained in place: and that the second can be as well accomplished by a single fold of cloth, or by the compresses, which ought generally, even when the roller is used, to underlie the splints. Nevertheless we should hardly feel authorized to reject these primary dressings solely because the splints and compresses furnish a convenient substitute, especially since we are compelled to admit that they are occasionally useful, unless objections of a more serious nature could be brought against them. Unfortunately this latter supposition is actually true. By ligating the limb completely, leaving no point of the tegumentary surface to which the pressure is not applied, they too often occasion congestions, inflammation and gangrene. It is not until lately that the attention of surgeons has been sufficiently called to this subject; but the records of surgery are to day filled with these terrible accidents, formerly attributed to the original injury or to the splints themselves, but now understood to be plainly traceable to the too common employment of the primary bandage. The roller is by far the most dangerous dressing of the two, since it does not yield to the swelling so readily as the bandage of strips, and it is more objectionable also on account of the inconvenience of applying and removing it; but even the bandage of strips may be so confined as to produce the same consequences, as I have myself seen in more than one instance. It is also all the more dangerous in the hands of the inexperienced surgeon, because he feels a confidence that it will not cause ligation.

Except in rare cases and for especial reasons, which we shall attempt to indicate in their appropriate places, we cannot recommend the employment of any kind of bandages next to the skin.

In order to fulfil the second indication, namely, to maintain the fragments in place, we employ usually what are called short or side splints, and long or extending splints.

Side splints may be constructed from various materials, according to the size and circumstances of the limb, or according to the convenience of the surgeon; and as the surgeon cannot be expected to have always on hand, at the bedside of the patient, such splints as he might prefer to use, it is well for him to understand how to avail himself of such materials as may be within his reach, in order that he may make the most of his sometimes imperfect resources.

Lead, sheet iron, zinc, and other metals have been occasionally employed, but especially tin and copper, which possess all of the requisite firmness and malleability to allow them to be hammered and thus moulded to the limb. In general, however, they are unnecessarily heavy, and demand too much labor to be wrought into shape. I have sometimes employed tin splints perforated with large fenestræ to diminish their weight and increase their flexibility, and found them to answer an excellent purpose.

Iron wire splints, made from wire cloth or coarse gauze, was first publicly mentioned, so far as I can learn, in a communication to the *Memphis Medical Recorder*, made by Dr. J. C. Nott, of Mobile; but it has been brought more particularly into notice, and its construction perfected by Louis Bauer, of New York.[1] These splints are moulded upon "gypsum or wooden casts," of different sizes, and surrounded with a stout iron wire frame in order to give them the requisite degree of firmness, and to preserve their forms; after which they are tinned by galvanism, and varnished, to prevent them from becoming rusted. When applied, Dr. Bauer recommends that they shall be filled with loose cotton, and that they shall be held in place by rollers. It is claimed for these splints that they are light, flexible, permeable to air and to the perspiration, and that they permit the application of cooling lotions without impairing their firmness; the last of which is a quality of questionable value, since lotions applied to permanent dressings of any kind are only warm fomentations, and do not, therefore, in this respect, serve the purpose for which they were intended; besides that they render the skin tender, and dispose it to vesicate, they give rise to a sensation of scalding, which is sometimes almost intolerable; they soak into the bed, and in many other ways render the patients uncomfortable. Cooling lotions are only applicable where the dressings are open, loose, and temporary.

The same objections hold also to this as to all other forms of moulded metallic or carved wooden splints, namely, that they seldom exactly fit the limb, even when the supply of assorted sizes is complete, and that they are not sufficiently flexible to adapt themselves to anything but the slightest irregularity of surface. They are not, however, without merit, and they deserve at least a qualified recommendation in many cases. I shall refer to them again when speaking of fractures of the thigh and leg.

Horn and whalebone may be employed in thin plates, or in the form of narrow strips quilted into cloth; but they are expensive and possess no special value except in an emergency. Reeds, the coarse rank grass which grows in swamps, flags, willow branches, and unbroken wheat straw, may be quilted between two thicknesses of cloth in the same manner, and form very excellent temporary splints. I have especially found it convenient to use wheat straw in the form of junks. Gathering up a bundle of unbroken straws of the size of my arm, I roll them snugly in a broad piece of cotton cloth, cut off the projecting ends and then stitch up the cloth neatly. We have thus a splint of considerable firmness, and one which is cool and especially adapted to the summer, allowing the perspiration to evaporate freely. Straw splints were employed sometimes by Ambrose Paré, by J. L. Petit, Larrey, and I have several times seen them in the wards of certain European hospitals, although I am unable now to say under whose

[1] Nott and Bauer, Buf. Med. Journ., vol. xii., April, 1857.

direction. Mr. Tuffnell, of Dublin, has especially recommended them in the form of junks.

Wooden splints, made of pine, white or linden wood, or of some other light and easily wrought timber, are probably of more universal application, and possess greater intrinsic value than splints constructed from any other material; but I wish at once, and for all, to disclaim any intention of giving even a qualified approval of any of those carved, polished, and generally patented wooden splints, which are manufactured and sold by clever mechanics, and which one may see suspended in almost every doctor's office, whether in the city or in the country. Constructed with grooves and ridges, and variously inclined planes, for the avowed purpose of meeting a multitude of indications, such as to protect a condyle, to press between parallel bones, to follow the subsidence of a muscular swelling, &c., they never meet exactly a single one of these indications, whilst they seldom fail to defeat some other indication of equal importance. They deceive especially the inexperienced surgeon into the belief that he has in the splint itself a provision for all these wants, and consequently lead him to neglect those useful precautions which he would otherwise have adopted.

If carved wooden splints are employed, they ought to be made especially for the case under treatment. But this requires time and some more mechanical skill than can always be commanded; and when accurately fitted, it is quite probable that the subsidence or increase of the swelling will, within the next forty-eight hours, render some change in the form of the splint necessary, or compel the surgeon to throw it aside.

We much prefer to use plain, straight strips of wood, of the requisite width and length, which may be cut at any moment from a shingle or a thin piece of board.

In order that these splints may adapt themselves to the inequalities of the limb, and properly support the fragments, they may be underlaid with pads or junks of a suitable thickness; or, what is still better, they may be covered with a muslin sack, open at both ends, into which, and on the side of the splint which is to be placed against the limb, bran, wool, cotton batting, or curled hair may be pressed, until it is made to fit accurately. I generally prefer cotton batting. Bran is liable to get displaced, and curled hair does not pack firmly enough. When the sack is sufficiently filled, the two ends must be stitched up. This mode of constructing the splint is simple and easy of accomplishment; the splint can be fitted very accurately; the pad never becomes displaced; and when the bandages are applied, they may be pinned or sewed to the cover in such a way that they shall not slide or loosen.

If pads are employed separate from the splint, and for this purpose, also, I generally prefer the cotton batting; they ought to be made and fitted with the same care, and neatly stitched together at their ends, rather than pinned. Cotton batting laid loosely next to the skin, or

[1] Tuffnell, New York Journ. Med., March, 1847, p. 264.

underneath the splints at any point, will not keep its place so well as when it is inclosed in covers—it is more liable to get into knots, and it has altogether a slovenly appearance. The pads may be stitched to the roller, and in this way secured effectually in place, but loose cotton is subject to no control.

When I speak of pads, it must not be understood that I intend to recommend them for compresses, or for the purpose of pressing fragments into place. Nothing could be a greater source of mischief in the dressing of a broken limb. I have only directed their employment as a means of adaptation, and to protect the skin against the direct pressure of the splint.

Dr. Jacob, of Dublin, says that he has seen an excellent splint made from the "fresh bark of a tree taken off while the sap is rising." "It fits admirably," says Dr. Jacobs, "just like pasteboard soaked in water."[1]

Undressed sole-leather, cut into shape and beaten with a hammer, adapts itself easily to the limb and is sufficiently firm. It is especially applicable to fractures of the larger limbs.

A splint is also occasionally made of thin calfskin veneered with some light timber, such as linden or white-wood, the latter being subsequently split into strips of from half an inch to one inch in width, so as to combine a certain degree of flexibility with the requisite firmness.

Fig. 9.

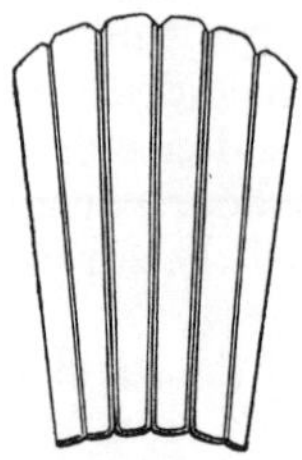

Wood and leather splint.

The Turks use, according to Sedillot, in a similar manner, the "nervures" of palm laid upon sheepskin and fastened with wooden thongs;[2] and Dr. Packard mentions that he has seen narrow slips of some light wood glued in the same way upon soft pieces of buckskin, and then fastened together with two strips of buckskin, which were also glued to the splints.[3]

Common pasteboard, cardboard, or the stout millboard used by bookbinders, constitute invaluable domestic resorts, since they can generally be found in the house of the patient; and if in no other way, pasteboard may generally be had at the expense of some paper box or of the loose cover of some old book. For small bones, the thinner sheets afford a sufficient support; but for large bones the thick binders' board is necessary. In preparing the latter for use, it ought to be moistened with water; but if soaked too much it will separate and fall into pieces, or lose its firmness when dry, in consequence of having parted with some of its paste. This splint may be applied to the limb without the interposition of anything but a few folds of muslin cloth, or a piece of flannel; or we may use instead a single sheet of cotton wadding. It must be bound to the limb by the roller while it is moist, and as it dries speedily it forms a smooth, firm, and reliable splint.

Felt, made of wool saturated with gum shellac, and pressed into

[1] Jacobs, New York Journ. Med., March, 1847, p. 265, from Dublin Med. Press.
[2] Amer. Journ. Med. Sci., vol. xxiii., Feb. 1839, p. 481.
[3] Packard's edition of Malgaigne, vol. i. p. 173.

sheets, makes an excellent moulding tablet for splints. This may be obtained at any hat manufactory. A much cheaper material, however, and which has nearly all of the qualities of the real felt may be made from old pieces of broadcloth, or from any similar closely woven texture, by saturating it thoroughly with gum shellac, the gum being dissolved in alcohol in the proportions of one pound of the former to two quarts of the latter. Thus prepared, it is to be spread upon both surfaces of the cloth with a common paint brush. When this first coat is well dried by suspending the cloth where the air will have free access to both surfaces, a second must be spread upon one of the surfaces; and then a third; the cloth being allowed to dry after each successive coat. Finally, the sheet is to be folded upon itself, so as to bring the most thickly covered surfaces together, and pressed with a hot flat.

If it is necessary to have greater strength, more gum may be laid upon the cloth, and it may be again folded and pressed.

When used, it is to be dipped into boiling water or held near the fire until it becomes flexible. It hardens very rapidly in cooling, and demands, therefore, some quickness in its application; but once applied and fitted, it forms a hard but smooth splint well adapted for all the purposes for which it is designed.

It is well to mention, if one wishes to keep any portion of the solution which is not used, that in order to prevent evaporation the vessel in which it is contained must be closely covered.

I have used this material for many years, both in hospital and private practice, and I can safely recommend it for all cases in which splints are required.

Dr. Jacob says he has sometimes found an old hat to furnish a very efficient splint in the small fractures of children, and I have no doubt from my experience with felt that it might prove a valuable resort in an exigency.

It has been objected to this splint occasionally, that it is impervious to air and moisture, and that it confines the insensible perspiration; an objection which may be obviated in some measure by rubbing the surface which is to be laid against the limb, with pumice-stone until it is roughened or until a short nap is raised. But as I never use splints of any kind without underlaying them with compresses which act sufficiently as absorbents, I have never been aware of any inconvenience from this source.

Within a few years, sheets of gutta percha have been brought into the market, varying in thickness from the one-sixteenth to one-quarter of an inch. For fractures of the thigh, and for the large bones generally, I prefer a thickness of about one-sixth or one-fifth of an inch; but for the fingers or toes, it need not be more than one-sixteenth of an inch in thickness. In its natural state, and at the ordinary temperature of the body, it is nearly as hard and as inflexible as bone; but when immersed in boiling water it almost immediately softens, and would melt completely unless soon removed. It can therefore be adapted to any surface, however irregular, and its form may be changed as often as may be necessary. It does not harden quite as rapidly as felt, and it possesses, therefore, in this respect an advantage, since it allows the surgeon more time for adjustment; while, on the other hand, it hardens much more rapidly than either starch, paste, or dextrine. Ten or twenty minutes is all the time usually required for gutta percha to acquire that degree of firmness which will prevent it from yielding under the pressure of a bandage.

To use it skilfully requires some experience, and I have known surgeons to reject it after a single trial; but by those who have acquired the necessary skill it is generally regarded as an invaluable resource.

When constructing from this material a thigh splint, we should order a very large tin pan, or some open, flat tray, in which we may lay the splint at full length. If the splint is required to be twelve inches long, and six inches wide, we must cut it about sixteen inches long by eight wide, so as to allow for the contraction which always takes place more or less when the hot water is applied. It is then to be laid upon a sheet of cotton cloth of more than twice the width of the splint, in order that the cloth may envelop it completely when it is folded upon it; and the cloth should be enough longer than the splint to enable us to handle and lift it by the two ends without immersing our fingers in the hot water. Beside, if the gum is not thus covered and supported it will adhere to the vessel, to the fingers, to the surface of the limb, and indeed to whatever else it comes in contact with; it may even fall to pieces, or become very much stretched and distorted by its own weight. The cloth cover will generally adhere to the splint, and may be permitted to remain upon it permanently.

Place the splint, thus covered, in the basin, and pour on the water at or near the temperature of boiling. As soon as it is sufficiently softened, lift it carefully, and lay it over the limb, and by its own weight it will adjust itself to the surface, or it may be moulded with the hands, or by pressing it against the limb with a pillow. If it does not harden rapidly enough, this process may be hastened by sponging the outer surface with cold water; and as soon as it has acquired sufficient firmness to support itself it may be removed and immersed in a pail of cold water or placed under a hydrant; after this, it is to be neatly trimmed and dried, when it is ready for use.

The same objection has been made also to gutta percha which is occasionally made to felt, namely, that it confines the perspiration, but to this we have already sufficiently replied.

There is scarcely any fracture demanding the use of a splint in which I have not demonstrated its utility, but it is especially valuable, as I shall have occasion to mention again, as an interdental splint in fractures of the jaw, and as a moulding tablet in all fractures occurring in the vicinity of joints.

Benjamin Welch, of Lakeville, Conn., has contrived a very ingenious application of gutta percha to the purposes of a splint, by veneering a thin plate of the gum with equally thin plates of elastic wood. The veneering is laid upon both sides, and then it is pressed into form in moulds. The elasticity of the wood, together with the plasticity of the gum, enables the surgeon to change its form somewhat at pleasure, by dipping it into hot water.

Fig. 10.

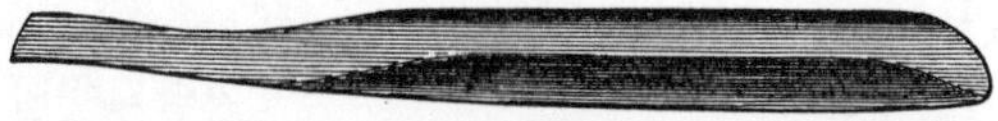

Fig. 11.

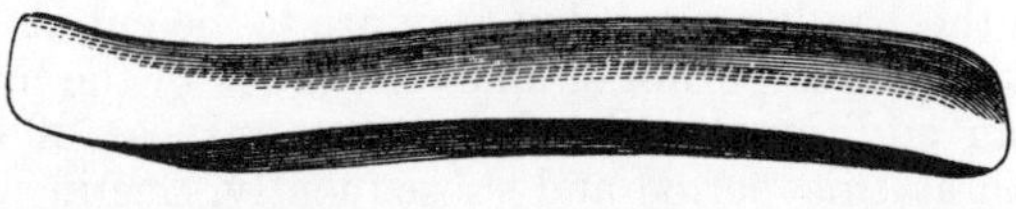

Welch's veneered gutta-percha, dorsal and palmar splints for forearm.

Its form cannot, however, be changed to any great extent, and by frequent immersion in hot water the veneering is apt to loosen from the gutta percha. Nevertheless it is a most excellent splint, and in very many respects it is superior to any of the carved wooden splints which we have ever seen.

Fig. 12.

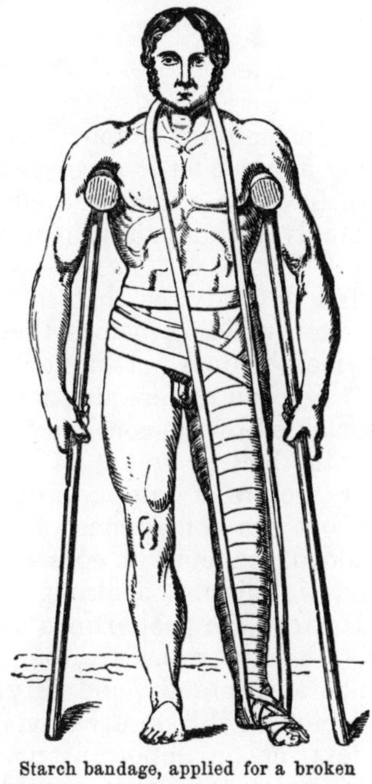

Starch bandage, applied for a broken thigh.

The moulding tablet of Alfred Smee, composed of gum Arabic and whiting, spread upon cloth,[1] has nothing special to recommend it, any more than the cloth splints, hardened with the whites of eggs and flour, used by Larrey.[2] Starch and alum, glue, pitch, and various other materials of a similar character deserve only to be mentioned as having been occasionally employed, but which have never succeeded in securing for themselves the confidence of surgeons.

In 1834, Suetin, of Brussels, introduced the use of starch as a means of hardening the bandages; his method of using which is essentially as follows. A dry roller is first applied to the skin, and then smeared with starch; all of the bony prominences and irregularities of the limb are filled up or covered with cotton batting, charpie, down, etc.; strips of pasteboard, or of binders' board, moistened and covered also with starch, are now laid alongside the limb, over which again are turned in succession one, two, or three layers of the starched roller; the number of rollers and the thickness of the pasteboard being proportioned to the size of the limb, or to the required strength of the

[1] Amer. Journ. Med. Sci., vol. xxvi. p. 220, May, 1840; from London Lancet, Jan. 25, 1840.

[2] Amer. Journ. Med. Sci., vol. ii. p. 216, May, 1828; from Journal des Progrès, vol. iv.

splint. The whole is completed by starching the outside of the last bandage.

This dressing will generally become dry within from thirty to forty hours; which process may be expedited by exposing its sides as much as possible to the air, or by the application of artificial heat with bags of dry sand, or with hot bricks. As a temporary support until the drying is completed, some surgeons lay upon each side of the limb additional splints, securing them in place with tapes.

As soon as the bandages are dry they are to be cut along the front to a sufficient extent to permit of an examination of the limb, and then closed with an additional roller. For the purpose of opening the bandages both at this period and subsequently, Suetin uses a pair of strong scissors or pliers, such as are represented in Fig. 13.

Fig. 13.

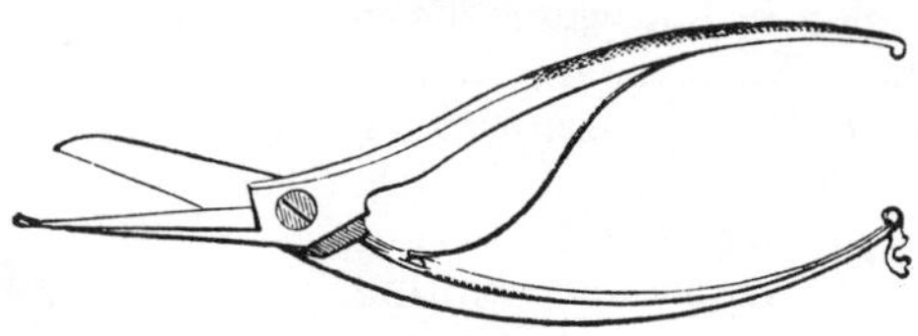

Suetin's pliers.

On the third or fourth day, or as soon as the subsidence of the swelling may render it necessary, the bandages should be cut open through their whole extent, the edges pared off and brought together again snugly with an additional roller.

Erichsen, who uses the starch bandage in all fractures and from the first day, advises that the limb shall be completely enveloped with cotton wadding before the first roller is applied; in consequence of which he does not think it necessary to apply the first roller dry.

Velpeau prefers dextrine ("British gum") a kind of glue or jelly obtained by the continued action of diluted sulphuric acid upon starch at the boiling point. It is prepared for use by dissolving it in alcohol or tincture of camphor, or camphorated brandy, until it has acquired about the consistence of honey; at this point hot water should be added, reducing its consistence to that of thin treacle, when, after one or two minutes' shaking, it is ready for application. According to F. D'Arcet, the proportions most favorable to the drying and solidifying of the apparatus are, one hundred parts of dextrine, sixty of camphorated brandy, and fifty of water. Malgaigne, to whom I am indebted for this observation of D'Arcet, says, also, in a note, "as regards dextrine, an important point was recently brought practically under my notice, viz., that as sold in the shops, it is often unfit for making an agglutinative mixture; it forms lumps with alcohol, as starch does with cold water, without cohering; and twice in succession I have been obliged to change the supply at the Hôpital Saint Antoine. The dextrine thus deteriorated is whiter and less saccharine; it crepitates more in the fingers; and on pouring a few drops of tincture of iodine into the solution, there is produced a violet tint, indicating the presence of fecula; while true dextrine, treated with iodine, gives a vinous red, or the color of onion peel."

Velpeau soaks his bandages with the dextrine before applying them, but like Suetin, he applies his first roller dry. He uses but one bandage, which he carries first from below upwards and then from above downwards; and he rarely thinks it necessary to employ the pasteboard as a collateral support.

For myself I am quite as much in the habit of using wheat flour paste as either starch or dextrine, and if properly made it dries about as quickly as the starch, and is equally firm.

Whatever material is used in the construction of what is now usually termed the "immovable apparatus," or as Suetin has more lately called it, the "movable immovable apparatus," ("movo-amobile") in reference to his practice of opening it at an early period, it is still the same apparatus in effect, and is liable to the same judgment—a judgment which we shall find it very difficult to declare, since, from the day in which this practice was first recommended by Suetin, to the present moment, it has been constantly experiencing the most extraordinary vicissitudes in the public favor. At one time, and by the most experienced surgeons, extolled as a method unequalled in its simplicity, efficiency, and safety, and at another, and by surgeons of equal experience, denounced as eminently lacking in all of the true essentials of an apparatus for broken limbs. These conflicting opinions, which it is impossible to reconcile, have nevertheless some foundation in truth. The immovable apparatus, of whatever materials constructed, is under some circumstances a very simple, safe, and efficient dressing, while under other circumstances it is, as we think, eminently unsafe and inefficient. Thus, in all of those fractures which are accompanied with such injury to the soft parts as to render subsequent inflammation inevitable or probable, this form of dressing exposes to congestions, strangulations, and gangrene. Whatever its advocates may say to the contrary, the simple fact is before us, that the number of accidents resulting from this practice is out of all proportion with any other yet introduced. I have met with them myself in all parts of my own country, and the journals abound with records of disasters from this source.[1] Nor is it a sufficient reply to this statement, that, with proper care and prudence, such accidents may be avoided. We think they could not always be avoided. But admitting that they could, it is still undeniable that in certain cases the immovable apparatus demands extraordinary attention; and what is the need of multiplying our cares when already they are more than sufficient? Many circumstances, over which he has no control, may prevent the surgeon from giving to the limb the full amount of attention which is required; and for this reason that apparatus is the best which, whilst it answers the indications equally well, exacts the least amount of skill and attention on the part of the surgeon.

Immovable dressings are not only liable to become too tight as the swelling augments, but, on the other hand, the surgeon may omit to notice that as the swelling has subsided it has become loose. Portions

[1] See Amer. Journ. Med. Sci., vol. xxv. p. 460, Feb. 1840; also vol. xxxi. p. 212.

of the limb may vesicate, ulcerate, or even slough, without the knowledge of the surgeon. If, however, the bandages are frequently opened and all the proper precautions are taken, it is possible that these accidents may also be avoided; but unfortunately experience has shown that they have not been avoided in too many instances.

The cases, then, to which this apparatus seems to be adapted, are a few examples of transverse or serrated fractures in which the bones have not become displaced, and in which little or no swelling is anticipated; and in certain fractures which were originally more complicated, but in which a partial union, and the subsidence of the inflammation, have reduced them to a more simple condition; and especially in cases of delayed union. If now the dressings are applied carefully, the bandage being only moderately tight, and a portion of the extremity of the limb is left uncovered so that we may observe constantly its condition, and at proper intervals the apparatus is opened completely in order that we may subject the whole limb to a thorough examination; in such cases as we have now indicated and with such precautions, we admit that the "apparatus immobile" constitutes an invaluable surgical appliance, and one of which no surgeon can well afford to be deprived.

Fig. 14.

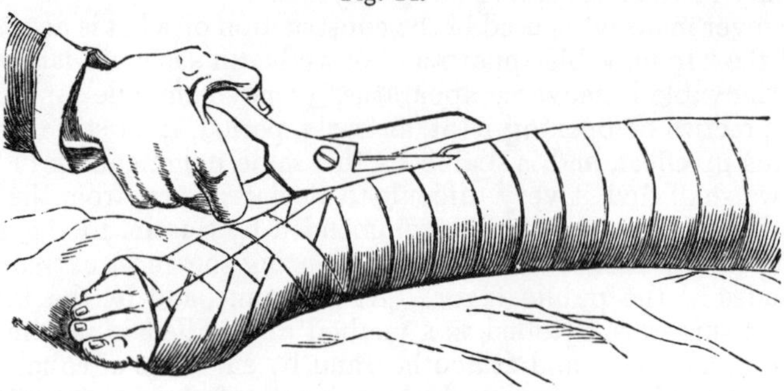

Opening the apparatus with Suetin's pliers.

Fig. 15.

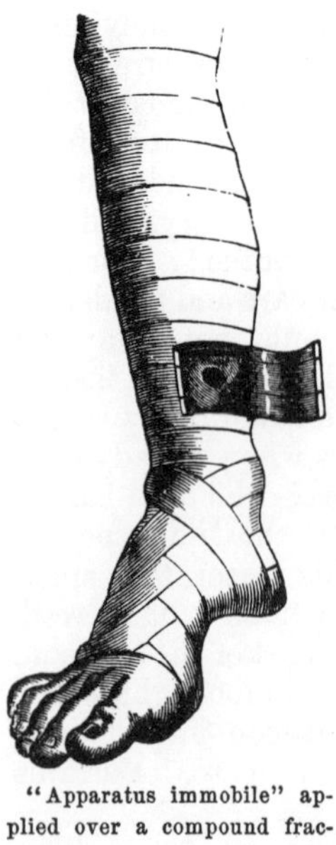

"Apparatus immobile" applied over a compound fracture.

I have even met with examples of compound fractures in which it has seemed proper to apply this dressing; but only when a sufficient time had elapsed to render it probable that there would be no sudden accession of swelling in the limb. In such cases I have preferred generally to lay the several turns of the roller directly over the suppurating wound in the same manner as if no wound existed, and to make a valvular opening, or window, with the scissors on the following day in order to allow the matter to escape, after which the valve may be laid down and stitched, or the piece may be removed entirely, and a new piece of bandage drawn closely around the limb at this point. This may be repeated once or twice daily. If an opening is left by the roller, and no additional bandage is laid over it, the margins of the wound soon become œdematous and protrude, making an ugly-looking and ill-conditioned sore.

Plaster of Paris moulds, employed occasionally from a very early period, and more lately recommended by Hendriksz, Hubenthal, Keyl, and Dieffenbach, are not entitled to serious consideration. Heavy stone coffins, they might serve well enough the purposes of interment, but they are wholly unsuited to the purposes of a splint.

Plaster of Paris has, however, been of late employed in another form, and in relation to which our judgment must be much more favorable. I allude to the so-called "plaster of Paris bandages," which were first introduced to notice by Mathiesen and Van der Loo, of Holland, but the value of which has been more especially brought to notice by Prof. Nicholas Pirogoff, of St. Petersburg, the late Surgeon-in-chief at Sebastopol.

The manner of using the gypsum bandages is as follows: A dry roller is first applied to the limb, or it may be covered with a single piece of cloth of any kind, and the irregularities are filled up and protected with cotton wool, the same as we have directed when about to apply the starch bandage. The remaining dressings being now at hand and ready for use, we proceed to mix the plaster. For this purpose we must select the fine, fresh, well-dried, white powder. The gray does not solidify well, nor that which has been a long time ground, or is moist. The proportions of water and plaster usually required are about equal parts by weight. For the thigh it may require, perhaps, seven or eight pounds of plaster, and for the leg or arm much less. It is probably a better rule to direct the gypsum to be added to the water until it is of about the consistence of cream. The water should be cold and the gypsum thrown in not too rapidly, at least not more rapidly than it can be thoroughly mixed, otherwise we shall not be able to determine precisely its consistence. If, while applying the paste, it begins to harden in the bowl, we must not add more water, as this will again interfere with its final solidification upon the limb. It must be thrown away and some fresh immediately prepared; or the crystallization may be retarded by throwing in a few drops of carpenters' glue. When the plaster is good, and it is properly mixed, we may allow ourselves from five to eight minutes in the application. A large paint brush is the most convenient thing for spreading it, but the hands will do very well in an emergency.

Everything being ready, the limb is to be seized by assistants at both of its extremities and held in a position of steady extension until the dressing is completed, and for one or two minutes longer, or until the plaster is hard. It will be sufficiently hard to support itself even when the dressings are quite moist. The surgeon then proceeds to lay a long piece of linen—old sack will answer as well as any—folded three or four times, and saturated with the paste, parallel to the two sides of the limb, around which are to be immediately placed horizontally, and at several points, short and wide strips of the same material. These latter are intended to increase the strength of the apparatus, and to bind on the side strips. Finally, the whole may be painted with the solution. It is very well, however, not to cover the front of the limb, or a narrow strip somewhere in the line of the axis of the limb, with the plaster, as this will not diminish materially its strength, and it will enable the surgeon to open it more easily with the scissors. Pirogoff accomplishes the same purpose by laying a piece of narrow tape, soaked in oil, along the line through which he wishes to make the section of the splint.[1]

Another mode of applying the gypsum is to employ common rollers, made of unglazed, open calico. The cloth, being torn into strips of a suitable width and length, is laid upon a table, and the dry plaster rubbed into it for several minutes, until its meshes are well and evenly filled. Each bandage is then rolled up closely, and immediately before being applied a little water must be dropped into the extremities of the roll to moisten the plaster, but not enough to soak through the plaster and thereby wash it out. Thus prepared, the gypsum roller is applied to the limb in circular turns, until the whole is completely encased with one or two layers. Reversed turns must be avoided as far as possible, and when they become necessary, the fold should not be made over a projecting ridge of bone.[2]

I have omitted to mention that the limb must be completely covered and protected with a dry roller and with cotton pads or compresses, before the gypsum roller is applied.

All that we have before said of the advantages and hazards of the "apparatus immobile," are equally applicable to this form of the apparatus, or at least with only slight modifications. It dries much more rapidly; but this apparent advantage is sometimes more than counterbalanced by the necessity of haste in its application, and the consequent danger of having done our work in a slovenly manner. No doubt, on the field of battle, and in army surgery generally, the speed with which it becomes hard and firm, would secure for it a preference over almost any other form of dressing.[3]

Professor B. W. Dudley, of Lexington, Ky., one of the most successful surgeons in this country, but especially distinguished as a lithotomist, has for many years employed in the treatment of fractures nothing but a roller, regarding both side splints and extending apparatus as not only useless but absolutely pernicious.[4] This practice, which seems to have originated with Radley, of England, has not found, hitherto, in this country or elsewhere, many imitators; and although one ought in general to speak very cautiously of a practice which he has never seen tried, and especially when it brings with it the au-

[1] Weber on Plaster of Paris Bandage, New York Journ. Med., May, 1856, p. 341.

[2] Gamgee's Researches, London, 1856, p. 154.

[3] Practical Lectures on Military Surgery, by Isidor Glück, of New York, chief surgeon to the Hungarian (Vilmos) Hussars, &c. &c., during the late war in Hungary. Amer. Med. Monthly, Dec. 1855, p. 449, &c., vol. iv.

[4] Dudley, Trans. Amer. Med. Assoc., vol. iii., 1850, p. 349.

thority of so distinguished a surgeon as Dr. Dudley, I do not hesitate to pronounce it irrational, and to declare my belief that it is in no way entitled to the confidence of the profession.

Still more unscientific, and absurd even, is the practice of Jobert, of Paris, who employs neither side splints nor bandages, but only extension, in the treatment of all, or of nearly all fractures of the long bones.

As to the question of permanent extension in fractures, and the means by which it may be most effectually accomplished, nothing need be said at this time, inasmuch as it relates only to the fractures of certain bones, and to certain forms of fractures; we must therefore refer its consideration to those chapters which treat of individual bones.

In the treatment of *comminuted* fractures, no pains ought to be spared to bring the fragments as nearly as possible into apposition; and if there exists at the same time an external wound, and the fragments are small and loose, they ought to be removed carefully. Nor, indeed, should we be deterred from the attempt to remove them by finding that they are adherent, if still they are easily moved about with the finger.

In *compound* fractures, not unfrequently the end of one of the fragments protrudes from the wound, and its reduction may be attended with considerable difficulty. My practice is usually in such cases to attempt the reduction first, by simple extension and counter-extension; but if this fails, I introduce my finger into the wound, and endeavor to stretch the skin over the sharp point of bone; or I make use of a spatula formed from a piece of shingle, or of any suitable piece of metal which may be at hand; finally, but not until all other expedients have failed, I enlarge the wound sufficiently to insure its return.

There are some cases, however, in which the surgeon may feel justified in sawing off the projecting end; as when the periosteum is completely torn from it by its having penetrated a boot, or even sometimes when its extremity is very sharp, and there is reason to suppose that it would prick and irritate the tissues.

If arteries bleed freely and for a long time, we may make some effort to find the open mouths in the wound, but in this we rarely succeed, nor is it prudent always to tie the main branch which supplies the limb. Fortunately this bleeding, although at first profuse, generally ceases in a few hours under the steady employment of cold lotions, moderate compression, and rest. If it does not, the chances are that the case will call for amputation.

The rule generally laid down by surgeons that we should at once close the wound in compound fractures, with sutures and adhesive straps if necessary, or with bandages, is far too absolute. This practice will do when there is no great contusion or extravasation of blood, but if blood is flowing it is much better to leave the wound open so as to permit it to escape freely; and if the severity of the injury warrants the supposition that much inflammation is to ensue, the danger of gangrene is greatly lessened by thus allowing the opening to remain as a channel of exit for the inflammatory effusions.

Many years since Dr. J. Rhea Barton introduced into the Pennsylvania Hospital what has since been called the "bran dressing" for the treatment of compound fractures of the leg; the limb being made to repose in a box filled with this material.[1] I have used it very frequently, and can speak of it as possessing many qualities of excellence, especially as a summer dressing. The particular mode of using this apparatus I shall describe more minutely when treating of fractures of the leg.

The treatment of inflammatory symptoms, and of the later accidents, such as suppuration, œdema, gangrene, &c., must be left mainly to the good judgment of the surgeon. Gentle manipulation, uniform support, rest and sometimes cooling lotions constitute the most important means by which inflammation is to be controlled. Bleeding is rarely necessary, and in a large majority of cases it might prove injurious by lowering too much the vital forces, which need to be husbanded in view of the requirements of the process of repair and of the long and exhausting confinement. Cathartics should also be administered cautiously for the same reason, and because they are liable, especially in fractures of the lower extremities, to occasion a serious disturbance of the limb.

CHAPTER VI.

DELAYED UNION AND NON-UNION OF BROKEN BONES.[2]

MOST surgical writers concur in the statement that non-union of broken bones is an uncommon event. Walker, of Oxford, affirms that of not less than one thousand fractures which have come under his treatment at some period of the repair, he does not recollect more than six or eight instances. According to Lonsdale, not more than five or six cases of false joint, excepting those within a capsule, have occurred out of nearly four thousand fractures treated at the Middlesex Hospital. In a table of 367 cases, collected and arranged by W. W. Morland, from the books of the Massachusetts General Hospital, extending through a period of nineteen years, only one example of

[1] Paper on Bran Dressings, by Reynell Coates. of Philadelphia. Amer. Journ. Med. Sci., April, 1842, p. 515; from the Med. Examiner, Nos 9 and 11, vol. i., New Series.

[2] I shall, in this chapter, avail myself freely of the labors of George W. Norris, of Philadelphia, whose paper, entitled "On the Occurrence of Non-union after Fractures, its Causes and Treatment," published in the *American Journal of Medical Sciences* for Jan., 1842, constitutes the most complete and reliable monograph upon this subject contained in any language.

false joint is recorded; but as only seventy-four days had elapsed when this patient was discharged, it is doubtful whether this might not have proved to be a case of delayed union simply.[1] Of 946 cases of recent fracture treated in the Pennsylvania Hospital between the years 1830 and 1840, no instance of false union followed the treatment pursued.[2] Sir Stephen Hammick, Mr. Liston, and Malgaigne affirm also the infrequency of these accidents in the cases which have come under their personal treatment. I have myself seen a considerable number of examples of non-union, but in not one of my own cases, whether in hospital or private practice, has the bone refused finally to unite; and my opinion is, that in proportion to the number of fractures everywhere, these cases are very rare, perhaps not in a larger proportion than one in five hundred.

Amesbury alone seems to have entertained a contrary opinion. His own experience having supplied fifty-six examples of what he has called "fractures of long standing." Norris remarks that he is "at a loss to account for its frequency in his practice, but a reviewer of his own nation observes of his statement that the surgery of fractures must be singularly bad, where one individual has had occasion to number fifty-six examples of non-union, even making allowance for the fact, that all the bad cases came to Mr. Amesbury." I notice, also, that at a later period Mr. Amesbury's experience in false joint extended to ninety cases.

The humerus and femur would appear to be the bones most liable to non-union, as shown by Norris's statistics; in which forty-eight belonged to the humerus, forty-eight to the femur, thirty-three to the leg, nineteen to the forearm, and two to the jaw. In my own experience, I have found the humerus ununited much more often than the femur.

Bérard has shown that in the growth of the long bones the period at which the epiphyses are united to the diaphyses depends upon the direction of the nutritive artery; for example, "it is found that in the humerus, where the direction of this vessel is from above downwards, consolidation takes place soonest at its inferior extremity. In the forearm, the course of the nutrient vessels is from below upwards, and here consolidation of the epiphyses is found to occur at the elbow sooner than at the wrist. In the inferior members, on the contrary, the epiphyses composing the knee are the last which become firm, because in the femur the nutritious artery runs upwards, and in the bones of the leg it courses from above downwards." A knowledge of these facts led Guéretin to inquire into the influence of these arteries upon the consolidation of fractures; and the cases collected by him did indeed seem to show a positive relation between the direction of the artery and the union of the bone; that is to say, the examples of non-union were chiefly found where the fracture had taken place on that side of the nutritious foramen, from which the artery entered, as if to imply that the non-union was in some measure due to the imperfect nutrition of this extremity of the bone. In thirty-five cases of

[1] Address on Fractures, by A. L. Peirson, read before the Massachusetts Med. Soc. May 27, 1840.

[2] Norris, loc. cit.

non-union analyzed by Guéretin, ten belonged to that portion of the bone which was traversed by the artery, and twenty-five to the other portion. But an analysis of forty-one cases, made by Norris, does not seem to confirm this observation of Guéretin, since twenty-seven were in the direction of the nutritious arteries, and only fourteen in the opposite portion, or in that which is supposed to be less nourished.

Another observation made by Curling, that in fractures of the long bones the portion below the entrance of the nutrient artery, or on that side of the nutritious foramen towards which the blood flows, being defrauded of its proper supply, is subjected to a species of atrophy, presenting a larger medullary canal, with thinner walls, and a spongy tissue less dense, also needs confirmation. Malgaigne has not noticed this fact in any of the specimens contained in the public museums of Paris; and we do not know that any other writer has made the question a subject of especial inquiry.

According to Norris, there are four principal kinds of false joint:—

In the first, the bones are united and completely enveloped in a cartilaginous mass or callous tumor, but in consequence of some retardation in the process bony matter is not deposited, and, as a consequence, it wants solidity, the part continuing easily movable. This may be regarded as a proper example of delayed union, as distinguished from complete non-union, or false joint.

In the second, there is entire want of union of any sort between the fragments, the ends of which seem to be diminished in size and extremely movable beneath the integuments. The limb in these cases is found wasted and powerless.

In the third and most common class, the medullary canal is obliterated in both fragments, and the ends are more or less absorbed, rounded, and covered, in part or in whole, with a dense tissue resembling the periosteum. A connection also exists between the opposing fragments in the form of strong ligamentous or fibro-ligamentous bands, which, if of any length, are quite flexible, and allow of considerable motion at the seat of fracture.

Fig. 16.

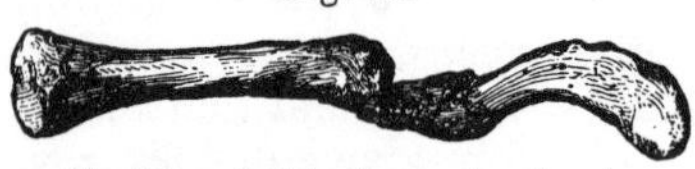

Clavicle united by ligamentous bands.

In the fourth, "a dense capsule without opening of any kind containing a fluid similar to synovia, and resembling closely the complete ligaments, is found." In these cases the points of the bony fragments corresponding to each other, are rounded, smooth and polished, in some instances eburnated, and in others covered with points or even thin plates of cartilage, and a membrane closely resembling the synovial of the natural articulation." It is in this kind of cases, Norris remarks, that the member affected may still be of use to the patient, the fragments being so firmly held together as to be displaced only upon the application of considerable force.

The existence of these newly formed joints, or true diarthroses, has been called in question by Boyer, Hewson, Chelius[1] and others;

[1] Malad. Chirurg., t. iii. p. 103, Paris, 1831; North Amer. Med. and Surg. Journ., No. ix. p. 7, 1828; Trait. de Chir., trad. par Pigné, p. 150, 1836. (Norris, loc. cit.)

but the observations of Sylvestre, Brodie, Beclard, Home, Howship, Otto, Kuhnholtz, Houston, Cooper, Langenbeck and Breschet prove that such examples are occasionally found.[1]

Norris is a disciple of Dupuytren, and accepts his doctrine of the formation of callus without reservation; consequently he finds no necessity for but one form of delayed union, namely, that which we have described as belonging to the first class. In all of this class he assumes the existence of a cartilaginous ring or ferrule; but we think the error of this exclusive theory has been sufficiently shown by the observations of Paget and others, and we should be warranted therefore in affirming the existence of as many varieties of delayed union as there are varieties in the manner and position of the deposit of callus, even if their actual existence had not been repeatedly demonstrated by dissections.

The causes of delayed union and of non-union, are either constitutional or local.

The constitutional causes are chiefly those conditions of the general system which manifest themselves by anemia, debility, or some peculiar dyscrasy.

Sanson, Beulac, Condie[2] and many others have mentioned cases in which the existence of syphilis in the system has seemed to prevent the formation of callus; but on the other hand Lagneau and Oppenheim[3] incline to the opinion that syphilis exerts in this respect but little influence; and even Bérard, who admits the pertinence of one case observed by Nicod, concludes, after numerous researches, that it has been very rarely shown to affect the formation of callus.[4]

Pregnancy and lactation have been known to interfere with the union of bones. Werner, Hildanus, Wilson, Hertodius, Alanson, Bard, of New York, and Condie, of Philadelphia,[5] have all reported examples, in some of which the process of union was resumed and brought to a rapid completion so soon as the period of pregnancy was closed, or when lactation ceased; but three cases reported by Sir Stephen Love Hammick, would seem to show, what, indeed, other evidences render probable, that the delay was less due to the fact of the pregnancy and the lactation, than to the debility occasionally consequent upon these conditions.[6]

As to the question whether cancer ever causes a delay in the union

[1] Nouvelles de la Répub. des Lettres de Bayle, p. 718, 1685; Lond. Med. Gaz., xiii. p. 57, 1833; Beclard, Gen. Anat., trans. by Hayward, pp. 149, 248; Transac. Med.-Chir. Soc. of Edinburgh, i. p. 233, 1793; Med.-Chir. Trans., viii. p. 517, 1817; Otto's Path. Anat., trans. by South, i. p. 138; Journ. Complément., iii. p. 291; Dub. Med. Journ., viii. p. 493; Cooper on Frac. and Disloc, fourth London ed., p. 508; Récherch. sur les Formation du Cal, 1819, p. 34. (Norris, loc. cit.)

[2] Dict. de Méd. et Chir. Prat., iii. p. 492; Journ. de Méd. Chir. et Pharm., t. xxv. p. 216. (Norris, loc. cit.)

[3] Exposé des symp. de la mal. Vén., p. 525; Oppenheim on False Joints, 1837. (Norris, loc. cit.)

[4] Op. cit., p. 21.

[5] Cooper's Dic., ed. 1838, p. 546; Opera Hild., 1681; Wilson on the Human Skeleton, p. 214; Bib. Choisie de Méd., xxiv. p. 595; Med. Obs. and Inquiries, 4, 1772; Philosoph. Trans., xlvi. p. 397, 1750. (Norris, loc. cit.)

[6] Practical Remarks on Amputations, Fractures, &c., p. 121. (Norris, loc. cit.)

of bones, Norris declares, that after a very careful examination of what has been written upon this subject, it is his opinion that where the fracture arises in consequence of a true cancerous deposit around, or in the interior of the bones, producing absorption of their tissue, no union takes place; but where, as is usually the case, the fracture is due to a fragility of the bones, occasioned by what Mr. Curling has denominated eccentric atrophy, it will be found to unite readily. Parker, of New York, relates the case of a girl only fifteen years of age, in whom the femur was broken from a very trivial cause; and in which case the autopsy, made at the end of five months from the time of the accident, furnished some confirmation of these views. The place of fracture was occupied by an irregular encephaloid mass. It is curious, however, that in this case, the callus was actually formed at first, and the bone seemed to be well united at the end of five weeks; but at the time of the autopsy no callus existed.[1]

Scurvy, fevers of a low type, and on the other hand, fevers of a highly inflammatory character, profuse uterine and vaginal discharges, and rachitis, conduce to the same result.

The withdrawal of a habitual stimulus, and especially a change from a good to a low diet, or copious bleedings, may either of them delay the deposit of ossific matter or prevent it altogether.[2]

Bonn has furnished two cases in which advanced age seemed to have retarded the formation of callus, but Horner saw a fracture of the humerus in a woman ninety years old, unite in five weeks.[3] I have myself noticed a good many similar examples in advanced life; and it is now rendered quite probable that surgeons have generally over-estimated the influence of age upon the formation of callus.

The local causes are, arrest of the arterial circulation, paralysis or impairment of the nervous circulation, the occurrence of the fracture within a capsule, obliquity of the fracture, overlapping of the fragments, interposition of a piece of bone, of a tendon, muscle, or of a clot of blood, or separation of the fragments from any cause whatever, erysipelas, acute phlegmonous inflammation, suppuration, necrosis, too much motion, compression, exclusion of light and air inducing local scurvy, wet and especially cold and moist dressings, too early use of the limb, &c.

In order to hasten the consolidation when it is simply delayed, we resort to all of those expedients which are calculated to invigorate the general system; and for this purpose the employment of a nutritious diet and the use of mineral or vegetable tonics may not be properly omitted; but in our experience nothing has proved so efficient as encouraging the patient to leave his bed and get out into the open air; for which purpose, if the fracture is in the lower extremities, crutches will be necessary.

As local means we may enumerate first the removal of those local causes which seem to have interfered with the consolidation or with the union. If the fragments have been officiously disturbed, it may

[1] Parker, New York Journ. Med., July, 1852, p. 97.
[2] Norris, loc. cit.
[3] Ibid., p. 29.

be sufficient to impose upon the limb absolute rest for a certain length of time; and the fragments may be more closely pressed against each other; in other cases it will be found necessary to expose the limb freely to the light and air at least once or twice daily, and to rub it gently with the dry hand or with some moderately stimulating oil, so as to induce a more healthy condition of the soft parts, and encourage the natural circulation.

Moving the fragments freely upon each other, sufficient to determine a degree of excitement in the adjacent tissues, and upon the opposing surfaces of the bones, and then confining them during one or two weeks in firm and well fitting splints, will often succeed when other means have failed.

Indeed I may say that by one or another of the simple methods now enumerated I have never failed sooner or later to effect consolidation, in recent fractures; and it has only been in fractures of at least four, six, or eight months' standing that I have been compelled to resort to more extreme measures.

As a means of combining immobility with compression and healthful exercise the "apparatus immobile," in many of its forms, is peculiarly adapted. White, of Manchester, employed a firm leather sheath for the thigh. H. H. Smith, of Philadelphia, recommends a more complex artificial support, upon which the limb may be allowed to rest while in the act of progression.[1] With some surgeons the object of allowing the patient to walk in fractures of the thigh or leg, is chiefly to excite in the tissues adjacent to the seat of fracture some degree of inflammatory action, but which, as the result in one of White's patients has sufficiently shown, may be carried too far, and even determine a suppuration.

Blisters, mustard cataplasms, the tincture of iodine,[2] caustics,[3] &c., applied externally over the seat of fracture, can have no other effect than to increase moderately the congestion of the tissues, and in so far they may aid in the accomplishment of the bony union; but in this respect they are inferior to the violent twistings, flexions, and rubbings of the broken ends of which we have already spoken.

Electricity was first employed by Mr. Birch, of London, but Dr. Mott obtained no effect from it in two cases where he seems to have given it a fair trial.[4] Lente, of the New York Hospital, has more recently furnished an account of three cases treated in that institution by electricity in connection with acupuncturation; the mode of using which was to pass a needle down to the periosteum on each side of the bone, and to attach the poles of the battery to these opposite points. Lente thinks that electricity employed in this way is much more efficient than when the poles are merely applied to the surface. He informs us also that other cases than these now reported have been treated successfully in this hospital by means of electricity.[5]

[1] H. H. Smith, Amer. Journ. Med. Sci., Jan. 1855.
[2] Hartshorne, Eclectic Rep., vol. iii. p. 114, 1813.
[3] Willoughby, Am. Journ. Med. Sci., Aug. 1834, p. 444.
[4] Mott, Med. and Surg. Rep., p. 21, p. 375.
[5] Lente, New York Journ. Med., Nov. 1850, p. 317.

Mercury, urged to ptyalism, will no doubt prove serviceable occasionally by virtue of its powers as an anti-syphilitic, but its beneficial influence in other cases is far from having been established.

The seton is said to have been first suggested by Winslow, in 1787; but what is of much more consequence, the credit of its first successful application and its general introduction into practice, is due to Dr. Philip Syng Physick, of Philadelphia, by whom it was employed in 1802.[1]

Physick used for his seton, generally, silk ribbon, or French tape; and this he introduced by means of a long seton needle, between the ends of the fragments. He recommended that the seton should remain in place four or five months, and longer if necessary, and it was his opinion that the failures were generally due to its being removed too early. At the present day, however, surgeons who employ the seton think it serves its purpose better when it remains in place but a few days, not longer, perhaps, than ten or fifteen, always taking care that it is removed before excessive suppuration is induced. It has been found especially valuable in fractures of the inferior maxilla, clavicle, and upper extremity generally; but in the case of the femur, it has so frequently failed that Dr. Physick himself did not recommend its use.

Fig. 17.

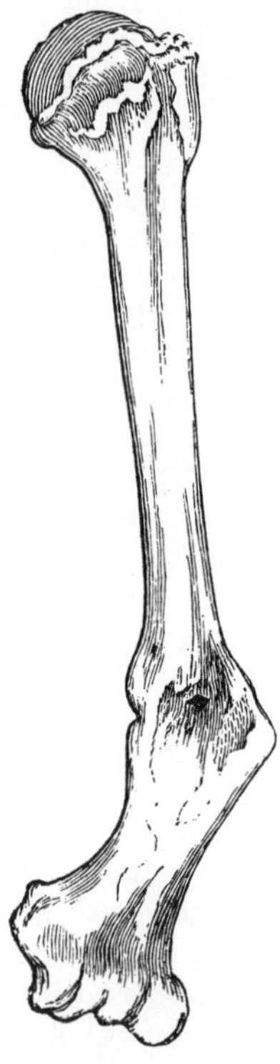

Physick's first case, after 28 years.

In case the seton cannot be passed directly between the opposing fragments, as recommended by Physick, we may adopt the practice suggested by Oppenheim, and carry two setons, one on each side, close to the bone.

Sommé, of Antwerp, preferred a loop of wire to the silk seton employed by Physick.[2] Seerig passed a ligature around the ligamentous mass connecting the two fragments, and then proceeded to tighten the ligature until it fell off.[3] Dr. Hulse, of the U. S. Navy, employed stimulating injections with success in a case of non-union, accompanied with an external and fistulous opening.[4] In 1848, Dieffenbach recommended that ivory pegs be introduced into holes previously made in the bone,[5] by means of a gimlet or drill, and Mr. Stanley has succeeded once by this method.[6]

Malgaigne, in 1837, tried to introduce acupuncture needles between the ends of an ununited fracture, but although he thrust the needle down to the bone thirty-six times, he was unable to make it pass once

[1] Physick, Med. Repository of New York, vol. i. 1804.
[2] Amer. Journ. Med. Sci., vol. vii. p. 497. [3] Norris, loc cit., p. 46.
[4] Hulse, Amer. Journ. Med. Sci., vol. xiii. p. 374.
[5] Malgaigne, trans. by Packard, op. cit., p. 258, note.
[6] Stanley, New York Journ. Med., Nov. 1854, p. 441, from Dublin Press.

between the ends of the fragments.[1] Wiesel succeeded better. In a case of ununited fracture of the ulna of nine weeks' standing, having passed two needles between the fragments, at the end of six days, the needles being removed, consolidation rapidly ensued.[2] This practice does not differ essentially from the metallic loop of Sommé. It is only a modification of the seton.

Fig. 18.

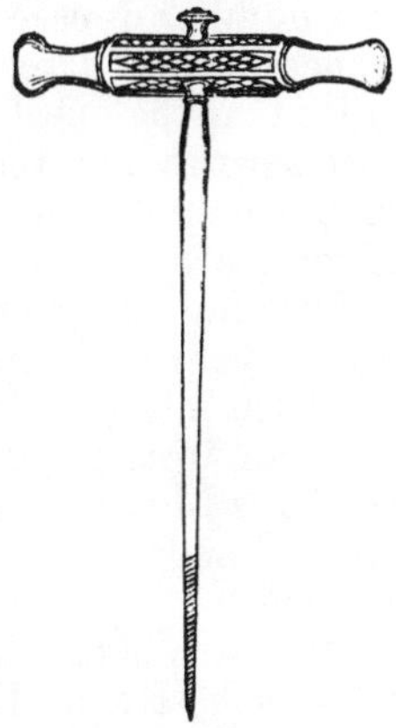

Dieffenbach's drill for ununited fracture.

Brainard, of Chicago, has attempted to show that setons of any kind, whether of wood, ivory, or metal, placed in contact with the bone, occasion absorption, caries, and necrosis, but that they never directly give rise to bony callus; and that the occasional success of the seton, which success he believes to have been greatly exaggerated, has not resulted from any tendency to favor the formation of callus, but from the induration and tenderness of the soft parts produced by it; circumstances which by conducing to rest, indirectly favor the consolidation.[3]

In May, 1848, Miller, of Edinburgh, reported five cases treated successfully by subcutaneous puncture. The operation consisted in passing the point of a needle or small tenotomy bistoury, down upon the ends of the bone, and freely irritating the surfaces at several points.[4] George F. Sandford, of Davenport, Iowa, has successfully imitated this practice in two cases.[5]

Brainard employs for this purpose a strong metallic perforator, consisting of a handle into which points of different sizes may be inserted, and which have been hardened so as to penetrate the hardest bone or even ivory in every direction easily. The points are "somewhat awl-shaped; but more pointed in the middle rather than like a drill, which leaves chips." His manner of using this instrument is as

Fig. 19.

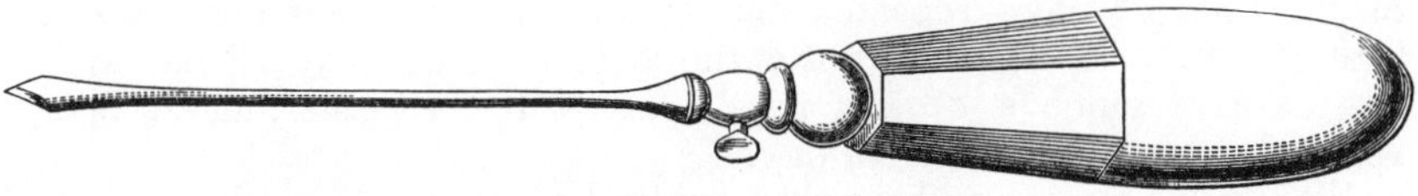

Brainard's perforator, reduced one-half.

follows: "In case of an oblique fracture, or one with overlapping, the skin is perforated with the instrument at such a point as to enable it to be carried through the ends of the fragments, to wound their surfaces, and to transfix whatever tissue may be placed between them.

[1] Malgaigne, op. cit.
[2] Wiesel, Amer. Journ. Med. Sci., vol. xxxiv. p. 254, July, 1844.
[3] Brainard, Trans. Amer. Med. Assoc., vol. vii., 1854: Prize Essay.
[4] Miller, New York Journ. Med., July, 1848, p. 134.
[5] Sandford, Trans. Amer. Med. Assoc., vol. iii. p. 355, 1850.

After having transfixed them in one direction, it is withdrawn from the bone, but not from the skin, its direction changed, and another perforation made, and this operation is repeated as often as may be desired." Dr. Brainard, who has already succeeded by this procedure in a number of cases of ununited fracture, thinks it is better to commence in most cases with not more than two or three perforations, in order that the effect produced shall not be too severe. It is scarcely necessary to add that, after the punctures have been made, the limb should be put completely at rest in appropriate splints, or in apparatus of some kind.

Scraping or rasping the ends of the bones is a practice which dates from a very early period. Mr. Brodie scraped the ends of the bones, and then interposed a bit of lint.[1] Mayor, in 1828, contrived to introduce an iron, previously heated in boiling water, through a canula, and thus brought the heat to bear directly upon the ends of the fragments; and by repeating the application several times a cure was effected.[2]

Resection of the ends of the bones, first brought into notice by White, of Manchester, in 1760,[3] and opposed by Brodie[4] as dangerous, and by Malgaigne regarded as generally useless or unnecessary, has still been practised a great number of times with more or less success. It is especially applicable to superficial bones, and in cases where the bones overlap.

Roux practised resection in one instance, and then managed to engage the point of one of the fragments in the medullary canal of the other.[5]

White, of Manchester, Henry Cline, of London, Hewson, Barton, and Norris, of Philadelphia, have applied caustics directly to the ends of the fragments, after having exposed them by a free incision.[6] Petit applied the actual cautery.[7]

Tying the fragments together by means of metallic ligatures, is as old as the days of Hippocrates; but in 1805 Horeau adopted the same procedure in a case of ununited fracture.[8] J. Kearney Rodgers, Mott and Cheeseman, of New York, Flaubert, of Rouen,[9] and N. R. Smith, of Baltimore,[10] have repeated the operation with complete success. The operation is, however, not without its hazards. Norris has seen one case in which a broken patella was wired together, and a fatal result followed on the fourth day.

Finally, having thus brought rapidly before us all of the various modes of treatment which have been suggested and practised for non-union of broken bones, we are prepared to affirm the following conclusions, or summary of what we believe ought to be the general course of procedure in these cases:—

First. Improve the condition of the general system.

[1] Brodie, Lond. Med. Gaz., July, 1834. [2] Norris, loc. cit., p. 48.
[3] Dict. de Méd., vol. xiii. p. 503.
[4] Brodie, New York Journ. Med., vol. viii. 1st ser., p. 133.
[5] Norris, loc. cit., p. 49. [6] Ibid. [7] Ibid. [8] Ibid.
[9] Rodgers, New York Journ. Med., vol. i. 1st ser., p. 343, 1839.
[10] Note to Packard's Trans. of Malgaigne, p. 255.

Second. Remove as far as possible the local impediments, such as a separation of the fragments, local paralysis, local scurvy resulting from long exclusion from light and air, congestions, &c.

Third. Increase the action of the tissues immediately adjacent to the fracture, upon which tissues rather than upon the bone, as Malgaigne thinks, the formation of callus depends. A theory which, as applied to old and ununited fractures, we are not prepared to deny. This may be accomplished by frictions, and violent flexions of the limb at the seat of fracture; possibly in some measure by the application of vesicants or of other stimulants, to the skin itself.

Fourth. Employ again compression and rest for a period of from two to four or eight weeks.

Fifth. Resort to the practice recommended by Brainard, namely, perforation of the soft parts and bone with an awl.

Sixth. If in the lower extremity, allow the patient to walk about, after the plan of White or Smith.

Seventh. If the fracture is not in the femur, and as an extreme measure, employ the seton.

Eighth. Resection is applicable only to superficial bones, and in cases of overlapping.

Where these measures have failed, after a fair trial, we should either abandon the case as hopeless, only supporting the limb by such apparatus as may be found most serviceable, or we should recommend amputation.

CHAPTER VII.

BENDING, PARTIAL FRACTURES, AND FISSURES OF THE LONG BONES.

§ 1. Bending of the Long Bones.

Strictly speaking, no bone can be much bent without being also more or less broken, and that, whether it immediately and spontaneously resumes its position or not; for, if the bending and straightening of the bone be repeated a sufficient number of times, the yielding of the fibres will become apparent, and at length the separation will be complete. The first of this series of flexions was quite as much responsible for this result as the last, and, no doubt, performed its share in the production of the complete fracture.

There could be no impropriety, therefore, in speaking of a bending of the bones as a variety of incomplete fractures, as I have done in the first section of my "Report on Deformities after Fractures," made to the American Medical Association in 1855.[1]

They have been called, not inappropriately, interperiosteal fractures, since in these cases the periosteum is not broken; M. Blandin thinks that the outer and semi-cartilaginous laminæ of the bone also do not break, while the deeper laminæ suffer an actual disruption.[2] But it is quite as probable that in a majority of cases the true pathological condition is a compression of the bony fibres upon one side, with a corresponding expansion upon the opposite side, with only a slight interstitial fracture, too trivial to be easily recognized even in the dissection. Sometimes, as I have several times observed in my experiments on the bones of chickens, when the bones are small, and the bending is near the centre of the shaft, the whole of the laminæ on the side of the retiring angle produced by the bending are doubled in, or indented toward the hollow of the bone, so that the fibres on the side of the salient angle are not even stretched, and much less broken. In such cases, the interstitial disruption, if it exists at all, and I think it does, first takes place in the deeper layers of the retiring angle.

I might, therefore, feel justified in continuing to call these cases partial fractures, or, perhaps, interstitial fractures, but I believe that the whole subject will be rendered more intelligible if I call them simply bending of the bones, as distinguished from those other and more palpably partial fractures of which I shall speak presently.

1. *Bending with an immediate and spontaneous restoration of the bone to its original form.*—The possibility of this accident, to which, however, surgical writers have hitherto made no distinct allusion, is rendered certain by the following experiments:—

Experiment 1.—July 16, 1857. I bent the tibia of a Shanghai chicken, four weeks old, at about the middle of the bone. It was bent to an angle of quite twenty-five degrees, but it was not felt or heard to break. It immediately and spontaneously resumed the straight position.

July 18, two days after the bending, I dissected the limb, and found no trace of the injury, either within or without the bone, unless I except a very minute blood-clot in the centre of the shaft.

Experiment 2.—I bent the leg of a chicken, four weeks old, at the same point and to the same degree. It immediately resumed the straight position.

Dissection after two days. Nothing abnormal except a small blood-clot in the centre of the bone, and a slight disorganization of the medulla.

Experiments 3 *and* 4.—Bent both legs of a chicken, four weeks old, at the same point and in the same manner. They immediately resumed their positions.

Dissection after two days. No lesions or morbid appearances which I could detect.

[1] Op. cit., pp. 421–422.

[2] Markham's Obs. on the Surg. Practice of Paris, London Med.-Chir. Rev., vol. xxxiv. p. 473, 1841.

Experiments 5 *and* 6.—Bent both wings of a chicken, four weeks old. Bent the right wing to an angle of thirty-five degrees. I did not feel them break. Both resumed their positions spontaneously.

Dissection after two days. No lesions or other morbid appearances.

Experiment 7.—July 16, 1857, I bent the leg of a Shanghai chicken, five weeks old, below the knee, and at about the middle of the bone. It was bent to an angle of about twenty-five degrees, but the bone was not felt or heard to break. It immediately and spontaneously resumed the straight position.

July 20, four days after the bending, I dissected the leg, but could not discover the slightest trace of the injury, unless it be that there was a very minute ossific deposit in the centre of the bone at the point at which I suppose it to have been bent.

Experiment 8.—July 16, 1857, I bent the right leg of a Shanghai chicken, five weeks old, at the same point as in the first experiment, and to the same extent. The bone did not seem to break, but it immediately and spontaneously resumed the straight position.

Dissection after four days. Nothing appeared to indicate the seat of the bending except a small clot of blood in the centre of the shaft.

Experiment 9.—Bent the leg of a chicken, six weeks old, in the same manner, and to the same degree, as in the other examples. It resumed its position spontaneously.

Dissection after ten days. No evidence of injury of any kind; the bone being sound and straight.

These experiments were made in connection with others, which I shall take occasion hereafter to mention. They are selected, and constitute the whole number of those in which I did not feel the bone break or crack under my fingers. In every instance the bone sprung back immediately and spontaneously to its natural form. In no instance could I afterward discover any trace of lesion, or sign indicating the point at which the bone had been bent before dissection; nor did dissection itself disclose anything but the most inconsiderable marks, and that in but three examples.

I infer, therefore, not forgetting the caution with which the conclusions from all such experiments ought to be applied to similar accidents upon the human skeleton, that whenever the bones of healthy infants have been forcibly bent, they will, probably, in all cases, unless prevented by causes foreign to the bones themselves, spontaneously and immediately resume their position; and that no sign will remain to indicate that a bending has occurred. The accident will not be recognized; and, as a farther inference, this bending does not belong to that class of cases which have been so frequently described as examples of bending without fracture.

2. *Bending without immediate and spontaneous restoration of the bone to its original form.*—"Dethleef, believing that he had broken the two bones of the leg of a dog, found the fibula bent, without a fracture. Similar results were obtained by Duhamel upon a lamb; by Troja upon a pigeon; and I have myself twice succeeded in bending the

fibula while breaking the tibia. The possibility of simple curvature is then not contestable" (the writer means to say that the possibility of a simple curvature *remaining permanently* bent, is not contestable), "but we must observe that they have never been obtained except upon young animals, and that they have been unable to maintain themselves permanently except through the aid of a fracture and displacement of a neighboring bone; and there is a wide difference between these and those pretended curvatures which some believe they have seen in man, in which the curved bone maintains itself, and resists perfect reduction until the fracture is complete."[1]

In this single paragraph Malgaigne seems to have given a fair summary of the testimony upon this point. With the exception of these and a few other similar examples, some of which I think I have observed myself, where one of the bones of the forearm has been broken and the other bent, I know of no well attested cases of a permanent bending; using the term bending in a sense distinguished from a partial fracture.

If, in numerous cases mentioned by surgical writers, there has seemed to be probable evidence that the permanent bending was unaccompanied with fracture, there has always been wanting, so far as I know, the positive evidence of dissection. The example of partial fracture mentioned by Fergusson, and represented by a drawing, is described as having also, "toward the lower extremity, a slight indentation and curve."[2] This was the radius of a child; but how long the child survived the accident, and what was the condition of the ulna, we are not informed. The observations made by Jurine, of Geneva, in Switzerland,[3] by Barton[4] and Norris,[5] of Philadelphia, all fail to furnish any such conclusive evidence of the correctness of their own views. Norris says that "Thierry, of Bordeaux, Martin, and Chevalier, had all met with and published cases of this kind prior to the appearance of Jurine's paper (in 1810), the former of whom asserts that Haller, in experimenting upon the subject, had been able satisfactorily to produce the same accident in young animals." For myself, I cannot say how much confidence we ought to place in these assertions of Thierry, Martin, and Chevalier, having never seen the papers referred to; but since Dr. Norris has neglected to inform us whether any dissections were ever made, we shall not be expected to regard their testimony as conclusive.

Fig. 20.

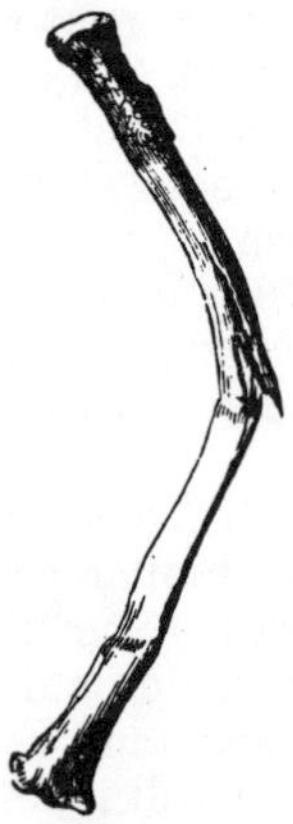

Case mentioned by Fergusson.

With the qualifications now made, Gibson was more nearly right when he said, "Dupuytren and Dr. John Rhea Barton have each furnished accounts of *bent* bones. There are no such injuries, however, in my opinion; such cases being, in reality, *partial*

[1] Traité des Frac., etc.; par L. F. Malgaigne, tom. i. p. 48.
[2] Practical Surgery; by Wm. Fergusson, 4th Am. ed., p. 208.
[3] Journ. de Corvisart et Boyer, tom. xx. p. 278, etc.
[4] Phila. Med. Recorder, 1821.
[5] Phila. Med. Journ., vol. xxix. p. 233, 1842.

fractures, from which deformities result, upon the same principle that a piece of tough wood, like oak or hickory, if broken half through, may be inclined to one side and shortened, although still held together by interlocking of fibres. Many specimens in my cabinet, and in the Wistar Museum, attest the accuracy of this assertion."[1]

In my own experiments upon the chicken, the bones uniformly resumed their original position as soon as the restraining force was removed, unless a fracture occurred, and this notwithstanding the bones were bent quite abruptly and to an angle of twenty-five degrees. Certainly, if the bones of children may be bent during life and be made to retain this position without a fracture, then the same thing might be done upon the bones of children recently dead, and by successful experiments, this long agitated question might be easily and forever put to rest.

It will be understood that our observations are confined to the long bones. That the flat bones, and especially the bones of the cranium, in childhood, may be indented by blows, and remain in this condition, is undeniable. Scultetus says he had seen "the skull pressed down in children, without a fracture, so that those who touch or look upon it can perceive a small pit,"[2] and it has been mentioned by many writers since, and perhaps before his day. I have myself published two examples of it in the second volume of the *Buffalo Medical Journal*.[3]

§ 2. Partial Fracture of the Long Bones.

1. *Partial Fracture with immediate and spontaneous restoration of the bone to its original form.*—No writer seems to have given any special attention to the form of fracture now under consideration although its existence appears to have been occasionally recognized. In the case reported by Camper, in 1765, of a partial fracture of the tibia, the bone had regained its natural form, but whether immediately after the accident occurred, or at a later period, I am not able to learn.[4] Jurine, Gulliver, and others, have noticed a gradual straightening of the bone after a partial fracture, so that its complete restoration has been accomplished after several weeks or months; but this, although partly due to the same cause which produces occasionally an immediate restoration, namely, its elasticity, is in part also due to other causes, and will be more properly considered under the next division of partial fractures.

Says Malgaigne: "Finally, at other times the fracture takes place without opening and without curvature; the only sign which one can recognize is a yielding of the bone under the pressure of the finger, at the point of fracture; yet, upon the living subject, we may see the

[1] Institutes and Practice of Surgery, by Wm. Gibson, Phila., 1841, vol. i. p. 254.
[2] The Chirurgeon's Storehouse, by Johannes Scultetus, 1674, p. 126.
[3] Op. cit., p. 347, 1846, Cases 1 and 2.
[4] Essays and Obs. Phys. and Lit. of Soc. of Edinburgh, vol. iii. p. 537.

same symptom pertain to complete and simple fractures without displacement."[1]

Blandin has described the accident a little more distinctly: "In some cases of fracture of the clavicle occurring about the middle of the bone in young subjects, displacement of the fragments does not immediately take place, thus giving rise to a risk of an error in diagnosis, by which the ultimate probability of a cure is diminished. A lad seventeen years of age, was recently admitted into the Hôtel Dieu, under the care of M. Blandin, having, a few days previously, fallen upon one of his comrades while playing with him, when he instantly experienced pain and a cracking sensation about the middle of the left clavicle, where there soon formed a tumor, which, increasing, induced him to enter the hospital. On examination, the swelling was found to occupy the middle of the clavicle; it was about as large as half a hen's egg, ovoid in shape, well circumscribed, colorless, and hard, but sensible to pressure. There was not any deformity of the shoulder, nor any abnormal modification of the axis of the bone, to indicate the existence of a fracture; and although the different movements of the arm caused pain in the shoulder, yet they could be made without much difficulty.

"The symptoms in this case would lead to the belief that it was a case of simple periostitis, caused by external violence; but M. Blandin at once decided that there existed a fracture of the bone, having seen a similar case previously at the hospital Beaujon, where the tumor was treated as traumatic periostitis, the patient merely carrying his arm in a sling, until, by a sudden movement of the limb, displacement of the fragments was produced, and clearly demonstrated the existence of a fracture. A second case occurring soon afterward, M. Blandin profited by the experience gained from the preceding, and by moving the fragments of the broken clavicle on each other, obtained motion and crepitus. Still these indications were not so clear, that M. Marjolin could diagnosticate a fracture; he was of opinion that the case was one of exostosis, probably syphilitic, and the crepitus, he believed, depended on an erosion of the osseous surface. In consequence, the patient was left to himself, until a movement of the arm gave proof of the fracture by the displacement of the broken portions of the bones.

"Two other cases occurring in young subjects have been admitted since into the Hôtel Dieu, under the care of M. Blandin, one of whom was purposely left without surgical assistance, while Desault's bandage was applied to the other. The former soon showed evidences of consecutive displacement; the latter was cured without any deformity following.

"The surgeon may diagnose a fracture, without displacement of the middle portion of the clavicle, when a circumscribed tumor forms in that part in young subjects, consecutive on a fall on the shoulder, and motion of the fragments, with crepitus, can be detected, there not being any syphilitic taint in the constitution."[2]

[1] Op. cit., tom. i. p. 50.
[2] Am. Journ. Med. Sci., vol. xxxi. p. 473, from Journ. de Méd. et Chirurg. Prat., July, 1842.

Prof. Green, of Geneva Med. Col., N. Y., has furnished me the following account of a case which came under his observation.

"December 21, 1847, I was called to dress what was considered to be a fractured clavicle, of George Stone, a lad eight years of age. One of his playmates had tripped him in such a manner that he fell on his side, striking on the extremity of the left shoulder. I found that he was unable to raise the hand to the head. On examination, I discovered on the posterior edge of the clavicle, at the inner extremity of the external curvature, a point which was swollen, tender, and painful. The anterior edge of the clavicle was continuous, and there was neither crepitus nor displacement. Considering the age of the patient, and the appearance of the parts, I diagnosed bending of the clavicle forward, with a splitting out of the posterior edge, and that the bone, by its elasticity, had resumed its ordinary direction. In order to be safe, however, I dressed the shoulder as for actual fracture of the clavicle, lest the fracture might have extended nearly through the bone, and there be subsequent displacement. The swelling subsided in four or five days, and as all seemed secure, I removed the dressings, and heard no more of the matter until the 11th of May, ult., when I was called to see the patient again, and found that he had met, the day before, with precisely the same accident, at the old point, and by the same cause, being tripped down by a playmate. This time the swelling and other symptoms of inflammation were greater than before. The anterior edge of the clavicle was entirely continuous, but he could not raise the arm. I merely directed him to keep to his bed until the swelling and inflammation should in a measure subside. In three or four days he was about. The callus left is not large, still it is quite evident."

The following examples which have come under my own observation, will illustrate more completely their usual history and symptoms:—

A. B., aged three years, fell from the sofa on to the floor, striking, it is thought, on her right shoulder. Two days after this, she fell again, and then, for the first time, Mr. B. noticed the deformity. She was brought to me three days after the second fall. There existed then a round, smooth projection at the outer end of the middle third of the clavicle. It felt hard, like bone. The line of the clavicle was not changed. I advised a handkerchief sling, simply to steady and support the arm. Seven months after the accident, she fell sick and died. The projection continued at the time of death, only slightly diminished.

H. S., aged six years, was thrown from a horse, partially breaking his left clavicle, near its middle. Dr. Sprague, of Buffalo, was employed. The projection in front was for several days very apparent, and was examined by myself at Dr. Sprague's request. The bone did not seem to be out of line. Five years after the accident, I examined the lad, and could not find any trace of the original injury.

September 25, 1855. Mrs. T. C. brought to me her infant child, then but two weeks old. Upon the left clavicle, at a point a little nearer the acromion than the sternum, was an oblong swelling, three-quarters of an inch in length, smooth and hard like callus; the skin was not reddened, nor tender. There was no motion or crepitus, and the line of the axis of the bone was perfect. The mother, who had been put to bed by a midwife, thinks the injury occurred in the act of birth, although she did not notice the swelling until a week after.

October 20. Nearly one month later, I found no change in the condition of the bone; the hard lump remained, but it was still entirely free from tenderness. I have not seen the child since.

An infant boy, three years old, fell, August 12, 1857, from the hands of the nurse. The child cried, but the point of injury was not detected until the third or fourth day, although the mother examined the shoulders and neck carefully at the time. She is quite certain that if any swelling or discoloration had been present she would have seen it then, or on the subsequent days, while washing and dressing the child; when first seen it was very distinct, but not so large as at present.

August 19. The child was brought to me. A little to the sternal side of the middle of the right clavicle there was an oblong node-like swelling, of the size of the half of a pigeon's egg, hard, smooth, and feeling like bone; there was no discoloration or swelling of the integuments; no crepitus or motion; the line of the clavicle seemed nearly or quite unchanged.

I have not noticed this variety of accident in any other bone except the clavicle, yet it is not improbable that it happens occasionally, and perhaps quite as often, in other long bones, but that its existence is not elsewhere so easily recognized.

Of eighty-nine fractures of the clavicle, which have come under my observation, twenty-one were partial fractures; and of these six were spontaneously and immediately restored to their natural axes.

Experiment.—In fourteen experiments upon the bones of chickens, a partial fracture, with immediate and spontaneous restoration, has occurred but once. In nine of these cases the bones were only bent, and in five they were partially broken; an immediate restoration has occurred, therefore, in one case out of five of partial fracture; while in my reported examples of partial fracture of the clavicle it has been noticed about once in every four cases. The following is the experiment to which I have referred:—

I produced a partial fracture of the tibia in a chicken six weeks old. The fracture was near the middle of the bone. I felt it break under my finger; but on removing the pressure, it immediately and spontaneously resumed the straight position.

I dissected the limb on the tenth day. The line of the axis of the bone was perfect; but on the fractured side was a node-like enlargement, sufficient to be distinctly felt and seen before the soft parts were removed.

Pathology.—In no case, except in my single experiment upon the bone of a chicken, has the actual condition been determined by dissection, and if any question has existed heretofore as to the possibility of an immediate and spontaneous restoration after a partial fracture, this experiment ought to decide it in the affirmative; but then the first nine experiments already quoted have shown that a mere bending with immediate restoration leaves no such traces or signs as have been described as following these accidents. We have, therefore, the negative argument that, since a bending with restoration leaves no signs, these examples reported by myself and others as having occurred, and as having been followed by a node-like swelling, etc., must have been partial fractures. Moreover, in one of the cases reported by Blandin, there was a feeble crepitus; and in another, the subsequent displacement proved the correctness of his diagnosis.

We conclude, then, that these are examples of partial fracture, but that the number of bony fibres which have given way is too inconsiderable, as compared with those not broken, to affect materially the elasticity of the bone.

Diagnosis.—The diagnosis will depend somewhat upon the history of the accident as well as upon the present symptoms. In no instance, where I could ascertain the cause, have I known an incomplete fracture of this variety produced by any other than an indirect blow; and where the clavicle has been the seat of the curvature the counter-blow has been received upon the end of the shoulder. This fact possesses, therefore, equal significance in its relation to either of the varieties of partial fracture; but in the case of a partial fracture, with a permanent curvature, the diagnosis would be complete without the history, while in this case it might not be, and a knowledge of the manner in which the accident occurred would, therefore, be of great importance.

The signs, then, after a knowledge of the fact that a blow has been received upon the shoulder, are a node-like swelling upon the anterior or upper face of the clavicle, generally in its middle third, this swelling being hard, smooth, oblong; the skin only slightly or not at all swollen or tender, and in no way discolored, as it would have been had the swelling upon the bone been the result of a direct blow, and the line of the axis of the bone unchanged. I have never detected motion or crepitus at the point of injury, yet we have seen that Blandin was able to detect both in one instance; nor has it ever occurred to me to see the swelling upon the bone until two or three days after the injury was received. We are not likely, therefore, to recognize this accident immediately after its occurrence.

Treatment.—In the case of the clavicle, neither bandages, slings, compresses, nor lotions can be of much service. The utmost that can be necessary is to enjoin some degree of care in using the arm of the injured side. The consolidation will be speedily accomplished, and after a time the ensheathing callus will wholly disappear.

If a similar accident should occur in any other of the long bones, as retentive and precautionary means, splints might be applied, at least for a few days.

2. *Partial Fracture without immediate and spontaneous restoration of the bone to its natural form.*—The causes of this accident are the same with those which produce simple bending, or partial fracture with immediate and spontaneous restoration, from which latter they differ pro-

bably in the greater extent of the bony lesion. Perhaps, also, they differ sometimes in the peculiar form and degree of the denticulation at the seat of the fracture; in consequence of which an antagonism of the fibres takes place, preventing a restoration of the bone to its original form.

Fig. 21.

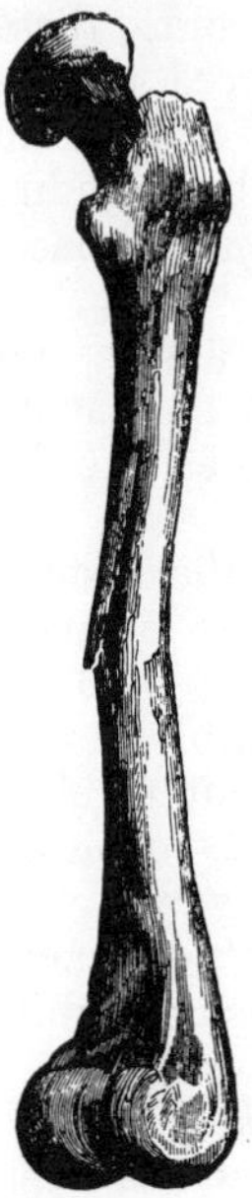

Partial fracture without restoration of the bone to its natural form.

They constitute a large majority of those examples of partial fractures which come under our observation in the various long bones. In eighty-nine fractures of the clavicle, it has been observed by me fifteen times, or once in about every six cases. In one hundred and eighty-eight fractures of the radius and ulna, it has occurred twelve times, or once in about fifteen cases. The following are the exact observations upon which this latter statement rests:—

Fractures of the radius alone, fifty-four; no partial fractures.

Fractures of the ulna alone, thirty; no partial fractures.

Fractures of both bones at once, fifty-two (one hundred and four fractures); twelve partial fractures.

The one hundred and four fractures last enumerated were as follows:—

Radius and ulna both partially broken five times; ten partial fractures.

Radius partially broken and ulna completely, once.

Ulna partially broken and radius completely, once.

It has not happened to me to meet with this fracture in any other bone; but examples have been mentioned as having occurred in the humerus, ribs, femur, tibia, and fibula.

Very few surgeons have spoken of partial fractures in the clavicle, while Jurine, Symes, Liston, Miller, Norris, and many others, have declared that it is much more frequent in the bones of the forearm than elsewhere. This does not agree with my experience, according to which it occurs oftener in the clavicle than in the forearm: a discrepancy which I cannot very well explain, except by supposing that, in the case of the clavicle, the accident has either been overlooked entirely or misapprehended. Blandin, who we have seen has reported five cases of partial fracture of the clavicle with immediate restoration, states distinctly that in two of these cases distinguished surgeons of Hôpital Beaujon and Hôtel Dieu failed to recognize it.

Fig. 22.

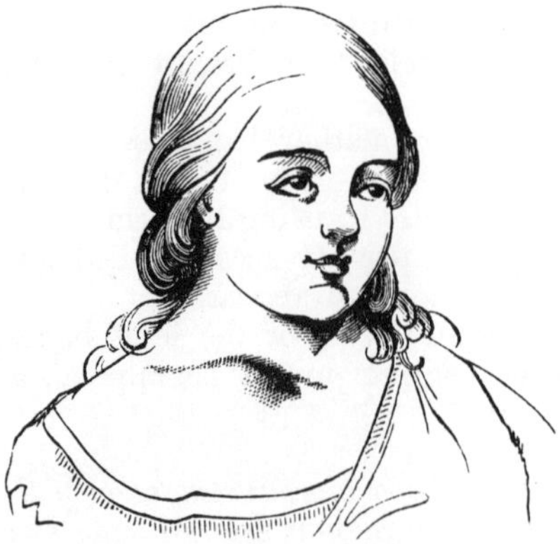

Partial fracture of the clavicle without spontaneous restoration. From nature; taken three weeks after the accident.

Says Turner: "The next I shall descend to is that of the clavicle, or collar-bone, which I have found the most frequently overlooked, I think, of any other, till it has been sometimes too late to remedy, especially among the children of poor people; for, though they find these little ones to wince, scream, or cry, upon the taking off or putting on their clothes, yet, seeing that they suffer the handling of their wrists and arms, though it be with pain, they suspect only some sprain or wrench, that will go away of itself, without regarding anything further or looking out for help; whereas, this fracture discovers itself as easily as most others. For not only the eye, in examining or taking a view of the part, may plainly perceive a bunching out or protuberance of the bones when the neck is bared for that purpose, with a sinking down in the middle or on one side thereof, which will be still more obvious on comparing it with its fellow on the other side; but when it is more obscure, and the bone, as it were, cracked only—a *semi-fracture*, as we say—yet, by pressing hard upon the part, from one extremity to the other, you will find your patient crying out when you come upon the place; and by your fingers, so examining, sometimes perceive a sinking farther down, with a crackling of the bone itself."[1]

Erichsen, who regards all of these cases as mere bendings of the bones, remarks that it "most commonly occurs in the long bones, especially the clavicle, the radius, and the femur."[2] He says, moreover, "fracture of the clavicle in infants not unfrequently occurs, and is apt to be overlooked. The child cries and suffers pain whenever the arm is moved. On examination, an irregularity, with some protuberance, will be felt about the centre of the bone."[3] The reader will not fail to recognize, in these symptoms, the incomplete fracture of which we are now speaking, although Erichsen evidently believes them to be examples of complete fracture.

In addition to this testimony as to the frequency of these fractures in the clavicle, I will only mention that Johnson, in his review of Markham's *Observations on the Surgical Practice of Paris*, says that "many surgeons have noticed the incomplete fracture of the clavicle as of other bones, which take place in the young."[4]

Pathology.—The following experiments will assist in the elucidation of this point of our subject:—

Experiment 1.—I bent the leg of a chicken five weeks old. It cracked under my fingers, and remained bent. Having waited a few seconds, and finding that it was not restored to position, I pressed upon it and made it straight. The chicken walked off without any limp.

On the fourth day, before dissection, the bone looked as if it was still bent; but on removing the soft parts, the line of the axis of the bone was found to be straight. The areolar tissue under the skin was infiltrated with lymph, which was most abundant near the fracture, and gradually diminished toward each extremity of the limb. This

[1] Art of Surgery, by Daniel Turner, London, 1742, vol. ii. p. 255.
[2] Science and Art of Surgery. Phila. ed., 1854, p. 180.
[3] Ibid., p. 205.
[4] Lond. Med.-Chir. Rev., vol. xxxiv. p. 474, 1841.

effusion was confined almost entirely to the front of the limb, or to that side which had been broken, and constituted the greater part of the enlargement which I had noticed before the dissection was commenced, and which then felt like bone.

On the front of the bone, also, underneath the periosteum, there was a loose, honey-comb deposit of ensheathing callus, about one line in thickness, and extending upward and downward about half an inch. This callus surrounded the bone in three-fourths of its circumference: but there was no callus on its posterior surface. It was also deficient exactly along the line of fracture, in front and on the sides, in consequence of which an oblique groove remained, indicating the seat of the fracture.

Experiment 2.—I produced a partial fracture at the same point, in a chicken five weeks old. The bone was felt to crack, and, as it would not straighten spontaneously, I immediately bent it back to its place.

On the eighth day I dissected the limb. The appearances, before and after dissection, were the same as in Experiment 1. No ensheathing callus on the posterior surface. The furrow over the line of fracture was not quite so deep as in Experiment 1. On opening into the centre of the shaft I found the canal nearly filled with bony matter opposite the fracture, and the broken ends were completely united.

Fig. 23.

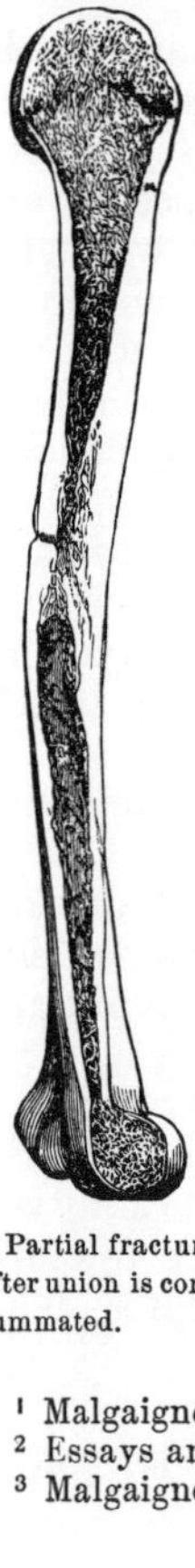

Partial fracture after union is consummated.

Experiment 3.—This was made upon the opposite leg of the same chicken, and with the same results.

Experiment 4.—Same as experiment 1, except that I supposed at first the bone was broken completely off. The dissection showed, however, that such was not the fact. The posterior wall was a little thickened, but the ensheathing callus was only in front and on the two sides. The medullary canal was closed with bone.

So early as the year 1673, a dissection made by Glaser, demonstrated incontestably the existence of partial fractures in the shaft, and in the direction of the diameter of long bones.[1] Camper, in 1765, again described a specimen which he had seen;[2] and Bonn, in 1783, added a third positive observation.[3]

M. Gimele is, therefore, in error when he ascribes to Campaignac the credit of having first proven by dissection their existence, in a paper communicated to the Academy of Medicine at Paris, in 1826. Campaignac, however, seems to have been the first who described very particularly the condition of this fracture. He has recorded the history and dissection of two cases, one of which occurred in the fibula, and one in the tibia. The first of these cases was a girl twelve years old, who survived the accident just eight weeks. The fracture had occurred near the

[1] Malgaigne, op. cit., p. 44, from Th. Boneti Sepulchretum, 1700, tom. iii. p. 424.
[2] Essays and Obs. Phys. and Lit. of Soc. of Edinburgh, 1771, vol. iii. p. 537.
[3] Malgaigne, op. cit., p. 44, from Descript. Thes. Ossium Morb. Hoviani, 1783.

middle of the bone, and upon the anterior and internal side; in which direction, resting against the tibia, the bone was found inclined. "The bony fibres had been broken at different lengths, almost exactly like what takes place in the branch of a tree which has been partially broken; and, as we see sometimes in this latter case, the bundles of splintered bony fibres abutted upon themselves, and did not take their places when we endeavored to restore them; so the abnormal angle which the fibula represented could not be effaced, the ends of the divided fasciculi not restoring themselves to their respective places. This disposition might be especially seen toward the anterior part of the internal face, where a packet of fibres, coming from below, was braced against the upper lip of the division, which it thus held open. This opening at first made me think that the fragments could not have been well consolidated; but I assured myself that it was, and the fact was subsequently confirmed by the Academy of Medicine; all the points which were in contact were found intimately united."[1]

Diagnosis.—The diagnosis is not difficult. The distortion indicates sufficiently the existence of a fracture, while the complete absence of crepitus in nearly all cases, and of either overlapping or lateral displacements, must, generally, especially where the accident has occurred in a child, sufficiently indicate that the fracture is incomplete. It will assist the diagnosis also to notice that these accidents are almost confined to the middle third of the long bones; and they are produced usually by a bending of the bones, the forces operating upon the extremities, and not directly upon the point which is broken.

In complete fractures, also, preternatural mobility is so constant a sign as to be regarded as diagnostic, while here there is almost always a great degree of immobility at the seat of fracture. The angle made by the projecting extremities is usually rather gentle and smooth; at other times it is abrupt, indicating a greater amount of fracture, or that the outer fibres are broken more irregularly. The power of using the limb is generally sensibly impaired, but not completely lost.

Treatment.—Jurine, Murat, Campaignac, Gulliver, Malgaigne, with some others, have noticed the fact that it is often difficult, and sometimes quite impossible, to restore these bones to position; a circumstance which they have justly ascribed to that condition of the fragments described by Campaignac. The broken extremities of the fasciculi become braced against each other, and effectually resist all efforts to straighten the bone; unless, indeed, so much force is used as to render the fracture complete; a result which, if it should chance to happen, need not occasion any alarm, since, while it enables us at once to restore the bone to line, does not much increase the danger of lateral displacement and overlapping. That the fracture has become complete we may know by a sudden sensation of cracking, by the increased mobility, and by the crepitus which is now easily developed.

But we need not, on the other hand, be over anxious to straighten

[1] Des Fractures Incompletes et des Fractures Longitudinales des Os des Membres; par J. A. J. Campaignac. Paris, 1829, pp. 9–10.

the bone completely, since experience has shown that after the lapse of a few weeks or months the natural form is usually restored spontaneously. I am not now speaking of those cases in which the restoration occurs immediately, where it is probable that the splintered fibres offer no resistance to the restoration; but only of those in which the bone straightens so gradually as to induce a belief that the broken ends are the cause of the resistance. To this variety of accident belong cases one, five, six, seven, and eight, published in my Report on Deformities after Fractures;[1] in one of which the natural axis was resumed in less than four weeks. In a case mentioned by Gulliver, it required about the same time to render the bones of the forearm perfectly straight; and in one case mentioned by Jurine, at the end of six months it was "difficult to say which arm had been broken, and at the end of one year it was impossible."

Jurine attributes this restoration to "muscular action, or more especially to the reaction of the compressed bony plates;" but while it is easy to understand how the reaction of the compressed fibres may accomplish the gradual restoration, I am unable to understand in what manner muscular action contributes to this result, since most of the muscles attached to the long bones operate so much more energetically in the direction of their axis than in the direction of their diameters. Indeed, we have often seen these bones bent after complete fractures, and before the union was consummated, by muscular action alone.

I repeat, then, that the gradual restoration of these bones is due to the same circumstance which produces at other times an immediate restoration, namely, the elasticity of the unbroken fibres, but which elasticity, in this latter instance, is, for a time, effectually resisted by the bracing of the broken fibres. At length, however, in consequence of the gradual absorption of the broken ends, this resistance is removed, and the bone becomes straight. If this absorption refuses to take place, and the fibres continue pressed forcibly against each other, as in the case described by Campaignac, then the bone remains permanently bent.

Having straightened the bone as far as is practicable, it only remains to secure the fragments in place by suitable bandages or splints. If the restoration is incomplete, these means may assist the efforts of nature in accomplishing a gradual restoration.

It is scarcely necessary to say that extension and counter-extension avail nothing in partial fractures.

§ 3. Fissures.

These constitute the second principal form of incomplete fractures, or those in which the fracture is accompanied with no appreciable bending, which occur almost exclusively in inflexible bones, such as the compact bones of adults, and more often in the direction of their

[1] Trans. Am. Med. Assoc., vol. viii., 1855, pp. 392-5.

axes than of their diameters. They are complete so far as they extend, but they do not completely sever the bone so as to form two distinct fragments. They have been most frequently observed in the flat bones, such as the bones of the skull, and in the upper bones of the face; occasionally in the long bones, both in their diaphyses and epiphyses, and rarely in the short bones.

M. Gariel has reported, in the *Bulletins de la Société Anat.*, for 1835, a case of fissure of the inferior maxilla, occurring in a lad sixteen or eighteen years old. Paletta found a fissure extending partly through the third dorsal vertebra, in a man who had fallen upon his back eleven days before; and M. Lisfranc has mentioned a remarkable case of fissure and partial fracture, with bending of five ribs in the same person.[1] Malgaigne believes that he has seen one example of this variety of incomplete fracture of the scapula, occurring through a portion of the infra-spinous region. I have myself elsewhere recorded another, as having been found in the skeleton of Nimham, an Oneida Indian, who was a great fighter, and who died when about forty-five years old, in consequence of severe injuries received in a street brawl; but his death did not occur until four or five months after the receipt of the injuries.

In addition to this fracture of the right scapula, five of his ribs were broken, and both legs, all of which, except the scapula, had united completely by intermediate and ensheathing callus.

The scapula was broken nearly transversely, the fracture commencing upon the posterior margin at a point about three-quarters of an inch below the spine, and extending across the body of the bone one inch and three-quarters, in a direction inclining a little upwards, being irregularly denticulate and without comminution. The fragments were in exact apposition, and, throughout most of their extent, in immediate contact. They were, however, not consolidated at any point, but upon either side of the fissure there was a ridge of ensheathing callus, of from one to three or four lines in breadth, and of half a line or less in thickness along the broken margin, from which point it subsided gradually to the level of the sound bone. The same was observed upon the inner as well as upon the outer surface of the scapula. This callus had assumed the character of complete bone, but it was more light and spongy than the natural tissue, and the outer surface had not yet become lamellated. Its blood-canals and bone-cells opened everywhere upon the surface.

Directly over the fracture, and between its opposing edges, no callus existed, but as the bone had lain some time in the earth before it was exhumed, it is probable that a less completely organized intermediate callus had occupied this space, and that, owing to the less proportion of earthy matter which it contained, it had become decomposed and had been removed.

M. Voillemier found the head of the humerus penetrated by two or three fissures;[2] and M. Campaignac has reported the case of a lad ten

[1] Des Fract. Incomplet. et des Fissures, par J. A. J. Campaignac, 1829, p. 20.
[2] Malgaigne, op. cit., p. 35.

or twelve years old, who was compelled to submit to amputation of his arm at the shoulder-joint, in consequence of a severe injury, in which the humerus was found fissured from the insertion of the deltoid to near the condyles, extending through the entire thickness of the bone, and the edges of the fissure so much separated toward its lower extremity as to admit the blade of a knife.[1] Chaussier has related a case in which a criminal, who died soon after having submitted to the torture, was found to have a nearly longitudinal fissure of the radius in its upper fourth, and which penetrated half way through the thickness of the bone.[2] Gulliver saw a fissure in the pelvis of an infant.[3] Malgaigne has seen two specimens of this fracture in the iliac bones, both of which belonged, as he thinks, to adults; in one, the fissure was limited to the internal table;[4] and in the case of the lad reported by Gariel, as having a fissure of the inferior maxilla, there was also found a fissure of the left ilium, but which was limited to the outer table.[5]

M. J. Cloquet has mentioned a case of fissure of the shaft of the femur passing through the condyles and extending upward to near the middle of the bone. The fissure was produced by a bullet, which had completely traversed the bone from behind forward, a little above the condyles.[6] M. Malgaigne has also represented, in one of his plates, a fissure of the femur extending along the front of the bone, somewhat irregularly, from a point a little below the trochanter minor to near the condyles.[7] The bone was presented to the Museum of Val-de-Grâce, by M. Fleury; but it is to be regretted that we have no farther account of this remarkable specimen. Certainly, in the complete absence of any farther history of the case, one might be justified in expressing a doubt whether it was not a fissure occasioned by the contraction consequent upon exposure and drying after death.

The following account of a fissure of the neck of the femur, of the same character with those which now occupy our attention, is copied from the proceedings of the "Boston Soc. for Med. Improvement," at its regular meeting in September, 1856:—

"*Partial Fracture of the Neck of the Femur in a man æt.* 44 *years.* Specimen shown by Dr. Jackson.—The fracture, which appears as a mere crack in the bone, commences anteriorly just above, but very near to, the insertion of the capsular ligament, runs along this insertion for about an inch, and then extends directly upward to the margin of the head of the bone. From this last point it crosses the upper surface of the neck almost in a straight line, and at a little distance from the margin of the head, but afterward approaches very closely to this margin posteriorly; it then turns downward and obliquely forward, and stops at a point about half way between the small trochanter and the head of the femur, and two-thirds of an inch or more anteriorly to the line of this trochanter. The fracture then involves

[1] Campaignac, Des Fract. Incomplet., &c., p. 24.
[2] Méd. Légale, p. 447 et seq.
[3] Gazette Méd., 1835, p. 472.
[4] Op. cit., p. 34.
[5] Bulletins de la Soc. Anat., 1835, p. 24.
[6] Thèse du Concours de Pathol. Externe, 1831, pl. xii., fig. 7. Also, Des Frac., etc., par Campaignac, 1829, p. 19.
[7] Op. cit., p. 37, pl. 1, fig. 1.

about three-fourths of the neck of the bone; the inner-anterior portion only being spared. There is considerable motion between the neck and the shaft, and the fracture could, undoubtedly, be completed without the application of any extraordinary force. Dr. J. referred to other causes of partial fracture; but a fracture of this sort, as occurring in this situation, and in a fully adult subject, he believed had never before been described. There was, also, in this case, a transverse fracture of the same femur midway, with a split extending upward nearly to the neck of the bone; and still further, a fracture of the spine. The patient, a laboring man, fell through two stories of a building and down upon a hard floor. On the same day he entered the Massachusetts General Hospital, and on the 18th day from the time of the accident he died. The femur is perfectly healthy in structure, and no changes are observable in the bone about the fracture."[1]

Whatever doubts may have been thrown upon the possibility of this accident, as applied to the neck of the femur, by the ingenious arguments of Robert Smith, of Dublin,[2] the question is now at least determined by an incontestable fact. Dr. Smith had rendered it quite probable that both Colles and Adams were mistaken, and that the cases described by them were examples of impacted fracture, and not of partial fracture; but, in arguing the improbability of its occurrence, from the infrequency of fractures of the neck of the femur in early life, he overlooked the fact that there were two forms of incomplete fractures, and that it was only the "green stick" fracture which belonged mostly to childhood; "fissures" being found most often in the bones of adults. Indeed, I think the example recorded by Tournel in the *Archives de Médecine*, had already, so early as the year 1837, established the possibility of a "fissure" in the neck of the femur; although by Malgaigne this case has been mentioned as an example of that other variety of partial fractures, which is almost peculiar to childhood, and in which the bones yield quite as much by bending as by breaking. But the man was eighty-five years old, and, having died three months and a half after the accident, a long crevice was found, extending nearly through the neck of the femur, partly within and partly without the capsule.

I have seen, in Dr. Mutter's valuable collection of bones at Philadelphia, a specimen of fissure of the trochanter major, which, it is believed, occasioned the death of the patient by hemorrhage.

Gulliver says there is an example of a fissure in a patella belonging to the museum of the Edinburgh College of Surgeons; the fissure traversing its articular face only.[3]

The first example of a fissure of the tibia is recorded by Corn. Stalpart Vander-Wiel, in 1687; and indeed this is, according to Campaignac, the first exact observation of this species of fracture which our science possesses, although its existence had been recognized by

[1] Bost. Med. and Surg. Journ., vol. lv. p. 351. See, also, Amer. Journ. Med. Sci. for 1857, p. 306; with engraving.

[2] Treatise on Fractures in the Vicinity of Joints, etc., by Robert Wm. Smith, Dublin, 1854, p. 44 et seq.

[3] Malgaigne, op. cit., page 35.

the most ancient authors. A servant had been kicked by a horse, and after a time, pain continued in the limb, his surgeon, Dufoix, suspected a fissure of the tibia, and having cut down to the bone, a cure was soon effected.[1]

In the Dupuytren Museum, at Paris, there are two tibiæ with linear fractures; one without history, and the other presented by MM. Marjolin and Rullier, "and which had been broken by a ball."[2] In the example related by Campaignac, a woman, having leaped from a second-story window, died immediately, and upon examination she was found to have three fissures in the upper portion of the left tibia, one only of which entered the articulation.[3]

The soldier spoken of by Bécane, having been struck upon the middle of the tibia, continued to march for some distance; but serious complications ensuing, he finally died. A fissure was found, after death, near the middle of the shaft of the tibia.[4]

Léveille relates that an Austrian soldier had his leg penetrated by a ball at the battle of Marengo; from thence he marched several miles, and then was transported to Pavia. Although the wound at first seemed very simple, graver symptoms soon followed, and it became necessary to amputate the thigh. Dissection showed that the ball had occasioned several oblique and longitudinal fissures, which extended nearly the whole length of the shaft of the bone.[5]

Duverney saw a priest who had fallen and bruised the middle of his left leg; the swelling and pain consequent upon which were subdued after a few days. The patient believed himself cured and acted accordingly. Suddenly, in the night, he was seized with an acute pain in the limb; and on cutting down to the bone, a bloody serum escaped from between it and the periosteum, and the bone was discovered to be fissured longitudinally. Subsequently the tibia was trephined, but the fissure did not reach the marrow. He recovered completely in less than two months.

The same writer mentions another case in which a soldier received the kick of a horse in the middle of his left leg which was followed immediately by great pain, and subsequently by much inflammation, and even gangrene of the skin. The wound, however, cicatrized kindly, but after three months he was seized suddenly with a severe pain in the limb; and, after the trial of many remedies, resort was finally had to the knife, when the tibia was seen to be discolored, and cracked longitudinally. On the following day the bone was opened over the course of the fissure with a chisel and mallet, and the patient was at once relieved by the escape of a yellowish and very offensive matter. At the next dressing, the bone was opened more freely by several applications of the trephine, and an abscess was exposed in the centre of the bone. The patient finally recovered after about four months.[6] M. Campaignac saw, also, at the hospital La Charité, the

[1] Campaignac, op. cit., p. 17.

[2] Malgaigne, op. cit., p. 36.

[3] Campaignac, op. cit., p. 21.

[4] Abrégé des Maladies qui attaquent la Substance des Os. Toulouse, 1775, p. 134.

[5] Malgaigne, op. cit., p. 39.

[6] Malgaigne, op. cit., p. 39 et seq.

tibia of a woman, æt. 38 years, upon which were found four fissures; the report of which case is accompanied with a wood-cut illustration.[1]

Fissures may occur probably at all periods of life, but they are more frequently found in the bones of adults. Campaignac, however, mentions a fissure of the humerus in a child ten or twelve years old, and Gulliver has seen a fissure in the pelvis of an infant.

Etiology.—They may be occasioned by most of those causes which produce fractures in general, such as direct or indirect shocks; but they are occasioned much more often by direct blows, especially when inflicted upon bones imperfectly covered by soft parts, such as the tibia. Bullets, having violently struck or penetrated the bone, have frequently occasioned fissures.

Their course may be parallel with the axis of the bone, oblique or transverse; they are often multiple; some merely enter the outer laminæ, others open into the cellular tissue, and others still divide both surfaces of the bone through and through; and, according as they penetrate more or less deeply the bone, their lips will be found to be more or less separated. They frequently extend into the joint surfaces.

Diagnosis.—The signs which indicate the existence of a fissure must, in a large majority of cases, be insufficient to determine fully the diagnosis during the life of the patient. It is not probable that such fissures could ever be clearly made out by the touch alone, where the skin is not broken, since the pain, swelling, suppuration, etc., are only characteristic of inflammation of the bone or of its coverings, and might be equally present whether a fracture existed or not. In those rare cases only in which the flesh is torn off, and the surface of the bone is brought directly under the observation of the eye, will the diagnosis become certain.

Treatment.—Fortunately, an error in judgment in this matter will not materially, if at all, prejudice the interests of the patient; since whatever may be the fact in other respects, if the bone, or its periosteum, or its medullary membrane, is inflamed, and rest, with antiphlogistics, does not accomplish its speedy resolution, incisions and perforations become inevitable, if we would give either safety or relief to the sufferer. Accordingly, in the inflammation and suppuration consequent upon these fractures, we have seen that it has been occasionally found necessary to lay open the soft tissues freely, and even to trephine the bone at one or more points.

Fissures in Cartilage.—I have once met with a fissure in the thyroid cartilage, which constitutes, so far as I know, the only example upon record of a fissure in cartilage.[2]

[1] Campaignac, op. cit., pp. 21–22.

[2] See Buffalo Med. Journ., vol. xiii. Article entitled Fracture of the Thyroid Cartilage.

CHAPTER VIII.

FRACTURES OF THE NOSE.

§ 1. Ossa Nasi.

Of twenty-two cases of fracture of the ossa nasi recorded by me only thirteen were seen by a surgeon in time to afford relief. It seemed to me necessary, therefore, that the student should be instructed how frequently the nature of this accident is overlooked by the friends, and even by the surgeon himself, to the end that he might be thus admonished of the necessity of always instituting in such cases, careful and thorough examinations. In some of the cases recorded in my notes, where surgeons were called in time, and a deformity remains, it is not improbable that the accident was not recognized. The rapidity with which swelling ensues after severe blows upon the nose, concealing at once the bones, and lifting the skin even above its natural level, explains these mistakes. The nose, also, is remarkably sensitive, and the patient is often exceedingly reluctant to submit to a thorough examination. It ought, however, not to be forgotten that the omission on the part of the surgeon to do his duty will not always be excused, even though the patient himself has protested against his interference, especially where an organ so prominent, and so important to the harmony of the face, is the subject of his neglect or mal-adjustment; since the most trivial deviation from its original form or position, even to the extent of one or two lines, becomes a serious deformity.

When the ossa nasi are struck with considerable force, from before and from above, a transverse fracture occurs usually within from three to six lines of their lower and free margins, and the fragments are simply displaced backwards, or if the blow is received partially upon one side, they are displaced more or less laterally. This is what will happen in a great majority of cases, as I have proven by examinations of the noses of those persons who have been the subjects of this accident, both before and after death, and by repeated experiments upon the recent subject.

These fragments are generally loose and easily pressed back into place by the use of a proper instrument. A silver female catheter, which we have seen recommended by surgeons, may answer well enough in a few instances, but it will more often fail. The diameter of the meatus at the point where the instrument must touch in order to make effective pressure upon the ossa nasi, is on the average not more than two lines, and when the membrane which lines it is injured, it becomes quickly swollen, and reduces the breadth of the channel to a line or less. Under these circumstances, any instrument of the size of a female catheter could only be made to reach and press against the nasal process of the superior maxilla, which is too firm and unyielding to allow it to pass without the employment of unwarrantable force. In this way it happens that the operator is occasionally surprised to find how much resistance is opposed to his efforts to lift the bones, and after repeated unsuccessful attempts the case is not unfrequently given over. If, however, he had used a smaller instrument, he would have found almost no resistance whatever. A straight steel director, or sound, or sometimes even a much smaller instrument, if possessing sufficient firmness, is more suitable than the catheter. For the same reason, also, one ought never to wrap the end of the instrument with a piece of cotton cloth as some have, I suspect, without much consideration, recommended.

What I have said of the facility with which these bones may be replaced, when a proper instrument is employed, is true only when the treatment is adopted immediately, or at most within a few days after the accident.

Boyer, Malgaigne, and others have noticed the fact that these fractures are repaired with great rapidity. Hippocrates thought the union was generally complete in six days; and in a case which has come under my own observation, the fragments were quite firmly united on the seventh day.

A lad aged eleven years had the right nasal bone broken through its lower third, and displaced to the right side. Seven days after the accident he was brought to me. I introduced a strong steel instrument into the right nostril, and pressed upward and to the left, while with my thumb I pressed forcibly upon the right side of the nose. My object was to lift the bone, and carry it a little over to the left side. During the effort, the bones were felt to crack and give way slightly, but not sufficiently. I then gave him chloroform, as the manipulation had proved very painful, and again pressed in the same manner with great force, until the restoration seemed complete.

Nor has Malgaigne, whose observations are always very accurate, overlooked the fact, also, that their repair is effected without the interposition of provisional callus, but as it were "*par premiere intention.*" My own observation confirms this statement. Among all the specimens which I have seen in the various college and private collections illustrating fractures of the ossa nasi, and amounting in all to over forty, in no instance has there been detected, after a careful examination, the slightest trace of provisional callus.

I am not certain that it will always be found so easy to retain these loose fragments in place, as it is to replace them. The very swelling which takes place so promptly under the skin tends to depress the fragments, unsupported as they are by any counter force; a tendency which, possibly, is in some instances increased by attempts on the part of the patient to clear his nostrils by snuffing and hawking. I have, in one instance, noticed very plainly a motion in the fragments when such efforts were made. How we are to remedy this I am not prepared to say. None of the plans which I have seen suggested possess, in my estimation, very much practical value. Few patients will consent to the introduction of pledgets of lint, or of stuffed bags, or, indeed, of anything else, sufficiently far up into the nostril to answer any useful purpose. The membrane is too sensitive and too intolerant of irritants to enable us to have recourse generally to such methods. Then, too, it would require on the part of the surgeon more than ordinary tact to accomplish so nice and delicate an adjustment of the supports from below as these cases demand, where the slightest excess of pressure or the least fault in the position of the compress must defeat the purpose of the operator.

Yet, if one were disposed to make the attempt in certain cases where the comminution was very great, or where for any other reason the fragments would not remain in place, I think there could be no better plan than to push up in succession a number of small pledgets of patent lint, smeared with simple cerate, to each one of which there has been attached a separate string, so arranged as that their relative position may be recognized, and that they may at a suitable time be removed in the order of their introduction.

The employment of canulas, as recommended by Boyer, B. Bell, and others, allows of the nostrils being stuffed, without interfering materially with the breathing; a provision, however, which is quite unnecessary with a majority of persons, so long as there exists no impediment to the free admission of air through the fauces.

With nicely adjusted compresses made of soft cotton or lint, and secured upon the outside of the nose with delicate strips of adhesive plaster or rollers, we shall be better able to prevent the fragments from becoming displaced outwards, than by moulds of wax, of lead, or of gutta percha, under which it is impossible to see from hour to hour what is transpiring.

The complicated apparatus devised by Dubois and recommended by Malgaigne, to lift the bones and retain them in place, seems to me indeed very ingenious, but destitute of a single practical advantage.

A more considerable force than that which I have first supposed, will break, generally, the ossa nasi transversely and a little above their middle, while, at the same time, the nasal processes of the superior maxillary bones may suffer slightly.

With neither of these accidents is the cribriform plate of the ethmoid likely to be broken or disturbed. Indeed, in numerous experiments made upon the recent subject, and in which the force of the blow was directed backwards and upwards, breaking and comminuting the nasal bones above and below their middle, with, also, the nasal processes of the superior maxillary bones, and the septum nasi, the cribriform plate of the ethmoid was, without an exception, uninjured. The exceeding tenuity and flexibility of the septum nasi at certain points, prevents effectually the concussion from being communicated through it to the base of the brain. If, therefore, after these accidents, cerebral symptoms are occasionally present, as I have myself twice seen,[1] they must be due rather to the concussive effects

[1] Report on Deformities after Fractures, Cases 16 and 18.

of the blow upon the very summit of the nasal bones, where they rest immediately upon the nasal spine of the os frontis, or to some direct impression upon the skull itself.

The amount of force requisite to break in the nasal bones, at their upper third, is very great; no less, indeed, than is requisite to fracture the os frontis. If they do finally yield at this point, then no doubt the base of the skull must yield also. Nor do I think patients could often be expected to recover from an accident so severe. To this class of fractures belongs the specimen contained in my museum, in which not only both of the nasal bones are sent in—the nasal spine being broken at its base—but also the os frontis is depressed, the nasal processes of the upper maxillary bones are broken and greatly displaced, and the anterior half of the cribriform plate of the ethmoid is forced up into the base of the brain. If it is meant that in *these* cases the patient is in danger from injury done to the base of the skull, through the fracture and depression of the ossa nasi, we can appreciate the value of the opinion; but we do not understand how this danger can exist when the nasal spine of the os frontis is not broken, and the upper ends of the nasal bones are not displaced backwards. But, admitting that it were possible in this way to force up the base of the skull, it does not seem to me that we ought to attach any value to the advice occasionally given, to attempt to restore the broken ethmoid by seizing upon the septum and pulling downwards. A force sufficient to break the base of the skull, never fails to comminute and detach almost completely the septum nasi. We are to proceed in such a case as we would in a case of broken skull. We must lay open the skin freely, and with appropriate instruments seek to elevate and remove, if necessary, the fragments. Indeed, after such accidents, we shall generally see plainly enough that death is inevitable, and that our services will be of no value.

Occasionally, I have observed, the bones are neither broken at their lower ends nor through their central diameters, but only at their lateral, serrated, or imbricated margins. This is rather a displacement, or dislocation, than a fracture. It is more likely to happen, I think, in childhood than in middle or old age, as in the following example:—

Thomas Kelley, aged four years, was kicked by a horse. Two hours afterwards, when he was first seen by a surgeon, the nose and face were much swollen, and the fracture was overlooked.

One year after the accident, I found both nasal bones depressed through nearly their whole length, and especially in their lower halves. The right nasal process was also much depressed, and the right nostril obstructed. The lachrymal canals upon this side were closed.

Sometimes the lower ends of the nasal bones are bent backwards, or laterally, constituting a partial fracture.

A lad, aged ten years, was hit by one of his mates, accidentally, with his elbow, upon the left side of his nose. I was immediately called, and found the lower end of the left os nasi displaced laterally and backwards, so that it rested under the lower end of the right os nasi. There did not appear to be any fracture beyond that which was inevitable by the mere separation of its serrated margins from the bone adjoining. The angle formed by the bone at the point where the bending had occurred, was smooth and rounded, and not abrupt as in a complete fracture.

With a steel instrument, introduced into the left nostril, I attempted to lift the bone to its place. The membrane was very sensitive, and the patient very restless under my repeated efforts. I pressed upwards with considerable force, and succeeded at length in bringing the bone nearly into position.

If there is more complete displacement, the upper ends are not usually forced backwards, but rather a very little forwards, from their articulations with the os frontis, and the bones then swing, as it were, upon the lower ends of the nasal spine, as upon a pivot. In this condition, they are very firmly locked, and it requires considerable force, applied under their lower extremities, to restore them to place.

Such seemed to be the position of the bones in the case of the lad Kelley, already mentioned, and also in a German, whose nose was flattened by a severe blow when he was eleven years old, whom I saw, thirteen years after the accident, in the Buffalo Hospital. In this last example the bones were very much displaced backwards.

In children, also, the nasal bones may be spread and flattened, the lateral margins not being depressed or displaced, but only the mesial line or arch forced back, so as to press aside the processes of the superior maxilla; which deformity may become permanent.

A block of wood fell upon a child three weeks old, as she was lying in the cradle. The nature of the injury was not understood by the parents, and no surgeon was called. The ossa nasi are now, twelve years after the accident, much wider than is natural, and depressed; the nasal processes of the superior maxilla appearing to have been spread asunder.

Jacob Kibbs, a German, aged seven years, fell from a height of forty feet, striking on his face. His parents did not suspect the injury, and no surgeon was called. Twenty-four years after this, I found the nose almost flat. The nasal bones appeared unusually wide, and were sunken between the processes of the upper maxillary bones, which latter might be recognized by two parallel ridges on each side, slightly rising above the level of the ossa nasi.

Benjamin Bell and others have spoken of tedious ulcers, polypi, necrosis, fistula lachrymalis, abscesses, impeded respiration, and impairment of the sense of smell and of speech, as circumstances apt to result from these injuries, and it is certain that such consequences have occasionally followed; but they must sometimes be regarded as accidents due to the state of the general system, and as having no connection with the fracture, except as this injury served to awaken certain vicious tendencies.

Two years ago, a gentleman, then twenty-five years old, was struck accidentally upon the right side of his nose by a board, and the ossa nasi were displaced to the left. A surgeon made an attempt to reduce them, but did not succeed, and they have remained displaced ever since.

The nose for a time was much swollen. A few months after the accident, a purulent discharge commenced from the right nostril, and at length an abscess formed in the right cheek. The abscess is now healed, but the nose continues to discharge pus, and occasionally it bleeds freely. There is a perforation of the septum, of the size of a three-cent piece, which is continuing to enlarge.

No hereditary maladies exist in the family, except that, on his father's side, it has been generally observed that wounds do not heal kindly. The same is the fact with him. When a child, he was also very subject to epistaxis; at sixteen, a pulmonary difficulty began, and he had more or less cough, with hæmoptysis, for two years. Since then, his health has been good. He is a lawyer by profession, but of late he has lived in the country, upon a farm, and has accustomed himself to much out-door exercise.

As to the prognosis in these fractures, I can only say that either owing to the ignorance and carelessness of the patients themselves, who neglect to call a surgeon in time, or to the difficulty of diagnosis, or to the greater difficulty in maintaining an adjustment of the fragments, it has hitherto happened that, after a fracture of the ossa nasi, more or less deformity has usually remained. I have never seen but four which could be said to be perfectly restored.

§ 2. Fractures and Displacements of the Septum Narium.

Fractures or displacements of the septum narium must occur to some extent in all fractures of the ossa nasi accompanied with depression; but they are also occasionally met with as the results of a blow upon the nose, which has been insufficient to break the bones, and in which only the cartilaginous portion of the nose has been bent inward upon the septum.

Of these simple, uncomplicated accidents, I have seen seven; in three of which no surgeon was employed, or surgical treatment of any kind adopted, and it is quite probable that only in a small proportion of all the cases was the nature of the accident recognized. Such, at least, has been generally the statement of the patients themselves. The same causes will explain this which have been invoked to explain similar oversights in cases of broken ossa nasi. To which we may add, as an additional reason why it may be overlooked, the frequency of lateral distortions or deviations in the natural development of this septum.

The cartilaginous portion of the septum is that which is most frequently displaced by violence, and then it is usually at the point of its articulation with the bony septum. Next, in point of frequency, the perpendicular nasal plate is broken, and especially where it approaches the vomer. We omit in this enumeration, of course, those cases where the nasal bones themselves are broken down, in most or all of which, as we have already said, the perpendicular plate is more or less fractured and displaced. We cannot say how often the vomer is broken, since it is beyond our observation, except in autopsies. It is probable, however, that the force of the concussion rarely reaches it, the cartilage or the perpendicular plate giving way first and easily.

Where the deviation is only lateral, the results are less serious, yet sufficiently so in a few instances to demand our attention. Lateral obliquity of the lower portion of the nose follows generally, but not uniformly, a lateral displacement of the cartilage, and when it does exist, it is not always proportioned to the amount of displacement existing in the septum, so that the septum is then made to project obliquely across the nasal passage, causing often a serious obstruction and permanent inconvenience. In one instance, also, I have known it to occasion a chronic catarrh.

A lad, æt. 15, was struck violently on the nose, which became immediately much swollen, but no surgeon was called. Eight years after, I found the septum displaced laterally, and to the left side, producing also a slight lateral inclination of the end of the nose. He was unable to breathe freely through the left nostril, and from the same side a catarrhal discharge had continued from the time of the accident.

The following example, in which the accident has been followed by a morbid condition of the cutaneous glands, is of more difficult explanation:—

A young man, æt. 23, called upon me, supposing that he had a polypus nasi. I found that in consequence of a fall upon the ice, seven years before, the septum narium had been displaced to the right so as to almost completely close this nostril. In very cold weather, when the vessels of the membrane are contracted, the passage is more free. The left nostril is proportionably wide.

During the last four or five years, the right side of his face has been subject to profuse perspiration. It is almost constant in summer, and only occasional in winter. The line of division between the perspiring and non-perspiring portions of the face passes perpendicularly from the top of the centre of the forehead, along the ridge of the nose, and down to the centre of the chin. The phenomenon is due, perhaps, to an increased vascularity in the right side of the face; possibly to some peculiarity in the condition of the nervous trunks, occasioned by the nasal obstruction.

A depression of the cartilage forming a portion of the ridge of the nose is necessarily accompanied with a corresponding degree of lateral displacement, with or without fracture, of its perpendicular portion, and produces, therefore, not only great deformity, sometimes a complete flattening of the end of the nose, but, also, in some instances, complete obstruction of the nostrils.

We conclude, from all that we have seen, that fractures and displacements of the septum narium are generally followed by permanent deformity, and occasionally with still more serious results. We suggest, therefore, a more careful examination in recent injuries, with a view to the ascertainment of its lesions, and it would be well, certainly, if we could devise some reliable mode of treatment.

It is doubtful whether a partition so thin and unsupported can ever be well adjusted and supported by artificial means. We possess, however, one advantage in the treatment of this accident which we do not in the treatment of broken ossa nasi, viz: facility of observation and of approach, and if we can do little with plugs and supports in the one case, we may possibly do more in the other. Nothing seems more rational, then, than to plug carefully and equally each nostril, with pledgets of lint, while we cover the outside of the nose completely with a nicely moulded gutta percha splint or case, which ought to be made to press snugly upon the sides, and permitting these to remain for several weeks, or until the cure is completed. The *papier machè* of Dzondi, employed by him in cases of broken ossa nasi, would be equally applicable here; but the gutta percha, as being more plastic, and hardening more quickly, ought to be preferred.

Attempts to remedy the deformities of the nose at a later period, belong to the department of anaplastic surgery, and the modes of procedure must be varied according to the circumstances of the case.

The following example will serve as an illustration of what may sometimes be accomplished in these cases:—

A young man fell from a two-story window, striking upon his face. A surgeon was called, but he did not discover the nature of the injury to the nose.

One year after the accident he called upon me for relief. The cartilaginous portion of the septum was broken just at the ends of the nasal bones, and forced backwards about three lines, producing a striking depression at this point of the ridge of the nose, while at the same time the end of the nose was thrown up. The deformity was very unseemly, and annoying both to himself and to his friends, who at first could scarcely recognize him.

I introduced a narrow, sharp-pointed bistoury through the skin of the nose on the right side, and resting its edge upon the ridge at the junction of the cartilage with the ossa nasi, I cut the cartilaginous septum directly backwards about three lines, and then making a gradual curve with my knife, I cut downwards about eight lines towards the end of the nose. The intercepted portion of cartilage could now be easily lifted with a probe, and the line of the ridge of the nose completely restored. It was at once apparent, also, that lifting the cartilage would depress the tip of the nose and restore its symmetry.

To retain the cartilage in place, I constructed a gutta percha splint, of the length and shape of the nose, but so formed along its middle as that it would not press upon the cartilage which I had lifted, resting well upon the ossa nasi, but not touching the ridge from the lower ends of these bones to the tip of the nose, at which latter point it again received support. I now passed a needle, armed with a stout ligature, through the upper end of the uplifted cartilage, transfixing, of course, the skin on both sides of the nose, and this I tied firmly over the splint. This accomplished the important object of pressing backwards and downwards the tip of the nose, and thus tilting up the upper part of the ridge and septum, and of more effectually securing the cartilage in place by lifting it directly with the ligature. On the second day the ligature was removed, but the splint was continued two weeks, during most of which time a band was kept drawn across the lower end of the splint, and tied behind the neck.

To prevent the cartilage from falling back when final cicatrization occurred, I pressed the sides of the splint firmly towards each other, just below the incision, so as to force as much as possible the walls of the nares into the fissure in the septum, made by lifting it up.

The result is a complete and perfect restoration of the nose to its original form.

CHAPTER IX.

FRACTURES OF THE MALAR BONE.

I HAVE been unable to find any records of a simple fracture of the malar bone, that is to say, of a fracture unconnected with a fracture of other bones of the face. It is probable, however, that it sometimes occurs, but that not being accompanied with much displacement, it is overlooked. I have myself seen a fracture of the upper margin, or of that portion which constitutes a part of the orbital border, in two or three instances, while I was unable to detect any other fracture among the bones of the face; but it is by no means certain that other fractures did not exist, perhaps in some of the bones which form the socket, or in the superior maxilla, as mere fissures, or as fractures with only slight displacement. The prominence of the malar bone and especially the sharpness of its orbital margin would enable the surgeon to detect easily the smallest displacement, or even a fissure, while a much more extensive displacement elsewhere would escape detection.

The following observations will illustrate these remarks:—

Observation First.—With a heavy steel hammer I struck the left malar bone of a naked skull, breaking the orbital margin near its middle, the line of fracture extending backward through the whole length of the orbital plate, and the outer half of the plate being pressed about two lines into the orbital cavity. There was no other fracture of the malar bone.

The nasal process of the superior maxilla was broken near its base, and the whole upper portion of this bone was thrown inward toward the nasal passages in such a manner as nearly to close them; while its lower margin was thrown out, separating the two upper maxillary bones from each other along the whole line of the inter-maxillary suture. This separation was about two lines in front and less toward the palatal bones.

The ethmoid was fissured through the whole length of its os planum, from before backward.

It is very easy to understand how a blow upon the malar bone, coming a little from one side, should produce this form of displacement of the superior maxilla.

The two upper maxillary bones form, as they are placed opposite to each other, an irregular arch, one end of which rests upon its fellow, at the intermaxillary suture, and the other end rests upon the nasal and frontal bones; while over the centre of the arch is situated the malar bone. The force of a side blow upon the malar bone will expend itself therefore chiefly upon the base of the maxillary apophysis, as being in the line of the direction of the force. The force continuing to act, after the apophysis is broken, the portion of the superior maxilla above the floor of the nares will fall inward toward the septum, while the portion below will tilt outward and open the inter-maxillary suture along the roof of the mouth. This suture will also open more widely in front than behind, owing to the greater depth of the suture in front.

One might suppose that it would be a very easy matter to restore these bones to place upon the naked skull, after such an accident. Certainly it would be very desirable to do so, were this accident to occur to any patient, since the malar bone is slightly depressed, the nostril upon this side is nearly closed, and the line of the teeth is disturbed, and it is possible also that an opening might be established between the nose and mouth immediately back of the incisors. In fact, however, I found the restoration impossible. It could not be accomplished by an instrument within the nose pressing outward, nor by pressing inward upon the teeth and alveoli; not certainly without very great and unwarrantable force. The difficulty consisted simply in the antagonisms of the serrated margins of the intermaxillary suture, which projecting one or two lines on each side, could not be made to interlock again, but were firmly braced against each other.

A repetition of the blow broke the malar bone completely in two, disarticulating it also at its zygomatic suture.

The superior maxilla was now separated wholly from the other bones of the face and skull, carrying the palate bone with it entire. The body and sinus of the upper maxilla still, however, remained unbroken.

Observation Second.—A blow inflicted with the hammer, square upon the malar bone, broke the malar bone on its orbital margin in the same manner as in Observation First. There was also a fissure on the upper and outer margin of the bone. There was no other fracture of the malar bone.

The zygoma was broken transversely near its middle, through that portion which belongs to the temporal bone.

The superior maxilla was broken through the antrum, a little below the base of the malar eminence, and the malar bone was forced into the antrum several lines. The dental arcade was not broken.

The ethmoid bone was fissured antero-posteriorly through its orbital plate.

In this example the walls of the antrum having at once given way, the force of the blow did not reach the nasal apophysis. It was found very easy to lift the malar bone to its place, with an instrument introduced through the broken walls of the antrum.

Observation Third.—The hammer falling upon the malar bone depressed it slightly, but did not break it.

The superior maxilla was found broken through the walls of the antrum a little below the malar apophysis. No other fracture.

The *second* blow broke the malar bone through its centre, breaking also the zygoma near its centre.

The *third* blow broke the nasal apophysis of the superior maxilla near its base, comminuting the antrum; into which the malar bone was forcibly driven. At the same time the orbital plate of the malar bone was thrown up into the socket. The ethmoid was also broken.

Observation Fourth.—The first blow did not fracture the malar bone, but broke the walls of the antrum, and at the same moment produced a fissure extending vertically through the dental arcade between the first and second molars, into the mouth.

The *second* blow broke the malar bone through its centre irregularly, and also the zygoma transversely, near the centre of its arch. The nasal process of the superior maxilla was broken at two points, one of the lines of fracture extending into the orbital socket.

The skull was also found broken at its base through the lesser wings of Ingrassias; the force of the blow having been conveyed, apparently, along the orbital plate of the superior maxilla and os planum.

This is the only example in which the fracture extended through the dental arcade, and it was the result of the first blow. The fracture of the base of the skull by the second blow indicates the possibility of producing a fatal lesion of the brain or of its bloodvessels by a blow upon the malar bone.

General Summary.—A fracture of the superior maxilla has occurred in every instance; and twice when the malar bone was not broken: in each of the two last cases the antrum alone was broken and the depression of the malar bone was scarcely noticeable. In the second of these cases, the fracture extended also through the dental arcade.

In three cases the nasal apophysis has broken near the base, and in one case at two points. One of the three fractures of the nasal apophysis was accompanied with a diastasis of the superior maxilla through its intermaxillary suture.

The malar bone has been broken twice by the first blow, and always when the blow has been repeated. The orbital margin and orbital plate have been fissured twice, the outer portion of the orbital plate being pushed a little into the socket. Once this plate has been pushed downwards.

The zygoma has been broken three times, and always transversely, a little beyond its centre, or where the bone is the most slender and most convex.

The ethmoid has been broken three times, and always longitudinally through the orbital plate.

The sphenoid has been broken once, at the base of the skull.

In addition to these observations upon the naked skull, I have seen two examples, which illustrate the relative infrequency of fractures of the malar bone, as compared with fractures of the superior maxilla and of the other bones of the face, even when the blow is received directly upon the malar bone.

Pat. Maloney, æt. 55, fell about twenty feet and struck upon his face. Six weeks after the accident, while an inmate of the Buffalo Hospital of the Sisters of Charity, I found the right malar bone depressed, but I could not trace any line of fracture in the malar bone. I think the antrum of the superior maxilla was broken and the malar bone forced in upon it.

Thomas Crotty, æt. 20, was struck with a hoop, August 15, 1855. He was seen immediately by a surgeon in Canada, but the fracture was not recognized. Five days after he called at my office. I found the outer portion of the right malar bone lifted slightly and the lower and anterior angle depressed about three lines, as if this portion had been forced in upon the antrum.

Prognosis.—The malar bone may be depressed, as we have seen, to the extent of two or three lines, without being broken. This accident will be more properly considered under fractures of the upper maxilla. A fracture of the malar bone implies, therefore, generally, that great force has been applied, and that other fractures exist as complications. This may not be true, however, when only the orbital margin of the socket is broken. If the orbital plate is broken, and a portion of it is pushed into the socket, it may occasion a slight protrusion of the ball, as in two cases related by Dr. Neill as fractures of the upper maxilla, and as has been noticed in the experiments already recorded. This protrusion of the eyeball will probably continue in some degree, as long as the bones remain displaced. It is quite probable, however, that in some cases, after severe injuries of the face, a moderate protrusion of the eyeball is due entirely to extravasation of blood in the socket; a circumstance which would be likely to follow a fracture of the bones of the socket, and to increase temporarily the protrusion of the eye.

If the body of the bone is broken entirely through, and coma supervenes upon the accident, there is some reason to fear that the skull is fractured at its base, and the prognosis ought to be grave.

Treatment.—If there is only a fissure of the orbital margin, it will not require attention; but if the fissure extends through the orbital plate and at the same time the anterior and inferior margin of the bone is depressed, in consequence of which the orbital plate is tilted upward and made to push forward the eyeball, the propriety of surgical interference may be considered. If this protrusion is considerable, and evidently due to the displaced bone, an attempt should be made to lift the body of the malar bone and thus to restore to position its orbital plate. The method of accomplishing this I shall describe particularly when speaking of fractures of the superior maxilla with depression of the malar bones.

CHAPTER X.

FRACTURES OF THE UPPER MAXILLARY BONES.

THESE fractures assume so great a variety in respect to form, situation and complications, that it would be impossible to speak of them systematically or to establish anything but very gêneral rules as to treatment and prognosis.

They may be broken, or loosened from each other or from the other bones with which they are articulated, with or without any farther fracture; the nasal processes may be broken, and generally this accident is accompanied with a fracture of the nasal bones also; the malar bones may be forced in, carrying with them a portion of the outer wall of the antrum; the alveoli may be broken and more or less completely detached; and either of these several fractures may be complicated with fractures of the other bones of the face or of the base of the skull even.

Treatment.—When the harmonies of the upper maxillary bones are only slightly disturbed, nothing but a retentive treatment is necessary.

A man was thrown backward from a loaded cart, one wheel of the cart passing over his face. He was taken up unconscious, but when I saw him on the following morning, his consciousness had returned. The right malar bone was broken and forced down upon the antrum about three lines. Both superior maxillæ were loosened from their articulations, and could be moved laterally, the motion producing a slight grating sound. The same motion and grating occurred whenever he attempted to swallow. No effort was made to elevate the malar bones, nor did I find any means necessary to retain the maxillary bones in place, the amount of displacement being very inconsiderable, and never sufficient to be observed by the eye. Cool lotions were applied constantly to the face, and the patient was sustained by a liquid diet. On the ninth day all motion of the fragments had ceased, and on the twenty-seventh day the patient was completely recovered, with only the depression of the malar bone remaining.

Sargent, of Boston, reports a similar case, in which a slight separation of the maxillary bones united promptly and without any retentive apparatus.[1]

But in a case in which the superior maxillary bones had been more completely torn from their connections, complicated with other severe injuries, I found it necessary to support the fragments by closing the lower jaw upon the upper, and by suitable bandages. The patient died, however, on the twelfth day.[2]

[1] Boston Med. and Surg. Journ., vol. lii. p. 378.

[2] Report on Deformities after Fractures. Trans. Amer. Med. Association, vol. viii. p. 375, Case IV.

Graefe recommends, where the bones are thus extensively separated and displaced, an apparatus made of steel, and suitably covered, which is to be applied against the forehead and buckled under the occiput. From the two sides descend a couple of steel plates, which, having arrived at the free border of the upper lip, are reflected upon themselves, and are made to support upon their extremities long silver gutters, intended for the reception of not only the displaced teeth and alveoli, but also those teeth which are firm.[1]

Wiseman having been summoned to a child with his whole upper jaw forced in, by the kick of a horse, "beating the ethmoides quite in from the os cribriform," and forcing the palate bone against the back of the pharynx, found great difficulty in securing a permanent readjustment. At first he attempted to introduce his finger back of the bone, but failing in this he bent an instrument into the form of a hook, and passing it between the bone and the pharynx, he easily replaced the fragments. But, on removing the instrument, they were again displaced. Immediately he had constructed an instrument by which the bones could be not only easily reduced, but also retained in place, extension being made by the hands of the child, his mother and others, alternately. In this way the reunion was finally effected, and "the face restored to a good shape, better than could have been hoped for."[2]

Harris, of New York, mentions a case in which a child, two years old, having fallen from a height of fifty feet upon the pavement, was found to have a diastasis of both the superior maxillary and palate bones; the separation being sufficient to admit the little finger, and extending from between the alveoli which supported the central incisors, to the soft palate. It is not said whether any efforts were made to reduce the bones, but six weeks after the injury was received, they were still open, and it was proposed to close the space by a plastic operation as soon as the condition of the patient would warrant such a procedure.[3]

I suspect that in this example, as in the first experiment quoted under fracture of the malar bone, it was found impossible to adjust the bones and close the intermaxillary suture, and for the same reasons.

If, in consequence of a blow received upon the ossa nasi, the nasal processes of the superior maxillæ are broken down, they may be lifted and adjusted in the same manner as the ossa nasi.

I have seen several examples of this accident, and I have in my cabinet a specimen, in which the nasal bones being driven in by the kick of a horse, the nasal process upon the left side is broken off just above the root of the cuspid tooth, and its upper end inclined inward toward the nasal passage and backward, until it is completely buried. In this situation it has become firmly united to the bony and soft tissues into which it was brought in contact.

The following example will illustrate some of the complications and

[1] Traité des Frac., etc., par L. F. Malgaigne, p. 373.
[2] Chirurgical Treatises, by Richard Wiseman, 1734, p. 443.
[3] New York Journ. Med., vol. xiii., 2d ser., p. 214.

difficulties connected with a depression of the malar bone, and consequent fracture of the antrum maxillare.

M. P., of Colesville, aged about 34 years, was thrown from a height, striking upon his face, forcing the right malar bone down upon the antrum of the superior maxilla. Dr. L. Potter, of Varysburg, and myself were called.

The deformity produced by the sinking of the malar bone was very striking, and both the patient and myself were very anxious to have it remedied if possible. We found some of the teeth upon the side of the fracture loose, and we determined to extract them and press up the bone with an instrument introduced through the empty sockets. The first attempt to extract a molar tooth, however, brought down several teeth, and the whole floor of the antrum. The detachment of this fragment was also now so complete that we believed it necessary to remove it entirely, a labor which was accomplished with infinite difficulty, and with no little hazard to the patient, as dissection had to be extended very far back into the throat, and in the end it was not effected without bringing out, attached to the fragment of maxillary bone, a considerable portion of the pyramidal process of the os palati.

The time occupied in this operation was at least one hour, during which we were every moment in the most painful apprehensions lest we should reach and wound the internal carotid, which lay in such close juxtaposition to the knife that we could distinctly feel its pulsation. After its removal, the hemorrhage was for an hour or more quite profuse, and could only be restrained by sponge compresses pressed firmly back into the mouth and antrum.

When the hemorrhage was sufficiently controlled, we proceeded to examine the antrum, the floor of which being removed entire, permitted the finger to enter freely. The restoration of the malar bone was now accomplished without much difficulty, and with only moderate force.

Two years after the accident, the face presented, externally, no traces of the original injury. The malar bone seemed to be as prominent as upon the opposite side, and there was no perceptible falling in where the teeth and alveoli were removed. During several months after the removal of the bone, the antrum continued to discharge pus, but at length a semi-cartilaginous production closed in the cavity below, entirely reconstructing its floor, and the discharge ceased. Since then he has experienced no further inconvenience.

I wish to propose two or three expedients for lifting the malar bone when it has been thrust down, which may in certain cases be substituted for the mode which has been heretofore generally adopted.

In many instances, no difficulty will be experienced in resorting to the usual method. The recent loss of one or more teeth opposite the floor of the broken antrum, or the complete displacement of a tooth by the accident itself, will give an opportunity for the perforation of the antrum through the open socket, and for the introduction of a suitable instrument for lifting the depressed bone. Unless, however, the opening is quite large, the instrument employed must be so small, such as a straight steel sound or a female catheter, as to expose the parts against which its end is made to press, to some risk of being broken and penetrated. It is even possible in this way to penetrate the socket of the eye, and thus inflict serious injury upon the eye itself. Yet, with some care, such accidents may be avoided, and it is probable that, in the cases supposed, where the sockets of the teeth opposite the base of the antrum are open, this method will continue to have the preference.

But if the teeth remain firm in their places, or if they have been some time removed, and the sockets are filled up, and we wish to enter the antrum at its base, we must either drill through its anterior wall above the roots of the teeth, or we must proceed to extract a tooth. The first method gives an inconvenient opening, and one through which it will be necessary to use a curved instrument; but yet it is a method far less objectionable than the extraction of a tooth which is firm, or which is even tolerably firm in its socket, and which may require the forceps for its removal. The objections to this latter procedure were suggested by the tedious and painful operation already detailed. The first attempt to extract a tooth brought down the whole floor of the antrum, with all its corresponding teeth and the pyramidal process of the palate bone. The tooth was already loose, and we thought it might easily be taken out, but it had not occurred to us that it was loosened by the comminuted condition of the walls of the antrum, and of the dental arcade. The experiments made upon the dead subject would seem to show that this fracture and comminution of the alveoli is not a very frequent result of a fracture of the antrum produced by a blow upon the malar bone, yet it may happen, and whenever it does the attempt to extract a tooth must always expose the patient to the same hazards. Certainly it is no trifling matter to pull away all of a man's upper teeth upon one side, and to open freely into a broad cavity which might never close again, and which, in this event, must always serve as a place of lodgment for particles of food, and for foul secretions, to say nothing of the external deformity which it is likely to produce, and of the severity and even danger of the operation.

I wish, then, to suggest certain procedures, the value of which I have not yet had an opportunity to determine by any experiment upon the living subject, but which I have carefully and frequently tested upon the dead.

First, we ought to attempt to lift the bone by putting the thumb under its zygomatic process and body within the mouth. If the bone is thrown directly downward, or downward and backward, this method can scarcely fail; and even when it is thrown downward and forward so as to press into the antrum, it is likely to succeed. If, however, for any reason, the thumb cannot be brought to bear upon its under surface, we may make a small incision upon the cheek over the anterior margin of the masseter muscle, where its insertion into the malar bone terminates, and pushing a strong blunt hook under the bone, we may lift it with ease.

Where the depression of the malar bone is in the direction of the anterior and superior angle these means may not be found available, and we may then employ a screw elevator, an instrument which I find already constructed in a case of trephining instruments made for me by Mr. Lüer, of Paris, and which I have often used and constantly recommended to my pupils, in certain cases of fractures of the skull. The instrument ought to be made of the best steel, and with a broad, sharp-cutting thread. A slight incision being made through the skin, and down to the centre of the malar bone, the elevator is then screwed firmly into its structure, and now its elevation and adjustment may be accomplished with the greatest ease.

Malgaigne remarks: "In all complicated fractures of the upper jaw, there is one principle which surgeons cannot too much study, namely, that all fragments, however slightly adherent they may be, ought to be most carefully preserved, and they will be found to unite with wonderful ease. This remark had already been made by Saviard. Larrey insists strongly upon it, and we have seen that M. Baudens, so great an advocate for the removal of loose fragments, has declared for these fractures a special exemption."[1]

Malgaigne has here especial reference to fractures of the dental arcade or to fractures implicating the alveoli and extending more or less into the body of the bone.

It would be an error, however, to suppose that a reunion will in these cases uniformly take place. Exceptions have occurred in my own practice, the fragments becoming loosened and completely detached after the lapse of several weeks. In the case related by Miller, the whole floor of the antrum having been broken off, in an unskilful attempt to extract the second right upper molar, it was found impossible to make it unite, and it was subsequently removed.[2] Such unfortunate results certainly may sometimes be reasonably anticipated. Yet they occur so seldom as to justify the opinions and practice advocated by Malgaigne.

In some instances, where fragments are displaced carrying with them several teeth, while others in the same row remain firm, it will be sufficient to close the mouth and apply a bandage as for fracture of the inferior maxilla; in others the teeth and their alveoli, ought to be fastened with silk, or gold or silver thread; or gold or silver clasps may be applied, or gutta percha moulded to the teeth and jaw.

In a case of fracture of the right superior maxilla, reported by Baker, of Norwich, N. Y., complicated with a fracture of the inferior maxilla, the alveoli were retained in place very perfectly by a mould of gutta percha.[3] Neill, of Philadelphia, has also reported three cases of fracture of the bones of the face, involving the superior maxilla, in two of which the eyes were made to protrude more or less from their sockets.[4] The loosened alveoli were made fast by wire. The subsequent deformity was inconsiderable, yet in no instance was the restoration complete.[5] The same method was adopted successfully by

[1] Op. cit., vol. i. p. 376. Paris ed.

[2] News Letter, April, 1854. Also, Bost. Med. and Surg. Journ., vol. li. p. 246.

[3] New York Journ. of Med., vol. i., 3d ser., p. 362.

[4] See Observations first and second, under Fractures of the Malar Bone; in which cases the orbital plate of the malar bone was pushed into the sockets.

[5] Phil. Med. Exam., vol. x., new ser., pp. 455–8.

a surgeon in Virginia, in the case of a negro fifty years old, where most of the teeth of the left upper jaw were forced into the mouth, carrying with them their corresponding alveolar processes. The teeth remained firm in their sockets, but the separation of the bone was complete, the fragment being held in place only by the mucous membrane of the mouth. On the eighth day the surgeon found that the negro had removed the wire, and also the cork from between his teeth, and the maxillary bandage; but the soft parts had already united, and the bones showed no tendency to displacement. His recovery was speedy, and it was accomplished without any farther treatment.[1]

CHAPTER XI.

FRACTURES OF THE ZYGOMATIC ARCH.

THE zygoma, strictly speaking, is formed in a great measure by the body of the malar bone, and it is broken whenever the malar bone is completely separated through any portion of its body; but I propose to confine my remarks to that portion only which is composed of the two processes, called respectively the zygomatic processes of the malar, and temporal bones.

Duverney relates a case in which a young child having in his mouth the end of a lace spindle, fell forwards and thrust the spindle through the mouth from within outwards, breaking the zygoma in the same direction, and leaving the fragments salient outwards.[2] To which case of outward displacement Packard, in a note to Malgaigne's work on fractures, &c., has added a second.[3]

I know of no other examples in which the fragments have been thrust outwards. A reference to my experiments upon the naked skull will, however, show that the zygoma may be broken and displaced in the same direction, by any force which shall fracture the superior maxilla, and depress the anterior margin of the malar bone. In my experiments this has happened three times, and always at the same point, viz., a little beyond the middle of the zygoma, near where the suture which joins the two processes terminates below. The fractures were always transverse, and not in the line of the suture. They were therefore fractures of that portion of the zygoma which belongs to the temporal bone.

I suspect, also, that to this class of cases belongs the example related by Dupuytren, in which the patient having died on the fifth day,

[1] Amer. Med. Gazette, vol. viii., new ser., p. 106.
[2] Bulletin de la Societé Anatomique, p. 138, 1810. [3] Op. cit., p. 289, vol. i.

from the effects of the cerebral concussion, the autopsy disclosed "a fracture through the zygomatic arch; and that part of the superior maxillary bone which constitutes the antrum was driven in."[1]

In another case mentioned by Dupuytren, produced by a direct blow, the fracture was compound and comminuted, and although the fragments were raised easily by an elevator, suppuration ensued beneath, and the matter was discharged within the mouth.[2]

Tavignot reports a case of fracture of this arch which was not discovered until after death, the fragments not being at all displaced.[3]

Dr. John Boardman, one of the surgeons to the Buffalo Hospital of the Sisters of Charity, informs me that he has lately met with a fracture of the zygoma in a man about thirty years of age, occasioned by a blow from a cricket ball. Dr. Boardman saw him on the fourth day, and ascertained that immediately on the receipt of the injury he felt slightly stunned, and that he soon recovered from this, but was unable to open his mouth except by pulling it open with his hand; neither could he close it except in the same manner. This immobility of the jaw continued several days with only very slight improvement; at the end of five weeks, however, when last seen, the mobility was nearly, but not quite restored. The depression, a little in front of the centre of the zygoma, was discovered by the patient himself immediately after the receipt of the injury, and he says he tried at once to ascertain whether he could not push the fragments back by moving the jaw. He was unable to make any impression upon them by this manœuvre. The depression still remains, but it is not so distinct as it was when first seen.

Symptoms.—An irregular projection or depression of the fragments is the only sign which can be relied upon to indicate the existence of this accident; and this must often be concealed by the swelling, which follows so rapidly wherever the integuments are severely bruised over a superficial bone. This displacement can scarcely occur in but two directions, either outwards or inwards; since the attachments of the temporal aponeurosis above, and of the masseter muscle below, must effectively prevent its descent or ascent.

Neither motion nor crepitus will often be present. In some few cases the difficulty in opening or shutting the mouth, occasioned by the projection of the fragments towards or into the tendon of the temporal muscle, may assist in the diagnosis.

Prognosis.—If the fracture has been produced indirectly by a depression of the malar bone, the prognosis must depend upon the amount of injury done to the other bones of the face; in itself, the fracture of the zygoma cannot be a matter of any moment. The same remark might apply also to any fracture of the zygoma in which the angles were salient outwards. If, on the contrary, the angle is salient inwards, the fracture having been produced by a blow inflicted directly upon the zygomatic arch, from without, or by a blow upon the outer por-

[1] Injuries and Diseases of Bones, by Baron Dupuytren. Syd. ed., London, 1847, p. 336.

[2] Op. cit., p. 335.

[3] Bulletins de la Soc. Anat., 1810, p. 138.

tion of the malar bone, it may, perhaps, occasion some embarrassment to the action of the temporal muscle.

If the force which produces the fracture has acted more upon the temporal portion of the arch, near where the process arises from the temporal bone, it may be accompanied with a fracture of the skull, and with serious cerebral lesions, as in one of the cases already alluded to as having been noticed by Dupuytren.

The abscess which followed in the case of the compound, comminuted fracture, quoted from the same author, indicates the danger of this complication; but it must be noticed that its evacuation resulted in a rapid cure, and that no deformity or difficulty in moving the jaw remained.

Treatment.—A fracture, accompanied with an outward displacement, and occasioned by a depression of the malar bone, will be adjusted by a restoration of the malar bone in the manner already described, when speaking of fractures of the superior maxillary, &c. If the fragments are displaced outwards, in consequence of a direct blow from within, then they may be replaced by pressing upon the projecting angle. In this way Duverney easily reduced the bones in the case which I have cited.

When the fragments, in consequence of a direct blow from without, have been driven inwards, and, as a consequence, serious embarrassment to the motions of the temporal muscle ensues, an attempt ought to be made at once to replace them; if, however, no impediment to the action of the muscle exists, it is scarcely necessary to say that no surgical interference will be required. It is quite probable, indeed, that a slight amount of embarrassment may be the result of the direct injury to the muscle inflicted by the blow, without reference to the displacement of the bone, and that a few days will suffice to remedy this evil entirely; and, moreover, experience teaches that in the case of a fracture in other bones, where the fragments actually penetrate the muscles and remain thus displaced, the points are gradually absorbed, and rounded, so that after a time they constitute no impediment to the action of the muscles. It is proper to infer that the same thing will occur here. The surgeon may be reminded, also, that it is not the muscle but only its tendon which is liable to be penetrated, and that even this is usually protected somewhat by a plate of soft adipose tissue.

If to these considerations we add the difficulties which we shall be likely to encounter in the reduction, we shall expect to find but few cases in which a resort to surgical interference will be necessary.

Duverney says that he restored a fracture of this arch, accompanied with depression, by pressing against the zygoma from within the mouth; but an examination of the interior of the buccal cavity will convince us that this is impossible when the fracture is at any point near the middle of the zygoma, and that it can be only when the fracture is at or near the junction of the zygoma with the body of the malar bone that any effective pressure can be made from this direction. In such a case, we may, perhaps, lift the portion of the zygoma remaining attached to the malar bone, by the same means which have already been suggested for lifting the bone itself.

If the bone is driven toward the tendon of the temporal muscle at or near its centre, as happens almost always, then if its restoration becomes necessary, it can be accomplished only by approaching the bone from without.

Dupuytren found an external wound through which, by the aid of a levator, he easily restored the fragments to place.

M. Ferrier, however, of the Hospital of Arles, in a case brought before him, made an incision through the integuments down to the bone, and then attempted to slide underneath the small extremity of a spatula; but the aponeurosis would not yield, and he was obliged to cut it also. He was now able to lift the fragments easily. The wound healed rapidly, and the patient was dismissed without any deformity.[1]

CHAPTER XII.

FRACTURES OF THE LOWER JAW.

Division.—Of 25 examples of fracture of this bone which have come under my observation, 24 were broken through some portion of the body, namely, 1 perpendicularly through the symphysis; 2 through the symphysis and through the centre of the body at the same time; 1 through the angle and centre of the body; 1 through the body and ascending ramus; 2 through the angle and centre of the body upon one side, and through the centre of the body upon the opposite side; 5 through the angle only, and 12 through the body only.

Of the whole number 11 were broken completely asunder at two or more points, constituting double and triple fractures; and of the remaining 14, 4 were accompanied with detachment of portions of the alveoli, and 1 with the detachment of a considerable fragment from the base.

Fig. 24.

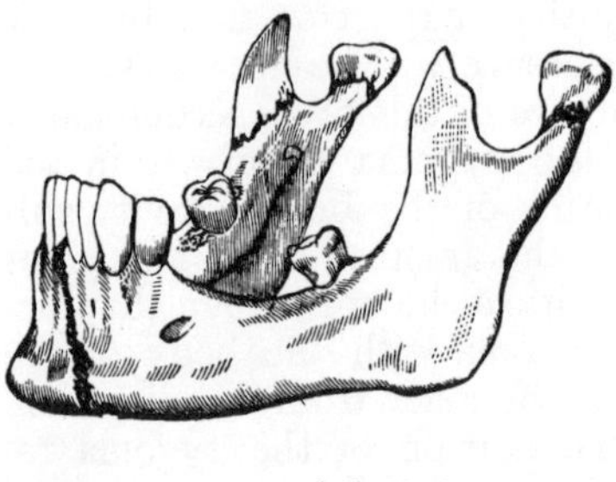

From this analysis it will be seen that 15 of the 25, or more than one-half, were comminuted fractures. 10 were compound; not to include in this enumeration several examples in which the partial or complete dislodgment of a tooth, might entitle them to be called compound.

[1] Bulletin des Sciences Méd., tom. x. p. 160.

The three fractures through or near the symphysis were vertical, and eleven of the remainder were known to be oblique. Malgaigne has remarked, also, that in fractures of the body of the bone the direction of the obliquity is generally such that the anterior fragment is made at the expense of the internal face of the bone, and the posterior fragment at the expense of the external face: this latter overriding the former. Buck, of New York, has seen the fragments in an opposite condition, requiring the use of the knife and the saw for their extrication.[1]

In eighteen examples of fractures through the body, not including fractures of the symphysis, the line of fracture has been observed to be twelve times at or very near the mental foramen; twice between the first and second incisor; three times behind the last molar, and once between the last two molars.

Syme, Liston, and Miller, have remarked, also, the greater frequency of fracture near this foramen, but Mr. Erichsen thinks he has seen it most frequently broken near the symphysis, between the lateral incisors or between these teeth and the canine. Boyer observes that it is generally somewhat in front of the foramen; for which reason, as he thinks, the dental nerve is rarely torn.

Says Boyer, in his *Traité des Maladies Chirurgicales*, "A fracture never takes place in the central point of the length of the jaw, called the symphysis of the chin; but when the solution of continuity occurs towards the middle of the bone, it is upon one or the other side of the symphysis, which remains always upon one of the fragments." An opinion which, however, he does not seem always to have entertained, since Richerand, in a report of his lectures, has made him say that a fracture sometimes takes place "near the chin, but seldom so as to produce the division of the symphysis of that part, though it be not impossible." But many surgeons since his time have noticed this fracture, and Malgaigne assures us that J. Cloquet has demonstrated its existence upon an anatomical specimen. In the two following cases the evidences were so complete that I do not myself entertain much doubt as to their character:—

An Irish laborer, aged seventeen years, was thrown from a wagon, breaking the inferior maxilla on both sides through the body, and, also, exactly in the centre, vertically, between the central incisors.

I dressed the jaw with a four-tailed bandage, but found great difficulty in bringing up the left fragment to a line with the right. I therefore closed the jaws; but finding that the left side still fell three lines below the right, I placed a pine wood wedge between the teeth on the right side, and drew the inferior maxilla up firmly. It now lacked only about half a line of being in place.

There did not appear to be, after this, much difficulty in maintaining quiet and apposition of the fragments; and I supposed, from repeated examinations, that they were in exact line, until four weeks after the fracture had occurred, when I discovered that the central fragments

[1] New York Journ. Med., March, 1847. Proceedings of N. Y. Med. and Surg. Soc., Sept. 19, 1846.

were lifted about two lines above the lateral, and, also, slightly carried back; and although union had not taken place, yet they could not be replaced by any moderate force. The bones united with this slight deformity. Four days later no motion was perceptible, and the displacement seemed to be rather less. From this time the dressings were discontinued.

A gentleman, aged twenty-five years, had his inferior maxilla broken by the kick of a horse. The left lateral incisor was completely displaced, and a large piece of the dental arcade detached.

Dr. S. G. Ellis, of Gowanda, N. Y., dressed the fracture, securing the loosened fragment by the main-spring of a watch, made fast to the teeth by a silver wire, and closing the mouth completely, without any interdental splint. Upon the outside he placed a pasteboard splint and bandages. On the fourth week a fragment exfoliated, and came out under the chin. The union was delayed some six or eight weeks.

I examined the jaw ten years after it was broken, and found the line of a vertical fracture exactly through the symphysis menti. The left half of the chin was slightly elevated, and the whole of that side of the shaft was smaller than the right. He could not close his teeth perfectly, yet he could close them sufficiently for the purposes of mastication.

Stephen Smith, of New York, has seen two examples,[1] Lonsdale mentions three,[2] and Gibson has seen one.[3]

One ought not to be too confident, however, of the exact line of the fracture unless its existence can be demonstrated upon the naked bone, since a slight deviation to the one side or the other of the symphysis might not be easily detected in the living subject.

Velpeau, Fergusson, Gibson, Henry Smith and others, have remarked that a separation at the symphysis takes place usually in infancy or childhood. But in the eight examples in which I find the ages reported, only one, a case mentioned by Lonsdale, occurred in a person as young as ten years; in one of the cases seen by myself the patient was seventeen years old, and the remainder have ranged from twenty-five years to sixty: and the average age of all is thirty-two years.

I have seen one example of a fracture of the ramus, in a man twenty-three years old, who had been struck by a wooden block on the side of his face. The ramus was broken just above the angle, and the body was broken, also, obliquely near the symphysis. The intercepted fragment was carried inwards.[4] Ledran mentions the case of a child, ten or twelve years old, in whom the fracture was double also; one fracture having taken place through the body, and one extending obliquely from the root of the coronoid process to the neck of the condyle. The intercepted fragment was, however, so little displaced that the fracture of the ramus was not discovered until after death.[5]

[1] New York Journ. Med., Jan. 1857, Hospital Reports.

[2] Practical Treatise on Fractures. By Edward F. Lonsdale. London, 1838, p. 226.

[3] Institutes and Practice of Surg. By Wm. Gibson. Philadelphia, 1841, p. 261.

[4] Trans. Amer. Med. Assoc. Report on "Deformities after Fractures," vol. viii. p. 385, Case 17.

[5] Malgaigne, op. cit., p. 377, from Ledran, Observ. Chirurg., tom. i. obs. viii.

Malgaigne refers to this as the only example recorded; but Stephen Smith, of the Bellevue Hospital, has met with it four times; in one case the ramus was broken on both sides; in two cases one ramus only was broken; and in one the body was broken on the right side and the ramus on the left.[1] In two of these examples the fragments were not displaced.

The coronoid process is so well protected by muscles and by the surrounding bony projections, that it is very rarely broken.

Houzelot mentions a case in which a fall from a height produced at the same time a fracture of both condyles, of both coronoid processes and of the symphysis.[2]

With this single exception, I am not able to find a recorded example of a fracture of this process.

At least nine cases have been reported of fracture of the condyles, in all of which the separation occurred through the neck, viz., three by Ribes, two by Desault, one by Bérard, one by Houzelot, one by Bichat, one by Packard, of Philadelphia, and two by Watson, of N. Y. The fracture always occurring through the neck and just below the insertion of the external pterygoid muscle.

According to Malgaigne, the analysis of these cases, excepting those mentioned by Packard and Watson, shows two classes of examples: the one occasioned by falls or blows upon the chin, and producing a simple fracture of the neck of the condyle; the other, occasioned by injuries inflicted upon the side of the face, and producing a fracture of the neck on the side corresponding to that upon which the injuries are received, and at the same time a fracture of the body upon the opposite side. These two varieties seem to be about equally common.

In the case mentioned by Houzelot, and already cited, there existed at the same time a fracture of both condyles, of both coronoid processes and at the symphysis. The man also whom Watson saw in the New York Hospital, had fallen from the yard-arm of a vessel, breaking his thigh and arm bones and both condyles of the lower jaw. "His face was somewhat deformed by the retraction of the chin; the mouth could not be opened so as to protrude the tongue to any great extent beyond the teeth, and the teeth of the upper and lower jaw could not be brought into contact. In attempting to move the jaw the patient experienced pain and crepitation just in front of the ears; the crepitation could easily be felt by placing the fingers over the fractured condyles. Nothing was done for the fractures of the jaw. In a few weeks the rubbing of the broken surfaces and attendant soreness ceased to trouble him; but the shape of the jaw and difficulty of opening the mouth, to any great extent, still remained unaltered."[3]

Etiology.—The causes, in such cases as I have myself investigated, seem generally to have been direct blows, in most instances inflicted by a club, or by the kick of a horse; in one instance the blow was inflicted by the fist. I have also seen a fracture immediately in front

[1] New York Journ. Med., Jan. 1857. Bellevue Hosp. Reports.
[2] Malgaigne, op. cit., p. 400.
[3] New York Journ. of Med., Oct., 1840. Hospital Reports.

of the right cuspid, in a lad eight years of age, produced by being pressed between two wagons, the pressure being made upon the two angles of the jaw. In ten of eleven cases mentioned by Stephen Smith, the causes were direct blows. Examples of fracture of the inferior maxilla from indirect blows have, however, been mentioned by other surgeons, the angles of the bone being pressed together by the passage of a wheel, and the fracture taking place usually towards the symphysis.

We have already alluded to the observation of Malgaigne, that fractures of the condyles belong to two classes: the one being occasioned by falls upon the chin, and the other by blows upon the side of the face: the former acting as a counter force and the latter as a direct.

The coronoid process can only be broken by a direct blow.

Symptoms.—Fractures of the body of the bone are characterized by the usual signs of fracture elsewhere, namely, displacement, mobility, crepitus, and pain.

The displacement is generally present; but its direction and amount vary according to the situation and course of the fracture, and also according to the violence and direction of the force producing the fracture. In one instance the displacement did not exist, and indeed I think it ought to be regarded as an example of a partial fracture.

A lad, æt. 9, was kicked by a horse on the 22d of June, 1858, the blow being received on the right side of the jaw. I saw him very soon after the accident, but could not detect any fracture, only the body of the jaw seemed to be bent in. On the third day, however, while endeavoring to straighten the jaw by violent pressure from within outwards I detected a feeble crepitus, which on more careful examination proved to be opposite the second incisor of the right side. I was also able to detect a slight motion at the same point. It was found impossible to rectify the bending, and no further efforts were employed. At this moment, after a lapse of nearly a year, the natural curve is partially but not completely restored.

Ledran and other surgeons have also seen examples where neither the periosteum nor mucous membrane was torn.

Generally, in fractures of the body, the anterior fragment is depressed; and Malgaigne affirms that where an overlapping occurs, the anterior fragment lies, generally, within the posterior; a fact which he explains by the direction which the line of fracture usually takes, namely, from without, inwards and backwards, as we have already mentioned. In one instance, reported by me to the Amer. Med. Assoc., where the jaw was broken at the symphysis and also on both sides through the body, the central fragments were found, after about four weeks, lifted two lines above the lateral fragments, and also slightly carried backwards.[1] I have twice also met with examples in which the posterior fragments were inclined to fall inwards toward the mouth, a circumstance which seemed to indicate that the course of the obliquity was in a direction opposite to that which Malgaigne has observed to be most frequent. In each of these examples the jaw was

[1] Trans. Amer. Med. Assoc., vol. viii. p. 380, 1855, Case 6.

broken upon both sides, by blows inflicted with a club, and the fractures were situated well back.[1] It is possible, however, that the position of the fragments was due rather to the direction and force of the impression than to the direction of the line of fracture.

As to the action of the muscles in the production of displacement, Boyer, S. Cooper, Erichsen, and Malgaigne, have observed that their action upon the anterior fragment is greater in proportion as the fracture is nearer the symphysis, and less in proportion as it approaches the angle. So that in the former case the attempt to close the mouth is sometimes attended with a depression of the anterior fragment, causing a separation of the fragments at their alveolar margins; while in the latter case, the attempt to close the mouth forcibly is occasionally attended with separation of the fragments along the line of the base.

While I am not prepared to deny the accuracy of these observations, it is proper to notice that Liston finds the greatest displacement when the fracture is opposite the first molar, and I must confess that the fact, as stated by Boyer and others, does not seem to admit of a satisfactory explanation; since the number, and consequently the power of the muscles which act upon the anterior fragment from below, is greatest at a point considerably remote from the symphysis. These muscles, namely, the digastricus, the genio-hyo-glossus, and the mylo-hyoideus, with several other muscles which act less directly, all tend to depress the anterior fragment, and in some slight degree to carry it backwards, a direction which, indeed, it usually takes, and which it would probably always take if left alone to the action of the muscles. If the fracture has occurred through the angle, or at any point within the attachments of the masseter muscle, the action of those fibres of this muscle which remain connected with the anterior fragment will sufficiently explain the fact that it is not now so easily depressed below the level of the posterior fragment; while the separation of the fragments along the line of the base when an attempt is made to close the jaw forcibly, is probably due to the loosening and partial dislodgment of some of the molars, which, being pressed upwards, act as a pivot upon which the fragments are made to bend.

Boyer affirms, also, that "the fractured portions are never deranged so as that one passes on the other, or in the direction of their length; for the action of none of the muscles of the lower jaw is parallel to the axis of that bone; besides, its extremities are retained in the glenoidal cavities of the temporal bones." But this theory is too exclusive, since the fragments may have become displaced in any direction independently of the muscular action. Moreover, the action of the muscles attached to the anterior fragment, although not parallel to the axis of the bone, does somewhat favor a displacement in this direction; and the action of the pterygoid muscles upon the posterior fragment still farther favors this form of displacement.

An overlapping of the fragments in the direction of the axis is, no doubt, exceptional, and in such examples as I have seen, it was very

[1] Ibid., Cases 1 and 10.

trivial. It occurred in case "three" of my "Report," the fracture being near the mental foramen; in case "two," the fracture being just anterior to the last molar; and also in case "six," where the bone had been broken through the centre of the body on both sides and through the symphysis; but in neither case did the overlapping exceed two or three lines, and it was always easily overcome.

The mobility of the fragments is not so striking in these accidents as in fractures of the long bones, yet it is generally sufficiently marked, and especially where the bone is broken upon both sides at the same time. If only one side is broken, both motion and crepitus will be most easily detected by lateral pressure upon the posterior fragment, which, being the smallest and the least supported by antagonizing muscles, will be found to be the most movable. If the fracture is upon both sides, mobility and crepitus will be most readily developed by seizing upon the anterior fragment and moving it gently up and down, while the finger rests upon the alveolus within the mouth.

Sometimes a slight swelling or tenderness at some point of the dental arcade, or the loosening or complete dislodgment of a tooth, will indicate the point of fracture.

Pain, especially when the fragments are moved, is here more constant than in most other fractures, owing, perhaps, in part to the superficial position of the bone which renders the soft parts lying over it more liable to injury from the causes of fracture; but also, in part, to the lesions which the inferior dental nerve may have suffered. It is, indeed, a matter of surprise that injury to this nerve does not oftener seriously complicate these accidents, coursing, as it does, through so large a portion of the angle and body of the bone. One might naturally suppose that its complete disruption would often occasion paralysis of those portions of the face to which it is finally distributed, and that its partial lesions and contusions would create, in many cases, the most acute and constant suffering. It is rare, however, that we have present an amount of pain which might not be attributed to a severe shock, or a slight strain upon its fibres. I have myself never seen any extraordinary suffering distinctly attributable to an injury of the dental nerve after fracture, nor any degree of facial paralysis. Rossi relates a case in which convulsions followed this accident, and in which, as a final remedy, he proposed to expose and bisect the nerve; and Flajani saw a patient whose jaw had been broken, die in convulsions on the tenth day, the muscular contractions having commenced as early as the fourth day after the accident. The autopsy disclosed a rupture of the dental nerve, but no injury to the brain.

These two examples are, as far as I know, all which our records supply, in which grave results have been attributed to lesions of this nerve; and even here some doubt must remain whether the symptoms were not quite as much due to the immediate injury done to the brain as to the nerve.

Boyer explained the infrequency of severe injury to the dental nerve by the supposition that the "greater part of these fractures takes place between the symphysis and the foramen by which this nerve comes out." An opinion which may be correct, but needs confirmation. I have seen the body or angle broken at points posterior to the mental foramen, and where the nerve lies within its bony canal, twelve times, and in front of the mental foramen, eight times, and twelve times the point of fracture has not been stated with such accuracy as to enable me to say whether it was in front of or behind the foramen; of these latter, ten were said to be near the foramen.

I suspect that a better explanation may be found in the fact that the fragments seldom overlap, to any appreciable extent, and that even the displacement in the direction of the diameters of the bone is generally inconsiderable, or if it does exist it is easily and promptly replaced.

If the displacement is sufficient to occasion a complete disruption of the nerve, some degree of temporary paralysis in the portions of the face supplied by it must be inevitable; and, perhaps, this occurs oftener than it has been noticed, since, during the confinement of the jaw by dressings, it is not likely to be observed, and after the lapse of a few weeks it will probably cease altogether.

Boyer remarks that when it is torn, "the square and triangular muscles of the chin are paralyzed. The skin of that part and the internal membrane of the under lip preserve their sensibility, which it appears they owe to some threads of the portio dura of the seventh pair; but the paralysis of these muscles does not prove of itself that the jaw is fractured." Boyer has, however, noticed this result but once, and then in a case where the bone was broken upon both sides and the soft parts greatly contused. The triangular and square muscles were paralyzed, in consequence of which there was a slight contortion of the mouth. A. Bérard has also mentioned a case of vertical fracture occurring between the second and third molars, without displacement, which was accompanied with complete insensibility of the lip on the same side throughout the space comprised between the commissure and the median line, and between the free border of the lip and the chin. The paralysis disappeared after a few days.[1]

To these signs now enumerated, we may add as occasional complications, rather than as diagnostic symptoms, salivation, swelling of the submaxillary and sublingual glands, abscesses, necrosis, &c. If the blow has been vertical upon the chin, and the direction of its force has been towards the articulations, the bony structure of the ear, and even the brain may have suffered serious lesions, which may be indicated by a deafness, or a roaring in the ears, by bleeding from the external meatus, and by fatal coma. Tessier saw a man who had received the kick of a horse exactly upon the centre of the chin, breaking the bone on both sides, and who, in consequence, bled freely from his ears;[2] and Alix relates the case of a young man who, falling from a height and striking upon his chin, had broken his jaw. Insensibility

[1] Malgaigne, from Gazette des Hôpitaux, 10 Août, 1841.
[2] Malgaigne, p. 383 and 386; from Journ. de Méd., 1789, tom. lxxix., p. 246.

immediately followed; convulsions also ensued upon the fourth day, and he died upon the sixth.[1]

If the fracture is at the symphysis, it is generally vertical, and either fragment may be found slightly displaced upwards or downwards. In one of the examples seen by myself, the left fragment fell three lines below the right, and in another the right side had fallen about one line. In a case mentioned by Syme there was scarcely any displacement.[2] Liston remarks that it is usually slight. Erichsen and B. Cooper have observed the same.

The signs which indicate a fracture through the angle have already been sufficiently considered when speaking of fractures of the body; from which it only differs in the less degree of displacement, and in the fact that the posterior fragments are a little more prone to fall inwards toward the mouth. I have noticed, also, that owing probably to the loosening and partial dislodgment of the last molar, it is sometimes difficult to close the mouth, the same as in the fractures a little farther forwards.

In the only example of fracture of the ascending ramus which I have seen, the bone being broken also through its body, the fracture of the ramus was easily recognized by both crepitus and mobility.

As to the signs which indicate a fracture of the coronoid process, I am only able to infer them from its anatomical relations. There must be some embarrassment in the motions of the jaw, occasioned by the detachment of a portion of the fibres of the temporal muscle; and it is probable that an examination by the finger, within the mouth, would readily detect mobility and displacement.

A fracture through the neck of the condyle is characterized by pain at the seat of fracture, especially recognized when an attempt is made to open or shut the mouth, by embarrassment in the motions of the jaw, by crepitus, which may usually be felt or heard by the patient himself, by mobility and displacement.

The upper fragment, if disengaged from the lower, is drawn forwards, upwards, and inwards, by the action of the pterygoideus externus; and it is felt not to accompany the movements of the lower fragment.

The lower fragment is at the same time drawn upwards, in consequence of which the lower part of the face is distorted: a circumstance first noticed by Ribes, and which supplies an important diagnostic mark between a fracture of one condyle and a dislocation. In dislocation, the chin is commonly thrown to one side, but it is to the side opposite that on which the dislocation has occurred, while in fracture the chin is drawn to the same side.

Prognosis.—Physick, of Philadelphia, saw a case of non-union of the body of this bone, which had existed nine months.[3] Dupuytren mentions a case which had existed three years.[4] Horeau has recorded one example in a man who had received a gunshot wound through

[1] Malgaigne, p. 386; from Alix, Observata Chir., fascic. 1, obs. 10.

[2] Amer. Journ. Med. Sci., vol. xviii. p. 243.

[3] Phila. Med. and Surg. Journ., vol. v.

[4] Leçons Orales.

his face.[1] Stephen Smith, of New York, reports a case of fracture of both the body and ramus, in a man forty-five years old. The severity of the injury, with the supervention of delirium tremens, prevented the application of dressings until the thirteenth day. On the twentieth day about a pint of blood was lost by hemorrhage from the seat of fracture. He remained in the hospital one hundred and thirty-seven days, and was finally discharged, the fragments not having yet united.[2] Malgaigne says that Boyer has seen several examples, but I know of no other cases which have been recorded. In no instance under my observation, has the bone refused finally to unite, although I have seen the union delayed six, seven, ten, and even eleven weeks or more.[3] In three of these cases the fractures were either compound or comminuted; but in one case the fracture was simple, the delay in the union being due to a feeble condition of the system, and in part, perhaps, to neglect of proper treatment.

The infrequency of non-union after this fracture, is a fact worthy of especial attention, because of the extreme difficulty, if not actual impossibility, in many cases, of preventing motion between the fragments, by any mode of dressing yet devised. Any one who has observed attentively, must have seen, not only that his dressings are more often found disturbed and loosened, than in the case of almost any other fracture, unless it be the clavicle, and thus the fragments have been through all the treatment subjected to frequent changes of position; but, also, that even while the dressings remain snugly in place, the patient seldom is able to perform the necessary acts of deglutition, or to speak, even, without inflicting some motion upon the fragments.

Indeed, the rapidity as well as certainty with which this bone unites, has, I think, been observed by other surgeons, and I have myself noticed one instance, in an adult person, in which the bone was immovable at the seat of fracture, on the seventeenth day, and, perhaps, earlier. In other instances, the union has been speedily effected after the removal of all dressings.

The amount of deformity resulting, also, from these fractures is usually very trifling, whatever treatment has been adopted. Ten of the twenty-five examples seen by me, are recorded as resulting in some degree of imperfection, but one of these cases was complicated with other injuries, of which the patient died in a few days, and one was a case of delayed union. Only eight of the united fractures are imperfect, and in none of these is the imperfection such as to be noticed in a casual examination of the face. The deformity which is usually found, is a slight irregularity of the teeth, produced, in most cases, by a falling of the anterior fragment, but in one case by a slight elevation of the anterior fragment. But even this does not always interfere with mastication, and would often pass unnoticed by the patient himself. It is probable, too, that time, and the constant use

[1] Malgaigne, from Journ. de Méd., par Corvisart, etc., tom. x. p. 195.
[2] Smith, New York Journ. of Med. and Surg., Jan. 1857.
[3] My Report on Deformities after Frac., Cases 2, 14, 15, 18.

of the lower jaw in mastication, will gradually effect a marked improvement in the ability to bring the opposing teeth into contact. I think I have observed this in several instances.

Chelius remarks that in "double or oblique fractures it is very difficult to keep the broken ends in their proper place; deformity and displacement of the natural position of the teeth commonly remain."

In the second example of fracture through the symphysis mentioned by me, the left fragment remained slightly elevated, and the patient could not close his teeth perfectly, yet he could close them sufficiently for the purposes of mastication. It is probable, however, that ordinarily no difficulty will be experienced in accomplishing a perfect cure, when the separation has taken place only at the symphysis.

In fractures of the condyles, more care is requisite to retain the fragments in apposition, and sometimes it may be found to be impossible. Richerand mentions the case of a man, who, having been three months in the "Hôpital de la Charité," for a double fracture of the lower jaw, one fracture being near the middle, and the other near the right condyle, left before the cure was complete. Seven or eight months after, he called upon Boyer, who extracted from a fistula in the meatus auditorius externus, a bony mass, which had evidently the form of the condyle.[1] Bichat mentions a similar case as having come under the observation of Desault;[2] possibly it was the same which Boyer saw. Ribes says that a Parisian surgeon treated a double fracture of the jaw in a gentleman, one fracture being through the body, and the other through the neck of the condyle; and in spite of the most assiduous and skilful attention, the patient recovered with a lateral distortion of the jaw, occasioned by the displacement of the fragments.[3] Ribes himself had to treat an accident of a similar character, and notwithstanding all his care, the result was the same as in the other example just cited.[4]

The proximity of this fracture to the articulating surface may occasion contraction of the ligaments about the joint: and a degree of embarrassment to the motions of the jaw has followed in the experience of Desault and others, even when the cure has been most complete; but this has usually remained only for a short period.

Sanson asserts that when the coronoid process is broken, the fracture never unites; but that mastication is performed very well, the masseter and pterygoid muscles then fulfilling the office of the temporal.[5]

Treatment.—The few attempts which I have made to restore a completely dislocated tooth to its socket, or to retain it in place when very much loosened, have generally resulted in its removal at some later day, and especially where the fracture has been near the angle, and a molar has been disturbed. I believe it would be better practice always to remove the molars under these circumstances, unless they

[1] Boyer, Lectures on Dis. of Bones, p. 53, Phila. ed., 1805.
[2] Desault, Treatise on Fractures and Luxations, Phila. ed., 1805, p. 3.
[3] Malgaigne, op. cit., p. 402.
[4] Ibid., p. 402.
[5] S. Cooper's First Lines, Amer. ed., 1844, vol. ii. p. 311.

remain attached to the alveoli, and cannot be removed without bringing them away also; and this, whether the loosened teeth are situated in the line of fracture or not. It is seldom that they can be made again to occupy their sockets perfectly, and where the teeth are in the line of the fracture, the attempt to restore them to place will sometimes prevent the proper adjustment of the fragments. In cases, also, in which the teeth farther forwards are completely dislodged at the seat of fracture, it is scarcely worth while to replace them.

As to those teeth whose loosened condition is due only to a splitting of the alveoli, the same rule will not always apply. Sometimes, after a careful readjustment, the fragments will reunite, and the teeth remain firm.

If the bone is chipped off upon the outside, through or near the line of the sockets, the teeth may not be always much disturbed, and the loss of the fragments may be of less consequence, nor have I generally succeeded in saving them; yet if they remain adherent to the soft parts, it is proper to make the attempt.

The expedients to which surgeons have resorted for the purpose of retaining in place the fragments, when the bone is broken through its body, may be arranged under the names of ligatures, splints, bandages, and slings.

The ligature has been applied both to the teeth and to the bone itself. Thus, in an oblique fracture near the angle, where the fragments could not otherwise be prevented from falling inwards, Baudens passed a strong ligature, formed of thread, around the fragments and in immediate contact with them, tying the ligature over the teeth within the mouth. No accident followed, and on the twenty-third day, when he removed the ligature, the bone had united firmly and smoothly.[1]

In the case of the fracture of the inferior maxilla, reported by Dr. Buck, to the New York Pathological Society, and already referred to, the bone "was broken between the two incisor teeth of the left side; the part of the bone on the left of the fracture was driven in, and interlocked behind the end of the right portion, so as to be separated by a finger's breadth. Finding it impossible otherwise to reduce the fracture, Dr. B. dissected off the under lip, so as to expose the fracture. He found that the right anterior portion of the fractured bone terminated in an angular projection as far as on a line below the left angle of the mouth. The lip was then divided to the chin, and the soft parts holding the fragments together incised. A chisel was then insinuated behind the projecting angle of the bone, while it was being excised by the metacarpal saw. When the bone was restored to its natural position, it was found so apt to become displaced, that holes were drilled at the lower angle of the fracture, and adjustment maintained by wiring them together, the wire passing out through the lower angle of the wound. Sutures and adhesive straps, with a bandage, were employed to maintain the adjustment of the parts. So far the patient has done well, being supported by liquid nourishment

[1] Malgaigne, op. cit., p. 398.

introduced through a tube, passed through the space left by one of the incisors, which, on account of its looseness, was removed."[1]

In May, 1858, while trephining at the angle of the jaw for the purpose of cutting out a portion of the dental nerve in a patient suffering from neuralgia, I accidentally broke the jaw in two at the point at which the trephine was applied. I immediately bored a hole in the opposite extremities of the two fragments, and fastened them together with a silver wire, by which I was able to maintain complete apposition, and in three weeks the union was accomplished, the wire separating and falling out of itself. No splints were ever used.[2]

With these exceptions, so far as I am aware, the ligature has been employed as a means of retention only by fastening it upon the teeth, either upon those which are situated on the opposite sides of the fracture, or upon others a little more remote, or upon the corresponding teeth of the upper jaw, or upon the teeth on the opposite sides of the same jaw.

Ordinarily the ligature, composed of either fine gold, platinum, or silver wire, or of firm silk or linen threads—(Celsus advised the use of horsehair)—has been applied to the two teeth on the opposite sides of the fracture, or if these have been not sufficiently firm, to the next teeth. This practice, recommended first by Hippocrates, has received the occasional sanction of Ryff, Walner, Chelius, Lizars, Erichsen, Miller, B. Cooper, Skey, and others, but by Boyer, Gibson, and Malgaigne, it has been reprobated.

Dr. S. G. Ellis, of Gowanda, N. Y., as we have already seen, has treated a fracture occurring through the symphysis, in an adult, by placing the mainspring of a watch within the dental arcade, and securing it in place with silver wire. The mouth was kept closed by bandages carried under the chin. The fragments united with only a slight vertical displacement.[3]

Dr. George Haywood, of Boston, surgeon to the Massachusetts General Hospital, says: "When the bone is not comminuted and there are teeth on each side of the fracture, the ends of the bone can be kept in exact apposition by passing a silver wire or strong thread around these teeth and tying it tightly. In several cases of fracture of the jaw, in which the bone was broken in one place only, I have in the course of the last few years, adopted this practice with entire success, and without the aid of any other means. It will be found very useful, also, as an auxiliary, in more severe cases, in which it may be required to use splints and bandages, or to insert a piece of cork between the jaws, as recommended by Delpech. It requires some mechanical dexterity to apply the thread neatly; but in large cities we can avail ourselves of the skill of dentists for this purpose."[4] I have myself in two or three instances used a linen thread with excellent results.

Guillaume de Salicet advises to secure, with a silk thread, at the

[1] New York Journ. of Med., &c., March, 1847, p. 211.
[2] Buffalo Med. Journ., vol. xiv. p. 148.
[3] Trans. Amer. Med. Assoc. My report on "Defor.," &c. vol. viii. p. 383, Case 14.
[4] Boston Med. & Surg. Journ., vol. xix. p. 133, 1838.

same moment the teeth belonging to the two fragments, and the corresponding teeth of the upper jaw;[1] while the dentist Lemaire, being applied to by Dupuytren to secure in place the ununited fragments of a broken jaw, fastened the two left canine teeth to each other by a wire of platinum, as had been already suggested by Guillaume de Salicet; to these he added two other modes of ligature which were altogether original. One wire, made fast to the last molar upon one side, traversed the mouth and was secured to one of the bicuspids upon the opposite side; the other was stretched from the first inferior bicuspid on the right to the first superior bicuspid on the left. A cure was accomplished at the end of two months, but one of the wires had nearly bisected the tongue; and as it had gradually become imbedded, the flesh had closed over it until it rested like a seton through the middle of the tongue![2]

None of these various methods recommend themselves very satisfactorily to the practical surgeon; for besides that they are all of them, in a large majority of cases, wholly unnecessary, and in other cases, owing to the absence of the teeth, or to their loosened or decayed condition, or to the closeness with which they are set against each other, absolutely impossible, it must be seen, also, that they will generally prove feeble and inefficient. The wires act only upon the upper extremity of the line of fracture, leaving its lower portions liable to be disturbed by trivial causes; they tend gradually to loosen even the firm teeth which they embrace, and not unfrequently, after having been made fast with much labor, they soon become disarranged or break. They require, therefore, always the additional protection afforded by bandages. Alone they are insufficient, and if properly constructed bandages or slings are employed, they are not needed. Sometimes, moreover, they are actually mischievous, as when they loosen a sound tooth or press upon and inflame the gums. A. Bérard passed a silver wire twice around the necks of two adjoining teeth on the opposite sides of a fracture. It retained the fragments perfectly in apposition during several days; but soon the gums swelled and became painful; the teeth loosened, and it was found necessary to remove the wire. Chassaignac sought to avoid these evils by placing the wire upon the middle of the crown, free from the gums, and by including four teeth instead of two. A waxed linen thread was made fast in this manner, in a case of simple fracture, on the seventh day. On the following morning the thread was found broken. He applied then a silk ligature in the same manner. On about the third day this also was disarranged; the ligatures were now discontinued until the eighteenth day, when he renewed the experiment with a piece of gold wire. Fourteen days after this the ligature remained firm, but the gums were red and bleeding. The patient not having again returned to Chassaignac, the result is not known.[3]

As to the method suggested by Guillaume de Salicet, it presents no advantages to compensate for its inconveniences; while that actually

[1] Malgaigne, op. cit., p. 392.
[2] Jour. Univer. des Sci. Méd., tom. xix. p. 77.
[3] Lond. Med. & Phys. Journ., Nov. 1822, p. 401.

practised by the dentist Lemaire, successful, indeed, threatened to substitute a loss of the tongue for an ununited fracture of the jaw.

Splints have been employed in various ways. First, simple interdental splints, laid along the crowns of the teeth and only sufficiently grooved to be easily retained in place; Second, clasps, which are applied over the crowns and sides of the teeth, operating chiefly by their lateral pressure; Third, splints applied to the outer and inferior margin of the jaw; Fourth, interdental splints or clasps, combined with outside splints.

Interdental splints have been recommended by many surgeons from an early day, and they continue to be employed occasionally up to this moment.

Boyer advises the use of cork splints placed one on each side between the upper and lower jaws, in a few exceptional cases. Miller recommends the same in all cases, the "two edges of cork sloping gently backwards, with their upper and under surfaces grooved for the reception of the upper and lower teeth." Fergusson also has usually adopted the same practice. Muys and Bertrandi employed ivory wedges.[1]

On the other hand they are rejected entirely by Syme, Chelius, Skey, Erichsen, and Gibson.

The objections which have been stated to their use are: that they are unsteady and become easily loosened and disarranged; that they occasionally press painfully upon the inside of the cheeks; that they accumulate about themselves an offensive sordes, and finally that they are unnecessary, since experience has proven, says Gibson, that "there is always sufficient space between the teeth to enable the patient to imbibe broth or any other thin fluid placed between the teeth."

It is not strictly true, however, that in all cases there will be found sufficient space between the teeth, when the mouth is closed, for the imbibition of nutrient fluids. I have myself seen exceptions, and in such a case the patient, if the mouth were closed in the usual way, would have to be fed through a tube conveyed along the nostrils into the stomach, as suggested by both Samuel and Bransby Cooper in certain bad compound fractures, or through an opening made by the extraction of one of the front teeth; neither of which methods ought to be preferred to the interdental splints; but then the separation of the front teeth for the purpose of receiving food, is by no means the only object to be gained by their use, nor indeed the principal object. Their great purpose is to act as splints whenever the absence of teeth either in the upper or lower jaw renders the two corresponding arcades unequal and irregular and prevents our making use of the upper jaw as a kind of internal splint for the lower jaw.

It is with a view to the accomplishment of this important end that they are often valuable, and ought sometimes to be considered as indispensable. I believe, also, that many of the inconveniences which have been found to attend the use of cork or wood, are obviated by the substitution of gutta percha in the manner which I have already recommended in my report to the American Medical Association,

[1] Lond. Med.-Chir. Rev., vol. xx. p. 470.

made in the year 1855. I have employed this method several times myself, and my suggestions have been followed by Stephen Smith, of the Bellevue Hospital, New York, who, after having used the gutta percha in four cases, affirms that nothing can surpass it in efficiency.

The mode of preparing gutta percha, and of adapting it between the teeth, is as follows: Dip a couple of pieces of the gum, of a proper size, into boiling water, and when they are sufficiently softened, mould them into wedge-shaped blocks, and, having wrapped each block with a piece of cotton cloth, carry them to their appropriate places between the back teeth; immediately press up each horizontal ramus of the jaw until the mouth is sufficiently closed, and the line of the inferior margin is straight; in this position retain the fragments a few minutes, until the gum has sufficiently hardened. Meantime, it will be practicable, generally, to introduce the fingers into the mouth, and to press the gutta percha laterally on each side towards the teeth, and thus to make its position more secure. When it is sufficiently hardened, remove the splints for the purpose of determining more precisely that they are properly shaped and fitted.

The superiority of this splint is now at once perceived. If properly made, it is smooth upon its surface, and not, therefore, so liable to irritate the mouth as wood or cork, and it is so moulded to the teeth that it will never become displaced.

The clasp, applied over the crowns and sides of the teeth is not intended to act as an interdental splint; but by its lateral pressure it is expected to hold the fragments in apposition upon nearly the same principle with the ligature.

Mütter, of Philadelphia, employs for this purpose a plate of silver folded snugly over the tops and sides of two or more teeth adjacent to the fracture, which apparatus he calls a "clamp."[1]

Fig. 25.

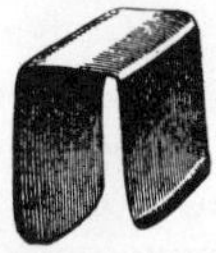

Mütter's clamp for fractured jaw.

Nicole, of Nuremburg, employed for the same purpose a couple of steel plates fitted accurately along the anterior and posterior dental curvatures, secured in place by a steel clasp, the clasp being furnished with a thumb-screw, in order the more effectually to accomplish the lateral pressure.

Malgaigne has extended the idea of Nicole, by substituting for the two steel plates, a single plate composed of flexible and ductile iron, which is fitted accurately to all the irregularities of the posterior dental arch. From the two extremities of this plate, and from two other intermediate points, four small steel shafts arise perpendicularly, cross the crowns of the teeth at right angles, and then fall down again perpendicularly upon the anterior dental arcade. Each steel shaft being furnished with a thumb-screw, the iron plate can now be made to bear against the teeth so as to form a posterior dental splint. The teeth are also protected in front against the direct action of the thumb-screw by the interposition of a leaden plate.

I am not aware that either of these modes has ever been practically tested; and I confess that I can see many disadvantages and incon-

[1] Trans. Am. Med. Assoc., vol. viii. p. 391.

veniences which would be likely to arise from their use. With the exception of Mütter's "clamp," they are all complex and must be liable to disarrangement; while thumb screws in the mouth cannot but inflict serious injury by their pressure and friction against the mucous membrane.

Gutta percha employed in the manner which I have recommended, is capable of giving no inconsiderable degree of lateral support to the teeth, and I suspect quite as much as the comfort or interest of the patient will permit, and without many of the inconveniences of the other modes, while it possesses the additional advantage of serving also, where this is needed, as an efficient interdental splint.

External splints, applied along the base or outside of the jaw, were first recommended by Paré, who used, for this purpose, leather; and they have been employed in some form, occasionally, by most surgeons. Generally they have been composed of flexible materials, such as wetted pasteboard, first recommended by Heister, felt, linen saturated with the whites of eggs, paste, dextrine or starch; plaster of Paris has also been used: and they have been retained in place by either bandages or the sling. I have myself used for this purpose, gutta percha, but I shall speak of it as one form of the sling dressing.

Undoubtedly useful, and even necessary in some cases, especially where there exists a great tendency to a vertical displacement, they will be found, also, in many cases, to render no essential service, and may properly enough be dispensed with.

Whatever objections hold to the use of metallic clasps, must hold equally to the use of those forms of apparatus in which it is attempted to secure the fragments by means of a combination of these clasps with outside splints, and in which it is proposed to dispense with all bandages or slings, the mouth being permitted to open and close freely during the whole treatment. They are liable, moreover, to additional objections, which will be readily suggested by an explanation of their mode of construction.

Chopart and Desault originated this idea as early as 1780, for fractures occurring upon both sides; in which cases they advised "bandages composed of crotchets of iron or of steel, placed over the teeth, upon the alveolar margin, covered with cork or with plates of lead, and fastened by thumb-screws to a plate of sheet iron, or to some other material under the jaw."

The apparatus invented by Rutenick, a German surgeon, in 1799, and improved by Kluge, is thus described by Dr. Chester: "It consists, 1st, of small silver grooves, varying in size according as they are to be placed on the incisors or molars, and long enough to extend over the crowns of four teeth; 2d, of a small piece of board, adapted to the lower surface of the jaw, and in shape resembling a horseshoe, having at its two horns, two holes on each side; 3d, of steel hooks of various sizes, each having at one extremity an arch for the reception of the lower lip, and another smaller for securing it over the silver channels on the teeth, and at the other end a screw to pass through the horseshoe splint, and to be secured to it by a nut and a horizontal branch at its lower surface; 4th, of a cap or silk nightcap to remain on the head; and 5th, of a compress corresponding in shape and size with the splint. The net or cap having been placed on the head and the two straps fastened to it on each side, one immediately in front of the ear and the other about three inches farther back, which are to retain the splint in its position by passing through the two holes in each horn; a silver channel is placed on the four teeth nearest to the fracture, on this the small arch of the hook is placed, and the screw end having been passed through a hole in the splint, is screwed firmly to it by the nut, after a compress has been placed between the splint and the integuments below the jaw.

"If there is a double fracture, two channels and two hooks must of course be used."[1]

Bush invented a similar apparatus in 1822,[2] and Houzelot in 1826; since which the apparatus has been variously modified by Jousset, Lonsdale, Malgaigne, and perhaps others.

Lonsdale says he has employed his instrument in numerous cases and with complete success.[3] Rutenick succeeded with his apparatus in a case where the displacement persisted in spite of all other means.[4] Jousset was also successful in two cases.[5]

But others have not been equally fortunate; or if they have succeeded in holding the fragments in apposition, and in securing a bony union, other serious accidents have followed.

In the first case mentioned by Houzelot, the instrument was kept on thirteen days, after which an attack of epilepsy deranged everything, and the patient was transferred to Bicêtre. The second patient complained immediately of an intense pain under the chin and a profuse salivation followed. These symptoms were subdued by the sixth day, but, for some reason, the apparatus was finally removed on the tenth day. The fragments hereafter showed no tendency to derangement. Seven days after its removal an abscess, which had formed under the chin, was opened. In the third case the apparatus was left in place thirty days, and an abscess formed also under the chin. Neucourt applied it in a double fracture where the central fragment was much displaced. The apposition was well preserved, but he was obliged to remove it on the seventeenth day on account of a phlegmon which was forming under the chin. The patient to whom Bush applied his apparatus, would wear it but a few days. Malgaigne had the same experience with Bush's apparatus.

In addition to the pain and inflammation, followed by submaxillary abscesses, which have been such frequent results of its use, Malgaigne has noticed that it is exceedingly inclined to slide forwards and become displaced.

In short, notwithstanding the unqualified testimony of Lonsdale in favor of this method of treatment, especially in fractures at the symphysis, and in fractures through any portion of the shaft anterior to the masseter muscle, it is, in my judgment, sufficiently plain that it is

[1] London Med.-Chir. Rev., vol. xx. p. 471, from Monthly Archives of the Medical Sciences, 1834.

[2] Malgaigne, op. cit., p. 395.

[3] Lonsdale: Practical Treatise on Fractures; London, 1838, p. 234.

[4] Malgaigne, op. cit., p. 396.

[5] Ibid., p. 396.

applicable to only a very limited number of cases, and I am not certain but that it would be better to reject it altogether; and I should scarcely have thought it worth while to notice these modes of treatment at all were it not for the respectability of the gentlemen who have given them their countenance, and perhaps to show how fruitful and exhaustless in resources is the genius of our profession.

The treatment of fractures of the inferior maxilla by a single-headed bandage or roller, numbers among its distinguished advocates the names of Gibson and Barton; indeed, I think the practice is at the present time peculiar to a few American surgeons. Gibson gives the following directions for applying his roller: "A cotton or linen compress, of moderate thickness, reaching from the angle of the jaw nearly to the chin, is placed beneath and held by an assistant, while the surgeon takes a roller, four or five yards long, an inch and a-half wide, and passes it by several successive turns under the jaw, up along the sides of the face and over the head; now changing the course of the bandage, he causes it to pass off at a right angle from the perpendicular cast, and to encircle the temple, occiput and forehead, horizontally, by several turns; finally, to render the whole more secure, several additional horizontal turns are made around the back of the neck, under the ear, along the base of the jaw, over the point of the chin. To prevent the roller from slipping or changing its position, a short piece may be secured by a pin to the horizontal turn that encircles the forehead, and passed backwards along the centre of the head as far as the neck, where it must be tacked to the lower horizontal turn —taking care to fix one or more pins at every point at which the roller has crossed."

Fig. 26.

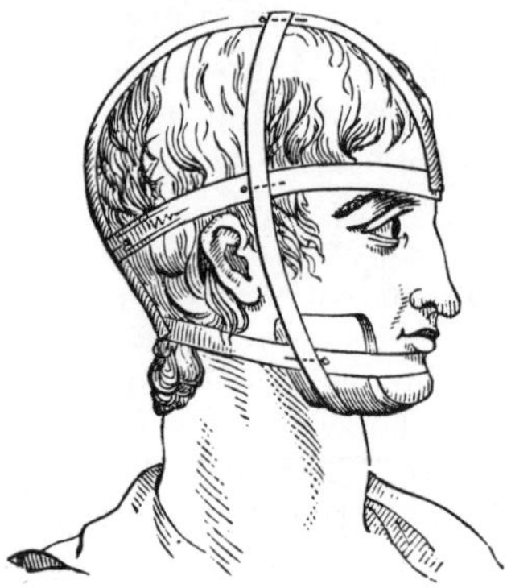

Gibson's bandage for a fractured jaw.

Barton employs, also, a compress, and a roller five yards long; the application of which is thus described by Sargent: Place the initial extremity of the roller upon the occiput, just below its protuberance, and conduct the cylinder obliquely over the centre of the left parietal bone to the top of the head; thence descend across the right temple and the zygomatic arch, and pass beneath the chin to the left side of the face; mount over the left zygoma and temple to the summit of the cranium, and regain the starting-point at the occiput by traversing obliquely the right parietal bone; next wind around the base of the lower jaw on the left side to the chin, and thence return to the occiput along the right side of the maxilla; repeat the same

Fig. 27.

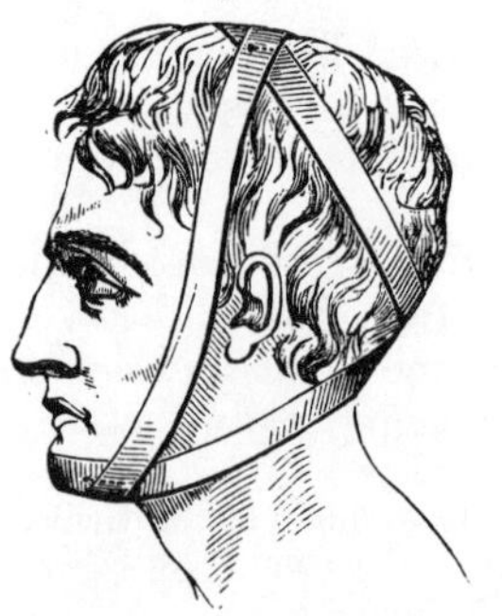

Barton's bandage for a fractured jaw.

course, step by step, until the roller is spent, and then confine its terminal end.

These bandages possess the advantages of being easily obtained, of simplicity and facility of application, and in general, we may add, of complete adaptation to the ends proposed. The only objections to their use which I have ever noticed, are occasional disarrangements, and the tendency, as in all other continuous rollers, to draw the fragments to one side or the other, according as the successive turns of the bandage are carried to the right or left. There is one other objection, having reference to the occasional inadequacy of this dressing to prevent an overlapping of the fragments, to which objection also the sling, as usually constructed, is equally obnoxious, and of which I shall speak presently.

Finally, it is to the sling, in some of its various forms, that surgeons have generally given the preference. The sling is known, also, by the name of the four-headed or the four-tailed roller or bandage.

Fig. 28.

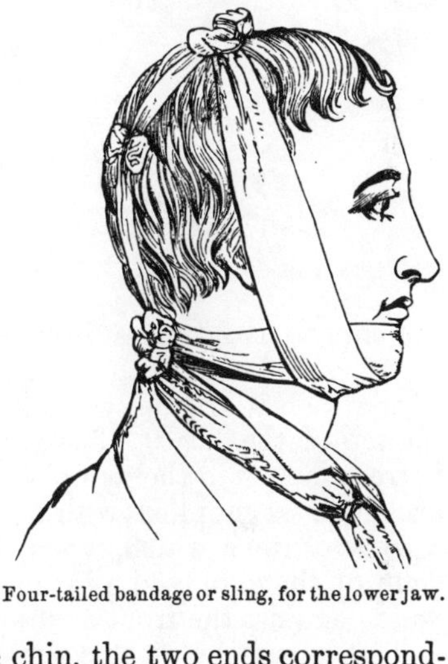

Four-tailed bandage or sling, for the lower jaw.

B. Bell, Boyer, Skey, S. Cooper, B. Cooper, Syme, Fergusson, Mayor, Lizars, and Chelius, employ the sling usually; and the favorite mode is to use for this purpose a piece of muslin cloth about one yard long and four inches wide, torn down from its two extremities to within about three or four inches of the centre. Others have used leather, gutta percha, adhesive straps, gum-elastic, etc.

Where the muslin is used, it is quite customary to lay against the skin a piece of pasteboard, wetted, and moulded to the chin, or simply a soft compress; and some choose to open the centre of the bandage sufficiently to receive the chin. The middle of this bandage being laid upon the chin, the two ends corresponding to the upper margin of the roller are now carried across the front of the chin, behind the nape of the neck, and made fast; while the two lower heads are brought directly upwards from under the sides of the chin, along the sides of the face, in front of the ears, and made fast upon the top of the head. The dressing is completed by a short counter-band extending across the top of the head from one bandage to the other; or the several bands may be made fast to a nightcap, in which case the counter-band will be unnecessary.

Fig. 29.

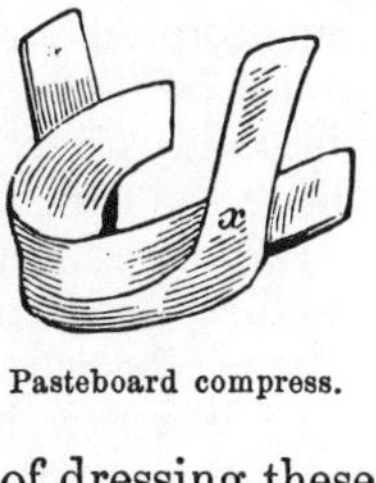

Pasteboard compress.

It only remains for me to describe my own method of dressing these fractures with the sling.

Having frequently noticed the tendency of the sling, as ordinarily constructed, and of Gibson's roller, to carry the anterior fragment backwards, especially in double fractures where the body of the bone is broken upon both sides, I devised, some years since, an apparatus intended to obviate this objection, and which I have used now several times with complete success.

It is composed of a firm leather strap, called maxillary, which, passing perpendicularly upwards from under the chin, is made to buckle upon the top of the head, at a point near the situation of the anterior fontanelle. This strap is supported by two counter-straps, called, respectively, occipital and frontal, made of strong linen webbing. One of these, the occipital, is attached to the posterior margin of the maxillary strap about half an inch above the ear, and being carried around behind and *under* the occiput, it is finally buckled to the maxillary strap upon the opposite side, and at a point exactly corresponding to its origin. The frontal stay simply antagonizes the occipital; and having its origin and termination at the anterior margins of the maxillary strap, it is buckled horizontally across the forehead, and just above the eyebrows.

Fig. 30.

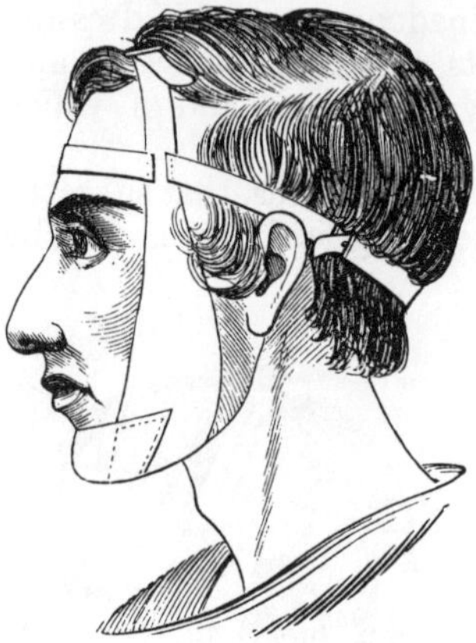

The author's apparatus.

The maxillary strap is narrow under the chin to avoid pressure upon the front of the neck, but immediately becomes wider so as to cover the sides of the inferior maxilla and face, after which it gradually diminishes to accommodate the buckle upon the top of the head. The anterior margin of this band, at the point corresponding to the symphysis menti, and for about two inches on each side, is supplied with thread holes, for the purpose of attaching a piece of linen which, when the apparatus is in place, shall cross in front of the chin, and prevent the maxillary strap from sliding backwards against the front of the neck.

The advantage of this dressing over any which I have yet seen, consists in its capability to lift the anterior fragment almost vertically, and at the same time it is in no danger of falling forwards and downwards upon the forehead. If, as in the case of most other dressings, the occipital stay had its attachment opposite to the chin, its effect would be to draw the central fragment backwards. By using a firm piece of leather, as a maxillary band, and attaching the occipital stay above the ears, this difficulty is completely avoided.

Having removed such teeth as are much loosened at the point of fracture, and replaced those which are loosened at other points, unless it be far back in the mouth, and adjusted the fragments accurately, the lower jaw is to be closed completely upon the upper, and the apparatus snugly applied. It is not necessary in most cases, to buckle the straps with great firmness, since experience has shown that a sufficient degree of immobility is obtained when the apparatus is only moderately tight. In this matter I am sustained also by the opinion of Mr. Fergusson.

If the integuments are bruised and tender, a compress made of two or more thicknesses of patent lint should be placed underneath the chin, between it and the leather.

If the inability to introduce nourishment between the teeth when the mouth is closed, or the irregularity of the dental arcade renders the use of interdental splints necessary, gutta percha, as I have already explained, ought to be preferred to any other material.

The patient must be forbidden to talk, or laugh, and when he lies down his head should rest upon its back, for whatever mode of dressing is employed, and however carefully it is applied, it will be found that a slight motion and displacement will occur whenever the weight of the head rests upon the side of the face.

Occasionally, indeed, as often as every two or three days, the apparatus may be loosened or removed, only taking care generally not to disturb the interdental splints, when they are used, and to support the jaw with the hand, during its removal; and, at the same time, the face may be sponged off with warm water and castile soap. It should not be left off entirely, however, in less than three or four weeks, even where the fracture is most simple, nor ought the patient to be allowed to eat meat in less than four or five weeks.

To cleanse the mouth and prevent offensive accumulations, it should be washed several times a day with a solution of tincture of myrrh, prepared by adding one drachm to about four ounces of water.

The same apparatus, and without any essential modification, is applicable to fractures of the symphysis and of the angle of the inferior maxilla, as well as to fractures of the body of the bone.

Instead of the leather, I have in a few instances, especially of compound fractures, where it became necessary to allow the pus to discharge externally, used a sling or a splint composed of gutta percha, suspended by bands carried over the top of the head. The piece from which this splint is made should be two or three lines in thickness, covered with cloth, and padded under the chin. It will be found convenient to cover it with cloth before immersing it in the hot water. The water should be nearly at a boiling temperature, so that the splint may become perfectly pliable; and it should be laid upon the face and allowed to mould itself while the patient lies upon his back.

Having thus fitted it accurately to the face, it may be removed and openings made at points corresponding with the wounds upon the skin, before it is reapplied.

In fractures of either condyle, unaccompanied with displacement, the simple leather or muslin sling will sometimes accomplish a perfect and speedy cure, as the two cases reported by Desault will sufficiently demonstrate. But if the fragments have become separated, the replacement is difficult, and the retention uncertain.

Ribes was the first to suggest and to practice the only rational method of reduction in these cases. Having seen two examples which had resulted in deformity under the usual treatment, which consisted in simply pressing forwards the angle of the jaw, it occurred to him that while the upper or condyloidean fragment was not acted upon at the same moment by pressure from the opposite direction, a reduction must be impossible. The case of a cannonier whose jaw was broken through the neck of the condyle on the right side, and through its body on the left, afforded him an opportunity to determine the practicability of a method of which he had as yet only conceived the idea. Malgaigne thus describes his procedure: "With the left hand seize the anterior portion of the jaw, for the purpose of drawing it horizontally forwards, while you carry the index finger of the right hand to the lateral and superior part of the pharynx. You will meet at first the projection formed by the styloid process, but moving your finger forwards you will find soon the posterior border of the ramus of the jaw; and following this border from below upwards, you will arrive at the inner side of the condyle, which you will push outwards in such a manner as to engage it upon the other fragment. This manœuvre cannot be made without causing nausea, as the finger always does when carried into the posterior part of the pharynx; but this is a slight inconvenience. The reduction obtained, bear the jaw upwards and backwards in order to press and fix the condyle between it and the glenoid cavity, then fasten it in place with the sling." The fragments were thus easily brought into apposition in the case reported by Ribes, and the patient was cured without any deformity.

In addition to these means, the angle of the jaw ought to be pressed permanently forwards by means of a compress placed between it and the mastoid process, and held in place by a suitable bandage.

If the coronoid process be alone broken, it is sufficient to close the mouth with any form of sling or bandage which may be most convenient.

CHAPTER XIII.

FRACTURES OF THE HYOID BONE.

M. ORFILA has reported the case of a man, aged sixty-two years, who had been hanged, and whose os hyoides was broken through its body on its right side.[1] M. Cazauvieilh has also seen a fracture of this bone in two persons who had been hanged: in one of which the fracture was probably in the body of the bone, and in the other through one of its cornua.[2]

Lalesque published in the *Journal Hebdomadaire*, for March, 1833, a case which occurred in a marine, sixty-seven years old, "who, in a

[1] Traité de Méd. légale, troisième éd., tom. ii. p. 423.
[2] Cazauvieilh, du Suicide, etc., p. 221.

quarrel, had his throat violently clenched by the hand of a vigorous adversary. At the moment there was very acute pain, and the sensation of a solid body breaking. The pain was aggravated by every effort to speak, to swallow, or to move the tongue, and when this organ was pushed backwards, deglutition was impossible. The patient could not articulate distinctly; and he was unable to open his mouth without exciting a great deal of pain. He placed his hand upon the anterior and superior part of his neck to point out the seat of the injury. This part was slightly swollen, and presented on each side small ecchymoses, one above, more decided, immediately under the left angle of the lower jaw. "The large cornua of the os hyoides was very distinctly to the right side," and it could be felt on the left deeply seated by pressing with the fingers; in following it in front toward the body of the bone, a very sensible inequality near the point of junction of these two parts could be perceived. By putting the finger within the mouth, the same projections and cavities inverted could be felt, and even the points of the bone which had pierced the mucous membrane, &c., were evident. Having bled the patient, and placed a plug between his teeth to keep the mouth open, the broken branch was brought by the finger back to the surface of the body of the bone, and easily reduced. The position of the head inclined a little back; rest, absolute silence, diet and some saturnine fomentations, composed the after-treatment. To avoid a new dislocation, by the efforts of swallowing, the œsophagus tube of Desault was introduced, to conduct the drinks and liquid aliments into the stomach; this sound was allowed to remain until the twenty-fifth day; at this time the patient could swallow without pain, and began to take a little more solid nourishment, and at the end of two months the cure was complete. By placing a finger within his mouth, a slight nodosity could be felt in the place where, in the recent fracture, the splintered points were perceptible.[1]

Dieffenbach has also recorded a fracture of the great right horn, produced in the same manner, by grasping the throat between the thumb and fingers, which occurred in a girl only nineteen years old. Very slight pressure upon the side of the bone was sufficient to move the fragment inwards, and to produce a crepitus, but it immediately resumed its place when the pressure was removed. There being, therefore, no displacement, the cure was effected in a short time without resort to any remedies except tisans and antiphlogistics. She was not even forbidden to speak.[2]

Auberge saw a similar case, in a person fifty-five years old, occasioned by grasping the throat. The fracture was in the great horn of the right side, and the displacement was so complete that crepitus could not be felt, and the mucous membrane of the pharynx was penetrated by the broken bone.[3]

The following example is reported by Dr. Wood, of Cincinnati, Ohio, as having come under his observation in the year 1855:—

[1] Amer. Journ. Med. Sci., vol. xiii. p. 250.

[2] Medic. Vereinszeitung für Preussen, 1833, No. 3; Gazette Méd., 1834, p. 187.

[3] Revue Méd., July, 1835.

"Through the kindness of our friend Dr. P. G. Fore, of this city, we were invited to examine a case of fracture of the os hyoides, that had occurred about one week before we saw it, in one of his patients. The patient was a female, about thirty years of age, who had fallen down the cellar steps, striking the prominent parts of the larynx and hyoid bone against a projecting brick, severely injuring the larynx as well as fracturing the bone.

"The fracture was on the left side, and near the junction of the great horn with the body of the bone. Crepitation was distinctly felt on pressing the bone between the thumb and finger; or when the patient would swallow; though, at this time, the severe symptoms that followed the accident, and continued for several days, had somewhat subsided.

"Immediately after the accident, there was profuse bleeding from the fauces, and she experienced great difficulty and pain in the act of swallowing, and the power of speech was almost entirely lost. On attempting to depress or protrude the tongue, she felt distressing symptoms of suffocation. Considerable inflammation and swelling of the throat and larynx ensued, and continued in some degree up to the time of our visit.

"To-day (about four weeks since the accident) Dr. F. informs us that the patient has so far recovered as to be able to converse, though the voice is somewhat impaired. She is yet unable to swallow solid food, and is wholly sustained by fluids."[1]

Marcinkovsky saw a woman in whom both the lower jaw and the left horn of the os hyoides were broken by a fall from her carriage against a wall. She died in about twenty-four hours from suffocation.[2]

Dr. Gründer reports the following:—

"A laborer, æt. 63, fell from a wagon on his face, and discharged a large quantity of blood by the mouth. He found he could not swallow, and when seen twelve hours afterward, complained of severe pain in the neck and nape, with inability to turn his head, though no injury of the vertebræ could be detected. His voice was hoarse and difficult. On attempting to drink, the fluid was rejected with violent coughing, the patient declaring he felt it as if entering the air-passages. An examination of the fauces led to no explanation of this condition. The epiglottis did not, however, appear to completely close the larynx, or to be in its exact position. The tongue was movable in all directions, and pressing it down with a spatula caused no inconvenience. The hyoid seemed to possess its continuity. No crepitation or abnormal movability could be perceived, and no pain at the root of the tongue occurred on attempting to swallow. After repeated examinations, the case was concluded to be one in which the functions of the nervus vagus had undergone great disturbance, or the muscles of the larynx had become torn or paralyzed. Medicine and food were administered by means of an elastic tube. The patient had a good appetite and slept well; the pain of the neck was lost, and its motion recovered;

[1] Western Lancet; also N. Y. Journ. Med., vol. xv. p. 152.

[2] Medic. Vereinszeitung, für Preussen, 1833, No. 15; Gazette Médicale, 1833, p. 354.

a hectic cough, from which he had long suffered, alone remaining. After continuing, however, to go on thus well for six days, the cough increased; the appetite failed; strength was lost; the voice was scarcely audible; and in five more days the patient died exhausted. At the autopsy a fracture of the os hyoides was found. One of the large cornua was broken, and had become firmly imbedded between the epiglottis and rima glottidis, inducing the raised position of the epiglottis, loss of voice, and difficulty in swallowing. The fracture was probably produced by muscular action, a cause first assigned in a case occurring to Ollivier d'Angers."[1] I think it more probable, however, that this fracture was the result of a direct blow, than of muscular action.

In the case referred to, however, as having been reported by Ollivier, there can be no doubt that the fracture was due to muscular action alone.

A woman, fifty-six years old, made a misstep and fell backwards, and at the same moment that her head was thrown violently back, she felt distinctly a sensation as if a solid body had broken in the upper part of her neck, and upon its left side. An examination showed that she had fractured the great left horn of the os hyoides. Inflammation and suppuration followed, and finally, after about three months, the posterior fragment made its way out in a condition of necrosis, and the fistula promptly healed, but there remained for many years a sense of uneasiness about these parts when she swallowed, sometimes amounting to pain.[2]

Etiology.—Of the ten cases which I have found upon record, three were produced by hanging; three by grasping the throat between the thumb and fingers; three by direct blows, or by falls upon the front of the neck; and one by muscular action alone.

The observation of Mr. South that fracture of the bone "is almost invariably found"[3] in persons executed by hanging, is probably incorrect, since although a large proportion of these subjects are submitted to dissection both in this and other countries, yet I know of but these three examples which have been published.

Pathology, Symptomatology, and Diagnosis.—The body of the bone seems to have been broken in all of those cases which resulted from hanging: while in all of the other examples the fracture has occurred in one of the great horns, or at the junction of the horns with the body. Generally the displacement inwards of one of the fragments has been so complete that crepitus could not be detected. It was present, however, in the examples mentioned by Dieffenbach and Wood. In two instances the mucous membrane has been penetrated, and in one the fragment was projected between the epiglottis and rima glottidis.

The accident has been characterized by a sudden sensation as if a bone had broken; in a few instances, by profuse bleeding from the fauces; by difficulty in opening the mouth; by impossibility of deglutition, and by loss of voice in others; with great pain in moving the

[1] Schmidt's Jahrbuch., vol. lxviii.; also Amer. Journ. Med. Sci., vol. xlix. p. 253, Jan. 1852.

[2] Malg., op. cit., p. 405.

[3] Note to Chelius' Surgery, Amer. ed., vol. i. p. 581.

tongue, the pain being especially at its root; in one instance the tongue was perceptibly drawn to one side. There is also usually more or less swelling and soreness about the neck, with ecchymosis; and at a later period, cough, expectoration, hoarseness, &c. The circumstances which, however, indicate certainly the nature of the accident, are preternatural mobility of the fragments, with or without crepitus, and the angular, inward projection, which may in most cases be distinctly felt in a careful examination of the pharynx.

In the case related by Grüner, the only symptoms were a loss of voice, difficulty of deglutition, and a sensation when the attempt was made to swallow, as if the fluids passed into the windpipe; with also an imperfect closure of the epiglottis upon the rima glottidis. No preternatural mobility or irregularity in the fragments could be detected, nor was there crepitus, and it was concluded that the bone was not broken, yet the autopsy showed that the fragment was imbedded deeply between the epiglottis and the rima glottidis.

Prognosis.—It is only in view of its complications that this accident can be regarded as serious; where the severity of the injury has been such as to fracture the lower jaw at the same time, as in the case related by Marcinkovsky, or such as to bury the fragment deep in the tissues about the rima glottidis as in the case mentioned by Grüner, a favorable termination could scarcely have been expected; and these are the only cases yet published in which the death was in any way connected with the fracture. One-half of the whole number have died, but of these, three have died by hanging, and the remaining two from the causes named. Of the three in which the accident resulted from a direct blow, only the patient of Dr. Fore, of Cincinnati, has survived; while of the three whose fractures resulted from lateral pressure upon the cornua, all recovered; so, also, did the patient in whom the fracture was produced by muscular action.

Treatment.—No doubt when the fragments are displaced an attempt ought to be made to replace them by introducing one finger into the mouth, while with the opposite hand the fragments are supported from without. Lalesque found this a matter of some difficulty, but Auberge experienced no difficulty at all. I suspect, however, that the amount of difficulty will very much depend upon the degree of displacement, and the consequent laceration of the soft tissues about the bone. But however this may be, it must be altogether another thing to be able to keep in exact apposition the broken ends of a bone whose diameter is so inconsiderable and upon which it is quite impossible to apply any apparatus or dressings to retain the fragments in place. Lalesque threw the head of his patient slightly back, with the view of making "permanent extension" upon the fragments through the action of the muscles and ligaments attached to the bone, and he recommends this position as that which is best calculated to preserve the coaptation. Malgaigne on the contrary, without having himself seen any example of this fracture, believes that the position of flexion of the neck, with entire relaxation of the muscles, would be most suitable.

In all cases it will be proper to enjoin silence, and to adopt suitable measures to combat inflammation: such as general or topical bleeding, fomentations, moistening the mouth with cool water, or permitting small pieces of ice to rest in the mouth until dissolved, without in general allowing the fluid to be swallowed; but in some examples, no doubt the patient may be permitted to swallow.

CHAPTER XIV.

FRACTURE OF THE CARTILAGES OF THE LARYNX.

§ 1. Thyroid Cartilage.

The examples of fracture of the larynx which may be found upon record, are also very few. M. Ladoz examined the larynx of a man who had been assassinated, and upon whose neck he found a handkerchief bound so tightly as to leave, after its removal, a deep furrow; but the neck showed also distinct marks produced by the fingers and thumb. There was a fracture of the thyroid cartilage which extended obliquely downwards and outwards through its right wing. The whole of the larynx was very much ossified, although the subject was only thirty-seven years old.[1]

In 1823, M. Ollivier communicated to the Academy of Medicine a case in which, this cartilage being broken, the patient died of suffocation.[2]

M. Marjolin says, "Two women at the hospital being engaged in a quarrel, one of them seized her antagonist by the throat, and griped her so strong that she broke the thyroid cartilage from its upper to its lower margin. You will imagine that it was not very difficult to determine the existence of a fracture, and that no retentive apparatus was demanded. Silence, regimen, a small bleeding, and the cure was accomplished."[3]

These are the only cases of fracture of the cartilages of the larynx of which we have any precise account, in which the thyroid cartilage was alone involved.

§ 2. Thyroid and Cricoid Cartilages.

Plenck saw a fracture of both the thyroid and cricoid cartilages produced by falling upon the rim of a pail.[4] Morgagni also says that he had seen fractures of the larynx; and Remer mentions a fracture of

[1] Gazette Médicale, 1838, p. 698.
[2] Archives Générales de Médecine, tome ii. p. 307.
[3] Marjolin, Cours de Patholog. Chir., p. 396.
[4] Malg., op. cit., p. 409.

the larynx found in a person who had been hanged;[1] but in neither case is it said in which cartilage the fracture occurred, or whether it had not occurred in both.

I am able, however, to furnish from my own observation another example of fracture of both cartilages:—

John Calkins, of Collins, Erie Co., N. Y., æt. 41, is supposed to have been kicked by a young horse on the 10th of Nov., 1856. He was alone in the stables when the accident occurred, and being stunned by the blow, he could not himself give any account of the manner in which the injury was received. When found he was sitting upright, but unable to articulate, except in a whisper. Drs. Barber and Davis, of Colden, saw him about two hours after. His countenance was anxious; his pulse feeble; extremities cold; and he was breathing with great difficulty. A small quantity of blood was issuing from his fauces. His upper lip was cut and a few of his teeth dislocated: the wound appearing as if inflicted by one of the corks of the horse's shoes. There was no other wound; but over the left wing of the thyroid cartilage there was a slight discoloration, pressure upon which produced intense pain and suffocation, and disclosed the fact that the thyroid prominence was depressed very much and broken. Cold lotions were directed to be applied, and as the thirst was excessive, but deglutition impossible, he was permitted to hold pieces of ice in his mouth. This plan, with but slight modifications, such as the substitution of warm fomentations to the neck for the cold lotions, was continued until the following evening, when, at the request of the attending physician, Dr. Barber, I was called to see him. The symptoms remained nearly the same as at first. He was unable to speak audibly, or perform the act of deglutition; his breathing was difficult and at times threatened suffocation. The lateness of the hour, with other circumstances, determined me to defer surgical interference until morning. At daybreak of the 12th I made the operation of laryngotomy, and introduced a large double canula into the crico-thyroidean space. This operation was rendered difficult by the great amount of swelling about the neck, due both to emphysema, and bloody with serous infiltrations. The breathing immediately became easy, and gradually the appearance of asphyxia disappeared from his face; but after about six or seven hours, he began perceptibly to fail in strength, and died at 3 o'clock P. M., of the following day, apparently from exhaustion rather than from suffocation: having survived the accident about seventy-two hours, and the operation about thirty-four hours.

The autopsy disclosed a comminuted fracture of the thyroid cartilage, with a simple fracture of the cricoid. The thyroid was broken almost perpendicularly through its centre; the line of fracture being irregular, and inclining slightly to the left side. The left inferior horn was broken off about three lines from its articulation with the cricoid cartilage. The right ala was broken also in a line nearly vertical, but irregular, at a point about six lines from its posterior margin. The pomum Adami was depressed to the level of the cricoid cartilage, and

[1] Morgagni, de Sedibus, etc., Epist. 19, num. 13, 14 et 16; Remer, Annales d'hygiene, tome iv. p. 171; from Malg.

the left ala, being completely detached, was thrown inwards and upwards several lines. Underneath the perichondrium, especially upon the inner side, there was pretty extensive bloody infiltration. Ossification of the cartilages had commenced at several points, but it had made but little progress. The central fracture of the thyroid was through cartilage alone. The fracture of the right ala was through cartilage until it reached a bony belt comprising the two inferior lines of its course. The left lower horn was ossified, and the fracture was through this bony structure. The fracture through the cricoid cartilage commenced close upon the margin of a bony plate, but in its whole course it traversed only cartilage. It was on the left side. There was also an incomplete fracture on the right ala of the thyroid cartilage, commencing in the line of the principal fracture and extending obliquely downwards about three lines, until it was arrested by the bony plate which constituted the lower margin of this wing.

A ragged, lacerated wound in the back of the larynx, above the cricoid cartilages, communicated directly with the œsophagus.

§ 3. Cricoid Cartilage.

Both Valsalva and Cazauvièilh have each met with a single example of this fracture, without fracture of the thyroid cartilage; and Weiss has found the cricoid cartilage broken into numerous fragments, and at the same time separated from the trachea.[1]

General Etiology of Fractures of the Laryngeal Cartilages.—As a predisposing cause, advanced age, with its usual concomitant, partial or complete ossification of the cartilages, has been thought to occupy a prominent place. The number of recorded cases is, however, too small to establish its actual value. In the case reported by Plenck, the cartilages were already very much ossified, although the subject was only thirty-seven years old. Morgagni observed that in his experience it had occurred always in advanced life. In my own case, however, the cartilages were only slightly ossified, the patient being forty-one years old; nor did the lines of the several fractures indicate a preference for the bony plates; but it seems to me that they rather avoided them, and in the case of the incomplete fracture, the bone appeared to have arrested the fracture. In fact, a few experiments have satisfied me that the adult laryngeal cartilages are quite as brittle as bone, and, consequently, that ossification in no way increases their liability to fracture.

The immediate causes have been direct blows, as falling upon the edge of a pail, a kick from a horse, or pressure, as in hanging, or in grasping the larynx strongly between the thumb and fingers.

General Symptomatology, etc.—The signs of this accident are such as usually attend any severe injury of this organ, whether accompanied with a fracture or not, such as pain, swelling, difficult degluti-

[1] Malg., op. cit., p. 408.

tion, embarrassed respiration, a loss of voice, cough, and perhaps bloody expectoration, with emphysema, &c.

But none of these can be regarded as diagnostic; although, when taken in connection with the history of the accident, especially if a very severe and direct blow has been received, or more certainly still, when symptoms so grave and complicated have followed an attempt at strangulation by grasping the throat, they may be regarded as probable or presumptive evidences.

A positive diagnosis must depend upon the presence of a sensible displacement, or motion of the fragments, with crepitus.

In the case related by Plenck, death followed almost immediately, with convulsions, and without any outcry; indicating, probably, some severe lesion of the spinal marrow; while in M. Ollivier's patient suffocation ensued, at first intermittent, and finally permanent.

In my own case, suffocation was throughout a prominent symptom, with only such slight intervals of amelioration as might have been occasioned by the extrication of the blood or mucus from the larynx.

GENERAL PROGNOSIS.—The prognosis ought to depend rather upon the complications and upon the gravity of the symptoms, than upon the simple decision of the question of fracture. A fracture produced by grasping the wings of the thyroid cartilage, and without any great contusion or laceration of the soft parts, might reasonably be expected to terminate favorably under judicious management; but when, on the contrary, the fracture is the result of great violence inflicted directly upon the front of the cartilages, producing severe contusion and laceration, and is followed by great swelling, very difficult respiration, complete aphonia, impossibility of deglutition, &c., the prognosis cannot but be unfavorable—and indeed the woman spoken of by Marjolin, whose larynx was broken by grasping the neck, is the only one, so far as we know, whose recovery has been mentioned.

GENERAL TREATMENT.—In examples of simple, uncomplicated fracture, "silence, regimen and a small bleeding," may suffice; but in other cases, it may become necessary to introduce a tube into the stomach to supply the patient with food and drinks, since deglutition may be impossible. If also, suffocation is imminent, there may remain no alternative but a resort to tracheotomy, or to laryngotomy. I am not aware that this has ever been practised except by myself, yet its propriety, under certain conditions, is sufficiently manifest.

As to a "reduction" of the fragments, by manipulation, I believe it will be found generally, if not always, impracticable. Whatever displacement exists must be mostly inwards, and we can have no means of forcing them again outwards. Nor if once replaced, do I see any reason to suppose that they would not become immediately displaced.

Chelius has suggested the propriety, in such cases, of cutting open the coverings of the larynx freely in the mesian line, and after stanching the bleeding, proceeding at once to divide the larynx itself in its whole length and then replacing the broken cartilages[1]. The pro-

[1] System of Surgery, Philadelphia ed., vol. i. p. 581, 1847.

cedure has an aspect of severity, but I can well conceive of circumstances which would justify its adoption; not, however, so much for the purpose of replacing the cartilages, as for the purpose of arresting a fatal internal hemorrhage, and of giving a free admission of air to the lungs. If this operation were to be practised, the wound ought to be left open for a sufficient length of time to allow of the subsidence of the inflammation, and then permitted to close with such precautions as experience teaches are usually necessary after the windpipe has been opened.

Active antiphlogistic measures, combined with fomentations to the neck, so far as these latter are found to be agreeable and practicable, are important measures, and not to be overlooked in the general plan of treatment.

My own patient, also, found small pieces of ice, permitted slowly to dissolve in the mouth, very grateful; but he preferred very much as an external application, the warm fomentations to the cold lotions.

CHAPTER XV.

FRACTURES OF THE VERTEBRÆ.

It will be convenient to divide fractures of the vertebræ into fractures of the spinous processes, transverse processes, vertebral arches and bodies.

§ 1. Fractures of the Spinous Processes.

Fractures of the spinous apophyses, independent of a fracture of the arches, may occur at any point of the vertebral column; and they may be occasioned by a blow received upon either side of the spinal column; or by a force directed from above or from below.

Fig. 31.

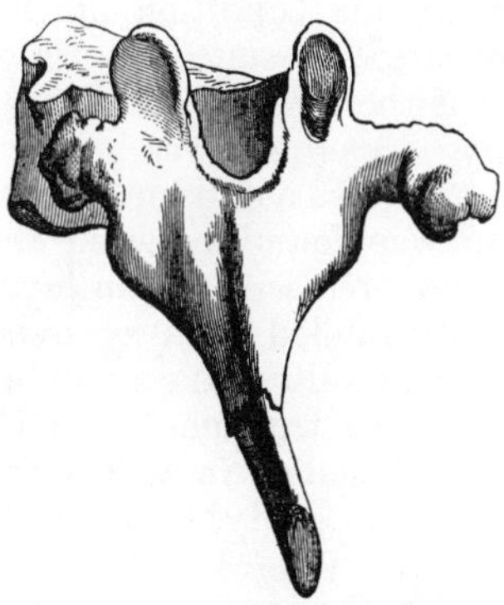

Fracture of the spinous process.

Symptoms and Pathology.—These accidents may be recognized by the lively pain at the point of fracture, produced especially when the patient bends forwards, which position renders the skin and muscles tense and drives the fragments into the flesh; by the swelling, tenderness and discoloration; but chiefly by the lateral displacement of the broken process, and the mobility.

Duverney met with a fracture of two of the processes in the same person, and which could only be recognized by the mobility, since, as the autopsy proved, there was no displacement. Nor would it be surprising if the displacement was absent in a majority of these accidents, inasmuch as the attachment of the ligaments from above and below with the strong and short muscles upon either side, must prevent a deviation in any direction until these tissues were more or less torn. Sir Astley mentions a case in which, however, such lacerations did occur, and the lateral deformity was quite conspicuous.

A boy had been endeavoring to support a heavy weight upon his shoulders, when he fell, bent double. Immediately he had the appearance of one suffering under a distortion of the spine of long standing. Three or four of the processes were broken off and the corresponding muscles were detached so as to allow the processes to fall off to the opposite side. There was no paralysis, and he was soon discharged with the free use of his limbs, but the deformity remained.[1]

If the fragment is thrown directly downwards, as it possibly may be, especially in the cervical or lumbar region, yet not without a rupture of the supra-spinous ligaments, or of the ligamentum nuchæ, then the displacement will be more difficult to detect, and it may require some more care not to confound it with a fracture of the vertebral arch or of the plates from which the spinous processes arise. The process not being felt in its natural position, nor upon either side, it may seem to have been forced directly forwards, when in fact it is only thrown downwards towards its fellow. The danger of error in the diagnosis will be increased when to these conditions are added paralysis of those portions of the body which are below the seat of the fracture, and which, in this case, may be the result of an extravasation of blood or of simply a concussion of the spinal marrow. Nor do I think it would be possible now to determine positively whether it was simply a fracture of a spinous process, of the arch, or of the body itself of the vertebra. In case, however, the paralysis results from concussion, the fact will in most cases soon become apparent by a return of sensation and of the power of motion.

Prognosis.—Hippocrates affirmed that here, as in fractures of other spongy bones, the union took place speedily. It is quite probable that this venerable father of surgery has stated the fact correctly, and yet in the only example known to me where the condition of this process, as proved by dissection, has been carefully stated, the fragment had not united by bone at all. This is the case related by Sir Astley as having been examined by Mr. Key. A subject was brought into the dissecting room in which one of the processes had been broken, and, on dissection, a complete articulation was found between the broken surfaces, which surfaces had become covered with a thin layer of cartilage. The false articulation was surrounded with synovial membrane and capsular ligaments, and contained a fluid like synovia.[2]

Ordinarily the displacement continues, whatever treatment may be adopted; but Malgaigne says he has seen one instance in which the twelfth dorsal spine being broken and displaced laterally, resumed its

[1] Sir Astley Cooper, op. cit., p. 459.

[2] A. Cooper, op. cit., p. 459.

place spontaneously after a few days. Aurran mentions a similar example.[1]

Treatment.—If in any case it should be found possible to act upon the fragment, an attempt might be made to press it into place, and to retain it there by means of a compress and bandage; but even this would not be admissible so long as any doubt remained whether it was not a fracture of the vertebral arch, since if it were, any attempt to restore the bone to place by pressure would be likely to drive it more deeply upon the spinal marrow. Yet what need is there of surgical interference of any kind? If the apophysis remains displaced it cannot result in any serious, perhaps we may say in any appreciable deformity. The surgeon has therefore only to lay the patient quietly in bed and in such a position as he finds most comfortable, enjoining upon him perfect rest, and employing such other means as may be proper to combat inflammation.

§ 2. Fractures of the Transverse Process.

A fracture of a transverse process can scarcely occur except as a consequence of a gunshot wound. Dupuytren relates a case of this kind in which the ball had penetrated the transverse process of the second cervical vertebra. The man bled very little at the time, and his symptoms progressed favorably for ten days; after which secondary hemorrhage occurred, of which he ultimately died. The autopsy showed that the vertebral artery had been injured, and that the inflammation of its coats being followed by a slough, caused his death.[2]

I have also elsewhere reported the case of Charles Harkner, of this city, who was shot with a pistol on the 21st of Jan., 1851. I did not see him until the following day. The ball had entered the chin, a little to the left side and below the inferior maxilla, but its place of lodgment could not be discovered. He lay with his face constantly turned to the right. The left side of his neck was swollen and crepitant; the left arm and leg were paralyzed; he slept most of the time, but could be easily aroused, and when aroused he seemed to be conscious, but was unable to speak. By signs he indicated to us that he was suffering no pain. He gradually sank, without hemorrhage, and died in thirty-six hours from the time of the receipt of the injury.

The autopsy, made four hours after death, enabled us to trace the wound from the chin, through the left ala of the thyroid cartilage, and also through the roots of the transverse process of the fourth cervical vertebra; immediately behind which, lying embedded in the muscles, was the bullet. The cavity of the tunica arachnoides contained considerable serous effusion.

The emphysema in the neck was occasioned, no doubt, by the wound of the larynx, the ball having opened freely into its cavity. This circumstance also explained the aphonia; but the immediate

[1] Malgaigne, op. cit., p. 412.
[2] Dupuytren, Diseases, &c., of Bones, Syd. ed., p. 360.

cause of his death seems to have been arachnoid effusion as a result of meningeal inflammation.

The symptoms arising from this accident can only refer to the complications, since a mere fracture of the process is not likely to present any peculiar signs which could be recognized. Concussion or bloody effusions may take place so as to occasion more or less paralysis, or, at a later period, inflammation and its consequent effusions may give rise to the same phenomenon.

In itself considered, and independent of these complications, it is sufficiently trivial, but inasmuch as it has not been known to occur except from gunshot wounds, nor is it likely to occur except from penetrating wounds of some kind, the accident must always be regarded as exceedingly grave, if not actually fatal.

As to the treatment, nothing but strict rest and antiphlogistic remedies can prove of any service.

§ 3. Fractures of the Vertebral Arches.

The vertebral arches, upon which both the spinous and transverse processes have their principal support, may be broken at any point of their circumference, by a blow received upon the spinous process; but generally it is the lamellar portion, or the "vertebral plate," which gives way rather than the neck or pedicle of the arch; and in all of the cases recorded the plates have been broken upon both sides.

Fig. 32.

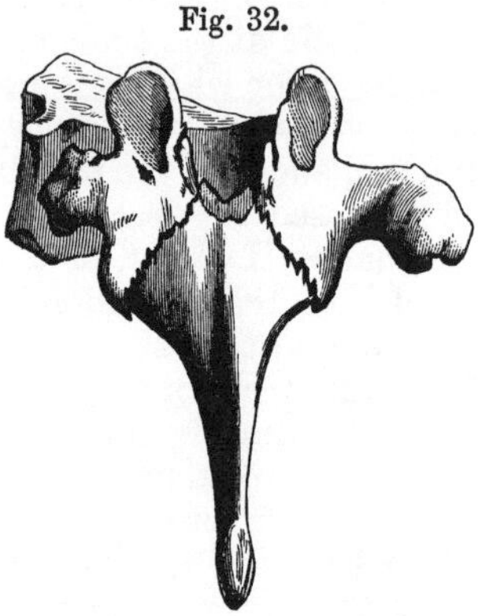

Fracture of the vertebral arches.

On the first of May, 1851, during a violent storm of wind and rain, a balustrade fell from the top of a high building, striking a man named John Larkin, who was about forty years of age, upon the back of his head and neck. He fell to the ground instantly, and did not again move his feet or legs, although he never lost his consciousness until he died. I found the bladder paralyzed also, and his left arm, but his right arm he could move pretty well. He conversed freely up to the last moment, and said that he was suffering a good deal of pain, which was always greatly aggravated by moving. His death took place thirty-six hours after the receipt of the injury.

Dr. Hugh B. Vandeventer, who was the attending surgeon, made a dissection on the following day in my presence, which disclosed the fact that the plates of the sixth cervical vertebra were broken upon each side, and that the spinous process with a small portion of the arch attached was forced in upon the spinal marrow. There was no blood effused, or serum at this point, but about one ounce of serum was found in the cavity of the tunica arachnoides at the base of the brain. The bodies of the vertebræ were not broken. It was our opinion, therefore, that the immediate cause of his death was the direct pressure of the spinous process.

In the case related by Prout, of Alabama, the man having died within forty-eight hours after the receipt of the injury, the arch of the fifth cervical vertebra was found to be broken in three places, and the spinous process was driven in upon the spinal marrow. There was a slight effusion of blood between the sheath of the spinal marrow and the bone, and a considerable effusion between the sheath and the cord. There was no material lesion of the cord or of its membranes, and the body of the bone was neither broken nor dislocated.[1]

It is probable, also, that in the following example the arch was broken, but that the force of the blow having been somewhat oblique, the process was but little if at all thrown in upon the spinal marrow.

R. L., of this county, aged about forty years, was thrown from a loaded wagon in February of 1851, striking, as he thinks, upon the back of his neck. He was stunned by the injury, and remained insensible several hours; on the return of consciousness, he found that his lower extremities and bladder were paralyzed. During four weeks his bladder had to be emptied by a catheter. Nine months after the injury was received he consulted me, and I found the spinous process of the last cervical vertebra pushed over to the left side. His head was strongly bent forwards, and he was unable to straighten it. He could walk a few steps, but not without great fatigue; and he suffered almost constant pain in his lower extremities, accompanied with excessive restlessness and watchfulness, for which he was obliged to take morphine in large quantities.

In the case related by Alban G. Smith, of Kentucky, to which I shall refer again presently, the deviation was lateral, and so also in Ollivier's case, mentioned by Malgaigne.

Symptoms.—We can imagine a case of fracture of the vertebral arch, with a lateral displacement only, in which the symptoms might not differ essentially from a simple fracture of the spinous process; and it is quite possible that some of the cases which have been supposed to be examples of this latter accident, and in which a speedy recovery has taken place, were really examples of fracture of the arches; yet it must be admitted that such a fortunate result is only possible, since the arches can hardly be broken without communicating a severe concussion to the marrow, nor without lacerations, inflammation, and effusions, which will be most certain to produce compression and paralysis, and probably death.

If, however, it is possible for us to confound a fracture of the process with a fracture of the arches, it is still more possible for us to confound a fracture of the arches with a fracture of the bodies of the vertebræ. If, as is usually the fact, the process, in case of a fracture of the arch, is less prominent than natural, and that portion of the body receiving its nervous supply from below this point is paralyzed, we may have

[1] Prout, Amer. Journ. Med. Sci., Nov. 1837, vol. xxi. p. 276, from Western Journ. of Med. and Phys. Sci.

reasons to believe that the arch is broken and the process driven in upon the spine; but dissections have shown that in many of these cases, or in most of them indeed, the bodies of more or less of the vertebræ are broken also, and in still other cases the bodies were alone broken.

If, as in the case mentioned by Ollivier, we can feel the plates move separately, the diagnosis might be made out, so far at least as to determine that the plates were broken; but we should be still unable to say that the bodies of the vertebræ were not broken also.

Something perhaps may be inferred from the direction and manner of the blow which has produced the fracture. Thus a fall upon the top of the head would most often produce a comminution of the bodies by crushing them together, while a blow upon the back could scarcely break one of the vertebræ without breaking the corresponding arch also. We might thus be led to infer, in the first instance, that the arches were not broken; and, in the second instance, if we could convince ourselves that the arches were not broken, we might rest pretty well assured that the bodies were not.

In the case related by Prout, there was no external mark of injury over the point of fracture, but a distinct crepitus was perceptible on pressure.

Treatment.—If the fragments are not displaced, nothing but rest and a cooling regimen are indicated; but if they are forced in upon the marrow, an important question is presented, and which has received from different surgeons different solutions. Shall an effort be made to reduce the fragments? and if so, by what means shall the indication be attempted?

It will be remembered that in nearly all of these cases we must remain in doubt, even after the most careful examination, as to the actual condition of the fracture. It may be that what we suppose to be a fracture of the arch is only a fracture of the apophysis, or that on the other hand it is a fracture of the body of the bone itself, and if we are expert enough to make out clearly a fracture of the arch, it is not possible for us to say that the body is not broken also, indeed it is quite probable that it is broken. With a diagnosis so uncertain, can we ever find a justification for surgical interference? Mr. Cline and Mr. Cooper thought that we might. According to them, the case presents in no other direction a point of hope or encouragement. Death is inevitable, sooner or later, if the fragment is not lifted, and we can scarcely make the matter any worse by interference. If it proves to be a fracture of the apophysis, as happened to be the case in a patient upon whom Sir Astley operated,[1] our interference was unnecessary, but it has done no harm. If the body of the bone is broken, the operation affords no resource, but the patient is probably beyond suffering damage at our hands. If the diagnosis is correctly made out and the arch only is broken, and if, as was the fact in the case of Larkin already mentioned, there is no bloody effusion, or laceration of the membranes or of the marrow, and if the concussion was not sufficient to deter-

[1] Chelius, Surgery, Amer. ed., note by South, vol. i. p. 592.

mine much inflammation of the cord, then it would seem possible that an operation might save the patient.

Paulus Ægineta first suggested that the compressing fragments ought to be removed by excision; and in 1762 Louis removed from a man who had received a gunshot wound in his back, after the lapse of five days, several loose pieces of bone belonging to the arch of the vertebra, and the patient recovered, but not without a partial paralysis of his lower extremities. Of course nothing could be more rational or simple than this procedure, adopted by Louis, in any case of an open wound, where the fragments could be easily reached; but the younger Cline was the first, in the year 1814, to put into practice the more ancient suggestion of Paulus Ægineta, namely, to attempt the removal of the fragments in a case of simple fracture. He made an incision upon the depressed bone as the patient was lying upon his face, raised the muscles covering the spinal arch, applied a small trephine to the arch, and cut it through on each side, so as to remove the spinous process, and the arch of the bone which pressed upon the spinal marrow. This patient died on the 4th day. Mr. Oldknow repeated this operation in 1819 in a case of fracture of the arch of the sixth vertebra. The patient died on the 7th day. In 1822, Mr. Tyrrell operated at St. Thomas Hospital on a man who had just been admitted with a fracture through the arches of the ninth and tenth vertebræ. The operation was accomplished with considerable difficulty, and resulted in only a partial return of sensibility. He died on the twelfth day.[1] In 1827, Tyrrell operated a second time, and death resulted on the fifth day. On the 30th of August, 1824, Dr. J. Rhea Barton, of Philadelphia, operated upon a man who had been received into the Pennsylvania Hospital twelve days before, with a fracture of the arch of the seventh dorsal vertebra, and the lower part of whose body was at the time completely paralyzed. On removing the spinous process, it was discovered that the seventh and eighth dorsal vertebræ were dislocated upon each other. No immediate relief was afforded by the operation, but sensibility began to return in the lower extremities after about forty-eight hours. On the third day he was attacked with a violent chill, and death took place twelve hours after. The dissection showed about half a gallon of blood in the posterior mediastinum, and bloody effusions existed along the whole length of the spinal canal.[2] Dr. Potter, of New York, who operated three months after the receipt of the injury, lost his patient on the eighteenth day.[3] The patient whom Laugier trephined at the base of the spinous process of the ninth dorsal vertebra, died on the fourth day. Chelius says that the operation has been repeated unsuccessfully by Wickham, Attenburrow, and Holscher.[4]

February 5th, 1834, Dr. David L. Rogers, of New York, operated upon a man who had fallen two days before, breaking the arch of the first lumbar vertebra, and forcing the spinous process upon the cord.

[1] Sir A. Cooper, op. cit., pp. 478–80.
[2] Barton, Godman's ed. of Sir A. Cooper on Disloc., &c., p. 421.
[3] Potter, Malgaigne, translated, note by Packard, p. 344.
[4] Chelius's Surgery, Amer. ed., vol. i. p. 590.

In the first steps of the operation several fragments of bone were removed which had been broken from the spinous process, and only those portions of the arch remained which were attached to the oblique processes. An effort was made to separate these processes by the knife, but this was found to be impossible; and an attempt to use Hey's saw caused great pain accompanied with convulsive actions of the muscles of the back. Having finally made the bone fast by the aid of a double hook and elevator, the saw was again applied successfully on one side. The opposite side was also at length removed at the articulations of the oblique processes by the cautious use of the knife and by tractions. About two inches of the spinal cord was now exposed, covered with coagulated blood. The cord itself did not seem to be injured. In about fifteen minutes after the operation, this patient expressed himself as being much relieved; sensibility returned to his lower extremities; respiration became easy, and with the assistance of an anodyne he slept for several hours. Subsequently he became worse, and on the eighth day he died; when the autopsy revealed a fracture of the body of the vertebra from which the spinous process and arch had been removed, but no displacement of the fragments.[1]

These are all of the cases of which we have any very accurate information in which this operation has been made, and they have all terminated fatally in a very few days. The case reported by Alban G. Smith, of Kentucky, is not related in such a manner as to enable us to make use of it safely, nor is it stated how long the patient survived the operation; Gibson says it gave no permanent relief. The example mentioned by an English writer is equally unreliable, inasmuch as it is given only upon rumor, and but a "few months" had elapsed since the operation was performed. It was said to have been made in the year 1838, by a surgeon of the name of Edwards, in South Wales; and it was affirmed that the compression was relieved and that the patient "did well."[2] So unique a case would certainly have found before this an ample confirmation.

Experience, then, seems to have sufficiently shown that we have no right to expect anything from this surgical expedient; and notwithstanding the strong hope expressed by Sir Astley, that Mr. Cline's operation might hereafter prove a valuable resource, and contrary to the conclusions which we in common with many other surgeons had drawn from the anatomical relations of these parts, we are compelled reluctantly to declare that the expedient is no longer worthy of a trial. To the same conclusion also many of the most distinguished surgeons have arrived; among whom we may mention, as especially entitled to confidence, Brodie, Liston, Malgaigne, and Gibson.

What more can be said of the attempt to raise the depressed bone by seizing the spinous process with the fingers, or with a pair of strong hooked forceps passed through the skin, or finally if this cannot be done, by laying bare both sides of the process and seizing upon it with a pair of firm tenacula? This is the alternative presented to

[1] Rogers, Amer. Journ. Med. Sci., May, 1835, vol. xvi. p. 93.
[2] Edwards, British and Foreign Med. Rev., 1838, p. 162.

Malgaigne, and which he ventures to recommend as deserving a trial. In the absence, however, of any testimony in its favor, beyond the mere rational argument adduced by this distinguished writer, we must waive any farther consideration of the subject; only expressing our well-established conviction that it will be found, after a fair trial, as useless and as inexpedient as the more severe operation of Cline.

As to the therapeutical treatment of the various symptoms belonging to this accident, and in relation to the prognosis, the remarks which we shall make will be found equally applicable to fractures of the bodies of the vertebræ, and we shall reserve the consideration of these topics for the following section.

§ 4. Fractures of the Bodies of the Vertebræ.

The same causes which produce fractures of the arches produce also fractures of the bodies of the vertebræ, that is, blows received directly upon the extremities of the spinous processes; but in these cases the arches are generally broken at the same time.

In other cases the bodies of the vertebræ are broken by falls upon the top of the head, by which the vertebræ are not only driven forcibly together, but often doubled forwards upon each other; or the patient may have alighted upon his feet or upon his sacrum.

Reveillon has reported a case of fracture of the fifth cervical vertebra from muscular action, which occurred in diving. The man was taken out of the water unconscious, and died in a few hours, having declared before death that his head did not strike the bottom, although he had jumped from a height of seven or eight feet, and the water was only three feet deep.[1] The statement of the sufferer under such circumstances could not really possess much value, and we think we see good reasons to suppose that he was mistaken. South also relates a case of fracture of the fourth and fifth cervical vertebræ occasioned by diving, in which it was supposed that the fracture was caused by the concussion of the head upon the water.[2]

Malgaigne says the spine bends at three principal points; comprised, the first between the third and seventh cervical vertebræ, the second between the eleventh dorsal and second lumbar, the third between the fourth lumbar and the sacrum; and that a majority of the fractures of the vertebræ occur at these points of flexion. He makes an argument from this also that these fractures "are generally the result of counterstrokes as the effect of forcible flexion of the column either forwards or backwards." Malgaigne observes moreover that dislocations follow the same rule.

The direction of the line of fracture varies greatly in the different examples which we have seen; some are crushed, and more or less comminuted. In some cases a narrow piece is chipped from the margin, others are broken transversely, and others obliquely. In oblique

[1] Reveillon, Chelius's Surg., note by South, vol. i. p. 584.
[2] South, ibid., p. 583.

fractures the line of the fracture is generally from behind forwards and from above downwards. Malgaigne thinks that a crushing or comminution can only occur from a forcible flexion forwards; but I have seen at least one example in which this was not the fact; the patient having fallen so as to strike with the back of his neck upon an iron bar. This was the case of the sailor, to which I shall again refer more particularly.

The upper fragment is almost always that which suffers displacement; sometimes being simply driven downwards and thus made to penetrate more or less the lower fragment; at other times, as in certain transverse fractures, it is only displaced forwards, and in still other examples, where the fracture is oblique, the upper fragment is displaced both downwards and forwards.

Fig. 33.

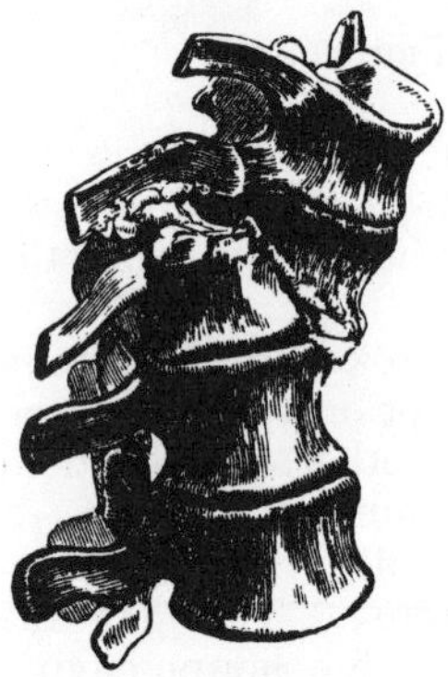

Oblique fracture of the body of a vertebra.

In the first and last of these examples the spine becomes bent forwards at the point of fracture, producing an angle of which the most salient point posteriorly is represented by the extremity of the spinous process belonging to the broken vertebra; in the second example the spinous process of the broken vertebra is depressed, and the process of the vertebra next below is relatively prominent.

In a pretty large proportion of cases also the fracture of the body of the vertebra is complicated, as we have already stated, with a fracture of the arches, in some instances with a fracture of the oblique processes and with a dislocation.

Symptoms.—Severe pain at the seat of fracture, felt especially when the part is touched or the body is moved, tenderness, swelling, ecchymosis, occasionally crepitus, a slight angular distortion of the spine, or simply a trifling irregularity in the position of the processes, and paralysis of all the parts whose nerves take their origin below the fracture, are the usual signs of this accident.

The paralysis may be due to the mere pressure of the displaced fragments, but it is much more often due to a severe and irreparable lesion of the cord itself. I have in one instance seen the cord almost completely separated at the point of fracture although the displacement of the fragments was inconsiderable.

Accompanying the paralysis of the bladder, there has been generally observed an alkaline state of the urine, and subacute inflammation of the coats of the bladder. Priapism is present in a certain proportion of cases.

Those who die immediately seem to be asphyxiated; while those who die later seem to wear out from general irritation, this condition being frequently accompanied with an obstinate diarrhœa and vomiting. A few become comatose before death.

It will be seen, moreover, that a certain proportion finally recover;

but scarcely ever are all the functions of the limbs and of the body completely restored.

We shall render this part of our description of these accidents more intelligible if we regard them as they occur in the various portions of the spinal column, since the symptoms, prognosis, and treatment, have reference mainly to the point at which the fracture has occurred.

1. *Fractures of the Bodies of the Lumbar Vertebræ.*

The nerves which emerge from the intervertebral foramina below the fourth and fifth lumbar vertebræ, join with the sacral nerves to form a plexus, which supplies the sphincter and levator ani, the perineal muscles, the detrusor and accelerator urinæ, the urethra, glans penis, and a great proportion of the lower extremities.

A fracture, therefore, of the third, fourth or fifth lumbar vertebra, produces more or less complete paralysis of the lower extremities, paralysis of the bladder, indicated by retention of the urine, and paralysis of the rectum, the latter being accompanied sometimes by involuntary discharges from the bowels and at other times by constipation. These patients generally die after a few months or years from a general nervous irritation with consequent exhaustion of the system. The following case, related by Sir Benjamin Brodie, illustrates, probably, a more favorable termination.

A boy was admitted into St. George's Hospital, in Sept. 1827, with a fracture and considerable displacement of the third and fourth lumbar vertebræ, the displacement being sufficient to cause a manifest alteration in the figure of his spine. His lower limbs were paralytic. An attempt was made to restore the displaced vertebræ, but it was attended with only partial success. At the end of a month he had slight involuntary motions of the lower extremities, and at the same time he began to recover the power of using them voluntarily. Three or four months after the receipt of the injury he left the hospital, and the history of his case was interrupted at this date.[1]

In case the fracture is at a point higher up, in the first or second lumbar or last dorsal vertebra, the whole of the lumbar nerves are cut off, producing a more complete paralysis of the lower extremities, accompanied with the same paralysis of the bladder and rectum. Death also ensues at a somewhat earlier period and from the same causes.

A few years since a Mrs. Squires, of Rochester, N. Y., was shot in her back, the ball lodging in the body of one of the lumbar vertebræ, from which it was found impossible to extract it. Her lower extremities were completely paralyzed, and also the sphincters of her bladder and rectum; a pin thrust into the body at any point below the middle of the abdomen was not felt. She survived the accident several months, and died at last covered with bed sores and exhausted with pain and watchfulness.

On the 11th of Oct., 1851, Alfred McCarty, æt. 47, residing at Fort Erie, C. W., was struck upon the back with a falling timber weighing

[1] Brodie, Sir Ast. Cooper on Disloc., op. cit., p. 471.

half a ton or more, fracturing four ribs upon the left side, and probably the lower dorsal vertebræ. The right leg was also badly broken at the same time. He was taken up insensible, but soon recovered his consciousness, when it was ascertained that the lower half of his body was paralyzed. I saw him a few days after the accident in consultation with Dr. Cronyn, a very intelligent surgeon residing at Fort Erie. We agreed that the treatment ought to be sustaining and expectant mainly. Constantly during the first three or four months, and occasionally for some time longer, the urine had to be drawn off with a catheter. A large bed-sore soon formed upon his sacrum. There was, however, in the main, a steady improvement, so that in April, six months after the accident, he was able to sit with his back supported; the bed-sore had healed; sensation had in a great measure returned to his lower extremities, but motion only slightly; he had gained flesh and strength. He now only rarely required the use of the catheter, but as soon as the desire to urinate was experienced he was compelled to discharge it, having lost the power of retention. It was the same with his fecal discharges. The urine was alkaline. About this time he began to experience a stiffness in one of his hands, inability to close the fingers upon the palm, and slight uneasiness in the neck. Gradually both arms became completely paralyzed, vomiting and purging supervened, and after repeated attacks in the last month of his life of laryngo-tracheal constriction, on the 20th of Sept., 1852, he sank into a state of complete paralysis and insensibility, and died.

A patient in Guy's Hospital, under Mr. Key, with a fracture of the first lumbar vertebra, lived one year and two days. On examination after death it was ascertained that bony union had occurred between the fragments, and that the spinal marrow was completely separated at the point of fracture.[1]

Fig. 34.

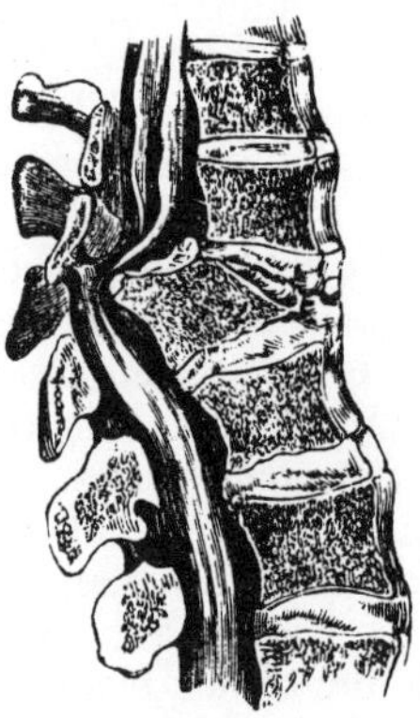

Key's case of fracture of the first lumbar vertebra.

Mr. Harrold relates a case of fracture of the first and second lumbar vertebræ, in which the patient survived the accident one year lacking nine days; death having resulted finally from a sore on the tuberosity of the ischium and disease of the bone. After death it was ascertained that the fracture had united by ossific matter, and that the spinal marrow was almost completely cut in two, the divided extremities being enlarged and separated nearly an inch from each other.[2]

Dr. Thompson, of Goshen, N. Y., has seen a partial recovery after a fracture of the third or fourth vertebra of the loins. The patient fell from the roof of a house striking first upon his feet and then upon his buttocks. This occurred in Oct. 1853. The usual signs of a fracture were present, such as paralysis, &c. A bed-

[1] Key, A. Cooper on Disloc., &c., op. cit., p. 467.
[2] Harrold, A. Cooper, op. cit., p. 464.

sore formed above the top of the sacrum, and a piece of bone exfoliated which seemed to belong to the last lumbar vertebra. He was confined to his bed seven months. After eighteen months he began to use crutches. At the end of about three years all improvement ceased; at which time he could not quite stand alone, yet with the aid of apparatus he was able to get about the country and peddle books, prints, &c. This was also his condition one year later.[1]

2. *Fractures of the Bodies of the Dorsal Vertebræ.*

In these examples, the same organs are paralyzed as in the fractures lower down, in addition to which there is generally considerable disturbance of the functions of respiration, irregular action of the heart, indigestion accompanied with a tympanitic state of the bowels.

Dupuytren, who reports several examples of fractures of the dorsal vertebræ, has not taken the pains to record the length of time they survived the accident except in two instances, both of which were fractures of the eleventh vertebra. One died of suffocation on the tenth day, and the other on the thirty-second. In Sir Astley Cooper's cases, mention is made of a fracture of the twelfth dorsal vertebra, which the patient survived fifty-two days, one of the tenth dorsal, which terminated fatally in six days, and another of the ninth dorsal, which did not result in death until after nine weeks.

In 1853 Dr. Parkman presented to the Boston Society for Medical Improvement a specimen of fracture of the fifth dorsal vertebra, the bodies of the third and fourth being also displaced forwards, in which position they had become firmly ossified. The spinal cord had been completely separated, yet the patient survived the accident two months.[2]

Dupuytren has related also two examples of fractures, one of the tenth and the other of the last dorsal vertebra, from which the patients completely recovered after from two to four months' confinement.[3] A similar case is related by Lente, of New York. Barney McGuire, having fallen a distance of twelve or fifteen feet upon his back, was found with nearly complete paralysis of his lower extremities, and of his bladder. Swelling existed over the lower dorsal vertebræ, and this point was very tender. Subsequently, when the swelling subsided, the prominence of the spinous processes of the tenth and eleventh dorsal vertebræ put the question of a fracture beyond doubt. Gradually under the use of cups, strychnia, mineral acids, laxatives, buchu, and electricity, his symptoms improved. In six months he was able to walk about the streets, and four years after the accident he was employed in a foundry under regular wages, being able to stand fifteen or twenty minutes at a time, and to walk half a mile without resting. At this time there remained no tenderness in the spine, but the projection of the process was the same as at first.[4]

[1] Thompson, Amer. Journ. Med. Sci., Oct. 1857. Lente's paper.
[2] Parkman, New York Journ. Med., March, 1853, p. 286.
[3] Dupuytren, op. cit., pp. 356–7.
[4] Lente, Amer. Journ. Med. Sci., Oct. 1857, p. 361.

3. *Fractures of the Bodies of the five lower Cervical Vertebræ.*

We shall now have added to the symptoms already enumerated, paralysis of the upper extremities, greater embarrassment of the respiration, and more complete loss of sensation and volition in the lower part of the body. In general also the eyes and face look congested, owing to the imperfect arterialization of the blood, and death is more speedy and inevitable.

In eight recorded examples of fractures of the five lower cervical vertebræ, one died within twenty-four hours, four in about forty-eight hours, one in eleven days, one lived fifteen weeks and six days, and one about four months. The most common period of death seems therefore to be about forty-eight hours after the receipt of the injury.

The example of the patient who survived the accident fifteen weeks and six days, is recorded by Mr. Greenwood, of England. A woman, Mary Vincent, æt. 47, was injured by a blow on the back of her neck, but she was not seen by Mr. Greenwood until after eleven days, at which time she was breathing with difficulty, occasioned by paralysis of the intercostal muscles, respiration being carried on by the diaphragm and abdominal muscles alone. This was the extent of the paralysis. There seemed to be a depression opposite the fourth and fifth cervical vertebræ, and pressure at this point occasioned universal paralysis, as did also the action of coughing and sneezing. About three weeks after the accident, she attempted for the first time to move, in order to have her clothes changed, when she was immediately seized with paralysis in the right arm and hand. After this she lost her appetite, had frequent attacks of purging, and thus she gradually wore out.[1]

The patient who survived about four months, was admitted into Hôtel Dieu, under the care of Dupuytren, in 1825, on account of a fracture of the fourth cervical vertebra, caused by a fall on the back of his neck, and suffering under paralysis of the bladder and extremities. After two months and a half of entire rest, he was convalescent and quitted the hospital, with only slight weakness in his left leg, and with his head a little bowed forwards. In returning from a long walk he fell paralyzed, and remained in the open air all night. From this time he continued to fail, and died thirty-four days after the second fall. On examination after death, the body of the vertebra was found to be broken, and also the processes of the fifth, allowing the fourth to slip forwards and compress the cord. A true callus existed in front of these bones, which looked as if recently broken. The cord itself exhibited an annular constriction, which Dupuytren conceived to be the seat of the original lesion narrowed by cicatrization.[2]

The following example furnishes a fair illustration of the usual phenomena which accompany fractures of third or fourth cervical vertebra.

[1] Greenwood, Sir A. Cooper on Disloc., p. 472.
[2] Dupuytren, op. cit., p. 358.

On the 25th of July, 1857, a sailor fell backwards from the wharf, striking with the nape of his neck upon a bar of iron. I saw him on the following day in consultation with his attending physician, Dr. Edwards, of this city. He was lying upon his back breathing rapidly. His lower extremities were completely paralyzed; legs and feet swollen and purple; right arm completely paralyzed, and his left partially; from a point below the line of the second rib, there was no sensation whatever; his bowels had not moved, although he had already taken active cathartics; the urine had been drawn with a catheter; the pulse was slower than natural, and irregular. He was constantly vomiting. In reply to questions, he said that he felt well, articulating distinctly and with a good voice. His eyes and face were somewhat congested, but with this exception his countenance did not betray the least physical disturbance. He lived in this condition about forty hours, only breathing shorter and shorter, and his consciousness remaining to the last moment.

In proceeding to examine the spine a few hours after death, and before any incision was made, we were unable, upon the most minute examination, to detect any irregularity of the processes of the cervical vertebræ, or any crepitus, but on dissecting the neck we found that the arches of the third and fourth vertebræ were broken, and the spinous processes slightly depressed upon the cord. The bodies of the corresponding vertebræ were comminuted and the vertebræ above were driven down upon them, carrying the processes in the same direction. The theca and the spinal marrow were almost completely severed upon a level with the fourth vertebra.

About one year since, a man was thrown backwards suddenly from the back end of a wagon, alighting upon the top of his head. Dr. Mixer, of this city, having requested me to see this patient with him, I found the symptoms almost an exact counterpart of those which belonged to the case which I have just described, except that a crepitus and a mobility of the fragments could be distinctly felt in the upper and back part of his neck. His death occurred in very much the same manner after about forty-eight hours. No autopsy was allowed. We noticed in this case, also, that whenever he was turned over upon his face respiration almost entirely ceased, but it was immediately restored by laying him again upon his back.

Dupuytren, Sir Astley Cooper, South, and other surgeons, have related cases simulating fracture, but which proved to be strains of the ligaments uniting the cervical vertebræ, accompanied with more or less injury to the spinal marrow. In one instance, I have met with what has seemed to be a strain of the ligaments and muscles of the neck, but which presented no symptoms of serious injury to the spinal marrow.

John Neuman, of Canada West, æt. 25, fell head foremost from a height of fourteen feet, striking upon the top of his head. He was taken up insensible, and remained in this condition six hours. When consciousness returned, his head was very much drawn backwards, and it was impossible to move it from this position. There was no lack of sensibility or of the power of motion in his limbs, and all the functions of his body were in their natural state; but he has suffered with occasional severe pains in his arms ever since. The accident happened on the twenty-fourth of November, 1857, and he called upon me eight months after. His head was then forcibly bent forwards instead of backwards, into which position it had gradually changed. In the morning he generally was able to erect his head completely, but after a few hours it was constantly drawn forwards, as when I saw him. There was no tenderness or irregularity over the cervical vertebræ, and he was so well as to be regularly employed as a day laborer.

Sir Astley Cooper has collected four examples of what he terms "concussion of the spinal marrow," all of which recovered after periods ranging from a few weeks to many months; but in only one case is it stated that the recovery was complete.[1] Boyer also enumerates three cases of concussion which came under his own observation, all of which terminated fatally in a short time. In the first example mentioned by Boyer, the autopsy disclosed neither lesion nor effusion of any kind; in the second case, it does not appear that any autopsy was made. The third is related as follows: "A builder fell from a height of fourteen feet, and remained for some time senseless; and, on recovering from that situation, found that he had lost the use of his inferior extremities. He had at the same time a retention of urine, an involuntary discharge of the feces, and some disorder in the function of respiration. Death followed on the twelfth day after the accident. The body was opened, and the vertebral canal was found to contain a sanguineous serum, the quantity of which was sufficient to fill a little more than its lower half."[2]

Treatment.—In a few instances, I have noticed among the recorded examples of fractures of the bodies of the vertebræ, that surgeons have made some slight attempt to reduce the fracture, or rather to rectify the spinal distortion, generally by the application of moderate extension to the limbs, and by laying the patient horizontally upon a hard mattress. But I have not been able to discover that in any case the patients have derived benefit from the attempt, although it has been said occasionally by the gentlemen making the report, that the deformity was slightly diminished. Nor am I aware that in any instance the patient has suffered any damage from the attempt; at least the reporter has in no case thought it necessary to make this observation. I am confident, however, that such manipulation can never serve any useful purpose; and I very much fear that it has been frequently a source of mischief. Although in cases so generally fatal, it might be very difficult to estimate with much accuracy the amount of injury done. If by any possibility the fragments could be replaced, I know of no means by which they could be kept in place; and in truth we are much more likely to increase the penetration of the spinal cord and the general disturbance, than to diminish it by extension or pressure. Moreover, it inflicts upon the unfortunate sufferer great pain, and for this reason, unless it can be shown to have

[1] A. Cooper, op. cit., p. 454.
[2] Boyer, Lectures on Diseases of the Bones, Amer. ed., 1805, p. 55.

heretofore accomplished some good purpose, it ought to be discouraged.

When treating of fractures of the arches of the vertebræ, I took occasion to call attention to Mr. Cline's operation, occasionally recommended and practised in such cases. I was not ignorant, however, that Mr. Cline and several other of the advocates of this operation had recommended it especially for fractures of the bodies of the vertebræ when accompanied with displacement. Even Malgaigne has preferred to consider the merits of this operation in its relations to these latter fractures; but while I am prepared to admit the propriety of an argument as to the value of Cline's operation considered in reference to fractures of the arches, I cannot admit its propriety in reference to fractures of the bodies of the vertebræ. The proposition appears to me too absurd to be entertained for a moment.

The treatment, then, ought to be, in a great measure, expectant. The patient should be laid in such a position as he finds most comfortable, and, as far as possible, the spine should be kept at rest, since the most trivial disturbance of the fragments and even that which may cause no pain to the patient, is liable to increase the injury to the spine, and prevent the formation of a bony callus. Especially ought the surgeon to be careful while making the examination, not to turn the patient upon his face, in which position the spine loses its support and a fatal pressure may be produced. The urine should be drawn very soon after the accident, and at least twice daily, for the next few weeks. Indeed, it is a better rule to draw the urine as often as its accumulation becomes a source of inconvenience, or whenever the bladder fills, which will in some cases be as often as every four or six hours. It is especially necessary to attend to these urgent demands of the patient during the first few weeks, when the paralysis is most complete generally, and the mucous surface of the bladder, already irritated and inflamed by the excessively alkaline urine, suffers additional injury from any degree of painful distension of its walls. It is unnecessary to say that the frequent introduction of the catheter may itself prove a source of irritation unless it is managed carefully and skilfully. This duty ought never to be intrusted to an inexperienced operator.

I do not see what advantage the surgeon can expect to derive from the administration of drastic purgatives, such as full doses of jalap, castor oil, or spirits of turpentine, at any period. If in the first instance the bowels are so completely paralyzed as that they seem to demand such violent measures to arouse them to action, we may be quite certain that the spinal cord is suffering from a pressure, or from some lesion which these agents have no power to remedy. The bowels may possibly be made to act, but it would be difficult to show how this is to relieve the suffering cord. So far from affording relief, these measures add directly to the nervous irritation and prostration, provoke vomiting and general restlessness. It is not desirable, we think, to obtain a movement of the bowels during the first few days by any means, however gentle. The effort to defecate, and the consequent motion, will probably do much more harm than the evacuation can do good; and especially for the same reason ought we to avoid putting into the stomach anything which will occasion nausea and vomiting.

After the lapse of a few days, if reasonable hopes begin to be entertained of a recovery, it will become important to establish regular evacuations of the bowels, either by a judicious management of the diet, by gentle laxatives, or by enemata. At a still later period, when the inflammatory stage is past, and the nerves remain inactive or paralyzed, nothing could be more rational than the employment of strychnia in doses varying from the one-twelfth to the one-eighth of a grain three times daily. Nor do I think that any single remedy has more often proved useful in my own practice, or in the practice of other surgeons with whom I am acquainted. In order, however, to derive benefit from this or from any other remedy, it must be continued for a long time; perhaps for a year or more. Electricity, setons, issues, and blisters are no doubt also sometimes useful. Care must be taken that setons, &c., do not produce bed-sores. Passive motion and frictions, good fresh air and nourishing diet, become at last essential to recovery.

During the whole course of the treatment great attention should be paid to the prevention of bed-sores, by supporting all of those parts of the body upon which the pressure is considerable. For this purpose we may employ circular cushions, air-cushions and water-cushions or water-beds; but with the utmost diligence they cannot generally be wholly prevented. When the sores have formed they should be treated, if sloughing, with yeast poultices, or the resin ointment. I find also the resin ointment an excellent dressing for the sores after the sloughs have separated. In case the surface is only slightly abraded, simple cerate forms the best application.

§ 5. Fractures of the Axis.

The phrenic nerve is derived chiefly from the third and fourth cervical nerves. If, therefore, the second cervical vertebra is broken and considerably depressed upon the spinal cord, respiration ceases immediately, and the patient dies at once, or survives only a few minutes. In such examples of fracture of this bone as have not been attended with these results, the displacement and consequent compression, have been inconsiderable, or there has been no displacement at all.

Mr. Else, of St. Thomas's Hospital, says that a woman in the venereal ward, and who was then under a mercurial course, while sitting in bed, eating her dinner, was seen to fall suddenly forwards; and the patients, hastening to her, found that she was dead. Upon examination of her body, it was discovered that the processus dentatus of the axis was broken off, and that the head in falling forwards had driven the process backwards upon the spinal marrow so as to cause her death.[1]

Sir Astley also relates the case of a man who was shot by a pistol through the neck, breaking and driving in upon the spinal marrow

[1] Else, A. Cooper on Disloc., &c., op. cit., p. 462.

both the "lamina and the transverse process" of the axis. He died on the fourth day.[1]

Malgaigne has collected three cases of fracture of the odontoid apophysis, all of which were accompanied with a displacement of the atlas. The first, reported by Richet, died on the seventeenth day; the second, reported by Palletta, died after one month and six days; and the third, by Costes, lived four months and two weeks.

In no case upon record has the patient survived this accident so long as in the case reported by Bigelow, and published by Parker, of New York. Says Dr. Parker—

"The patient, Mr. G. B. Spencer, was a man forty years of age, a milkman by occupation, of medium height, nervo-sanguine temperament, of active business habits, and capable of great endurance. His life was one of constant excitement, and he was addicted to the free use of liquors. He suffered, however, from no other form of disease than occasional attacks of rheumatism, for which he was accustomed to take remedies of his own prescribing, which were generally mercurials followed by liberal doses of iodide of potassium, 'to work it all out of the system.'

"On the 12th of August, 1852, while driving a 'fast horse' at the top of his speed on the plank road near Bushwick, L. I., he was thrown violently from his carriage by the wheel striking against the toll-gate. He alighted upon his head and face about fifteen feet from the carriage. Upon rising to his feet he declared himself uninjured, but soon after complained of feeling faint; after drinking a glass of brandy he felt better, got into his carriage with a friend, and drove home to Rivington Street in this city, a distance of more than two miles. There was so little apparent danger in his case that no physician was called that night. Early on the morning of the following day, Dr. B. was called to visit him. He found his patient reclining in his chair, in a restless state, and learned that he had suffered considerable pain in the back part of his head and neck during the night. He was entirely incapacitated to rotate the head, which led to the suspicion of some injury to the articulations of the upper cervical vertebræ; but so great a degree of swelling existed about the neck as to prevent efficient examination. There was no paralysis of any portion of the body, his pulse was about 90, and his general system but little disturbed. Warm fomentations were applied to the neck, and a mild cathartic administered. On the following day there was no particular change in his symptoms, but as there existed considerable nervous irritability, tinct. hyoscyami was prescribed as an anodyne, and fomentations of hops applied locally. On the third day, leeches were applied to the neck, and after this the swelling so much subsided, that on the fifth day an irregularity was discovered to exist in the region of the axis and atlas, which had many of the features of a partial luxation of these vertebræ.

"At this time he began to walk about the room, having previously remained quiet on account of the pain he suffered on moving. He persisted in helping himself, and almost constantly supported his head

[1] A. Cooper on Disloc., etc., op. cit., p. 476.

with one hand applied to the occiput. He often remarked, if he could be relieved of the pain in his head and neck he should feel well. He began to relish his food, and the swelling nearly disappeared at the end of a week, leaving a protuberance just below the base of the occiput, to the left of the central line of the spinal column, with a corresponding indentation. Notwithstanding strict orders to remain quietly at home, on the ninth day after the accident he rode out, and in a day or two after returned as actively as ever to his former occupation of distributing milk throughout the city to his old customers. During the following four months no material change took place in his symptoms, although he constantly complained of pain in his head. For this period he did not omit a single day his round of duties as a milkman, which occupied him constantly and actively from five o'clock in the morning to nearly noon. On the first of November, Prof. Watts examined him, and inclined to the opinion that there was a luxation of the upper cervical vertebræ.

"About the first of January, 1853, the pains, from which he had been a constant sufferer, became more severe, and he was heard to complain that he could not live in his present condition; he remarked, also, that he had heard a snapping in his neck. After going his daily round on the eleventh of January, he complained of feeling cold, and afterwards of numbness in his limbs. In the evening he had a chill and complained of a pain in his bowels. He passed a restless night, and arose on the following morning about six o'clock; he was obliged to have assistance in dressing himself, and experienced a numbness of his left, and afterwards of his right side. He attempted to walk, but could not without help, and it was observed that he dragged his feet. He sat down in a chair and almost instantly expired, at eight o'clock A. M., on the 12th of January, precisely five months from the receipt of the injury.

"The autopsy was made thirty hours after death by Dr. C. E. Isaacs, in presence of several medical gentlemen. Muscular development uncommonly fine. An unusual prominence discovered in the region of the axis and atlas. On making an incision from the occiput along the spines of the cervical vertebræ, the parts were found to be very vascular. These vertebræ were removed *en masse*, and a careful examination instituted. The transverse, the odontoid (ligamenta moderatoria), as also all the ligaments of this region, excepting the occipito-axoideum, were in a state of perfect integrity; this latter was partially destroyed. A considerable amount of coagulated blood was found effused between the fractured surfaces, some of it apparently recent, but much of it was thought to have occurred at the time of the accident, and afterwards to have prevented the union of the bones. The spinal cord exhibited no appearances of any lesion. The odontoid process

Fig. 35.

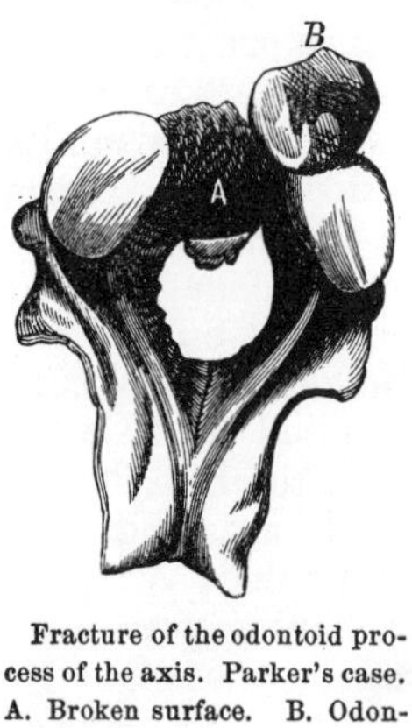

Fracture of the odontoid process of the axis. Parker's case. A. Broken surface. B. Odontoid process.

was found in the position well represented in the accompanying illustration, completely fractured off, and its lower extremity inclining backwards towards the cord. Death finally took place, doubtless, from the displacement of the process during some unfortunate movement of the head, by which pressure was made upon the cord. The destruction of the occipito-axoid ligament, which would otherwise have protected the contents of the spinal cavity, must have favored this result."[1]

§ 6. Fractures of the Atlas.

I have been unable to find but one example of a fracture of the atlas alone, and this is the case related by Sir Astley Cooper as having come under the observation of Mr. Cline.

A boy, about three years old, injured his neck in a severe fall; in consequence of which he was obliged to walk carefully upright, as persons do when carrying a weight on the head; and when he wished to examine any object beneath him, he supported his chin upon his hands, and gradually lowered his head, to enable him to direct his eyes downwards. In the same manner, also, he supported his head from behind in looking upwards. Whenever he was suddenly shaken or jarred, the shock caused great pain, and he was obliged to support his chin with his hands, or to rest his elbows upon a table, and thus support his head. The boy lived in this condition about one year, and after death Mr. Cline made a dissection and ascertained that the atlas was broken in such a manner that the odontoid process of the axis had lost its support and was constantly liable to fall back upon the spinal marrow.[2]

§ 7. Fractures of the First two Cervical Vertebræ (Atlas and Axis) at the same time.

A woman, æt. 68, fell down a flight of steps, striking upon her forehead, and died immediately. Upon making a dissection, it was found that the atlas was broken upon both sides near the transverse processes, and the odontoid process of the axis was broken at its base. These fractures were accompanied with a rupture of the atloido-odontoid ligaments, and a dislocation of the atlas backwards.[3]

South says there is a specimen in the museum of St. Thomas's Hospital, showing this double fracture. The man had received his injury only a few hours before admission to the hospital, and died on the fifth day. On examination the atlas was found to be broken in two places, and the odontoid process of the axis at its root. The fifth vertebra was also broken through its body. With neither fracture was there sufficient displacement to produce pressure, but a small quantity

[1] Bigelow, New York Journ. Med., March, 1853, p. 164.
[2] Cline, Sir Astley Cooper, op. cit., p. 459.
[3] Malgaigne, op. cit., tom. ii. p. 333.

of extravasated blood lay in the substance of the spinal marrow, and its tissue was at one point broken down and disorganized.[1]

Mr. Phillips relates that a man fell from a hay-rick, striking upon the occiput; after which, although momentarily stunned, he walked half a mile to the parish surgeon, and in two days more he returned to his occupation. About four weeks after the accident he was seen by Mr. Phillips, who discovered a small tumor over the second cervical vertebra, pressure upon which caused a slight pain. He complained also that his neck was stiff, and that he was unable to rotate it. No other disturbance of the functions of the body could be discovered. After a time the tonsils became swollen and the patient experienced some difficulty in deglutition, and upon examining the throat, a slight projection or fulness was discovered at the back of the larynx, opposite the second cervical vertebra. Subsequently he became affected with general anasarca and pleuritic effusions, of which he finally died. Up to the last week of his life he was able to walk about his bed-room, and his condition presented no other evidence than has been mentioned, that he was suffering from an injury of the spine. He died forty-seven weeks after the receipt of the injury.

The autopsy disclosed a fracture with displacement of the atlas and a fracture of the odontoid process of the axis. The two vertebræ were united to each other firmly by complete bony callus.[2]

CHAPTER XVI.

FRACTURES OF THE STERNUM.

FRACTURES of the sternum are of rare occurrence, owing, probably, to the elasticity of the ribs and their cartilages, upon which it mainly rests, and also, in part, to the softness of its structure. In advanced life, the ossification and fusion of all of its several portions becoming more complete, and the cartilages of the ribs also becoming more or less ossified, its fracture is relatively more frequent.

Causes.—They are generally the result of direct blows inflicted upon the part, such as the passage of a loaded vehicle across the chest, the fall of a tree or of some heavy timber upon the body; the fracture implying always, that great force has been applied.

Indirect blows, and voluntary muscular action alone have been known also occasionally to produce this fracture.

David, in his *Mémoire sur les Contrecoups*, published as a prize

[1] Chelius's Surgery, note by South, vol. i. p. 588.
[2] Phillips, Med.-Chir. Trans., vol. xx. 1837, p. 384.

essay by the Academy of Medicine, mentions the case of a mason, who, in falling from a great height, struck upon his back against a cross-bar which intercepted his fall, in consequence of which the abdominal and sterno-cleido-mastoidean muscles were so stretched that the sternum broke asunder between its upper and middle portions.[1] Sabatier reports another case of fracture at the same point, produced in a similar manner;[2] and Rolland has described a third example in a woman sixty-three years old, who, falling from a height backwards and striking upon her back, broke the sternum near its centre.[3]

Cruveilhier saw a man who, having fallen from a height of twenty feet upon his nates, was found to have a fracture of the sternum.[4] Cussan saw the same result in a person who fell from a third story, striking first upon his feet and then pitching over upon his back.[5] Maunoury and Thore have reported an analogous case, where a man fell from a height of twelve or fifteen *mètres*, first striking upon his feet and then falling over upon his back and head.[6] Mr. Johnson, late editor of the London Med.-Chir. Rev., reports a case of this kind, also, as having been received into St. George's Hospital, in London; the man, a healthy laborer, from the country, had fallen from the top of a hay cart, striking only upon his head. He walked with his head much bent forwards, and was incapable of either flexing, extending, or rotating it any farther. The fracture was transverse, and about three inches below the top of the sternum, opposite the centre of the third rib, the lower fragment projecting in front of the upper. The fragments were easily replaced by simply throwing the head back, and they fell into place with an audible snap, but they immediately resumed their unnatural position when the head was flexed. They finally united, but with a slight projection and overlapping.[7]

Malgaigne expresses a doubt whether all these can be considered as the results of muscular action, since in a certain number of the examples cited, the head seems to have been thrown forwards by the concussion, and in others, also, there is no evidence that the muscles attached to the sternum were put upon the stretch. The only remaining explanation is that in such cases the sternum has been broken by the violent shock, or *contrecoup*.

Seat and Direction of Fracture.—The sternum is separated most frequently either in the long central portion, or at the junction of this with the upper portion, where the bone is weakest. In fact a separation at this latter point may be regarded frequently as a diastasis or dislocation rather than as a fracture, since the two portions do not become firmly united by bone until late in life. The very late ossification and fusion of the xiphoid cartilage with the central piece, also, will explain the infrequency of its fracture.

1 Boyer on Bones, p. 57.
2 Malgaigne, from Sabatier, Mém. sur la Fract. du Sternum.
3 Ibid., from Bull. de Thérap., tom. vi. p. 288.
4 Ibid., from Bull. de la Soc. Anat., Juin, 1826.
5 Ibid., from Archiv. de Méd., Janv., 1827.
6 Ibid., from Gaz. Méd., 1842, p. 361.
7 London Med.-Chir. Rev., vol. xvii. new series, p. 536, 1832.

Boyer believed that the xiphoid cartilage was not susceptible of being permanently displaced backwards, except in aged persons after it had become ossified, "for," he says, "though violently struck and driven backwards by a blow on what is vulgarly termed the pit of the stomach, yet it restores itself by its own elasticity."[1]

The following case, however, which has come under my own observation, is conclusive as to the possibility of this accident:—

A man, twenty eight years old, fell forwards, striking the lower end of his sternum upon the top of a candlestick, breaking in the xiphoid cartilage. During two years following the accident he had frequent attacks of vomiting, which were excessively violent and distressing. The paroxysms occurring every five or six days. Both Dr. Green, of Albany, and Dr. White, of Cherry Valley, upon whom he called for relief, recommended excision of the cartilage, but the patient would not submit to the operation. Twelve years after the accident, in the year 1848, while he was an inmate of the Buffalo Hospital of the Sisters of Charity, I examined his chest and found the xiphoid cartilage bent at right angles with the sternum, pointing directly towards the spine. He now suffered no inconvenience from it, except that it hurt him occasionally when he coughed.[2]

The upper portion of the sternum is rarely broken, unless at the same time the central portion is broken also.

The direction of these fractures is generally transverse, or nearly so; occasionally a slight obliquity is found in the direction of the thickness of the bone. In three or four examples upon record the direction of the fracture was longitudinal. It is not so unfrequent, however, to find the bone comminuted. Compound fractures are exceedingly rare.

When the fracture is transverse, the lower fragment is almost always displaced forwards, and sometimes it slightly overlaps the upper fragment.

In one instance mentioned by Sabatier, where the separation had taken place at the point of junction between the first and second piece, the lower fragment was displaced backwards, and was also carried upwards under the upper fragment to the extent of twenty-eight *millimétres*.

Diagnosis.—In a few cases the patients have felt the bone break at the moment of the accident. When displacement exists it may generally be easily recognized, and the lower fragment will often be seen to move forwards and backwards at each inspiration and expiration. Crepitus may also be detected in some of these examples, but it is less often present where no displacement exists. To determine the existence of crepitus the hand should be placed over the supposed seat of fracture, while the patient is directed to make forced inspirations and expirations, or the ear may be applied directly to the chest.

Emphysema has, also, occasionally been noticed, indicating usually that the lungs have been penetrated by the broken fragments.

[1] Boyer on Diseases of Bones, p. 59.

[2] Buffalo Med. Journ., vol. xii. p. 282, Cases of Fractures of the Sternum.

The frequent occurrence of congenital malformations of the sternum should warn us to exercise great care in our examinations lest we mistake these natural irregularities for fractures. Bransby Cooper mentions a remarkable instance of malformation of the xiphoid cartilage which he at first suspected to be a fracture. It was so much curved backwards that, as Mr. Cooper thinks, its pressure upon the stomach produced a constant disposition to vomit whenever he had taken a full meal, or had taken a draught of water.[1]

Prognosis.—In simple fracture of this bone, uncomplicated with lesions of the subjacent viscera, and especially where the fracture is the result of muscular action or of a counter stroke, no serious consequences are to be apprehended. The bone unites promptly even where it is found impossible to bring its broken edges into apposition. Indeed, generally, where the fragments have been once completely displaced, although it is not difficult to replace them momentarily, a re-displacement soon occurs, and they are found finally to have united by overlapping; but no evil consequences usually result from this malposition. In nearly all of the cases reported in which palpitations, difficult breathing, &c., have been charged to the persistence of the displacement, the injuries were of such a character as to furnish for these unfortunate results other and much more adequate explanations. In one instance only, already mentioned, serious inconveniences followed from a displacement of the cartilage backwards.

In other cases, however, where the fracture is the result of a direct blow, constituting a large majority of the whole number, the prognosis is often very grave: a conclusion to which one would naturally arrive from the fact already stated, that the fracture of the sternum thus produced, in itself implies the application of great force.

An abscess occurring in the anterior mediastinum, and caries or necrosis of the bone, are among the most common results of a blow delivered directly upon the sternum; complications which generally end sooner or later in death. Blood may be also extensively effused into the anterior mediastinum.

Where emphysema is present we may anticipate inflammation of the pleura and of the lungs.

In several instances, where death has occurred speedily after the injury, the heart has been found penetrated and torn by the fragments. Sanson and Dupuytren have each reported one example of this kind. Duverney has mentioned two, and Samuel Cooper says there is a specimen in the museum of the University College, exhibiting a laceration of the right ventricle of the heart by a portion of fractured sternum. Watson mentions a case in which the pericardium was torn, but the heart was only contused.[2]

Treatment.—When the fragments are not displaced, the only indications of treatment are to immobilize the chest, and to allay the inflammation, pain, &c., consequent upon the injury to the viscera of the chest. The first of these indications is accomplished, at least in some

[1] B. Cooper, Princ. and Prac. of Surg., p. 359.

[2] New York Journal Med., vol. iii. p. 351.

degree, by inclosing the body, from the armpits down to the margin of the floating ribs, with a broad cotton or flannel band. A single band, neatly and snugly secured, and made fast with pins, is preferable to, because it is more easily applied than the roller which surgeons have generally employed; it is also much less liable to become disarranged. It should be pinned while the patient is making a full expiration. To prevent its sliding down, two strips of bandage should be attached to its upper margin and crossed over the shoulders in the form of suspenders.

Generally the patients prefer the half sitting posture, with the head and shoulders thrown a little backwards; and this is the position which will be most likely to maintain the fragments in place, and also to secure immobility to the external thoracic muscles, while it leaves the diaphragm and the abdominal muscles free to act.

The second indication may demand the use of the lancet; but more often it will be found necessary to allay the pain and disposition to cough by the use of opium.

If, however, the fragments are displaced, it is proper first to attempt their reduction; which, as we have already intimated, is generally more easy of accomplishment than is the maintenance of them in place until a cure is effected.

The upper fragment may be thrown forwards, and made to resume its position sometimes by a single full inspiration; but then it usually falls back during expiration; or it may be reduced by straightening the spine forcibly and at the same time drawing the shoulders back.

Verduc and Petit proposed, in those cases in which it was found impossible to reduce the fragments by these simple means, to cut down and lift the depressed bone. Nelaton suggests the use of a blunt crotchet introduced through a narrow incision; and Malgaigne has thought of another plan, which is, to penetrate the skin with a punch, and directing it to the broken margin, to push the fragment into its place, but which he does not himself regard as a suggestion of much value, since the bone is too soft to afford the necessary resistance; and, moreover, this, in common with all of the other similar methods, is liable, in some degree, to the objection that it may increase the tendency to caries and suppuration, already imminent. If reduced, the fragments will probably immediately again become displaced; and more than all, it still remains to be proven conclusively, that the mere riding of the fragments is in itself ever a cause of subsequent suffering or even of inconvenience.

When an abscess has formed in the anterior mediastinum, surgeons have occasionally recommended the use of the trephine. Gibson has twice operated in this manner at the Philadelphia Hospital, but in each case the caries continued to extend and the patient died; an experience which has inclined him latterly to discountenance the operation.[1]

There are other considerations mentioned by Lonsdale, which ought to decide us never to use the trephine in these cases. "For the symp-

[1] Gibson, Institutes and Practice of Surgery, vol. i. p. 269.

toms denoting the presence of the abscess, when completely confined to the under surface of the bone, will be very uncertain; and when the matter collects in larger quantities, it will show itself at the margin of the sternum, between the ribs; when it can be let out by making a puncture with the point of a lancet, without the necessity of removing a portion of the bone."[1]

We have already said that a separation of the first from the second piece of the sternum, occurring before ossific union had taken place, might with some propriety be regarded as a diastasis, or as a dislocation even. Maisonneuve, Vidal (de Casis), Malgaigne, and other French surgeons speak of it as a dislocation, and Vidal has collected five examples, in all of which the lower bone occupied a position in front of the upper. Malgaigne enumerates ten examples. The points of difference between the dislocation and the true fracture are too small, however, to demand of us especial attention.

CHAPTER XVII.

FRACTURES OF THE RIBS AND THEIR CARTILAGES.

§ 1. Fractures of the Ribs.

FRACTURES of the ribs, observed more often than fractures of the sternum, are rare as compared with fractures of other long bones.

In my records only eighteen patients are reported as having had broken ribs; but as in several of the cases two or more ribs were broken at the same time, the total number of fractures is about thirty-six. If, however, I had always accepted the diagnosis made by other surgeons, the number would have been much greater, since I have been repeatedly assured that the ribs were broken where, upon the most rigid examination, no evidence, beyond the existence of a severe pain and of difficult respiration, has been presented to me.

Etiology.—The force requisite to break the ribs is scarcely less than what is requisite to break the sternum; and in childhood and infancy it is sometimes almost impossible to break them, so that children and even adults are often crushed and killed outright, where, although the pressure has been directly upon the thorax, the ribs have resumed their positions, and have been found not to be broken. I have met with several examples of this kind.

In old age, the cartilages ossify and the ribs themselves suffer a gradual atrophy, which renders them much more liable to break.

[1] Lonsdale, Practical Treatise on Fractures, London, 1838, p. 242.

The most common causes are direct blows, of very great force, in consequence of which sometimes the fragments are not only broken, but more or less forced inwards; occasionally they are the result of counter-strokes, and then the fragments, if they deviate at all from their natural position, are salient outwards; a species of fracture which I have not met with so often.

Malgaigne has collected eight examples of fractures of the ribs produced by muscular action, by the beating of the heart, &c., all of which occurred upon the left side. It is believed, however, that in all of these cases the ribs had previously become atrophied, and perhaps undergone other changes in their structure, rendering them liable to fracture from the action of trivial causes.

Pathology, Seat, &c.—The fourth, fifth, sixth, and seventh ribs are most liable to be broken; the upper ribs, and especially the first rib, being so well protected in various ways as to greatly diminish their liability, while the loose and floating condition of the last two ribs gives them an almost complete exemption.

In my own cases I have found the first, second, and third ribs each broken once, the fourth three times; the fifth and sixth, nine times; the seventh, six times; the eighth, ninth, and tenth, twice each.

Twenty-one were broken through their anterior thirds, generally at or near the junction of the cartilages with the ribs; five through their middle thirds; and ten through their posterior thirds. Malgaigne has noticed, also, contrary to the general opinion of surgeons, that the ribs are most often broken in their anterior thirds, whether the cause has been a direct or a counter blow.

The direction of the fracture is generally transverse or slightly oblique; sometimes it is quite oblique. It is often compound; and in a few instances I have found it comminuted or multiple. Where the fracture is compound, it is rendered so generally by the fragments having penetrated the lungs, and not by a tegumentary wound. In only nine of the eighteen cases seen by me, has the fracture been uncomplicated with fractures or dislocations of other bones.

Displacement cannot occur in the direction of the axis of the bone unless several ribs be broken at the same time. The fragments are therefore either not at all displaced, or they fall inwards toward the cavity of the chest, or outwards, or very slightly downwards, in the direction of the intercostal spaces. Sometimes the rib moves a little upon its own axis.

Prognosis.—Death occurs sooner or later in a pretty large proportion of the cases in which the ribs have been broken; yet not often as a direct consequence of the fracture, but only as a result of the injury inflicted upon the viscera of the chest, or of other injuries received at the same moment. The violent compression of the heart and lungs has frequently produced death, and sometimes, as I have more than once seen, almost immediately; or the patients have succumbed at a later period to acute pneumonitis.

Lonsdale saw a case in which the body of a man having been traversed by the wheel of a wagon, eight ribs were broken, and death having followed almost immediately, the autopsy disclosed a rent in the left auricle of the heart, produced by one of the broken ribs.[1]—South says there is such a specimen in St. Thomas's Hospital.[2]

Dupuytren reports a similar case. The same surgeon has also seen several deaths produced by the emphysema, independent of the fracture, two of which are particularly described in his Clinical Lectures.[3] Amesbury has seen a case of death from rupture of the intercostal artery, where there was no injury of the lungs.[4]

In several instances observed by me, patients have suffered from pains in the side, occasionally from cough, &c., after the lapse of two or more years, and I suspect it is no uncommon thing for these injuries to entail some such permanent disability, but which is a consequence rather of the injury to the viscera of the chest than of any condition of the broken ribs themselves.

In general, simple fractures of the ribs unite in from twenty-five to thirty days. Malgaigne has seen one case of non-union; Huguier met with another upon the cadaver, in which a complete false joint existed, furnished with a capsule and lined with synovial membrane;[5] Eve, of Nashville, Tenn., saw a case of non-union occasioned, probably, by a caries or necrosis of the bone, since it was accompanied with a discharge of matter, and in which a removal of the ends of the fragments resulted promptly in a cure of the sinus;[6] and Samuel Cooper says there is a specimen in the museum of the University College, of a fracture of six ribs, where the fragments are only connected by a fibrous or ligamentous tissue.[7]

The union generally occurs with only a slight degree of displacement.

After the union is completed, even where there is no displacement, a certain amount of ensheathing callus may generally be felt at the point of fracture. Of five cases which I have carefully examined after recovery, in only one instance was I unable to detect any irregularity at this point. I have in my cabinet nine specimens of fractured ribs, in four of which the ensheathing callus is completely formed, but the fragments are in perfect apposition: in one, apposition is preserved, but there is no ensheathing callus; and the remaining four, all occurring in the same person, are united with displacement, but without a proper ensheathing callus.

In some specimens I have observed sharp spiculæ of bone or osteophytes extending along the course of the intercostal muscles from one rib to the other, forming a species of anchylosis between their adjacent margins.

Symptomatology.—Acute pain, referred especially to the point of fracture, sometimes producing great embarrassment in the respiration, and crepitus, are the most common indications of a fracture. The pain and embarrassed respiration are, however, far from being diagnostic, since they are often present in an equal degree when the walls of the chest have only been severely contused.

[1] Lonsdale on Fractures, p. 258.
[2] Chelius's Surgery, by South, vol. i. p. 599.
[3] Dupuytren, op. cit., p. 79.
[4] Amesbury on Fractures, vol. ii. 612.
[5] Malgaigne, op. cit., p. 435.
[6] Eve, N. Y. Journ. Med., vol. xv. p. 136.
[7] S. Cooper's Surg., vol. ii. p. 321.

The crepitus, also, is often difficult to detect, owing to the thickness of the muscular coverings, or to the amount of fat upon the body, or to the fracture having occurred perhaps directly underneath the mammæ in the female. In three instances, where the presence of emphysema rendered the existence of a fracture quite certain, I have been unable immediately after the accident to discover crepitus.

The crepitus may be discovered sometimes by pressing gently upon the seat of fracture, or by applying the ear or the stethoscope over this point while the patient attempts a full inspiration, or coughs; or we may press upon the front of the chest with one hand, while the fingers of the other hand rest upon the fracture.

Occasionally the patient has felt the bone break, and very often he feels or hears the crepitus after it is broken and will himself indicate very clearly the point of fracture.

At the same time that we detect crepitus we are able also to discover motion in the fragments, but I have once or twice discovered preternatural mobility without crepitus.

Emphysema, which is almost certainly indicative of a fracture, is present in a pretty large proportion of cases. It has been observed by me in ten out of eighteen cases; generally it did not extend over more than two or three square feet of surface; but in one instance it finally extended over nearly the whole body. It is remarkable, however, that in only three of these ten cases did the patients expectorate blood, and then in a very small quantity, and not until the second or third day.

Desault observes that emphysema rarely succeeds to fractures of the ribs; an observation which, as will be seen, my experience does not at all confirm.

Treatment.—In simple fractures, where there is no displacement, or where the displacement is only moderate, the chest may be inclosed with a broad belt or band, as we have already directed in case of fracture of the sternum: provided always that it is not found to increase instead of diminishing the patient's sufferings. Some patients cannot tolerate this confinement at all, while with a majority, although it is at first uncomfortable and oppressive, after an hour or two it affords them great relief from the distressing pain, and they will not consent to have it removed even for a moment. In nearly all cases of comminuted, or multiple fracture, it is inadmissible, on account of its tendency to force the pieces inwards.

Hannay, of England, has suggested the use of adhesive straps as a substitute for the cotton or flannel band; the several successive pieces being imbricated upon each other until the whole chest is covered.[1] The same objection holds to this mode of dressing as to a similar mode of dressing a broken clavicle, which has been recently recommended. It will certainly become loosened after a few hours, by the slight but uninterrupted play of the ribs.

The forearm ought also to be brought across the chest at a right angle with the arm, and secured in this position with a moderately

[1] American Journ. Med. Sci., vol. xxxix. p. 198. From Lond. Med. Gaz., Nov. 1845.

tight bandage or sling, so as to prevent any motion in the pectoral muscles.

As to position, the patient generally prefers to sit up, or he chooses a position only partly reclining upon his back; but there is no positive rule to be observed in this matter, except that such a position shall be chosen as shall prove most comfortable to the patient.

If the fragments are salient outwards, the fracture having been produced by a counter-stroke, they may be reduced by pressing gently upon them from without. If, on the contrary, the fragments are salient inwards, they will be found, in a great majority of cases, to have resumed their positions spontaneously or through the natural actions of respiration; but if they have not, it will be exceedingly difficult to restore them. Possibly it may be accomplished by pressing forcibly upon the front of the chest, or upon the anterior extremity of the broken rib; yet if the fragments are comminuted, and the ends are much driven in, this method will avail little or nothing. In such cases several surgeons have recommended that we should cut down to the bone and elevate the fragments, but Rossi alone claims to have actually put the suggestion into practice.

No doubt, if the necessity was urgent, this method might be successfully adopted; or, instead of cutting down to the broken rib, we might even seize the fragment with a hook, as suggested by Malgaigne, or, what in some cases might be even more convenient, with a pair of forceps constructed with long teeth, obliquely set upon a firm shaft. Yet the exigency which will demand a resort to any of these measures will be exceedingly rare.

In no case do I attach any value or importance to the advice given by Petit, that we shall place a compress upon the front of the chest, underneath the bandage, in order to reduce the fragments, or to retain them in place after reduction. Lisfranc, who advocated this method, claimed that its advantage consisted in the increased length which was thus given to the antero-posterior diameter of the chest, and the consequent accumulation of pressure from the encircling band, in this direction.[1] The mechanical law is no doubt correctly stated, but its value in practice is too inconsiderable to deserve consideration.

The emphysema generally demands no especial attention, since it is usually too limited to occasion inconvenience, and when more extensive it generally disappears spontaneously after a few days, or a few weeks at most. The advice given by some surgeons, that we ought in these cases to cut down to the pleural cavity so as to allow the air to escape freely through the incision, seems thus far to have rested its reputation upon a more than doubtful theory rather than upon any testimony of experience. Abernethy alone, so far as I know, has actually made the experiment, and his patient died.

Dupuytren, in the two cases already alluded to, bled the patients and applied resolvent liquids, with rollers; he also made incisions with the lancet at various points of the body, more or less remote from

[1] Ranking's Abstract, vol. ii. p. 204, from Gaz. des Hôpitaux, July 8, 1845.

the seat of fracture, a practice, however, in which he confesses he has no confidence whatever. These patients both died.

Dr. Stedman, of the Massachusetts General Hospital, has reported the case of a man aged sixty-nine, of intemperate habits, who, in addition to a fracture of one of his ribs, had also a dislocation of the outer end of the clavicle. The emphysema commenced immediately and reached its acme on the twenty-second day. At this time it had extended over his whole body; his eyes were closed and he breathed with great difficulty; but on the forty-fifth day, the emphysema had entirely disappeared, and he was dismissed cured. The treatment consisted chiefly in the free internal use of stimulants, and in the application of bandages; but the bandages soon became disarranged, and after a few days they were entirely laid aside.[1]

In the case of my own patient, where the emphysema was almost equally extensive, the patient recovered after a few weeks, under the use of a simple diet, and without any special medication whatever.

§ 2. Fractures of the Cartilages of the Ribs.

Boyer was incorrect when he said that the cartilages of the ribs could not be broken until they were ossified. They are often broken when there is no ossification, at the same time that the ribs themselves are broken. Sometimes they are broken alone. Not unfrequently, also, the separation takes place at the precise point of junction between the two.

Pyper relates a case in which the sternum was broken in a man aged twenty-five years, and also the cartilages of the sixth, seventh, and eighth ribs of the right side, as was proven by the autopsy, yet the cartilages were not ossified. The vena cava ascendens was also ruptured by the force of the compression.[2]

Etiology.—The causes are the same as those which produce fractures of the ribs, yet it is generally understood that it will require greater force, and that consequently the injury done to the viscera of the thorax will be more complicated and intense.

In the reports of the Massachusetts General Hospital, an account is given of the case of a man aged thirty, who was crushed by the fall of a heavy weight upon his body, and who died after about sixty hours. An examination after death revealed a fracture of the cartilages of the third and fourth ribs, with a laceration of the intercostal muscles to such an extent that a hernia of the lungs had occurred at this point. This hernia had been discovered and recognized by Dr. Warren, soon after the accident occurred; the protrusion being at that time as large as the clenched fist and regularly rising and falling with each movement of respiration. It was accompanied, also, with a moderate emphysema.

Pathology.—The fracture is clean and vertical, or transverse; never irregular or oblique. The direction of the displacement varies as in

[1] Boston Med. and Surg. Journ., vol. lii. p. 316.

[2] Ranking's Abstract, vol. i. p. 147, from the Lancet, Oct. 1844.

fractures of the ribs, but the anterior or sternal fragment is generally found in front of the posterior or spinal.

Union takes place in these fractures, not through the medium of cartilage, but of bone. Sometimes the new bone being deposited only between the ends of the fragments, in the form of a thin plate, and at other times it is formed around the fragments as well as between them. The latter of these two processes has been most frequently observed. The ensheathing callus appears to be supplied by the perichondrium, while the experiments of Dr. Redfern render it probable that the intermediate callus may result from a conversion or transformation of the adjacent cartilaginous surfaces. Paget remarks, also, that the ossification extends to the parts of the cartilage immediately adjacent to the fracture.

I do not know that any observations have been made upon the repair of these cartilages in very early life, and it is possible that the process may differ from this which has been described as it has been observed in the adult.

Treatment.—The treatment need not differ from that already recommended for fractured ribs.

CHAPTER XVIII.

FRACTURES OF THE CLAVICLE.

For the sake of convenience, I shall divide fractures of the clavicle into those occurring through the inner, middle, and outer thirds. By the "outer third" is meant all that portion of the clavicle included between its scapular extremity and the internal margin of the conoid ligament. The remaining portion is intended to be divided equally into two separate thirds. The peculiarities of these several portions, in respect to anatomical relations, liability to fracture, results, etc., will explain the propriety of the divisions.

Causes.—The clavicle is broken, in a large majority of cases, by a counter stroke, such as a fall, or a blow upon the extremity of the shoulder.

Occasionally it is broken by a direct stroke, as when a blow aimed at the head is received upon the shoulder; it is broken sometimes by the recoil of an overloaded gun, especially when the person lies upon the ground with the but of the gun resting against the clavicle.

Gibson has seen a case in which it was broken in a child at birth, by an ignorant midwife pulling at the arm.[1]

I have once seen the clavicle broken by muscular action alone. A large, well-built and healthy man, aged thirty-seven, standing upon

[1] Gibson, Principles of Surg., sixth ed., vol. i. p. 272.

the ground, attempted to secure the braces of his carriage top with his right arm, when he felt a sudden snap, as if something about his shoulder had given way. He did not, however, suspect the nature of the injury, and did not consult any surgeon until eight days after, at which time I found the right clavicle broken near its centre, but rather nearer the sternal than scapular extremity. The fragments were but slightly, if at all displaced, but motion and crepitus at the point of fracture were distinct. The usual node-like swelling was also present, indicating the existence of a considerable amount of ensheathing callus. He had been unable to raise the arm to a right angle with the body since it was broken, but he had suffered no other inconvenience from it.

A similar case is reported in the number for January, 1843, of the *American Journal of Medical Sciences*, copied from the *Revista Medica.* The subject of this case was a colonel of cavalry, about sixty years of age. In mounting his horse, he experienced a sensation as if something had broken, followed by acute pain in his left shoulder, and, on examination, it was found that the clavicle was fractured in the middle. The health of this gentleman had been impaired, it is further stated, by repeated attacks of syphilis.

Malgaigne has recorded three other examples of fracture of this bone from muscular action; and Parker saw a case which was produced by striking at a dog with a whip; the bone had been previously somewhat diseased, yet it united favorably.[1]

Of these six cases, five occurred on the right side, and always near the middle of the bone, if we except one case reported by Malgaigne, in which the point of fracture is not mentioned. In neither case did the fragments become displaced, only as they were found, in some of the examples, inclined slightly forwards.

Pathology.—It has already been observed, in speaking of partial fractures, that this bone suffers an incomplete fracture more often than any other, and that in such cases, the lesion occurs generally in the middle third, or rather to the sternal side of the centre, and in a direction nearly or quite transverse. They are not usually accompanied with much displacement, but if a displacement exists, it is a slight forward inclination of the fragments.

Fractures which are complete occur mostly after the bones have become firm and unyielding. They are also generally oblique, seldom comminuted, still more rarely compound. The point of the clavicle at which a complete fracture usually occurs, is at or near the outer end of the middle third, and a little to the sternal side of the coraco-clavicular ligaments, near where the trapezius and deltoid cease their attachments. It might be more exact to say, that the fracture extends from this point downwards and inwards, toward the sternum, embracing one inch or less of its entire length. In some cases the obliquity is greater, and the amount of bone involved is much more considerable.

Why the bone should break more frequently at this point, especially in the adult and in the male, it is not difficult to understand. It

[1] Parker, N. Y. Journ. Med., July, 1852.

is smaller here than elsewhere, and less supported by muscular and ligamentous attachments. At this point, also, the axis of the bone begins pretty abruptly to curve forwards, and more abruptly in the adult and male, than in the child and female. When, therefore, the clavicle is broken, as it usually is, by a counter-stroke, the force of the blow, conveyed from the shoulder through the outer portion of the bone, is suddenly arrested, and expends itself upon the point where the direction of the axis is changed.

In a record of eighty-nine fractures, including partial and comminuted, the latter of which have always been broken twice, sixty-six have occurred through the middle third, and, with the exception of the partial fractures, the fracture has in nearly all of the cases taken place near the outer end of this third. Three have occurred through the inner third, two of which were within one inch of the sternum; and twelve through the outer third.

A more practical analysis can be based, however, upon the point of fracture with reference to its cause; and I have never seen a complete fracture of this bone produced clearly by a counter-stroke, which was not near the outer end of the middle third.

When the fracture is at this point, or in any portion of the middle third, the direction of the displacement is almost uniformly the same. The sternal fragment is slightly lifted by the action of the clavicular portion of the sterno-cleido mastoid muscle, notwithstanding the resistance of the rhomboid ligament, and the subclavian muscle. On the other hand, the acromial fragment is dragged downwards by the weight of the arm, aided by the conjoined action of a portion of the pectoralis major and the latissimus dorsi, feebly resisted by the trapezius and other muscles from above; by the action of the same muscles, aided by the pectoralis minor, and perhaps by some portion of the subclavius, it is drawn toward the body, diminishing thereby the axillary space, while by the preponderating strength of the pectoralis major and minor, the acromial end of the fragment, with the shoulder, is drawn forwards; the sternal end of the same fragment being rather displaced backwards, and at the same time resting at a point somewhat elevated above its acromial end.

Fig. 36.

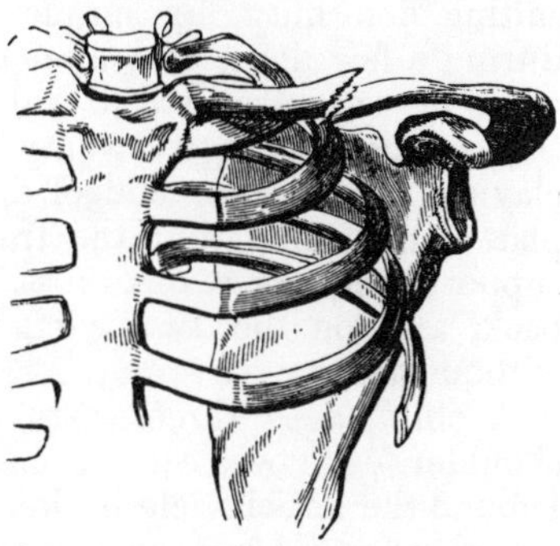

Complete oblique fracture, near the middle of the clavicle.

Desault has recorded one example of an overlapping by the elevation of the acromial fragment over the sternal;[1] and Bichat remarks, that Hippocrates speaks of the phenomenon as a thing which was familiar to him. Syme has mentioned a case of this kind which he had seen.[2] Guéretin, Malgaigne,[3] and Stephen Smith, have each re-

[1] Desault on Frac., op. cit., p. 16. [2] Amer. Journ. Med. Sci., vol. xvii. p. 251.
[3] Malgaigne, p. 461.

ported an example.[1] In Stephen Smith's case, the fracture occurred in a man thirty-eight years old. The bone was broken through the outer third, and transversely. He was treated at the Bellevue Hospital, but the overlapping, to the extent of one inch, remained after the cure was completed.

In nearly all the cases of oblique fractures occurring through the middle third, there follows immediately an overlapping, varying from one-quarter of an inch to an inch, and sometimes, though very rarely, exceeding this. There is a specimen in the Dupuytren Museum, in which the shortening equals one-third of its entire length.

Transverse fractures, wherever they may occur, are not so constantly found displaced, at least in the direction of the axis of the bone, as the following examples will illustrate:—

An old lady, aged eighty years, fell down a flight of stairs, breaking the right clavicle transversely, about one inch from the sternum. I saw her, with Dr. Trowbridge, on the day following the accident. Motion and crepitus were distinct, but there was scarcely any displacement. No dressings were applied, but she was directed to keep quiet in bed, and upon her back. In the usual time the fragments had united, without deformity.

A man about forty years old, fell backwards from a wagon, breaking the collar bone near the middle. The fragments were movable, but not displaced. He was treated successfully and without any resulting deformity, by simple confinement in the recumbent posture during a few days, and after this by suspending the arm in a sling, while he was permitted to walk about.

A young man, aged twenty-six, fell while wrestling, and broke the clavicle at the outer end of the middle third. There was some displacement at first, but the fragments being reduced, were found to support themselves. A cross, secured with straps, was applied to the back, and on the twenty-eighth day the union was complete, and without deformity.

A child, aged three years, fell about six feet, striking upon his shoulder. He was sent to me on the same day, by Dr. G. Burwell. I found the left clavicle broken off completely, about one inch from its scapular end. Crepitus and motion were distinct, but the fragments were not displaced. The arm was placed in a sling, and on the seventh day both motion and crepitus had ceased. The cure was accomplished without any degree of displacement.

The example of a fracture from muscular action, already mentioned as having been seen by me, was also probably transverse, and union has occurred without treatment and without displacement.

Stephen Smith, of New York, has met with two examples of transverse fractures without displacement, in a hospital record of eleven cases. Bichat says Desault has frequently observed the same, it having been seen three times at Hôtel Dieu, in the course of the year 1787.[2] Desault thinks, also, that sometimes the fracture, taking place

[1] N. Y. Journ. of Med., May, 1857.

[2] Desault on Fractures, op. cit., p. 15.

obliquely upwards and inwards, the usual form of displacement is prevented, and apposition is preserved.

If the fracture is near the sternum, and within the fibres of the costo-clavicular ligaments, as in the case of the old lady just cited, the displacement is inconsiderable. I have seen one other similar case in an adult also. Lonsdale mentions a case in a child, three years old, which came under his observation in Middlesex hospital,[1] which he regarded as a separation of the epiphysis; this bone, however, has no epiphysis, properly speaking, being formed entire from a single point of ossification. Malgaigne mentions two other examples, in one of which the fracture was so near the sternum that it was difficult to say whether it was not a partial dislocation. The displacement was only trivial.[2] But the only two specimens contained in the Dupuytren Museum offer a considerable displacement, and in both the external fragment is thrown downwards and forwards.

With regard to the amount of displacement usually attendant upon fractures near the outer end of the bone, surgical writers have generally united in declaring that it was in a majority of cases very inconsiderable, while some have even affirmed that there would be found no displacement whatever; neither of which opinions, according to the recent observations of Robert Smith, of Dublin, is strictly correct. He has examined eight specimens of fracture of the outer extremity of the clavicle, contained in the museum of the Richmond Hospital School of Medicine; three of which were broken between the conoid and trapezoid ligaments, and are united with very little displacement, while the remaining five, broken beyond the trapezoid ligament present a very marked deformity.

The following is a summary of the conclusions to which he has arrived:—

"When the clavicle is broken between the two fasciculi of the coraco-clavicular ligament, there is seldom any displacement of either fragment, and always much less than in fracture of any other portion of the bone. When displacement does occur, it is usually limited to a slight alteration in the direction of the bone, by which the natural convexity of this portion of the clavicle is increased.

"The explanation of which facts is found in the attachments of the ligaments from below to the two fragments; and, in the action of the trapezius from above, by which they are antagonized.

"But the case is very different when the bone is broken external to the trapezoid ligament. Here the coraco-clavicular ligaments can have no direct influence upon the outer fragment, which is displaced now partly by muscular action, and partly by the weight of the arm, the sternal end of the outer fragment being drawn upwards by the clavicular portion of the trapezius, while, by the action of the muscles passing from the chest, the entire outer fragment is drawn forwards and inwards,

Fig. 37.

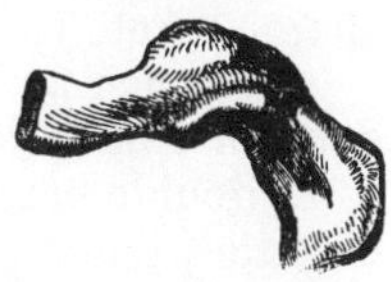

Fracture outside of trapezoid ligament. United.

[1] Lonsdale on Fractures, p. 206.

[2] Malgaigne, op. cit., p. 491.

so as to bring sometimes its broken surface into contact with the anterior surface of the inner fragment, and placing it nearly at right angles with this fragment, in which position it is generally united. The displacement in this direction, rather than any degree of overlapping, explains also the shortening which existed in all of these cases, varying in the different specimens from half an inch to one inch, and averaging about three quarters of an inch."

Such are the views of Mr. Smith; and I see no reason to call in question their correctness. In my own experience, a fracture occurring in a child three years old, within one inch of the acromial end, probably between the ligaments, was never displaced at all; a second, occurring somewhere in the outer third, presented, after many years, no displacement. Two recent cases were displaced each one quarter of an inch, and one old case, half and inch; these three latter cases occurred in adults, and always within an inch of the acromial end of the bone. In one of these last examples, the inner fragment was rather behind than above the outer fragment.

But it would be unsafe to draw conclusions from an experience which is confined entirely to living examples, and in which no dissections have been made, to verify the exact point of fracture, or the precise amount and character of the displacement. So far as they go, however, they seem to me to confirm the general correctness of the observations made by Robert Smith.

It has happened to me only six times to meet with a comminuted fracture of the clavicle, all of which fractures occurred through some portion of the middle third of the bone; the intercepted fragments being from one inch to one inch and a half in length, and lying obliquely, or, as in one case observed by me, at nearly a right angle with the main fragments.

I have never seen a compound fracture of this bone, although, in many cases, the sharp point of an oblique fracture has seemed just ready to penetrate the skin. One case is reported as having been presented at St. Bartholomew's Hospital. It occurred in a boy fourteen years old, and was produced by his having been drawn into some machinery while it was in motion.[1]

Lente also mentions a case, seen by himself, occasioned by the fall of a derrick upon the shoulder. The patient, twenty-four years old, was admitted into the New York Hospital in August, 1848. The left clavicle was broken at about its middle, and a large wound in the integuments communicated with the fracture. The fragments united firmly in about six weeks, after several pieces of bone had been discharged from the wound.[2]

Ayers mentions another case, the result of a severe gunshot accident, in which the bone was also very much comminuted.[3]

A double fracture, or a simultaneous fracture, occurring in both clavicles, seldom occurs. I have recorded two cases (*four fractures*, three of which are incomplete), both occurring in young boys.[4]

[1] London Med. Gaz., vol. ii. p. 382.

[2] Lente, N. Y. Journ. of Med., July, 1850.

[3] Ayres, ibid., Jan., 1857.

[4] Rep. on Def. after Frac., Cases 5, 6, 10.

Malgaigne says it has only happened to him to see it once in 2,358 cases, at the Hôtel Dieu, and he can recollect only five other examples. And of 158 cases of broken clavicles reported from the New York Hospital, it is stated to have occurred in only four. These gentlemen, however, only report hospital cases, and they have reference, doubtless, to complete fractures; while double fractures, according to my experience, occur more often in children than in adults, and are of the character of partial fractures, without usually much displacement; which facts, if sustained by subsequent observations, would sufficiently explain their infrequency in hospital, and their relative frequency in private experience.

Fig. 38.

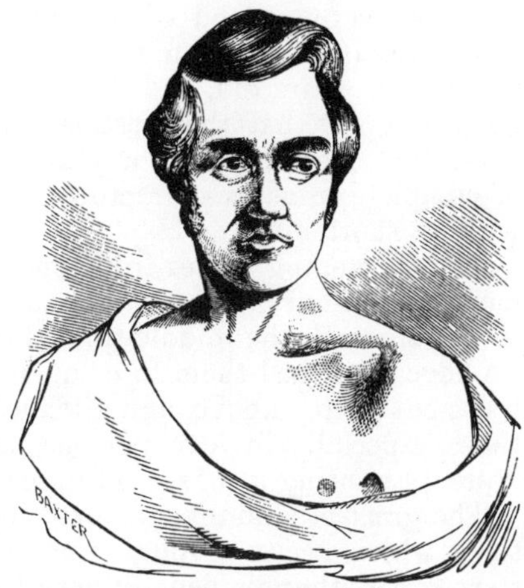

COMPLETE FRACTURE.—Oblique; at outer end of the inner two-thirds. (From nature.)

Symptoms.—In all cases of complete fracture with displacement, no difficulty will be experienced in deciding upon the nature of the injury.

The patient is found generally leaning toward the injured side, while the opposite hand sustains the elbow of the same side, to prevent its dragging downwards.

The shoulder falls downwards, forwards, and inwards; while, at the same time, the line of the bone is interrupted by the sharp and projecting point of the sternal fragment.

If the fracture is the result of a direct blow, a swelling and discoloration may be seen at the seat of fracture, but if it is the result of a counter-stroke, we must look to the top or point of the shoulder for the signs of a contusion.

The patient also experiences pain when an attempt is made to raise the arm at a right angle with the body, and especially in attempting to carry the arm across the body, by which the ends of the broken clavicle are driven into the flesh. In two cases (cases 19 and 50 of my Report on Deformities) of oblique fracture, accompanied with displacement, occurring in the middle third of the bone, I have particularly noticed that the patients could easily lift the hands to the head, and in one of these cases the patient, a boy, fourteen years old, raised his arm perpendicularly over his head. Such exceptions are not very uncommon.

Crepitus can be detected sometimes by simply pressing down the sternal fragment, but it is almost always present when we draw the shoulders forcibly back, so as to bring the broken fragments into more perfect contact.

If there is no displacement, still crepitus may generally be discovered by grasping the bone between the thumb and fingers, and moving it gently up and down, or by slight pressure upon the point of fracture.

When the fracture occurs close to the acromial extremity, external to the coraco-clavicular ligaments, although according to Robert Smith, there is usually considerable derangement, yet it is not accompanied with a corresponding amount of external deformity, and its diagnosis will require, therefore, more care and attention on the part of the surgeon.

Prognosis in this fracture deserves especial attention. In no other bone, except the femur, does a shortening so uniformly result. Of sixty-one complete fractures only fifteen united without shortening; and of twenty simple, oblique, complete fractures, which occurred at or near the outer end of the middle third, only one united without shortening (Case 46 of my Report), and in this case the patient was but fifteen years old, and the fragments were never much displaced; nor can I say that the treatment, a board across the back after the manner of Keckerly, had anything to do with the result. Five cases of complete transverse fracture, occurring at the same point, united without shortening.

The shortening varies from one-quarter of an inch to one inch, or more, and the fragments are almost always, especially when the fracture is through the middle third, found lying in the position in which we have described them to be at the first—the outer end of the inner fragment being above, and often a little in front of the outer: sometimes, especially in lean persons, and when the fracture is very oblique, presenting a sharp and unseemly projection.

The greatest amount of shortening is generally found in those fractures which occur through the middle third; in fractures near the sternal end there is usually very little permanent displacement; the same is true when the fracture is at the acromial end, and between the coraco-clavicular ligaments, as the observations of Robert Smith, already quoted, have sufficiently established, but if the fracture is beyond these ligaments, the final displacement and deformity may be very great.

The presence of a small amount of ensheathing callus soon after the cure is completed, sometimes increases the deformity. It is rarely seen to encircle the bone completely, but, if present, it appears to be most abundant in the direction of the salient points of the fracture, that is, above and below; so that, unless the examination is made with care, the projecting points of callus which remain, sometimes after many years, may be easily mistaken for an intercepted fragment turned at right angles to the axis of the bone. In the case of partial fracture, reported by Dr. Green, a similar circumstance was observed, which his natural shrewdness soon enabled him to explain.[1]

Robert Smith has observed, also, that in cases of fracture external to the conoid ligament, osseous matter is freely formed upon the under surface of each fragment, but there is seldom any deposited upon the upper surface of either. These osseous growths, occupying the situation of the coraco-clavicular ligaments, frequently prolong themselves as far as the coracoid process, and in some cases to the notch of the

[1] Transac. of Amer. Med. Assoc. for 1855, Case 13 of Frac. of Clavicle.

scapula. Still less frequently these osteophytes become fused with the coracoid process, and a true anchylosis exists.

In comminuted fractures the intercepted fragments generally fall off from the line of the other fragments, and cannot easily be restored.

The clavicle being a spongy and vascular bone, usually unites with great rapidity, generally within twenty days. In the fourth example of transverse fracture already mentioned as having been seen by me, the union seemed to be tolerably firm in seven days. Wallace reports one case from the Pennsylvania Hospital, which was cured in eight days, and another in nine days.[1] Velpeau says the clavicle will unite in from fifteen to twenty-five days; Benjamin Bell, in fourteen; Stephen Smith has seen it firm in fifteen days.

Fig. 39.

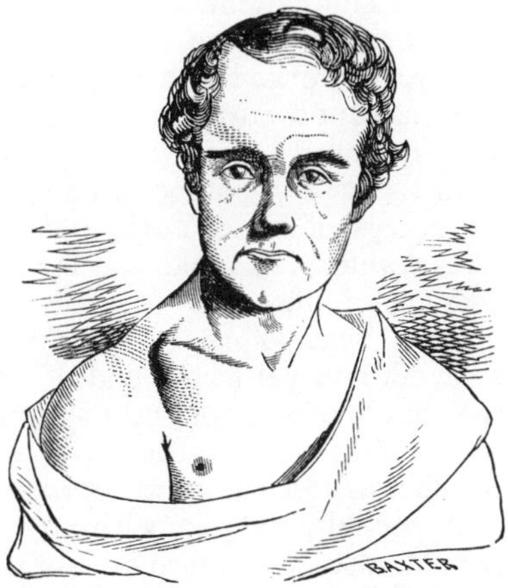

COMMINUTED FRACTURE.—United. (From nature.)

Whatever may be the degree of displacement, or the condition of the system, it is very seldom that it refuses to unite altogether or that the union is ligamentous: and in the few cases found upon record of a ligamentous union, the functions of the arm do not seem to have suffered any serious ultimate injury, as the following example, and the only one which has come under my observation, will illustrate:—

Edmund Nugent, a stout Irish laborer, now twenty-five years old, was received into the Buffalo Hospital of the Sisters of Charity, in March, 1854. He states that several years before, he fell from a horse and broke his left clavicle, at the outer end of the middle third. This was near Cork, in Ireland, and without consulting any surgeon or "handy man," he continued at work, holding the tail of the plough, nor from that day forward did he employ a surgeon, or dress his arm, or cease from his work.

The clavicle presents now the same deformity which nearly all other similar fractures present after what is usually termed successful treatment, except that it is not united by bone. The outer end of the inner fragment rides upon the inner end of the outer fragment half an inch. The ligament uniting the two extremities is so long and firm that it can be distinctly felt, and the fragments may be moved upon each other with great freedom.

In order that we might determine the amount of injury which he had suffered from the ligamentous union, we directed him to lift weights placed on a table before him, while he was seated upon a chair. We ascertained from this experiment that with his left arm he could lift

[1] Am. Journ. Med. Sci., vol. xvi. p. 115.

as much, within three ounces, as he could with his right, and he was not himself conscious of any difference. The muscles of the left arm seemed as well developed as those of the right.

Chelius also refers to two cases mentioned by Gurdy and Velpeau, in which, although an artificial joint remained, the use of the limb was but little impaired.[1]

Fergusson "once had occasion to remove various portions of this bone, which had become necrosed in consequence of neglected treatment. The patient, about twenty years of age, had the right collar bone broken by the fall of a tree; not knowing the nature of the injury, he worked as a reaper for several hours after; violent inflammation, suppuration, and necrosis followed; but after the dead pieces were removed he made a rapid and excellent recovery."[2]

In the case of compound and comminuted gunshot fracture reported by Ayres, of New York, and already referred to, the recovery was remarkable. The man was sixty-two years old, and in excellent health when the injury was received. The clavicle was so extensively comminuted that before the wound closed over one-third of the bone had escaped, and yet at the end of one year from the time of the accident the shoulder was perfectly symmetrical with its fellow, without drooping or falling forwards. Dr. Ayres thinks that all of the clavicle which was lost has been reproduced.

A partial paralysis, with atrophy of the muscles of the arm, accompanied, also, with more or less rigidity and contraction of the muscles, both of the arm and forearm, is, according to my observation, a more frequent result of these fractures.

Mr. Earle has recorded a case of comminuted fracture of the clavicle, in which the nerves converging to form the axillary plexus were so much injured that paralysis of the arm ensued; and it was noticed as an interesting fact, that the patient could not afterwards put her hand into even moderately warm water without the effects of a scald being produced, characterized by vesications, redness, etc.[3]

Desault saw a case at Hôtel Dieu, in which, although the clavicle was not broken, the force of the blow upon the clavicle was sufficient to produce a severe concussion of the brachial plexus, and paralysis of the arm. A timber had fallen from a building, striking upon the external part of the left clavicle. A considerable wound, followed by swelling, pointed out the place on which the blow had been received. No apparatus was applied, and on the third day a numbness and partial loss of the power of motion occurred in the arm of the affected side. Soon afterward an insensibility came on, and by the seventh day the paralysis of the arm was complete. It was not until after a tedious treatment that the limb recovered in part its original strength.[4]

In Case 23 of my report to the American Medical Association, which was followed by paralysis of the opposite arm, and spinal curvature, these results were probably due to some injury of the back received

[1] Chelius, Amer. ed., vol. i. p. 603.
[2] Fergusson, System of Practical Surgery. Amer. ed., p. 215.
[3] S. Cooper's First Lines, fourth Amer. ed., vol. ii. p. 323.
[4] Désault on Frac. and Disloc., Amer. ed., 14, 1805.

at the time of the accident; but one cannot avoid a suspicion that the apparatus, Brasdor's jacket, contributed somewhat to the unfortunate result. No axillary pad was employed, but the straps over each shoulder were buckled so tight that he was compelled to incline his head constantly to the right side. He was unable to lie down, and could only recline in a half sitting posture. This treatment was continued four weeks; and two months after its removal the paralysis and spinal distorsion commenced.

In Case 38, also, of the same report, a comminuted fracture, paralysis with contraction of the muscles extending to the wrist and fingers, existed, but whether it was due to the severity of the original injury or to the treatment, could not be satisfactorily ascertained.

Gibson relates a remarkable instance of this kind. A young man was struck on the clavicle by the falling limb of a tree, breaking it into numerous pieces, and bruising the parts so severely as to give rise to violent inflammation. "The fragments had been driven behind and beneath the level of the first rib, and so compressed the plexus of nerves as to wedge them into each other, and by the subsequent inflammation to blend them inseparably together. Complete paralysis and atrophy of the whole arm ensued, and the patient's object in visiting Philadelphia was to submit to an operation, in hopes of elevating the clavicle to its natural height, and taking off pressure from the nerves." Dr. Gibson, however, did not believe that the prospect of success was sufficient to warrant the operation, and the young man was sent home.[1]

Lizars says the callus is sometimes secreted so profusely, as by pressing upon the brachial plexus, to render the arm paralytic for a time; and he affirms that as a consequence of this pressure he has seen it remain in this condition three months. The statement, however, is made in a manner too vague, and needs confirmation.

It will not do to deny, therefore, the possibility of a paralysis as resulting from a concussion of the axillary nerves, produced by a blow upon the clavicle, nor of a paralysis resulting from a direct injury inflicted by the points of the fragments upon this plexus in certain very badly comminuted fractures; but it is certain that these conditions will not satisfactorily explain all of the other examples in which paralysis has followed simple fractures. In some cases it is no doubt due rather to the injudicious mode of using an axillary pad, by means of which the arm is converted into a powerful lever, and thus the brachial nerves are made to suffer from compression along the inner side of the arm itself. In short, it must be confessed that it is sometimes due to the treatment alone, and not to the original injury.

Parker, of New York, in a note to the edition of S. Cooper's Surgery, just quoted, declares that he has seen one patient who had lost the use of his arm from the pressure upon the nerves by the wedge-shaped pad, over which the limb was confined, in order to pry the shoulder outwards. Stephen Smith mentions a case of partial paralysis from the same cause.[2]

[1] Gibson, op. cit., vi. p. 271.

[2] New York Journal of Medicine, May, 1857.

A similar case has come under my own observation. A lady, aged fifty-one years, was thrown from her carriage, breaking the right clavicle obliquely at the outer end of the middle third. During the first three weeks the arm was dressed with Fox's apparatus, which was at no time particularly painful. She was then placed under the care of another surgeon, who, finding the fragments overlapped, applied very firmly a figure-of-8 bandage, with an axillary pad, securing the arm snugly to the side of the body; hoping by these means to restore the fragments to their place. The pain which followed was excessive, and notwithstanding the free use of anodynes, it became so insupportable that at the end of fourteen hours the dressings were removed by another surgeon, and Fox's apparatus again substituted. These were also applied much more snugly than at first, and during the four weeks longer that they remained on, repeated attempts were made to reduce the fragments.

Forty-eight days after the accident, she consulted me. The clavicle was then united, and overlapped half an inch. The whole arm was swollen, painful, and very tender, with total inability to move it.

I removed all the dressings, and, during the time she remained under my care, in a private room at the hospital, there was a gradual improvement in the condition of her arm, in respect to swelling and tenderness, but the paralysis did not much abate.

Erichsen thinks he has seen one case of comminuted fracture, produced by a direct blow, in which the subclavian artery was ruptured; great extravasation of blood resulted, and the arm was threatened with gangrene. The patient having recovered, however, the diagnosis could not be determined by actual dissection.[1]

Since among surgeons some difference of opinion seems to exist as to the practicability of overcoming the displacement in certain fractures of the clavicle, it is proper that I should defend the accuracy of my own observations by a reference to the observations of others.

In nine of eleven cases reported by Stephen Smith, one of the surgeons at Bellevue Hospital, New York, more or less deformity remained after the cure was completed. In the two remaining cases the actual results are unknown.[2]

"Great difficulty has been experienced in treating this fracture."[3]

"The indications of treatment are plain, but, unfortunately, not very easily fulfilled."[4]

"Fractures of the clavicle will often cause greater trouble than those which are considered of a more serious character, and the utmost pains will not, on all occasions, suffice to prevent a slight prominence of the inner fragment."[5]

"Setting of this fracture is easy, yet only in very rare cases is the cure possible without any deformity."[6]

[1] Erichsen, Surgery, Amer. ed., p. 205.
[2] New York Journ. Med., May, 1857, p. 382.
[3] Syme's Principles of Surgery, p. 266, Philadelphia ed., 1832.
[4] Miller's Practice of Surgery, 3d Amer. ed. from 2d Edinburgh, p. 309.
[5] Practical Surgery. By Wm. Fergusson. 4th Amer. ed., from 3d London, p. 215.
[6] System of Surgery. By J. M. Chelius, of Heidelberg, with notes by South. First Amer. ed., vol. i. p. 603.

"It is considered, also, that the close union of the fracture of the collar bone depends less on the apparatus than on the position and direction of the fracture; (therefore, in spite of the most careful application of this apparatus, some deformity often remains.")[1]

Fig. 40.

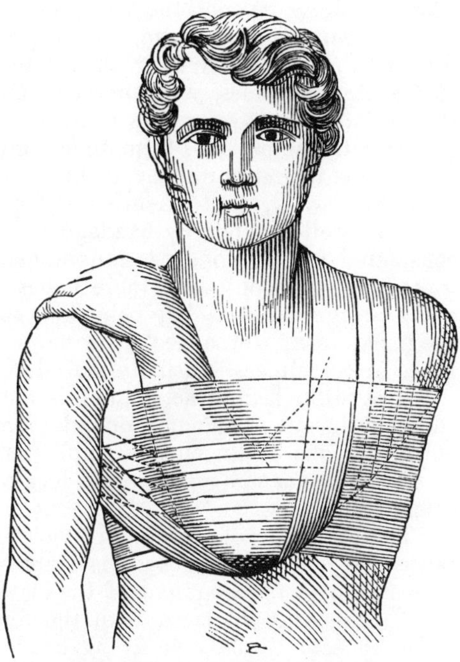

Velpeau's dextrine bandage; no axillary pad.

The following statements of M. Velpeau are found in a letter addressed to the editor of the *Boston Medical and Surgical Journal*, by J. Willis Fisher, dated Paris, Sept. 16th, 1846.

Mr. Fisher remarks that the report is drawn in part from his own notes, and partly from "the report published in the *Gazette des Hôpitaux*." It is the annual summary of M. Velpeau's practice at La Charité, for the year ending Sept. 1846.

"The fractures of the clavicle, less numerous than ordinarily, have been only four. They have proved these three often repeated propositions: First, that contrary to the general opinion, the patients can carry the hand to the head when they have a fractured clavicle. Secondly, that the consolidation of the bones demands only from fifteen to twenty-five days, and not six weeks or two months. Thirdly, that with all the bandage imaginable, we cannot prevent fracture of the two internal and oblique thirds from leaving a deformity."[2]

"Fracture of the clavicle is almost always followed by deformity, whatever may be the perfection of the apparatus and the care of the surgeon."[3]

"Hippocrates has observed that some degree of deformity almost always accompanies the reunion of a fractured clavicle; all writers since his time have made the same remark; experience has confirmed the truth of it."[4]

[1] Chelius, op. cit., vol. i. p. 605.

[2] Bost. Med. and Surg. Journ., vol. xxxv. p. 212. This is evidently a misprint. Instead of "fracture of the two internal and oblique thirds," the writer means to say an oblique fracture at the junction of the two internal with the outer thirds.

[3] Vidal (de Cassis), Paris ed., vol. ii. p. 105.

[4] Treatise on Fractures and Luxations. By J. P. Desault. Edited by Xav. Bichat, and translated by Charles Caldwell, M. D. Philadelphia, 1805, p. 9.

"As to the reduction of this fracture, it must be owned the same is often easier replaced than retained in its place after it is reduced; for its office being principally to keep the head of the scapula, or shoulder, to which, at one end, it is articulate, from approaching too near, or falling in upon the sternum, or breast bone, it happens that, on every motion of the arm, unless great care be taken, the clavicle therewith rising and sinking, the fractured parts are apt to be distorted thereby. Besides, even in the common respiration, the costæ and sternum aforesaid, where the other end of this bone is adnected, together with the motion of the diaphragm, rising and falling, especially if the same be extraordinary, as in coughing and sneezing, are able to undo your work, not to mention the situation thereof, less capable of being so well secured by bandage as many others. All which, duly considered, it is no wonder that upon many of these accidents, although great care has been taken, these bones are sometimes found to ride, and a protuberance is left behind, to the great regret particularly of the female sex, whose necks lie more exposed, and where no small grace or comeliness is usually placed."[1]

"Restituitur facile tractis humeris a ministro posterius, dum simul suo genu locato ad spinam dorsi, dorsum sustentet minister, nam tunc chirurgus folis digitis claviculam fractam reponere potest. *Difficilius autem in reposita sede retinetur*, sed loca cava supra et infra claviculam spleniis implenda."[2]

"The reduction of a broken clavicle is not very hard to be effected, especially when the fracture is transverse; nor is it usual for the humerus, with the fragment of the clavicle, to be so far distorted as not to be easily replaced with the fingers; *but the difficulty is much greater to keep the bone in its place when the fracture is once reduced, especially if the bone was broken obliquely.*"[3]

Amesbury, after having exposed the inefficacy of all previous modes of dressing, and especially of the figure-of-8 bandage, Desault's, Boyer's, and an apparatus recommended by Sir Astley Cooper, proceeds to describe his own apparatus and to affirm its excellence. It is, however, not much unlike a multitude of others, and is liable, I have no doubt, to the same objections. But the author thus writes:—

"The clavicle bandage, once properly applied, enables the surgeon to resist the action of all those powers which tend to produce displacement, and puts the fractured bone entirely under his control, without being productive of any of those evils which, I have endeavored to show, arise from the usual modes of treatment. I am not prepared to say that every fracture of the clavicle, treated in the manner which I have thought it expedient to advise, admits of being united without deformity; but, I am fully convinced that, if such cases should occur, they will be found very rare. I have had this bandage in use now about eight years, and, in the course of this time, I have used it in a large number of cases, many of which have occurred in the St. Thomas

[1] The Art of Surgery, by Daniel Turner, vol. ii. p. 256. London ed., 1742.
[2] Johannis de Gorter: Chirurgia Repurgata, p. 79. Lugduni Batavorum, 1742.
[3] Heister's Surgery, vol. i. p. 134. London ed., 1768.

Hospital. The result of these cases has been very satisfactory to myself, and to those surgeons by whom the treatment was witnessed.[1]"

"The direction the fracture takes is generally oblique, and in one place only, more particularly when it is caused by the indirect force; and this obliquity is one great reason why it is so difficult to treat this kind of injury without some slight deformity (and often a very great one) existing afterwards." * * * "One satisfactory result in the treatment of fracture of the clavicle is that, although it is very difficult to prevent deformity afterwards, the motion and free use of the limb do not become much impaired; for the bone is often shortened an inch or more, and still the limb possesses free motion and strength. This shortening causes the neck of the scapula to fall forwards, and makes the base of it project backwards, giving the person the appearance of having the chest contracted in front, by which the extent of range of action in the upper extremity will be diminished, although sufficient motion remains for the ordinary uses of the upper extremity. Where the fracture occurs in females, in whose dress the clavicle is exposed to view, it becomes an additional object to get the bone to unite as evenly as possible, to guard against the formation of an unsightly lump that will remain forever afterwards. The more the deformity is prevented in these cases, the more credit the surgeon will get for the cure."[2]

Fig. 41.

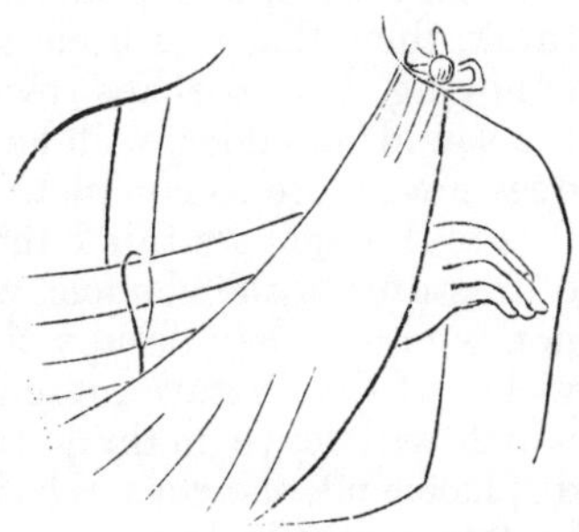

Lonsdale's apparatus; with axillary pad.

M. Mayor, of Lausanne, thinks that up to this day no successful mode of treatment has been devised. "Here everything appears as yet so little determined that each day sees some new propositions and different procedures," etc. He believes, however, that in his simple handkerchief bandage, with straps across each shoulder, the indications are most fully accomplished and the most successful results are obtained. If, however, it were to be treated *without* apparatus, the horizontal position, lying upon the back, would, in the end, make the most perfect unions.[3]

Says M. Malgaigne: "The prognosis, considering the trivial character of this fracture, is sufficiently difficult. For, little as may be the displacement, the surgeon ought not to promise a reunion without deformity; and certain successful results, proclaimed from time to time, betray, on the part of those who relate them, the most extravagant exaggerations."[4]

[1] Treatment of Fractures, by Joseph Amesbury, vol. ii. p. 527. London ed., 1831.

[2] Practical Treatise on Fractures, by Edward F. Lonsdale, pp. 207 and 209. London ed., 1838.

[3] Nouveau Système de Déligation Chirurgicale, par Mathias Mayor, de Lausanne, p. 384, etc.: (also Atlas, plate 3, fig. 23.) Paris ed., 1838.

[4] Traité des Fractures et des Luxations, par J. F. Malgaigne, tome premier, p. 473, Paris ed., 1847.

M. Nélaton having spoken of the various plans which have been suggested to retain this bone in place, and of their inefficiency, comes at last to speak of the handkerchief bandage of M. Mayor, and remarks:—

"This apparel is very simple; but neither will it remedy the overlapping." * * * * "Of all the apparels which we have passed in review there is, then, not one which fills completely the three indications usually present in the fracture of a clavicle. None of them oppose the displacement; they have no effect, with whatever care they may be applied, but to maintain immobility in the limb. We think, then, that it is useless to fatigue the patient with an apparatus annoying, and, perhaps, even painful; a simple sling, secured upon the sound shoulder, will be sufficiently severe. Nevertheless, as this does not assure so complete immobility as the bandage of M. Mayor, it is to this that we think the preference ought to be given in all cases of fractures of the clavicle, whether accompanied with displacement or not, whether they occupy the middle or the external part of the clavicle. If the fracture presents no displacement, we shall obtain a cure which will leave nothing to be desired. If there is a tendency to displacement, the consolidation will be effected with a deformity more or less marked; but since this deformity is inevitable, at least with adults, whatever may be the apparel which we employ, it is evident that the apparatus which causes the least constraint ought to have the preference. We may remark, farther, that this union with deformity in nowise impairs the free exercise of all the movements of the member."[1]

"The venerable gentleman who stands at the head of American surgery, and whose manipulations with the roller approach very nearly to the limits of perfection, informed us, in 1824, that he had never seen a case of fractured clavicle cured by any apparatus, without obvious deformity."[2]

I need not say that the "venerable gentleman" to whom Dr. Coates refers in this passage, was the late Dr. Physick, of Philadelphia.

Treatment.—If evidence were needed beyond that which has been furnished, of the difficulty of bringing to a successful issue the treatment of this fracture, it might be supplied, one would think, by a reference merely to the immense number of contrivances which have been at one time and another recommended.

A catalogue of the names only of the men who have, upon this single point, exercised their ingenuity, would be formidable, nor would it present any mean array of talent and of practical skill.

All these surgeons, however, have admitted the same indications of treatment viz., that in order to a complete restoration of the outer fragment, which alone is supposed to be much displaced, we are to carry the shoulder upwards, outwards, and backwards. But as to the means by which these indications can be most easily, if at all, ac-

[1] Elémens de Pathologie Chirurgicale, par A. Nélaton, tome premier, p. 720, Paris ed., 1844.

[2] Reynal Coates, Amer. Med. Journ., vol. xviii. p. 62, old series. It is probable that Dr. Physick here referred to complete and oblique fractures of the middle third, or that Dr. Coates has forgotten the precise language employed on this occasion.

complished, the widest differences of opinion have prevailed; and, in the debate, it may be seen that, while on the one hand, no invention has wanted for both advocates and admirers, on the other hand, no method has escaped its equivalent of censure.

Hippocrates, Celsus, Dupuytren, Flaubert, Lizars, Pelletan, and others, directed the patients to lie upon their backs, with little or no apparatus, but generally with the spinal column so supported and lifted with pillows, as that the shoulders would by their own weight fall backwards. S. Cooper and Dorsey also recommend that the patients should be confined in this position during most of the treatment; and, from the account given by Dr. Lente, it may be inferred that a similar plan is generally adopted in the New York City Hospital. "But this result (deformity) rarely happens when the patient has strictly followed the directions of the surgeon, as to position especially, for it is by position more than by any other remedial means, that a good result is to be effected. * * * * * The persevering continuance of the supine position in bed, with the head low, and, if necessary, a pad between the shoulders. This is the treatment uniformly adopted by Dr. Buck, in the hospital, and the results of his treatment are certainly such as to recommend it highly."

Nearly the same method we find recommended by Alfred Post, in 1840, then one of the surgeons of that hospital; the arm being merely kept in a sling and bound to the side, with the patient lying upon his back; and Dr. Post mentions a case treated in this manner, which terminated with very little deformity.[1]

Dr. Eve, of Nashville, Tenn., and Dr. Eastman, of Broome County, N. Y., have also employed this method successfully;[2] while Malgaigne declares it to be the most reliable means of obtaining an exact union.

Albucasis, Lanfranc, Guy de Chauliac, Petit, Parr, Syme, Skey, Brunninghausen, Parker,[3] and very many others, especially among the English, have preferred, in order to carry the shoulders back, a figure-of-8, while Desault, Colles, South, and Samuel Cooper, have represented this bandage as useless, annoying, and mischievous.

Heister, Chelius, Miller, Breffield, Keckerly,[4] Coleman,[5] Welch,[6] Hunton,[7] prefer, for this purpose, some form of back-splint, extending from acromion to acromion, against which the shoulders may be properly secured. Parker says that splints of this kind, with a figure-of-8 bandage, are "better than all the apparatus ever invented." While Mr. South gives his testimony in relation to all dressings of this sort, as follows: "I do not like any of the apparatus in which the shoulders are drawn back by bandages, as these invariably annoy the patient,

[1] N. Y. Journ. of Med., vol. ii. p. 266.

[2] Boston Med. and Surg. Journ., vol. lvi. p. 468.

[3] Parker, Samuel Cooper's First Lines, Amer. ed., vol. ii. p. 325.

[4] Keckerly, Amer. Journ. of Med. Sci., vol. xv. p. 115; also, my Report on Deformities after Fractures, in Trans. of Amer. Med. Assoc., vol. viii. p. 440.

[5] Coleman, New York Journ. of Med., second series, vol. iii. p. 274, from New Jersey Med. Rep.

[6] Welch, Trans. of Amer. Med. Assoc., vol. viii.; my Report on Deformities after Fractures, appendix, p. 441.

[7] Hunton, ibid.; also, New Jersey Med. Rep., vol. v. p. 146.

often cause excoriation, and are never kept long in place, the person continually wriggling them off to relieve himself of the pressure."

Fox,[1] Brown,[2] Desault, and others bring the elbow a little forwards, and then lift the shoulder upwards and backwards. Wattman and

Fig. 42.

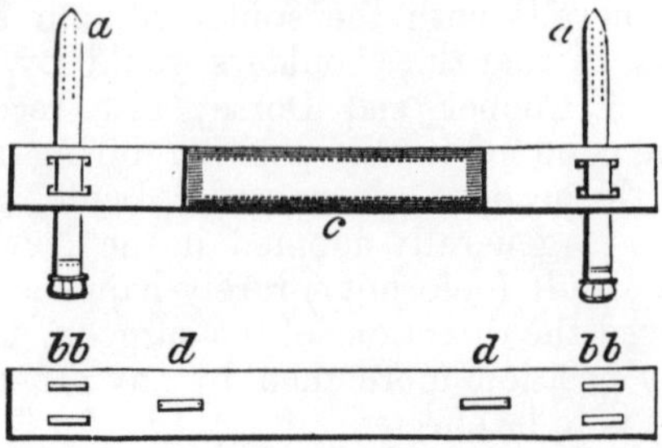

E. C. KECKERLY'S APPARATUS.—"The upper figure exhibits a front view, and the lower a back view of the splint. *a, a.* Are two bandages with buckles attached to one end of each. *bb, bb.* Are four mortised holes for the passage of the two bandages, *a, a. c.* A portion of the splint padded, to prevent its bruising the patient. *d, d.* Two loops of leather, tacked on the back of the splint, for the passage of the bandages, where the mortised holes are too far apart for the breadth of the patient from shoulder to shoulder.

"*Mode of Application.*—The end of the splint corresponding to the uninjured side is to be pressed close to the back of the shoulder, and retained so by drawing the bandage tight, and retaining it by means of the buckle. Previous to fixing the bandage, it should be passed through two loops on a small pad, which is to be placed in the axilla. This pad is used for the purpose of preventing the cutting of the bandage. After passing the other bandage through two loops, on a large, cuneiform pad, which is placed in the axilla of the injured side, it is drawn sufficiently tight and secured by the buckle. The last thing to be done is to place a handkerchief, doubled into a triangular form, in such a manner over the arm, the front and back parts of the thorax, as that it shall draw and confine the arm of the injured side close to the body, give it support, and prevent its falling down."

Fig. 43.

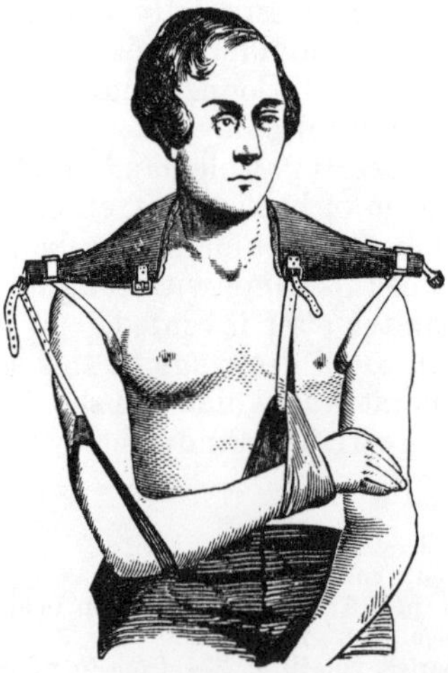

Hunton's "yoke splint," modified by Day.

Fig. 44.

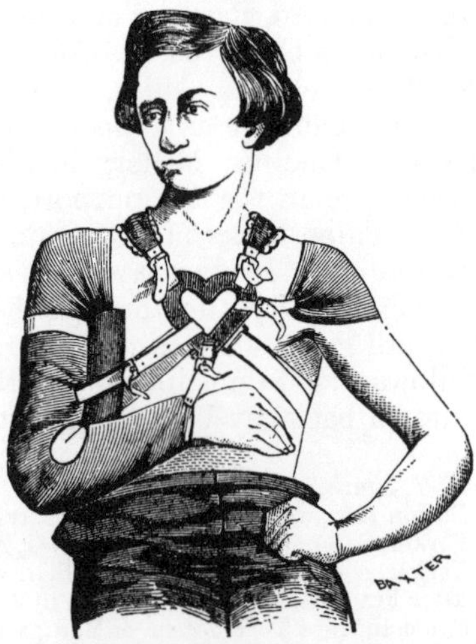

Front view of Welch's apparatus.

[1] Fox, Liston's Practical Surgery, Amer. ed., p. 47.
[2] Brown, Sargent's Minor Surgery, p. 132.

Fig. 45.

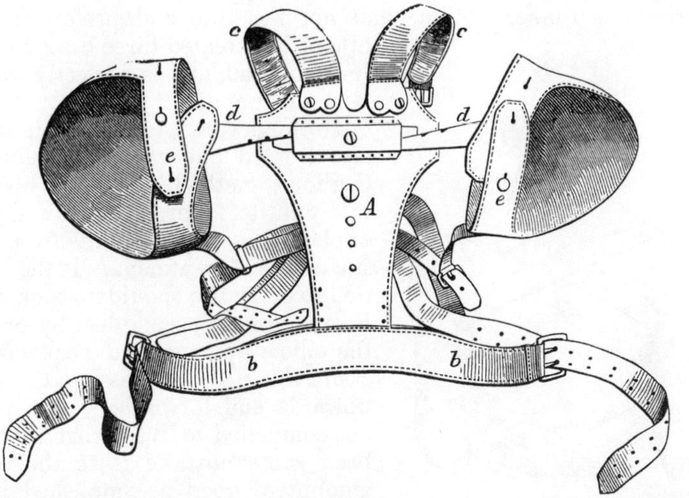

BACK VIEW OF WELCH'S APPARATUS.—*A*. Vertical or dorsal piece. *b*, *b*. Lateral or thoracic arms. *c*, *c*. Oblique or cervical arms. *d*, *d*. Transverse or acromial arms. *e*, *e*. Leather shoulder-caps and straps.

The frame, consisting of the dorsal piece with the thoracic and cervical arms, is formed of flexible metal, which yields sufficiently to adapt it always to the motions of the spine and chest. The lateral or thoracic arms encircle the body, and the vertical or cervical arms, passing upwards, outwards, and forwards, conform to the sides of the neck. The whole are well and thickly padded.

The transverse or acromial arms, running parallel with the spine of the scapula to the acromion process, are made of elastic steel, slightly curved backwards at their outer extremities, so that, when the shoulders are made fast to them by the shoulder-straps, they will tend constantly to pull the shoulders outwards and backwards.

The several parts of the apparatus are adjusted to persons of different sizes.

1st. The cervical arms can be made to approach or to separate from the arch, and they can also be made longer or shorter.

2d. The acromial arms can be lengthened or shortened upon either side, and when in use the arm opposite the broken bone should be longer than the one opposite the sound bone, to give greater freedom to the arm upon this side.

In the front view of the apparatus is seen "a padded metallic ring, the upper edge of which is placed nearly as high as the upper edge of the sternum. Above are straps connecting it with the cervical arms. Laterally is a strap connecting with the shoulder-cap of the sound side, to prevent the central ring from inclining toward the injured side; opposite this is another strap attached also to the sling supporting the arm and drawing the arm of the injured side inwards;" below these are straps connecting with the thoracic arms, and at the inferior point of the ring is a strap designed to support the hand and forearm.

"The sling in which the arm rests has thin strips of metal sewed into the cloth, at the sides of the arm both above and below the elbow, with rings for the straps, in order to give a uniform and unyielding support to the arm the entire length of the sling."

The axillary pad may be made in the usual form, and secured in the ordinary mode.

Lonsdale carry the elbow still further forwards, so as to lay the hand across the opposite shoulder, while Guillou carries the hand and forearm behind the patient, and then proceeds to lift the shoulder to its place.

Thus Desault, Fox, and Wattman accomplish the indication to carry the shoulder back, by lifting the humerus while the elbow is in *front* of the body, and Guillou accomplishes the same indication by lifting the humerus when the elbow is a little *behind* the body. Chelius also says: "The elbow, as far as possible, is to be laid backwards on the body."

Sargent, who believes that with Fox's apparatus "the occurrence of deformity is the exception," and not the rule, and prefers it to all others, has treated three cases by Guillou's method, and is perfectly satisfied with its operation.

Fig. 46.

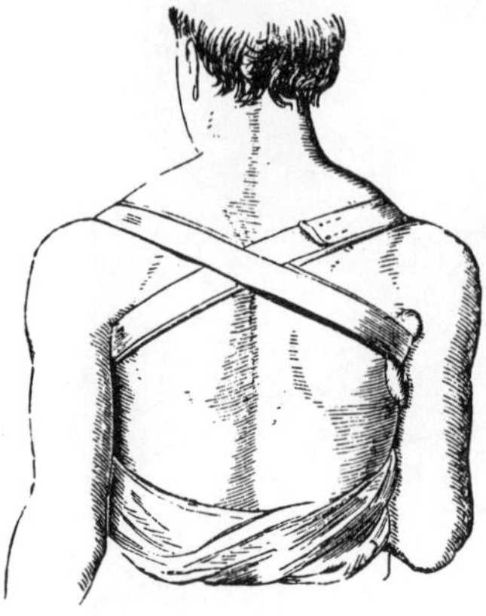

Figure-of-8.

Hollingsworth, of Philadelphia, has also treated one case successfully by Guillou's method, and adds his testimony in its favor. But how shall we explain these equal results from opposite modes of treatment? Is the indication to carry the shoulders back, which Fox sought to accomplish by pressing the elbow upwards and backwards, as easily attained by pressing the elbow upwards and forwards? Or are we not compelled to infer that there has been some mistake as to the precise amount of good accomplished by the apparatus in either case? Moreover, Coates,[1] Keal, and others, instruct us that the only safe and proper position for the humerus is in a line with the side of the body, and that it must neither be carried forwards nor backwards.

Paulus Ægineta, Boyer, Desault, Pecceti, Liston, Fergusson, Samuel Cooper, Erichsen, Miller, Skey, Dorsey,[2] Gibson,[3] Fox, H. H. Smith,[4] Norris,[5] Sargent, Eastman,[6] recommend an axillary pad, while Richerand, Velpeau, Dupuytren, Benjamin Bell, Syme, deny its utility, or affirm its danger. Dr. Parker has seen one patient in whom paralysis of the arm resulted from the pressure upon the brachial nerves, in the attempt "to *pry* the shoulder out;" and I have myself recorded another.

Cabot, of Boston, Massachusetts, has recommended a mould of gutta percha laid over the front and top of the chest.[7]

Desault's plan, which took its origin, as Velpeau thinks, in the spica of Glaucius, under various modifications, is recommended by Delpech, Cruveilhier, Lasere, Flamant, Samuel Cooper, Fergusson, Liston, Cutler, Physick, Dorsey, Coates, and Gibson; while by Velpeau, Syme, Colles, Chelius, Samuel Cooper, and Parker, it is regarded as inefficient and troublesome. Says Mr. Cooper: "In this country, many surgeons prefer Desault's bandages; but I do not regard them as meeting the indications, and consider them worse than useless."

[1] Coates, Amer. Journ. Med. Sci., vol. xviii. p. 62.
[2] Dorsey, Elements of Surgery, vol. i. p. 133.
[3] Gibson, Institutes and Practice of Surgery, vol. i. p. 271.
[4] H. H. Smith, Practice of Surgery, p. 354.
[5] Norris, Liston's Practical Surg., Amer. ed., p. 46.
[6] Eastman, Apparatus for Fractured Clavicle, by Paul Eastman, of Aurora, Ill.; Boston Med. and Surg. Journ., vol. xxiii. p. 179.
[7] Cabot, Bost. Med. and Surg. Journ., vol. lii. p. 232.

The dextrine bandages, or *apparatus immobile*, of Blandin, Velpeau, and others, constitute only another form of the bandage dressing of Desault. In this connection it ought to be noticed that Velpeau does not regard the employment of this apparatus, or of any other demanding great restraint, as imperative. In his great work on anatomy, referring to the fact that when the bone is broken and overlapped, the patient is still able, in many cases, to move the arm freely, he remarks: "Do not these cases give support to the opinion of those who admit that fractures of the clavicle do not actually require any other apparatus than the simple supporting bandage?" "It is necessary to observe," he adds, "that by thus acting we do not prevent an overlapping,"[1] etc.

The sling, in some of its forms, is employed by Richerand, Huberthal, Colles, Miller, Fox, Stephen Smith,[2] H. H. Smith, Bartlett,[3] Levis,[4] Dugas,[5] Benjamin Bell, Bransby Cooper, Earle, Chapman, Keal, and by a large majority of the English surgeons; while Dr. Gibson declares the sling bandage employed so much by the English, "the most inefficient, contemptible, and injurious of all contrivances for such purposes."

Fig. 47.

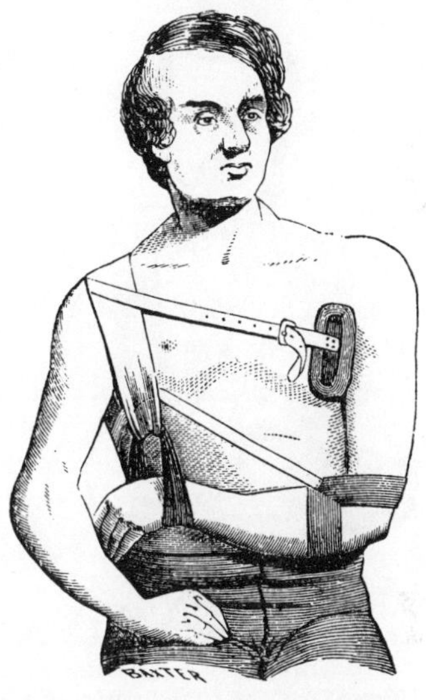

E. BARTLETT'S APPARATUS.—"For an axillary pad, roll a strip of woollen flannel, four or five inches wide, around the axillary strap, to the size required. The apparatus may be used for either side by changing the attachment of the sling." (*Bartlett.*)

No apparatus, perhaps, has been so generally employed, among American surgeons, as that form of the sling introduced by Dr. George Fox into the Pennsylvania Hospital in 1828; since which time no other has ever been used in that institution for the treatment of broken clavicles.

Sargent says of it: "Fractures of the clavicles, treated by this apparatus, are daily dismissed from the Pennsylvania Hospital, and by surgeons in private practice, cured without perceptible deformity."

Norris, in a note to *Liston's Practical Surgery*, affirms that "the chief indications in the treatment of fracture of the clavicle are perfectly fulfilled by the use of this apparatus."

Smith, in his *Minor Surgery*, declares that Fox's apparatus accomplishes "perfect cures" in very many cases, and that it is "a very rare thing for a simple case to go out of the house (Pennsylvania Hospital)

[1] Velpeau, Anatomy, Amer. ed., vol. i. p. 242.

[2] Stephen Smith, New York Journ. Med., vol. ii. 3d series, p. 384 (May, 1857).

[3] Bartlett, My "Report on Defor." etc., Appendix; also Bost. Med. and Surg. Journ., vol. li. p. 404.

[4] Levis, H. H. Smith's Practice of Surg., p. 365.

[5] Dugas, Report on Surgery.

with any other deformity save that which time cures, viz. the deposition of the provisional callus." He has also repeated substantially the same opinion in his larger work entitled *Practice of Surgery*.

Such testimony in favor of any dressing demands respectful attention; and I shall not be regarded as detracting from the respect due to these authorities, when I express my belief that it is in deference to the distinguished reputation of the surgeons who have during the last thirty years had charge of the services in that hospital, and who have been so loud in its praise, that the use of this apparatus has, with us, become so general. I believe, also, that, in some measure, this general preference is due fairly to the intrinsic excellence of the dressing. But I must be permitted to express a doubt whether it has made deformities of the clavicle "the exception, instead of the rule," with us. I have used this dressing oftener than any other form, and yet my success has by no means been so flattering as has been the success of these gentlemen. I have seen others employ it, also, and with pretty much the same results. Nor ought it to be forgotten that, in Great Britain, by far the greater majority of surgeons employ an apparatus essentially the same. I have seen it in many of the hospitals, and Mr. Bickersteth, one of the surgeons of the Liverpool Infirmary, informed me, in 1844, that it had been in use with them as long as thirty years. All that has justly been said against the English mode of dressing by slings, is equally true of this; and whatever has been affirmed of the danger of using an axillary pad applies as much to this as to any other mode of using the same.

Fig. 48.

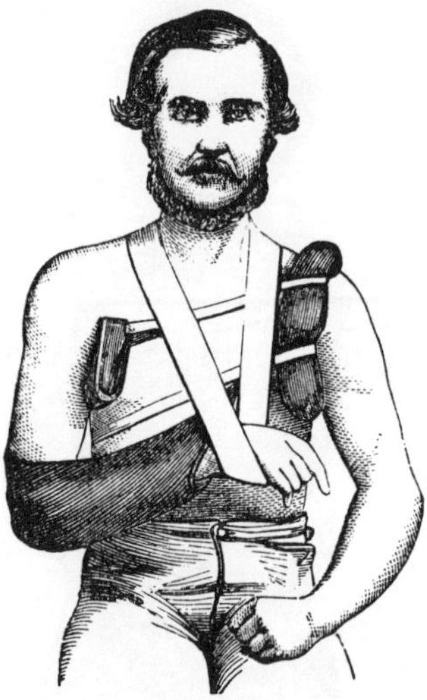

George Fox's Apparatus "consists of a firmly stuffed pad of a wedge shape, and about half as long as the humerus, having a band attached to each extremity of its upper or thickest margin; a sling to suspend the elbow and forearm, made of strong muslin, with a cord attached to the humeral extremity, and another to each end of the carpal portion; and a ring made of muslin stuffed with cotton to encircle the sound shoulder, and serve as means of acting upon and receiving the sling." (*Sargent.*)

I believe, however, that in the Pennsylvania Hospital, the axillary pad employed is not so large, and especially, not so thick, as that recommended by Desault, and in this respect it is plainly an improvement; but then, in the same proportion that it is made less thick, it is less powerful to accomplish the indication in question; and if it merely fills the axillary space, then it is no longer a fulcrum upon which the arm is to operate as a lever, but it is only, in its effect, "retentive."

Regarding, then, the importance of this question to the interests of surgery, and observing the wide differences of opinion which are entertained here and elsewhere as to the real value of this dressing, is it asking too much of these gentlemen that they will present us some more precise statistical testimony? It will be observed that its advocates claim for it what is not to-day, at least, claimed for any other apparatus, viz: that, under its use in the Pennsylvania Hospital, and in the hands of private practitioners, so far as they have seen, deformities have become the "exception." It is affirmed to answer "perfectly" *all* the indications. By which it must be intended to say, that, in addition to both of the other indications, that also, which has always heretofore been found so difficult, if not impossible, the carrying out of the shoulder, is in a majority of cases perfectly accomplished—the clavicles are not shortened.

If it is intended, however, to say that a shortening is not generally prevented, but only that no unseemly projection of the fractured ends will be found to result, I reply, that then it does not answer *all* the indications; and I beg, further, to suggest that the avoidance of an upward projection seems, to me, to depend much more upon that part of any apparatus which lifts the shoulder, and which belongs to a multitude of other forms of dressing as well as to that in question, than upon that which forces the shoulder out, and it may be accomplished, in a majority of cases, as well without an axillary pad, with a mere sling, as with it. But, in fact, my experience has convinced me that the absence or presence of such a projection, after union, is due much to the circumstances of the fracture, as to whether it is more or less oblique; and still more especially, to the degree of roundness, or emaciation of the patient, rather than to any form, or part, or condition of the apparatus. It will be found more distinct in oblique fractures than in transverse, and much more marked in thin persons than in plump, or fat persons, and more so in muscular than in non-muscular. In short, I affirm that such a projection has occurred as often under my observation, when this dressing has been used, as it has when other forms have been employed.

Finally, while I deprecate incautious assumptions in regard to the capabilities of any form of dressing for broken collar bones, a disposition to which is manifested by more than one advocate of special plans, I am ready to bear my humble testimony in favor of that one of whose claims I have taken the liberty to speak so freely, and which is usually known in this country by the name of Fox's apparatus, consisting essentially of a sling, axillary pad, and bandages to secure the arm to the chest, and to which the stuffed collar is a convenient accessory, but admits of various modifications, answering the same ends. Among the considerable variety of dressings which I have used, this, either with or without such slight modifications as I shall presently suggest, has seemed to be most simple in its construction, the most comfortable to the patient, the least liable to derangement (if I except Velpeau's dextrine bandage), and as capable as any other of answering the several indications proposed.

No apparatus is better able to answer the first indication, namely, "to carry the shoulder up," and thus to bring the fragments into line. If, as not unfrequently happens, the outer end of the inner fragment is also carried a little upwards and forwards, it may be, in some measure, replaced by inclining the head to the injured side, or by a carefully adjusted compress and bandage. But it is not probable that any patient will consent to remain a long time in a position so unnatural and constrained; nor is it very easy, as the experiment will show, to maintain a steady pressure upon this portion of the broken clavicle.

The second indication, "to carry the shoulder back," is certainly much more difficult of accomplishment than the first; and it does not seem to me to be fully met by the sling dressing, but, until some mode is devised less objectionable than any I have yet employed, or than any, the mechanism of which I have seen described, I see no alternative but to trust to that action of the muscles attached to the scapula, by which, as Desault first explained, when the shoulder is lifted perpendicularly, it is also in some degree carried backwards, and that, too, it has occurred to me frequently to observe, just as much as when the upward pressure is made with the elbow placed in front of the body.

It is my belief, however, from the evidences now before us, that the third indication, "to carry the shoulder out," still remains unaccomplished; that it cannot be claimed for this, or for any other apparatus yet invented, that, in a certain class of cases which I have sufficiently indicated, constituting a vast majority of the whole number, it is able to prevent a riding of the fragments. Nor, seeing the difficulties in the way, and the amount of talent which has been already devoted to their removal, have I much confidence that this end, so desirable, and so diligently sought, will ever be attained. Yet it is presumptuous, perhaps, to say what the skill and ingenuity of a profession whose labors never cease, may not hereafter accomplish.

Having already expressed my preference for the sling, I have only to add what I consider necessary modifications in the form of this dressing recommended by Dr. Fox.

Dr. Coates, in the excellent paper already referred to,[1] calls attention to the danger of making too much pressure upon the brachial artery and nerves, when the axillary pad is used, and the arm is, at the same time, carried forwards upon the body. In bringing the elbow forwards so as to lay the forearm across the body, the humerus is made to rotate inwards, and the brachial artery and nerves are brought into more direct apposition with the pad. The same objection must hold, only in a greater degree, to M. Guillou's method of carrying the forearm across the back.

The humerus ought then to be permitted to hang perpendicularly beside the body, and thus the nerves and bloodvessels will be removed in a great measure, yet not entirely, from pressure. The pad (to be employed only as a part of the retentive means, and not as a fulcrum) should be no thicker than is necessary to fill completely the axillary space when the elbow is made to press snugly against the side of the body.

In consequence of having placed the elbow farther back than is recommended by Dr. Fox, it will be necessary, also, to vary in some

[1] Am. Journ. Med. Sci., vol. xviii. p. 62.

way, the suspensory tapes; those coming from the humeral portion of the arm-tray must pass in equal numbers, and in opposite directions —before and behind the body—toward the stuffed collar; and each set of front and back tapes, attached to the humeral portion of the tray, must be in pairs, for the convenience of tying. I find it necessary also to secure the arm to the body by two or three turns of a roller, applied always lightly and with great care, so that its pressure shall be in no degree painful or uncomfortable.

Fig. 49.

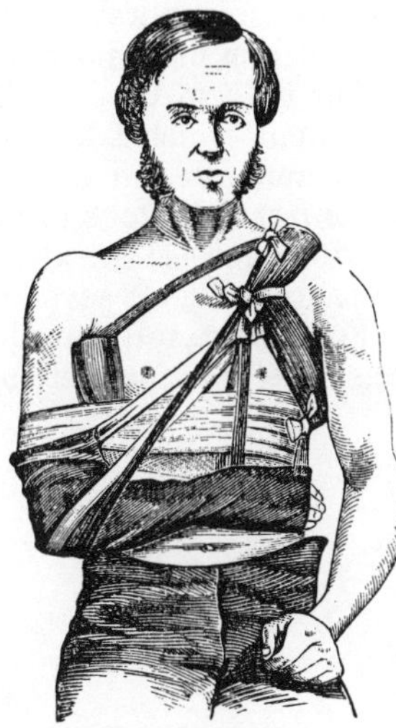

The Author's Apparatus.

An experience, limited to the two following examples, induces me to think that very many cases would be brought to a conclusion equally satisfactory without any form of apparatus, by retaining the patient a few weeks in the recumbent posture upon the back, as recommended by Hippocrates and others; and to which plan allusion has already been made.

Jan. 2, 1856—Mary Ann S., æt. 24, fell down a flight of stairs, breaking the right collar bone obliquely near its middle. She was unwilling to submit to bandages, and I directed her simply to lie upon her back in bed. On the fourteenth day the fragments had united; and at the end of the third week I dismissed her with an overlapping of the fragments of less than half an inch, and with scarcely any perceptible deformity.

Alexander Mooney, æt. 33, was admitted to the Buffalo Hospital, December 3, 1856, with an oblique fracture of the left clavicle, at the outer end of the middle third. On measurement we found the fragments overlapped nearly half an inch.

In presence of a class of medical students I applied Bartlett's apparatus, a very ingenious and convenient form of the sling dressing, and the same which is now in use at the Mass. General Hospital, in Boston. On the following day the apparatus was found to be loose, and it was carefully retightened. On the third and fourth day, also, it was found necessary to readjust it more or less, and the fragments of the broken clavicle continued to overlap.

On the fifth day Bartlett's apparatus was removed, and the patient laid upon his back in bed, with his arm simply tied to the side of his body by a few turns of a roller.

On the tenth day all motion had ceased between the fragments; but he was kept in bed three weeks.

Jan. 10, 1857, he was discharged from the hospital, with an overlapping of only about one quarter of an inch, and with scarcely any perceptible deformity.

In cases of partial fracture accompanied with a persistent bend in the line of the axis of the bone, it is proper to make some attempt by moderate pressure directly upon the salient fragments, to restore them to place; but I confess that I have never yet succeeded in accomplishing anything in this way. Nor is it a matter of much consequence, I imagine, since, as I have already explained when speaking of partial fractures in general, the line of the axis of the bone will eventually, at least in a majority of cases, be completely restored.

The only treatment which seems then to be indicated, and the only treatment which I have of late adopted in these cases, is to place the hand and forearm of the child in a sling, or I direct the mother to make fast the sleeve to the front of the dress in such a way that the child cannot use the arm until the union is consummated. Even this precaution I have several times omitted with no injury to the patient.

For a more full consideration of partial fractures of the clavicle, I beg to refer the reader to the chapter on "Partial Fractures," &c.

CHAPTER XIX.

FRACTURES OF THE SCAPULA.

FRACTURES of the scapula may be divided into those which occur through the body, the neck, the acromion, and coracoid processes.

§ 1. FRACTURES OF THE BODY OF THE SCAPULA.

Under this title I propose to consider not only fractures of the "body" properly speaking, but also fractures of the angles and of the spine.

Causes.—It is usually broken by the fall of some heavy body directly upon the bone, or by some severe crushing accident, by the kick of a horse, by a fall upon the back—in short, by direct causes alone, and by such causes as operate with great violence.

Malgaigne says that a Doctor Heylen has recently published a case of this fracture which he believes to have been the result of muscular action, occurring in a man forty-nine years old. The case, however, is not stated so clearly as to relieve us entirely of a doubt as to the nature and cause of the accident.

I have myself had occasion to treat but one case, and that was produced by a fall upon the back. It was a fracture of the body below the spine. Dr. Neill called my attention to a fracture involving the spine of the scapula then under treatment in the Pennsylvania Hospital, in the year 1855. I do not now remember to have ever seen another example. There are two cabinet specimens of fracture of the body of the scapula below the spine in the Pennsylvania

Medical College, and two involving the spine. Dr. Mütter has in his collection a fracture of the posterior angle, and Dr. March has a specimen of fracture of the body. I believe that Dr. Charles Gibson, of Richmond, has also one or two specimens of this fracture. I know of no other museum specimens in this country except my own of partial fracture, described in the chapter on Partial Fractures.

Ravaton, after a practice of fifty years, declared that he had never seen a fracture of the scapula, except as it had been produced by firearms. Among 2358 fractures reported from Hôtel Dieu during a period of twelve years, only four examples of fracture of the scapula are recorded; and at Middlesex Hospital, Lonsdale has noticed among 1901 fractures, only eight of the body of the scapula.

The infrequency of this fracture is no doubt due in a great measure to the elasticity of the ribs, to the mobility of the scapula, and to the softness of the muscular cushion upon which it reposes.

Symptoms.—Since this bone is seldom broken except by great force directly applied, the usual signs of fracture are likely to be concealed by the speedy occurrence of swelling. It is for this reason that it becomes necessary generally that the examination should be made with great care before we can safely determine upon the diagnosis. I have more than once had occasion to correct the diagnosis of other practitioners who believed they had discovered a fracture of the scapula.

When the line of the fracture has traversed the spine, and any considerable displacement has occurred, one ought to recognize the fracture easily by merely carrying the finger along the crest. In the example to which Dr. Neill called my attention in the Pennsylvania Hospital, although there was scarcely any displacement, the point of fracture could be distinctly felt. It is only when the swelling over the seat of fracture is very great that any difficulty in the diagnosis need to exist, or perhaps in the case of a patient who is very fat.

If the fracture has occurred through the body, below or above the spine, or through either of the angles, the displacement may not be so easily recognized. The surgeon ought then to trace carefully with his finger the outlines of the scapula, and this he will be able to do more satisfactorily if he places the scapula in such positions as elevate its margins and render them more prominent. In examining the posterior angle, the hand of the injured limb may be placed upon the opposite shoulder, the forearm being carried across the front of the chest; but in searching for a fracture below the spine, the forearm ought to be laid across the back.

Crepitus, which is not always present, owing to the fact that the fragments overlap completely, or because they have been widely separated by the action of the muscles, may generally be detected by placing the palm of the hand upon some portion of the scapula, so as to steady the fragment upon which it rests, while the arm is moved backwards and forwards, and in various other directions, until their broken surfaces are brought into contact.

Some degree of embarrassment in the motions of the shoulder and arm must always result from this fracture; sometimes this embarrassment is very great, but it ought not to be considered ever as diagnostic of a fracture, since it may be produced equally by a severe contusion; and even when it is accompanied with a fracture, it is due rather to the contusion than to the fracture.

Pathology, seat, direction, &c. Of incomplete fractures of the scapula, I have already mentioned that I have seen one example.

Malgaigne thinks that he has seen one case of incomplete fracture, which occurred in a man who was injured by the fall of a heavy block of stone, upon his back; but as the patient recovered, his diagnosis must remain doubtful. I know of no other recorded examples.

Complete fractures occur most often below the spine, and they are generally oblique or transverse, sometimes nearly longitudinal.

Fractures involving the spine are noticed occasionally, but I am not aware that any one has ever seen a specimen of a fracture of the spine alone, although many surgeons have spoken of them.

Fig. 50.

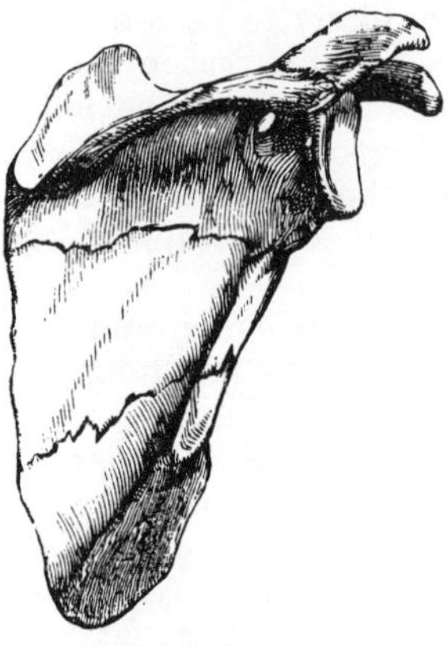

Fractures of the body and acromion process of the scapula.

I have mentioned one example of a fracture of the posterior angle as being in the cabinet of Dr. Mütter, of Philadelphia. Malgaigne seems to doubt its existence, but speaks of it as a fracture which surgeons have "imagined."

Occasionally the bone is broken into more than two fragments.

As a result of the fracture there is usually more or less displacement; generally, if the fracture is below the spine and transverse, and especially if its direction is oblique from before backwards and downwards, the inferior fragment is displaced forwards, or forwards and upwards, by the action of the serratus major anticus, or of the teres major, while the superior fragment is inclined to fall backwards, and sometimes it is carried upwards and backwards, following the action of the rhomboideus major.

In cases of comminuted fracture, and occasionally in simple fractures, the direction of the displacement is reversed, or altogether changed, so that the lower fragment instead of being in front is behind the upper fragment, and instead of overlapping, the two fragments are more or less drawn asunder. These are deviations which are not easily explained, but which depend, perhaps, rather upon the direction of the blow than upon the action of the muscles.

In a few cases there is no displacement in any direction, although the crepitus with mobility sufficiently demonstrates the existence of a fracture.

Prognosis.—If displacement actually has taken place, it will be found very difficult, as we shall see when we come to consider the treatment, to hold the fragments in apposition, until a cure is completed: so that they are pretty certain to unite with a degree of overlapping, or other irregularity.

Lonsdale, Lizars, Chelius, Nélaton, Gibson, Malgaigne, and others have spoken of the difficulty or impossibility generally of keeping these fragments in place. Nélaton and Malgaigne, indeed, confess that they have never succeeded; Gibson declares that it is scarcely possible; while Chelius affirms, that if the fracture is near the angle the cure is always effected with some deformity.

But then it is not probable that the patient will ever suffer any serious inconvenience from this irregular union of the fragments, since the perfection of its function depends less upon any given form or size than in the case of almost any other large bone; and if, as has been observed by Lonsdale, the free use of the arm is not recovered for some time, or if, as has been noticed by B. Bell, a permanent stiffness results, these should be regarded as due to the injury which those muscles have suffered which envelop the scapula, or to some injury of the ligaments and muscles which surround the shoulder-joint.

In some few examples upon record, the bone has been so comminuted, and the soft parts adjacent so much injured that suppuration and necrosis have ensued.

Treatment.—In the treatment of this fracture, the first object with all surgeons has been to restore the fragments to place, and this they have chiefly sought to accomplish by position; after which, they have endeavored to immobilize the fragments by bandages, &c.

In seeking to accomplish the first indication, they have placed the shoulder and arm in a great variety of postures. Nearly all seem to have regarded it as of some importance that the shoulder should be elevated, so as to relax the muscles attached to the upper and back part of the scapula, and thus permit the upper fragment to fall downwards and forwards.

If we confine our remarks first to fractures through the body, and do not include fractures of the inferior angle, this indication is the only one which Nélaton and Mayor have sought to accomplish, and for this purpose they employ a simple sling, while Amesbury, Liston, Lonsdale, S. Cooper, South, Skey, Miller, Pirrie, have added to the sling a bandage or roller, which is made to inclose snugly the body and arm.

Erichsen uses the body bandage alone, as in fractures of the ribs, while B. Cooper, Lizars, and Tavernier employ a bandage which incloses not only the body, but also the arm; neither of these last-mentioned surgeons recommends a sling, or any other means to elevate the arm.

Johannes de Gorter advises that a sling shall be used, but that the elbow shall be lifted away from the side of the body, so as to relax the deltoid. Chelius and Desault recommend the same position, but with the addition of an axillary pad, whose apex shall be directed upwards, secured in place with appropriate bandages.

Pierre d'Argelata used also an axillary pad, but instead of a wedge he recommended a simple roll; and instead of lifting the elbow away from the body, he directed that the elbow should be secured against the side, making use of the axillary roll as a fulcrum.

Petit and Heister advised that the elbow and forearm should be carried forwards upon the front of the chest, and secured in this position.

In the treatment of no other fracture perhaps have surgeons differed more widely as to the indications than in this, since, as we have seen, some recommend the elbow to be carried from the body, and some that it shall be made to approach the body; one directs that the elbow shall fall perpendicularly beside the chest, a second prefers that it shall be carried a little back, and a third that it shall be brought well forwards. In one thing alone have they nearly all agreed, namely, that the elbow shall be lifted; and generally also it has been recommended that the arm, forearm, and body shall be confined by sufficient bandages to insure quietude. It might be proper to conclude, therefore, that the sling and bandage constitute all of the apparatus which is necessary or useful; and that it is relatively unimportant whether the elbow is near or remote from the body, or whether it is in front of, or behind, or beside the chest.

Such, indeed, is the conclusion to which we have ourselves arrived; yet if, in relation to the position of the elbow, a choice were to be expressed, we would give the preference to that in which the arm is laid vertically beside the body, or, perhaps, with the elbow a little inclined backwards, so as to relax as completely as possible the teres major.

It is quite probable, however, that no single position will be found of universal application; and perhaps it would be more safe to advise the surgeon in any given case first to reduce the fragments as completely as possible by manipulation, and then to place the arm in such a position as, upon careful experiment in this particular instance, he shall find enables him to best retain them in place.

If, however, the fracture is such as to have separated the inferior angle from the body, it will be well to follow the advice of Boyer and of others, and to place a compress in front of the inferior angle to resist the greater tendency to displacement in this direction. This compress will more effectually accomplish this indication if the roller with which it is secured to the body, and with which we seek to immobilize the scapula and chest, is turned from before backwards, or in a direction of antagonism to the action of the muscles which produce the displacement.

Desault, with Chelius and Bransby Cooper, has recommended also, in the case of a fracture through the angle, that the forearm should be acutely flexed upon the arm, and that the hand should be placed in front of the chest, upon the sound shoulder, a position which is always irksome, and sometimes insupportable, and which does not offer in any case sufficient advantages to render it worthy of a trial.

§ 2. Fractures of the Neck of the Scapula.

If by "the neck of the scapula," surgeons mean that slightly constricted portion of this bone which is situated at the base of the glenoid cavity, and it is to this portion, we believe, that anatomists have generally applied the term "neck," then its fracture is certainly very rare. Indeed, its existence, uncomplicated with a comminuted fracture of the glenoid cavity, is denied by Sir Astley Cooper, South, Erichsen, and others. Mr. South says there is no such specimen in any of the museums in London; and I have not been able to find one in any of the American cabinets. Dr. Mott has said to me that he had never seen a specimen, and that in the natural condition of the bone he regards its occurrence as impossible. Such, I confess, also, is my own conviction.

Fig. 51.

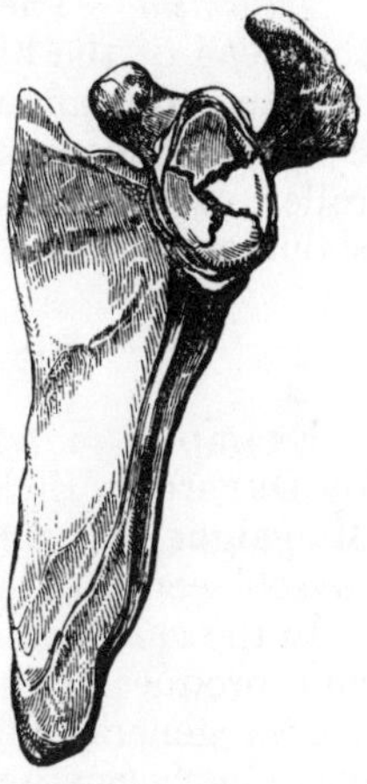

Comminuted fracture of the glenoid cavity.

If, however, it is intended, in speaking of fractures of the neck of the scapula, to refer, as Sir Astley Cooper has done, only to fractures extending through the semilunar notch, behind the root of the coracoid process, then its existence is certain; yet the fracture is not common. Duverney has reported one example, the existence of which he established by a dissection. The coracoid process was broken at the same time, but the fracture through what was called the neck, was distinct from this: and Sir Astley has recorded three examples in which the diagnosis was very clearly made out, yet not actually proven by an autopsy.

Symptoms.—Sir Astley justly remarks that "the degree of deformity produced by this accident depends upon the extent of laceration of a ligament which passes from the under part of the spine of the scapula to the glenoid cavity. If this be torn" (and to this we ought to add the ligaments passing from the coracoid process to the clavicle and acromion process) "the glenoid cavity and the head of the os humeri fall deeply into the axilla, but the displacement is much less if this remains whole."

Fig. 52.

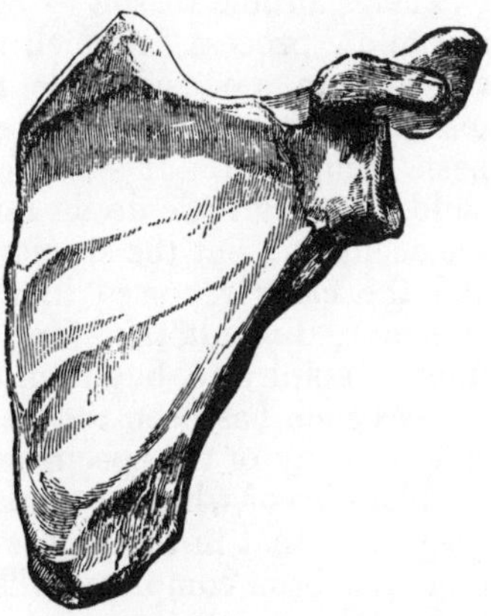

Fracture of the neck of the scapula; according to A. Cooper.

The usual signs are, a depression under the acromion process, the same as in dislocation of the head of the humerus downwards, but not so deep; the head of the humerus felt, perhaps, in the axilla; crepitus, and the immediate recurrence of the displacement whenever, after the reduction has been fairly accomplished, the arm is left unsupported. The crepitus is best discovered by resting one hand upon the top of the shoulder in such a manner as that a finger shall touch the point of the process, while the arm is rotated and moved up and down by the opposite hand. It may also be easily ascertained that the coracoid process moves with the humerus instead of the scapula. Occasionally, the accident is accompanied with paralysis of the arm, from pressure upon the axillary nerves, and a rupture of the axillary artery is also mentioned by Dugas.[1]

Treatment.—The indications of treatment are three, namely, to carry the head of the humerus, with the glenoid cavity, &c., up, to carry it out, and to confine the body of the scapula. The first is accomplished by a sling, the second, by a pad in the axilla, and the third by a broad roller carried repeatedly around the arm and chest and across the shoulder.

§ 3. Fractures of the Acromion Process.

Examples of fracture of the acromion process have been reported by Duverney, Bichat, Avrard, A. Cooper, Desault, Sanson, Nélaton, Malgaigne, West,[2] Brainard,[3] Stephen Smith,[4] and others. I have myself seen three examples.[5]

In the case seen by Cooper it entered the articulation of the clavicle, and produced at the same moment a dislocation. Malgaigne says it occurs generally farther up, and posterior to the attachments of the clavicle, "near the junction of the diaphysis with the epiphysis," and that the fracture is in most cases transverse and vertical; but Nélaton saw a case in which the fracture was oblique. In the case reported by C. West, of Hagerstown, Md., the fracture was through the base of the process. In two of the examples seen by me the fracture was in front of the clavicle; and in the third, occasioned by the fall of a barrel of flour upon the shoulder, the fracture occurred at the acromio-clavicular articulation, and was accompanied with an upward dislocation of the outer end of the clavicle.

There is some reason to believe, I think, that a true fracture of the acromion process is much more rare than surgeons have supposed, and that in a considerable number of the cases reported there was merely a separation of the epiphysis; the bony union having never been completed. If such fractures or separations occurred only in children, very little doubt might remain as to the general character of the accident: but the specimens which I have found in the museums, and the cases reported in the books, have been mostly from adults. It is more difficult, therefore, to suppose these to be examples of separations of epiphyses, but I am inclined to think that in a majority of instances such has been the fact. It is very probable, also, that in the case of many of the specimens found in the museums, called fractures, the histories of which are unknown, they were united originally by cartilage, and that in the process of boiling, or of maceration, the disjunction has been completed. The narrow crest of elevated bone which frequently surrounds the process at the point of separation, and which

[1] Remarks on Frac. of Scapula, by L. A. Dugas, Georgia. Am. Journ. Med. Sci., Jan. 1858.

[2] West, Penin. Journ. of Med., vol. v. p. 254.

[3] Brainard, Bost. Med. and Surg. Journ., vol. xxxi. p. 501.

[4, 5] S. Smith. Hamilton, Report on Deform., op. cit.

Malgaigne may have mistaken for callus, is found upon very many examples of undoubted epiphyseal separations which I have examined; and this circumstance, no doubt, has tended to strengthen the suspicion that these were cases of fracture.

This opinion is confirmed by the remark of Mr. Fergusson, that a fracture of this process is an accident "of rare occurrence." "I have dissected," he adds, "a number of examples of apparent fracture of the end of this process; but in such instances it is doubtful if the movable portion had ever been fixed to the rest of the bone." But the most complete explanation is furnished by that distinguished pathologist Dr. J. B. S. Jackson, of Boston, who observes that this process ossifies in two pieces, instead of one, as has usually been stated by anatomists; so that we may find an example of a short epiphysis or of a long one, a difference which many of the cabinet specimens present, although the usual length is about three-quarters of an inch. These two extreme points of ossification first coalesce, and then unite with the body. Dr. Jackson says, moreover, that there are four specimens in the museum of the Massachusetts Medical College, and in the museum of the Boston Society for Medical Improvement, which might easily be mistaken for fractures, but which only illustrate to how late a period the bony union is sometimes delayed. In one specimen the patient could not have been less than forty years of age; "the acromial process of each scapula was fully formed, but having no bony union whatever with the bone itself. The union was ligamentous, but strong and close."[1]

To the same class belong several specimens in my own collection; specimens 163 and 997 in Dr. March's collection; 707 in the Albany College collection; two specimens in the Mütter, and one in the Jefferson Medical College museums.

I wish to mention, also, that in the case of my own specimens of epiphyseal separation, as well as most of the specimens which I have examined, the ends of the fragments were closed with a compact bony tissue.

No doubt, however, a fracture of this process does occasionally take place. In addition to my own, I have already mentioned several other examples, some of which have been confirmed by dissection: and in the case mentioned by Stephen Smith, an autopsy, made three weeks after the accident, showed a fracture without displacement, the periosteum covering its upper surface not being torn; the fragment could be turned back as upon a hinge.

Prognosis.—The process generally unites with a slight downward displacement. This occurred in at least two of the examples seen by me; but in such cases the motions of the arm are not in consequence much, if at all, embarrassed; unless, indeed, it is so much depressed as to interfere with the upward movements of the arm; a result which Heister erroneously supposed was inevitable.

Sir Astley Cooper says that a true bony union is rare in these fractures, and that there generally results a false joint, the fragments

[1] The author's Report on Deform., &c., op. cit.

uniting by a fibrous tissue; but sometimes the surfaces, instead of uniting either by bone or ligament, become polished, and even eburnated.

Malgaigne has noticed, also, in a specimen contained in the Dupuytren museum, a hypertrophy of the lower fragment, this portion having a diameter nearly twice as great as that of the portion from which it was detached.

Symptoms.—Where no displacement exists, the diagnosis must always be difficult, if not impossible. In such a case we could only be instructed by the manner in which the injury had been received, by the contusion, and by the presence of mobility or crepitus.

In examples attended with displacement, if no swelling is present, the finger carried along the spine of the scapula to its extremity, will easily detect the fracture by the abrupt termination of the process, or by the presence of a fissure, or a depression; but as to the other symptoms, they must depend very much upon the point at which the fracture has taken place. If in front of the acromio-clavicular articulation, the position of the arm in its relations to the body will not be changed; but if the fracture is through the articulation, and a dislocation of the clavicle results, or if it is behind the acromio-clavicular articulation, the arm, having in either case lost the support of the clavicle, will assume the same position that it does in a fracture of the clavicle; that is, the shoulder will fall downwards, inwards, and forwards.

Treatment.—If the fracture has taken place in front of the acromio-clavicular articulation, no doubt the most rational plan of treatment is that recommended by Delpech; that is, placing the patient in bed, upon his back, and carrying the arm out from the body nearly to a right angle; since by this method the fragment is not only lifted, but the deltoid muscle is relaxed, and, consequently, the fragment is no longer forcibly drawn away from the spine of the scapula. If, therefore, the patient will submit to this treatment for a sufficient length of time, the union must be accomplished with the least possible amount of displacement. In case he will not consent to such confinement, I am confident no other plan which has been recommended merits a trial, unless it be simply to place the arm in a sling until the union is accomplished.

If, however, the fracture has taken place at, or behind the junction of the clavicle with the process, the indications of treatment must be in all respects the same as in a fracture of the clavicle.

§ 4. Fractures of the Coracoid Process.

I am surprised that Mr. Lizars should have never seen a case, or heard of a well authenticated example of a fracture of the coracoid process. "The coracoid process," he remarks, "is said to be broken off, but this I question very much; it must be along with the glenoid cavity, or there must be a fracture of the neck of the scapula."

Dr. Neill, of Philadelphia, has in his cabinet a specimen of separation of this process at about one inch from its extremity. The line of separation is somewhat irregular; there is no callus, but it is united to the upper portion by a dried tissue, half an inch in length, and continuous with the periosteum. This has been regarded as an example of fracture; but although the scapula is large and evidently belongs to an adult, the fact that the acromion process is not yet united by bone, renders it probable that this, also, is an epiphyseal separation. Prof. Charles Gibson, of Richmond, Va., informs me also that he has in his cabinet a dried specimen, from an adult, which has been broken obliquely near the end, but which is now united by a ligamentous or fibrous tissue of one line and a half in length. The fragment is displaced a little forwards, as well as downwards. Reuben D. Mussey, of Cincinnati, is in possession of a very remarkable and conclusive example of this fracture. The humerus is dislocated forwards, the head and neck being firmly united to the neck and venter of the scapula, while at the same time the coracoid process is broken and displaced. Dr. Jackson, of Boston, says that specimen No. 453 in the museum of the Massachusetts Medical College, seems clearly to have been a fracture involving the base of the coracoid process, and which, having taken place somewhere within a year of the death of the person, had become united by bone, and that just before death the process had broken off, and so completely, as to involve a portion of the glenoid cavity.[1]

Bransby Cooper relates a case of fracture through the base, which after eight weeks, when the patient died, was found to be united by a ligament. The acromion process was broken at the same time, and had united in the same manner. The head of the humerus was also broken and partly united.[2] One example is said to have occurred in the practice of Dr. Arnott, at the Middlesex Hospital, London, in consequence of which the patient died, when a dissection disclosed the true nature of the accident.[3] Mr. South has also reported a case resembling somewhat Mussey's, but much more complicated. The humerus was partially dislocated forwards, the clavicle, acromion process, and the olecranon were broken as well as the coracoid process. Neither the fracture of the clavicle nor of the coracoid process were made out until after the patient died, which was on the fourth day; the fact of the existence of these fractures being then ascertained by dissection.[4] Erichsen says there is in the museum of the University College, a preparation showing a fracture at the base of this process, the line of fracture extending across the glenoid cavity.[5] Duverney, Boyer, and Malgaigne, have also reported four additional examples confirmed by dissections.[6]

The existence of this form of fracture, established by at least nine or ten dissections, can no longer be denied; yet it is usually accompanied with serious complications, such as must in most cases prove

[1] The author's Report on Deformities, op. cit.
[2] B. Cooper, edition of Sir Astley on Frac. and Disloc., Amer. ed., p. 380.
[3] Arnott, Fergusson's Surg., p. 213.
[4] South, Lond. Med.-Chir. Rev., 1840, vol. xxxii., new ser., p. 41.
[5] Erichsen, Surgery, p. 207. [6] Malgaigne, op. cit., p. 512.

fatal. In the only case, however, in which I have had reason to believe that I had to deal with a fracture of this kind, the symptoms and termination were less grave, although it was complicated with an upward dislocation of the outer end of the clavicle. A gentleman residing in this county was struck by a board which fell edgewise upon his shoulder. The fracture of the coracoid process does not seem to have been recognized by his surgeon. An apparatus was applied to retain the clavicle in its place, but after three months, when he called upon me, it still remained displaced as at first. During all of this time the apparatus had been steadily kept on. On laying off the dressings I discovered that the coracoid process was detached, obeying constantly the movements of the head of the humerus, but being not at all subject to the movements of the scapula. Some months later I examined the arm again, and found the parts in the same condition as before, but the functions of the arm were not impaired.

It has been generally stated that when this process is broken off, it will be carried downwards by the united action of the pectoralis minor, the short head of the biceps, and the coraco-brachialis muscles; but this will depend upon whether the coraco-clavicular ligaments are ruptured also; a circumstance which is not very likely to occur, at least to any great extent; and in fact not one of the well-attested examples of this fracture have ever been accompanied with any considerable displacement in this direction.

Fig. 53.

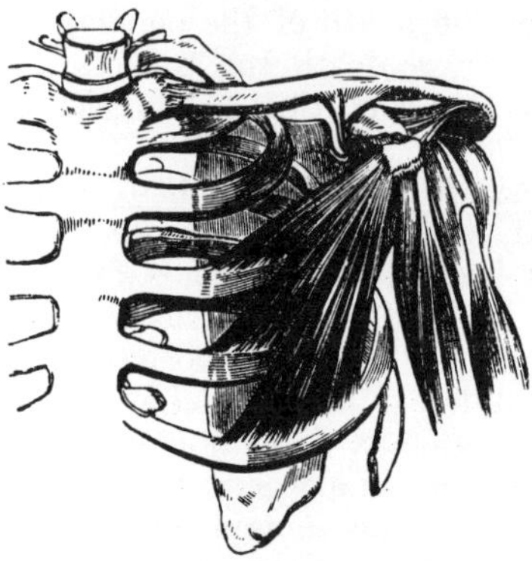

Fracture of the coracoid process.

Treatment.—In case of a simple fracture of the process unattended with any other lesions, it is sufficient to place the arm in a sling with the elbow advanced as much as possible upon the front of the chest; as by this position we relax somewhat all of the three muscles having attachments to this process. If we were to add anything to this simple procedure it would be merely to confine the scapula by a few turns of a roller. It is not probable, however, that by either, or both of these measures we should accomplish enough to justify their continuance if they were found to be painful, or even exceedingly irksome.

In the graver forms of the accident, where other bones about the shoulder are broken or dislocated, which, as we have seen, constitute the largest proportion of the whole number, the treatment must generally have little or no regard to this particular injury.

CHAPTER XX.

FRACTURES OF THE HUMERUS.

It is not sufficient to consider fractures of this bone as occurring through the shaft and its two extremities, as some systematic writers have done; since upon this simple arrangement it is impossible to base a natural division of their causes, symptoms, prognosis, and treatment.

We shall find it necessary to consider,

1. Fractures of the head and anatomical neck. (Intra-capsular; non-impacted and impacted.)
2. Fractures through the tubercles. (Extra-capsular; non-impacted and impacted.)
3. Longitudinal fractures of the head and neck, or splitting off of the greater tubercle.
4. Fractures of the surgical neck. (Including separations at the upper epiphysis.)
5. Fractures through the body of the shaft, or, of the shaft below the surgical neck and above the base of the condyles.
6. Fractures at the base of the condyles. (Including separations at the lower epiphysis.)
7. Fractures at the base, complicated with fractures between the condyles, extending into the joint.
8. Fractures or separations of the internal epicondyle.
9. Fractures or separations of the external epicondyle.
10. Fractures of the internal condyle.
11. Fractures of the external condyle.

Of 90 fractures of the humerus examined by me, 16 occurred through the upper third, 15 through the middle third, and 59 through the lower third. Or, if we reject fractures of the head and neck, and fractures of the condyles, and confine our analysis to the shaft, 12 belong to the upper third, 15 to the middle third, and 27 to the lower third. An observation which is in contrast with the statement made by Amesbury, and which has been repeated by Lizars, B. Cooper, Fergusson, Gibson, and others, that this bone is most often broken in its middle third.

Of the fractures belonging to the upper third, one was a separation at the junction of the epiphysis with the shaft, one was probably a fracture at or near the anatomical neck, with impaction and splitting of the tubercles, one was a fracture of the greater tubercle alone, and eight were fractures of the surgical neck.

Of the fractures belonging to the lower third, 14 were through the internal condyle and epicondyle, 14 through the external condyle, 14 were at the base of the condyles, and 4 through the condyles and across the base at the same time. The remainder, 13, being through the shaft, but above the base.

Unfortunately, surgical writers have not been agreed in the use and application of the terms "head," "neck," "anatomical neck," and "surgical neck" of the humerus; and, as a consequence, their meaning is often obscure, and their teachings are sometimes contradictory and absurd.[1] It is necessary, therefore, that we should define them more precisely.

The head of the humerus is that smooth, elliptical surface, covered by cartilage and synovial membrane, which articulates with, and is received into the glenoid cavity of the scapula.

The anatomical neck is the narrow line immediately encircling the head, and which receives the insertion of the capsular ligament.

The surgical neck is that portion which commences at the lower margin of the tubercles, or at the point of junction between the epiphysis and the diaphysis, and which terminates at the insertion of the pectoralis major and latissimus dorsi.

The neck is all of that portion included between the head and the insertion of the pectoralis major and latissimus dorsi, comprising not only the anatomical and surgical necks, but also the tubercles, which occupy the triangular space between these two.

§ 1. Fractures of the Head and Anatomical Neck. (*Intra-capsular; Non-impacted, and Impacted.*)

Causes.—The causes which have been found competent to produce fractures of the head and anatomical neck are, the penetration of balls or of other missiles directly into the joint, producing thus a compound, and generally comminuted fracture of the head; or falls, or direct blows upon the shoulder without penetration.

Fig. 54.

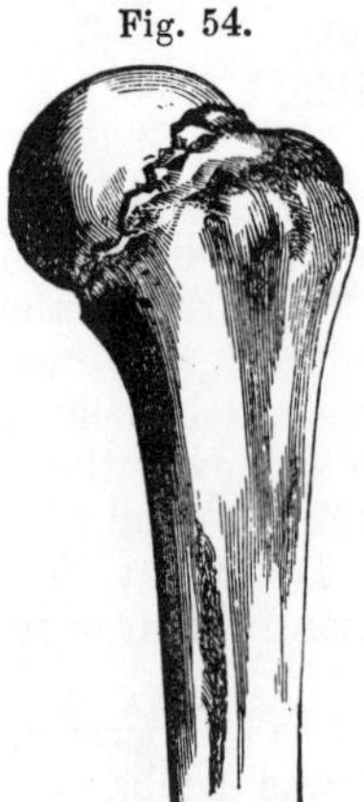

Fracture of the anatomical neck.

Pathology, Results, &c.—When the fracture results from the direct penetration of some foreign body into the joint, it is not only a compound fracture, but the head of the bone is almost necessarily broken into fragments. These accidents are generally fatal; not so much from the peculiar nature of the injury, as from the severity of the blow requisite for their production, and from the complications which usually attend them. If the patients recover, sooner or later the fragments have generally to be removed.

Fractures of the anatomical neck, produced by falls upon the shoulder without penetration, are, however, usually neither compound nor comminuted, but they often follow, with a remarkable degree of accuracy, the line of the insertion of the capsular ligament, being always, according to Robert Smith, within

[1] Boston Med. and Surg. Journ., June 24, 1858, p. 410.

the inferior or outer margin of this insertion. He calls them, therefore, intra-capsular. It is probable, however, since, as we shall presently see, bony union is not denied to this fracture, that the line of separation is not always, or generally, perhaps, completely within the insertion of the ligament, but that it is in some degree extra-articular, if not extra-capsular. If it is entirely intra-articular, no doubt union of the fragments can never take place, and generally suppuration will ensue, demanding, at a period not very remote, an operation for their removal, the same as in compound fractures. Dr. Daniel Brainard, of Chicago, informs me that he has twice had occasion to open the shoulder-joint for the removal of the head of the bone, rendered necessary by the suppuration resulting from severe injuries. In the first case, Dr. Brainard removed the fragment about one year after the accident. It was "loose, necrosed, and partly absorbed or macerated." In the second case the operation was made about three months after the receipt of the injury. Both have recovered, with pretty useful arms.

Gibson, however, thinks that the fragment occasionally remains, being gradually absorbed and changed in figure. He says that his museum contains three or four well-marked cases of this kind, in all of which the head has lost its spherical form, and is very much diminished, and rough and flattened next to the scapula.[1] Other cabinets contain similar specimens.

The displacements to which the upper fragment, or the head of the bone, is subject, are remarkable, and some of them do not seem to be satisfactorily explained. Frequently, indeed, its position is not sensibly disturbed, but at other times it is found impacted, or driven into the cancellous structure of the inferior fragment, in consequence of which one or both of the tubercles are frequently broken off.

Robert Smith relates the following case as having afforded him his first opportunity of ascertaining, by post-mortem examination, the exact nature of this form of displacement:—

"A female, æt. 47, was admitted into the Richmond Hospital under the care of the late Dr. McDowell, for an injury to the humerus, the result of a fall upon the shoulder. Five years afterwards, the woman was again admitted, under the care of Mr. Adams, with an extra-capsular fracture of the neck of the femur, one month after the occurrence of which she died, in consequence of an attack of diarrhœa.

"The shoulder was of course carefully examined; the arm was slightly shortened, the contour of the shoulder was not as full or round as that of its fellow, and the acromion process was more prominent than natural. Upon opening the capsular ligament, the head of the humerus was found to have been driven into the cancellated tissue of the shaft, between the tuberosities, so deeply as to be below the level of the summit of the greater tubercle; this process had been split off and displaced outward; it formed an obtuse angle with the outer surface of the shaft of the bone."[2]

The description is accompanied with two excellent drawings of the

[1] Gibson, Elements of Surgery, vol. i. p. 279.
[2] R. Smith, Fractures in Vicinity of Joints, pp. 191–3.

specimen, showing the distance to which the superior fragment had penetrated the inferior, and showing also complete union by bone.

I believe, also, that in the following example there was a fracture at or near the anatomical neck, with impaction, and splitting of the tubercles:—

January 12, 1858, a young man, aged about sixteen years, fell from a height in a gymnasium, severely injuring his left shoulder. I saw him, with Dr. Boardman, soon after the accident, and found him complaining very much of the shoulder, which was some swollen and tender. He could not tell us how he fell, nor could we discover any contusions by which to determine the point where the blow was received. All motions of the shoulder-joint were painful; and there was a remarkable fulness in front of the joint, feeling like the head of the bone, yet not such as is usually present in a forward luxation. To determine this more positively, however, the limb was manipulated as for the reduction of a dislocation. Once during the manipulation a feeble but distinct crepitus was detected; yet the position of the bone remained unchanged. The head was found to be in the socket, but the precise nature of the injury was not made out.

Fifteen days later, when the swelling had completely subsided, a careful examination was again made by Dr. Boardman and myself, when we arrived at the conclusion that it was a fracture through the bicipital groove, and that the lesser tubercle was carried forward half an inch or more from its fellow, while the head with the greater tubercle, occupied their natural positions opposite the socket. The fragment projecting in front presented a sharp point, and could not be confounded with any swelling of the soft parts. There was a distinct space between the tubercles, into which the finger could be laid. No depression existed under the acromion process behind, but on measurement the head of this humerus was found to be half an inch wider in its antero-posterior diameter than the opposite.

That this fracture was accompanied with impaction was rendered certain by the repeated and careful measurements of the length of the humerus, which constantly showed a shortening of half an inch.

Under these circumstances union generally takes place; but it is usually accompanied with the formation of an irregular mass of osteophytes, which encircle the head like a coronet; presenting in this respect again a remarkable resemblance to extra-capsular fractures of the neck of the femur. This ensheathing callus, as it may be called, is an outgrowth from the inferior fragment, and it sometimes incloses the upper fragment as the case of a watch incloses the crystal, only in a manner much more irregular, thus retaining it steadily in its place, although very little direct union has occurred. The cancellous tissue, nevertheless, is occasionally found united completely by a new and intermediate bony tissue, and at other times by a fibrous tissue, or by both fibrous and bony tissue.

In some cases a perfect false joint has been formed between the opposing surfaces, while in a few unfortunate examples the head not only refuses to unite, but by its presence, as we have already remarked, produces inflammation and suppuration, resulting in its final extrusion from the joint. The cases reported to me by Dr. Brainard, and already described, illustrate this latter class.

At other times the upper fragment turns upon its own axis, and is found more or less tilted or completely rotated in the socket; so that its cartilaginous or articulating surface rests upon the broken surface of the lower fragment, and its own broken surface presents toward the glenoid cavity.

Robert Smith has described a specimen of this kind, which he removed from the body of a woman, aged forty, who many years previous to her death fell down a flight of stairs, and struck her shoulder with great violence against the edge of one of the steps. Whether she applied to a surgeon or not at the time of the accident, Mr. Smith was not able to ascertain. After death the shoulder looked somewhat as if there was a dislocation of the humerus into the axilla, there being a marked depression under the acromion, but the shaft of the humerus was drawn upwards and inwards toward the coracoid process.

When the capsular ligament was opened, the head of the bone was found to have been broken from the shaft through the line of the anatomical neck, and to have completely turned upon itself; and the cartilaginous surface was actually driven one inch into the cancellated structure of the shaft, so as to split off the lesser tubercle with a portion of the greater. Only one-half of the upper fragment was thus impacted, the other half projecting beyond the margin of the lower fragment. Between the cartilaginous surface and the shaft no union had occurred; but there was complete bony union between the upper and lower fragment, beyond the limits of the cartilage.

The upper surface of the superior fragment rested in part against the inner half of the glenoid cavity and upon its inner margin, and in part it rested against the neck of the scapula in the direction of the coracoid process.[1]

Nélaton saw a similar specimen in the possession of M. Dubled, the revolution of the upper fragment being complete; but there was no lateral displacement, and the union had been accomplished in a manner similar to that which is seen after intra-capsular, impacted fractures, without reversion.[2]

I have also been permitted to examine a specimen belonging to Dr. Charles A. Pope, of St. Louis, Mo., which seems to have been broken not only through the line of the anatomical neck, but also through the surgical neck. Both fragments are united by bone, the lower fragment being carried in the direction of the coracoid process, while the upper fragment appears to be reversed, so that its articular surface is directed toward the shaft, and its broken surface articulates with the glenoid cavity. The history of this specimen is unknown.

It is possible, we think, that these extraordinary changes of position were not the direct result of the accident which broke the bone, but that they had been taking place gradually and through a long period. It is certainly quite as probable that the constant motions of the arm

[1] R. Smith, op. cit., pp. 193–6.
[2] Nélaton, Elémens de Pathol. Chirur., tom. prem. p. 730.

Fig. 55.

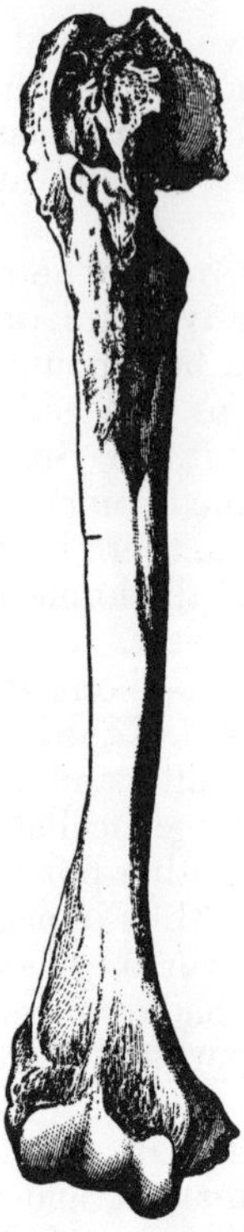

Fig. 56.

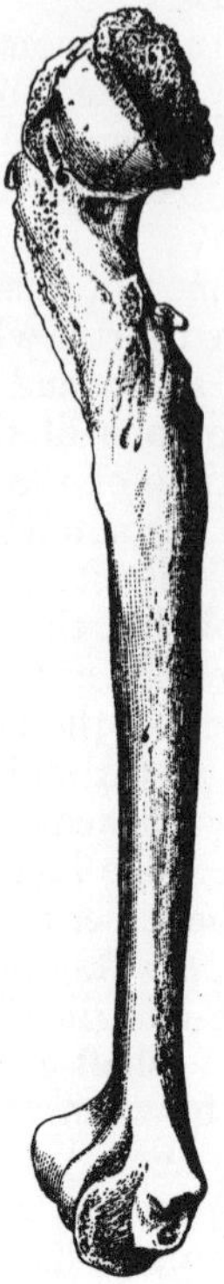

Dr. Pope's Specimen.

Front view. Side view.

should accomplish these displacements, as that they should be produced by a direct blow; indeed, the former supposition appears to us much the most probable.

There is another supposition which, in my opinion, is capable of explaining most of the phenomena usually present in these cases, and which, if admitted, renders the supposition of a fracture unnecessary. It is, that these are all of them examples of softening of the neck of the bone, as a result of chronic inflammation, ulceration, &c.; and that the changed position of the head is due to pressure alone, being acted upon by the muscles which surround the joint, and which act all the more vigorously because they partake also of the inflammation which has invaded the bone. This view of these specimens, which had already more than once suggested itself to me, was very strongly confirmed by its having occupied the mind also of Dr. Neill, of Philadelphia, and who at his own instance stated to me that he believed this was their true explanation. We were, at the time, examining Dr. Pope's specimen, already alluded to, and on comparing it with a specimen of dislocation and partial absorption of the head of the humerus, contained in Dr. Neill's Museum, the points of resemblance were so numerous and striking that we felt compelled to doubt whether Dr. Pope's specimen, together with those seen by Smith and Nélaton, did not belong to the same class with this of Neill's.

In a case of fracture of the "cervix humeri within the capsular ligament," examined by Sir Astley Cooper, there was also a complete forward luxation of the head; but ligamentous union had occurred between the fragments.[1] Many similar cases have been reported by other surgeons.

§ 2. Fractures through the Tubercles. (*Extra-capsular; Non-impacted and Impacted.*)

Under this division we intend to speak of all fractures traversing the upper end of the humerus, and involving the tubercles, or of all

[1] A. Cooper on Dislocations, &c., p. 372.

those which occur between the anatomical neck on the one hand, and the epiphyseal junction, or surgical neck, on the other hand, and which may be more or less oblique as well as transverse. Fractures of the greater or lesser tubercles are of course excepted, since they are more properly longitudinal fractures, and do not completely traverse the diameter of the bone. Nor do we intend to include those fractures which occur at the epiphyseal junction, since, being below the principal insertion of those muscles which are attached to the tubercles, they present very peculiar and distinctive features which will demand for them a separate classification.

Causes, Pathology, and Results.—Fractures through the tubercles, like fractures through the anatomical neck, are the results generally of direct blows received upon the shoulder. They are not usually accompanied with much lateral displacement at the point of fracture; a circumstance which finds a partial explanation in the fact that the line of fracture is through the insertions of the muscles converging upon the tubercles and not entirely above or below them, so that they continue to act nearly equally upon both fragments; but it is also sometimes due in a measure to impaction: the head being forced downwards toward the axilla, and upon the shaft until it is made to ride upon its inner or axillary wall like a cap; the compact bony tissue of the shaft penetrating the reticular structure of the head. These fractures generally unite by bone; yet more or less impairment of the motions of the limb results from the inflammation which occurs in and about the joint, or from the irregular deposits of callus in the vicinity of the fracture.

§ 3. Longitudinal Fractures of the Head and Neck; or Splitting off of the Greater Tubercle.

Causes, Pathology, Symptoms, and Results.—Mr. Guthrie seems to have been the first to call attention to this peculiar injury of the shoulder. In a lecture delivered in November, 1833, he described four cases which had come under his observation, and which he regarded as examples of separation of the small tuberosity, accompanied with more or less of the head, the fracture extending along a portion of the bicipital groove.[1]

Robert Smith, however, believes that it was the greater and not the lesser tuberosity which was thus detached in the cases mentioned by Mr. Guthrie, since the external signs were so nearly like those which were present in a woman seen by himself, and in whom an autopsy enabled him to verify his diagnosis. The following is the case as related by Mr. Smith:—

"In July, 1844, I was requested to examine the body of Julia Darby, æt. 80, who had died of chronic pulmonary disease. Upon entering the room, the appearances of the left shoulder-joint at once attracted my attention, and struck me as being different from those which attend the more common injuries of this articulation.

[1] Robert Smith, p. 181, from London Med. and Phys. Journal.

"The shoulder had lost, to a certain extent, its natural rounded form; the acromion process, although unusually prominent, did not project as much as in cases of dislocation of the head of the humerus. The breadth of the articulation was greatly increased, and upon pressing beneath the acromion, an osseous tumor could be distinctly felt, occupying the greater part of the glenoid cavity; it formed a prominence which was perceptible through the soft parts; it moved along with the shaft of the humerus, but was manifestly not the head of the bone.

"A second and larger tumor, presenting the rounded form of the head of the humerus, lay beneath the base of, and internal to, the coracoid process, and between the two the finger could be sunk into a deep sulcus, placed immediately below the coracoid process. The elbow could be brought into contact with the side, and there was no appreciable alteration in the length of the arm.

"Upon removing the soft parts, the head of the bone presented itself, lying partly beneath and partly internal to the coracoid process. The greater tuberosity, together with a very small portion of the outer part of the head of the bone, had been completely separated from the shaft of the humerus. This portion of the bone occupied the glenoid cavity, the head of the humerus having been drawn inwards so as to project upon the inner side of the coracoid process; it was still, however, contained within the capsular ligament.

"The fracture traversed the upper part of the bicipital groove, which, in consequence of the displacement which the head of the bone had suffered, was situated exactly below the summit of the coracoid process. A new and shallow socket had been formed upon the costal surface of the neck of the scapula, below the root of the coracoid process, and the inner edge of the glenoid cavity corresponded to the posterior part of the sulcus, which separated the head of the bone from the detached tuberosity. The latter was united to the shaft only by ligament.

"The capsule had not been injured, but was thickened and enlarged, and bone had been deposited in its tissue. The injury had evidently occurred many years before the death of the patient, but the history connected with it could not be precisely ascertained."[1]

Mr. Smith relates one other case, in the living subject, which he saw, in connection with Mr. Adams, at the Richmond Hospital, and he adds that "numerous" other living examples have fallen under his observation.

Sir Astley Cooper has also published the particulars of a case of fracture of the greater tubercle, which was communicated to him by Mr. Herbert Mayo.[2]

The following I believe also to have been an example of this rare accident:—

John Hill, æt. 78, fell upon the side-walk, striking upon his right shoulder. The physician to whom he was sent thought the humerus

[1] Robert Smith, op. cit., p. 178.

[2] A. Cooper, on Dislocations and Fractures of the Joints. Edited by B. Cooper. American edition, p. 384.

was dislocated, and directed him to the Buffalo Hospital of the Sisters of Charity, but he did not apply for admission until eight days after, Oct. 14, 1857, when Dr. Boardman and myself examined the limb carefully.

Although we placed him under the influence of chloroform, the diagnosis was not satisfactorily made out. We inclined, however, to the opinion that it was a fracture of the greater tubercle. The antero-posterior diameter of the upper end of the bone was greatly increased; there was occasional distinct crepitus, but the limb was not shortened.

Subsequently, the examinations were repeated many times, and the depression between the fragments becoming more palpable, the diagnosis was at length confirmed.

No treatment was adopted, except confinement in bed, and stimulating embrocations. Two months after the accident he still remained an inmate of the hospital, his shoulder being quite stiff, and the projection continuing in front.

Mr. Robert Smith thinks that when the displacement is considerable, the fragments generally unite by ligament rather than by bone.

§ 4. Fractures through the Surgical Neck. (*Including Separations at the Upper Epiphysis.*)

I have already defined the "Surgical Neck" as all of that narrow portion commencing at the epiphysis and terminating at the insertion of the pectoralis major and latissimus dorsi. It seems proper, therefore, that we should include under this division, both fractures and separations occurring at the epiphysis, especially since, owing to their anatomical relations, they are subject to the same displacements as fractures occurring half an inch or one inch lower down. The capsular muscles, with the exception of the teres minor, having no more influence over the lower fragment when a separation occurs at the epiphysis, than when a separation occurs at any other point of the surgical neck.

Fig. 57.

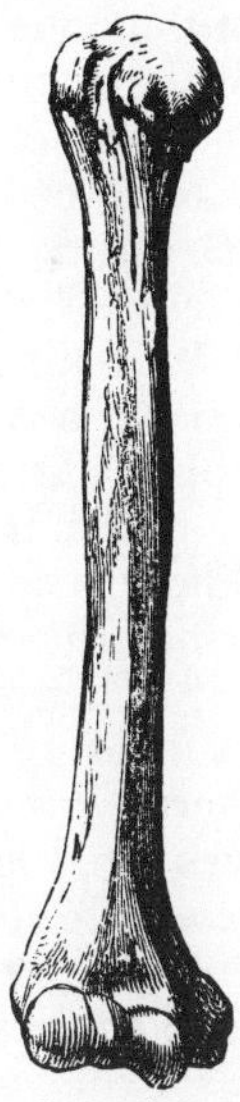

Separation of upper epiphysis.

The following is an account of the only case of separation at the epiphysis which I have ever recognized:—

Mike Bovin, æt. 13 months, fell sideways from his cradle in November, 1855. He was taken to an empiric, who called it a sprain, and applied liniments. Three weeks after the accident he was brought to me, and I found the arm hanging beside the body, with little or no power, on the part of the child, to move it. There was a slight depression below the acromion process, and considerable tenderness about the joint; but the shoulder was not swollen, nor had it been at any time. The line of the axis of the bone, as it hung by the side, was directed a little in front of the socket.

On moving the elbow backwards and forwards, the upper end of the shaft moved in the opposite directions with great freedom, and could be distinctly felt under the skin and muscles. This motion was accompanied with a slight sound, or sensation, a sensation not like the grating of broken bone, but much less rough. There was no shortening of the limb. When the elbow was carried a little forwards upon the chest the fragments seemed to be restored to complete coaptation; and of this I judged by the restoration of the line of the axis of the shaft to the centre of the socket, and by the complete disappearance of the depression under the point of the acromion process.

I applied suitable dressings to retain the arm in this position; but five months after the injury was received the fragments had not united, and the child was still unable to lift the arm, although the forearm and hand retained their usual strength and freedom of motion. The same crepitus could occasionally be felt in the shoulder, and the same preternatural mobility. The shoulder was at this time neither swollen nor tender.

Robert Smith and Sir Astley Cooper both speak of it as a frequent accident in early life, but the recorded cases are very few. The case mentioned by Mr. Smith has been given very much at length, and, as a characteristic example, deserves to be repeated:—

"During the early part of last year, a boy, eight years of age, was admitted to the Richmond Hospital, under the care of Dr. McDowell. About a week previous to his admission he had fallen upon the shoulder, and at once lost the power of using his arm.

"It was at first sight evident that there did not exist any luxation of the head of the humerus, and it was equally obvious that the case was not an example of any of the ordinary fractures to which the neck of the bone is liable. There was no diminution of the natural rotundity of the shoulder, nor any unusual prominence of the acromion process; the head of the bone could be distinctly felt in the glenoid cavity, and it remained motionless when the arm was rotated; there was very little separation of the elbow from the side, but it was directed slightly backwards.

"About three-quarters of an inch below the coracoid process there existed a remarkable and abrupt projection, manifestly formed by the upper extremity of the shaft of the humerus, every motion imparted to which it followed. Its superior surface, which could be distinctly felt, was slightly convex, and its margin had nothing of the sharpness which the edge of a recently broken bone presents in ordinary fractures.

"When this projecting portion of the bone was pushed outwards, so as to bring it in contact with the under surface of the head of the humerus (previously fixed as far as it was possible to do so), a crepitus was produced by rotating a shaft of the bone. It did not, however, resemble the ordinary crepitus of fracture, but it would be extremely difficult, by any description, to convey a clear idea of what the difference consisted in.

"From a careful consideration of the symptoms and appearances above mentioned (taking into account also the age of the patient), the diagnosis was formed, that the injury consisted in a separation of the superior epiphysis of the humerus from the shaft of the bone. Various mechanical contrivances were employed in this case, but all proved ineffectual in maintaining the fragments in their proper relative position."[1]

Sir Astley Cooper has also briefly described one example.

"Its age was ten years. The symptoms of the injury were, inability of moving the elbow from the side, or of supporting the arm, unless by the aid of the other hand, without great pain. The tension which succeeded filled up the hollow which was at first produced by the fall of the deltoid muscle. When the head of the bone was fixed, the fractured extremity of the humerus could be tilted under the deltoid muscle, so as to be felt, and even shown, by raising the arm at the elbow. Crepitus could be perceived, not by rotating the arm, but by raising the bone and pushing it outward. The cause of the fracture was a fall upon the shoulder into a saw-pit of the depth of eight feet."[2]

It will be necessary, in order to a full understanding of the various aspects of this fracture, to relate several illustrative examples.

CASE 1. *Simple fracture; never displaced. Union without deformity.*—Alexander Balentine, æt. 62; admitted to the Buffalo Hospital of the Sisters of Charity, December 19, 1851. He had fallen upon the sidewalk, striking upon his right arm. Dr. Johnson, of Buffalo, had reduced the fracture and applied appropriate dressings. No union of the fragments had yet occurred; but as the surfaces were in apposition, it was only after considerable manipulation, and not until we bent the forearm upon the arm, and rotated the humerus by means of the forearm, that the crepitus became distinct, and gave unequivocal evidence of the existence of a fracture, and of its situation.

The treatment, after admission, consisted in the application of one gutta percha splint, accurately moulded, and extending from above the shoulder to below the elbow, and encircling one-half the circumference of the arm; the splint being secured with the usual bandages, &c.

The result is a perfect limb.

CASE 2. *Simple fracture. Union with displacement and deformity.*—White, of Buffalo, æt. 12, fell fourteen feet, striking on the front and outside of the left shoulder. Dr. P., of Erie County, saw the lad within three hours (July 19, 1853). He was brought to me on the fourth day after the accident. The upper part of the arm was then very much swollen. I found the arm dressed as for a fracture of the middle or lower third of the humerus. It was shortened one inch. The elbow was inclined backwards, and there was a remarkable projection in front of the joint, feeling like the head of the bone. The hand and arm were powerless. I suspected a dislocation of the head of the humerus forwards; and, having administered chloroform, I attempted its reduction with my heel in the axilla. While making extension, I felt a sudden sensation like the slipping of the bone into its socket, but on examination I found the projection continued as before. I then repeated the effort, with precisely the same result.

I now applied an arm sling, and directed leeches and cold evaporating lotions.

[1] Robert Smith, op. cit., p. 201.

[2] A. Cooper, op. cit., p. 382.

On the 25th, five days after the accident, it was examined by Drs. Mixer, McGregor, Joseph Smith, with myself. We still believed it was a dislocation, and having administered chloroform, we again attempted its reduction. The same slipping sensation was produced as before, and the deformity was repeatedly made to disappear; but, on suspending the extension, it as often reappeared.

The character of the accident was now made apparent, and we proceeded at once to apply the splint and bandages suitable for a fracture of the surgical neck of the humerus, namely, a gutta percha splint, extending, on the outside, from the top of the shoulder to below the elbow, with an arm and body roller secured with flour paste.

On the 31st, twelve days after the accident, Dr. Wilcox, Marine Surgeon at Buffalo, saw the arm with me. The fragments were displaced the same as when I first saw it, and the same as when no apparatus was applied. We examined it again carefully, and attempted to make the fragments remain in place, but we were unable to do so, except while holding them and making extension.

August 9 (twenty-first day). I removed all the dressings. Motion between the fragments had ceased, but the projection and shortening remained as before; now, also, the irregular projections of the fractured bones were more distinctly felt. The dressings were never reapplied. Three months later no change had occurred. He could carry the elbow forwards freely, as well as backwards, the motions of the shoulder-joint being unimpaired.

CASE 3. *Simple fracture, with displacement; resulting in deformity and non-union.*—L. B., of Lockport, æt. 43, was thrown from his horse in February, 1854, striking upon his right elbow.

Dr. Maxwell, an experienced surgeon of Lockport, examined and dressed the fracture. Dr. Fassett was present and assisted at a subsequent dressing. Three surgeons who examined the arm before Dr. M., called it a dislocation.

Twelve weeks after the accident, Mr. B. called upon me. The right arm was shortened one inch; the elbow hung off slightly from the body; the upper end of the lower fragment was distinctly felt in front of the shoulder-joint under the clavicle, feeling very much like the head of the bone. The fragments were not united, but they could be seized easily, and made to move separately and freely. He stated to me that he was subject to rheumatism, and especially in the shoulder and arm of the side injured. He wished to know whether it could not be "re-set."

Two years after, I found the bone still ununited. He was, however, able to write with that hand, having first lifted his arm with the other hand and laid it upon the table.

CASE 4. *Simple fracture, probably impacted; resulting in deformity.*—Wm. A., of Buffalo, æt. 15, fell backwards, June 4, 1855, striking on his back and left shoulder. Dr. L. saw it immediately, and, regarding it as a dislocation, attempted its reduction. He subsequently repeated the attempt. I saw the patient with Dr. L. on the tenth day. The arm was shortened one inch and a half. The fragments were displaced forwards, projecting in front of and a little below the joint. As in

Case 3, it might easily be mistaken for the head of the bone; but the difficulty of diagnosis had been very much lessened by the subsidence of the swelling. There was no motion between the fragments; nor could the deformity, by any manipulation or extension, be made to disappear. It was probably impacted.

March 23, 1856, nearly ten months after the accident, I found the fragments remaining as when I first examined the limb, and the arm shortened one inch and a half. The elbow hung a very little back from the line of the body. The upper end of the lower fragment was lifted to within one inch of the head of the humerus; the upper fragment having its head in the socket, with its lower end downwards and forwards. The arm was, however, in every respect as useful as before it was broken. It was equally strong, and he could raise his arm as high, and move it in every direction as freely, as he could the other.

Causes.—Epiphyseal separations belong almost exclusively to children, but true fractures at the surgical neck occur most often in adult life; with the exception of the two lads, one of whom was twelve years old, and the other fifteen, all of the examples of this latter accident seen by me occurred in adults, and of twenty cases in which I find the ages recorded, the average age is forty-three years; yet Sir A. Cooper declares these fractures to be most common in infancy, while Malgaigne has never seen a case in a person under fifty-three years.

Both epiphyseal separations and fractures at this point are occasioned, in most cases, by direct blows or falls upon the shoulder. Of nineteen examples in which I find the cause recorded, fourteen were from direct blows, four from indirect blows, and one from muscular action, as in throwing a ball. Of the four resulting from indirect blows, one was from a fall upon the hand, seen by Desault, and three were from falls upon the elbow, of which two were seen by Desault, and one (Case 4) by myself.

Pathology.—I have found the fragments sensibly displaced in five cases out of seven; a proportion much greater than has been observed by Malgaigne, who has only seen a displacement twice in more than twenty cases. It is certain, however, that complete or sensible displacement is less common in this fracture than in most other fractures, the broken ends being retained in place, probably, by the long tendon of the biceps.

As to the direction of the displacement, I have seen the upper end of the lower fragment drawn forwards and upwards toward the coracoid process three times, in one of which examples the upper fragment plainly followed in the same direction. Sir Astley Cooper declares that with infants this direction is constant, and in museum specimens I have seen but one exception. In the specimen of fracture of the surgical neck, with also displacement of the head, belonging to Dr. Pope, this direction of the fragments is plainly seen, as also in a specimen belonging to Dr. Neill, of the Pennsylvania Medical College, where the lower fragment almost reaches the coracoid process, and in a specimen contained in one of the cabinets of the University of Pennsylvania, where the upper end of the lower fragment has become united by bone to the coracoid process.

The only exception which I have met with is in the possession of Dr. Neill. In this example the two ends are tilted toward the axilla. In the recorded examples, also, I find the displacement forwards mentioned four times, and the displacement toward the axilla but once. I am compelled, therefore, to doubt the accuracy of Malgaigne's observations, who thinks he has seen the lower fragment most often drawn toward the axilla, as well as the observations of those who think that the upper fragment is generally displaced outwards; yet, no doubt, they do sometimes assume this position. Desault has seen them both thrown backwards; while Dupuytren, Paletta, and others have seen them pushed outwards; and I have in my cabinet the copy of a specimen in which both fragments are drawn outwards, but the lower fragment is to the inner side of the upper.

When the fracture occurs at or near the epiphysis, it is sometimes accompanied with impaction, of the same character as we have already described when speaking of fractures through the tubercles. Robert Smith has given, in his treatise, an engraving intended to illustrate the relative position of the fragments in extra-capsular impacted fractures, and the line of separation very nearly corresponds to the line of junction of the epiphysis with the shaft.

But in a majority of cases no impaction occurs. Dr. Charles A. Pope, of St. Louis, Mo., has two specimens of this kind, in which no union has taken place, nor is there any evidence that impaction had ever occurred. In one case the line of fracture commences at the junction of the head with the shaft, and extends thence irregularly across to a point half an inch below the greater tuberosity. In the second specimen the fracture commences at the same point and terminates three-quarters of an inch below the greater tuberosity. In relation to these bones, Dr. Pope remarks: "These are not cases of detachment of the epiphyses, as the bones are evidently those of adults, and there is, at their lower extremities above the condyles, no trace of an epiphyseal line."

Results.—Four of the examples of fracture of the surgical neck seen by me resulted in perfect limbs, and three are more or less deformed; but it has already been noticed that of the whole number only five were ever displaced, and of these five, only two are completely restored. In one of these no bony union has taken place after the lapse of two years or more. It is satisfactory, however, to know that, with the exception of this last (Case 3), all of the patients have recovered the free and complete use of their arms.

Symptoms, or Differential Diagnosis of Accidents about the Shoulder-joint.—No place could be more appropriate than this to call attention to the difficulty of diagnosis in the case of accidents about the shoulder-joint, a difficulty which surgeons have constantly recognized, and which has sometimes rendered diagnosis impossible.

In presenting an epitome of the prominent diagnostic signs, I would refer the reader who seeks further information to my report to the American Medical Association, where the subject is treated more elaborately than is consistent with the design of the present volume.

Let us first study the ordinary signs of a dislocation at the shoulder-joint, regarding this as the type with which the other accidents are to be compared.

a. *Signs of a Dislocation.* (*Cause*, generally a fall upon the elbow or hand.)

1. Preternatural immobility.
2. Absence of crepitus.
3. When the bone is brought to its place it will remain without the employment of force.

These three are common signs, which apply to any other joint as well as the shoulder.

4. Inability to place the hand upon the opposite shoulder, or to have it placed there by an assistant, while at the same time the elbow touches the breast. This is a sign common to all of the dislocations of the shoulder.[1]

The following are special signs, or such as belong only to particular dislocations of the shoulder.

5. Depression under the acromion process; always greatest underneath the outer extremity, but more or less in front or behind, according as the dislocation may be into the axilla, forwards or backwards.
6. Round, smooth head of the bone felt in its new situation, and very probably removed from its socket; moving with the shaft. Absence of the head of the bone from the socket.
7. Elbow carried outwards, and in certain cases forwards or backwards, and not easily pressed to the side of the body.
8. Arm shortened in the dislocation forwards, and slightly lengthened when in the axilla.

b. *Signs of a Fracture of the Neck of the Scapula.* (*Cause*, generally a direct blow.)

1. Preternatural mobility.
2. Crepitus, generally detected by placing the finger on the coracoid process and the opposite hand upon the back of the scapula, while the head of the humerus is pushed outwards and rotated.
3. When reduced it will not remain in place.
4. The hand may generally, but with difficulty, be placed upon the opposite shoulder.
5. Depression under the acromion process, but not so marked as in dislocation.
6. Head of the bone may be felt in the axilla, but less distinctly than in dislocation. Never much forwards or backwards. Head of the bone moves with the shaft. Head of the bone not to be felt under the acromion process, although it has not left its socket.
7. Elbow carried a little outwards, but not so much as in dislocation. Easily brought against the side of the body.
8. Arm lengthened.
9. The coracoid process carried a little toward the sternum, and downwards.

[1] Report on a New Principle of Diagnosis in Dislocations of the Shoulder-joint, by L. A. Dugas, Prof. of Surgery in the Medical College of Georgia. Trans. Amer. Med. Assoc., vol. x. p. 175.

10. Pressing upon the coracoid process it is found to be movable, and it is also observed that it obeys the motions of the arm.

c. *Signs of Fracture of the Anatomical Neck of the Humerus. Intra-Capsular.* (*Cause*, a direct blow; generally opening to the joint, but not always.)

1. Mobility not increased, nor diminished.
2. Crepitus, generally discovered by pressing up the head of the bone into its socket and rotating; or, when the tubercles are also broken, by grasping the tubercles and rotating the arm.
3. Fragments not generally displaced.
4. The hand can be placed easily upon the opposite shoulder.
5. Very slight, if any, depression under the acromion process.
6. Head of the bone generally in its socket, but not felt so distinctly as before the fracture.
7. Elbow falls easily against the side of the body, or is easily placed there.
8. Arm not lengthened, nor appreciably shortened, unless the head be driven so much into the body as to separate the tubercles.
9. In this latter case there are present also the signs of fracture of the tubercles.

d. *Signs of Fracture of the Humerus through the Tubercles. Extra-Capsular.* (*Cause*, direct blows.)

1. Generally, there is neither marked mobility nor immobility, except what immobility may be due to a contusion of the muscles.
2. Crepitus, discovered, but not so easily as in intra-capsular fractures, by rotating the arm while the tubercles are grasped firmly.
3. If displacement exists, the fragments are not always easily kept in place when once reduced.
4. The hand can be placed upon the opposite shoulder.
5. No depression under the acromion process.
6. Head of the bone in its socket, and moving with the shaft, when, as is usually the case, it is impacted.
7. Elbow hangs against the side of the body.
8. Arm shortened when impacted, but not very appreciably.

The signs which characterize this accident are more obscure than in either of the other shoulder accidents. They are mostly negative, and will not generally be determined positively except in the autopsy.

e. *Signs of a Longitudinal Fracture of the Head and Neck, or splitting off of the Greater Tubercle.* (*Cause*, direct blow upon the front of the shoulder.)

1. Mobility of the limb natural.
2. Crepitus; elicited especially by grasping the tubercles and rotating the arm, or by carrying it up and back and then rotating.
3. When reduced, the fragments will not remain in place.
4. The hand can be placed upon the opposite shoulder.
5. Some depression under the acromion process.
6. A smooth bony projection directly underneath the coracoid process, or close upon its inner or outer side, moving with the shaft. The head of the bone cannot be felt in the socket, yet the space under the acromion is not entirely unoccupied.

7. Generally, but not always, the elbow hangs against the side. Sometimes it inclines a little backwards. It can always be easily brought to the side.

8. Arm generally neither lengthened nor shortened.

9. A remarkable increase in the antero-posterior diameter of the upper end of the bone.

10. A deep vertical sulcus between the tubercles, corresponding with the upper part of the bicipital groove.

f. *Signs of a Fracture through the Surgical Neck.* (*Cause*, direct blows.)

1. Preternatural mobility often, but not constantly present.

2. Crepitus, produced easily when there is no impaction, or when the displacement is not complete, but with difficulty when impaction exists or the displacement is complete.

3. When once the fragments have been displaced, it is exceedingly difficult ever afterward to maintain them in place.

4. If the fragments remain in place, the hand can be easily placed upon the opposite shoulder. When completely overlapped it is difficult.

5. A slight depression below the acromion, not immediately underneath its extremity, but an inch or more below.

6. Head of the bone in the socket, and moving with the shaft when impacted, but not moving with the shaft when not impacted. The upper end of the lower fragment being often felt distinctly pressing upwards toward the coracoid process; its broken extremity being easily distinguished by its irregularity from the head of the bone.

7. Elbow hanging against the side when the fragments are not displaced, but away from the side when displacement exists.

8. Length of arm unchanged unless the fragments are impacted or overlapped; or both fragments are much tilted inwards. If the fragments are completely displaced, the arm is shortened.

g. *Signs of a Separation at the Epiphysis.* (*Cause*, direct blows.)

1. Preternatural mobility.

2. Feeble crepitus; less rough than the crepitus produced when broken bones are rubbed against each other.

3. Fragments replaced are not easily maintained in place.

4. Same as in preceding variety of fracture.

5. The depression is not immediately under the acromion, yet higher than in most fractures of the surgical neck, perhaps three-quarters of an inch below the acromion process.

6. Head of the bone in its socket, and not moving with the shaft. Upper end of lower fragment projecting in front, when displacement exists, and feeling less sharp and angular than in case of a broken bone; indeed, being slightly convex and rather smooth, it may easily be mistaken for the head of the bone.

7. Same as in preceding variety.

8. Length of arm not changed unless the fragments are overlapped, or both fragments are tilted upon each other. When the fragments are overlapped, the arm is shortened.

9. This accident is almost peculiar to infancy and childhood. It seldom occurs after the fifteenth year.

There are other accidents about the shoulder-joint, such as a pathological partial luxation of the humerus, dislocation of the tendon of the biceps, &c., which might possibly be confounded with fractures, but the consideration of which I shall reserve for another time.

Treatment.—I have already spoken of the treatment of fractures of the neck of the scapula, and my remarks will now be confined to fractures of the upper end of the humerus.

Fractures of the Anatomical Neck; Intra-capsular.—As has already been stated, these are generally compound fractures, and from the extent of the injury often demand amputation of the entire arm. If an effort is made to save the arm, splints will not be applied, and the treatment will have little or no reference to the existence of a fracture; it will be directed only to the reduction or prevention of the inflammation, &c. At a later period the head of the bone may escape spontaneously, or it may become necessary to remove it by an operation.

Simple fracture of the anatomical neck, without any external wound communicating with the joint, and accompanied, as it often is, with impaction, frequently unites, or the upper fragment becomes encased in the lower.

It is not proper in such cases to employ great violence for the purpose of detecting crepitus, lest the fragments should become displaced; and if the arm should be found to be a little shortened, it must not be extended, with a view to overcoming the shortening, since upon the impaction probably depends, in a great measure, the chances of union.

The elbow and forearm may be suspended in a sling, while the arm is gently supported against the side, merely to insure quietude. No splints are necessary or useful.

Treatment of Fractures through the Tubercles (Extra-capsular); Non-impacted and Impacted.—In these cases, also, the fragments being seldom displaced, very little if any mechanical treatment is demanded. A sling is all that is usually required. If, however, on account of displacement of the fragments, a splint is thought necessary, it must be applied in the manner hereafter to be directed in cases of fractures of the surgical neck.

If impaction, with shortening, exists, the same remarks are applicable here as in intra-capsular impacted fractures, namely, that we ought not to rotate the limb much, nor violently, in order to discover crepitus, nor make extension with the view of overcoming the shortening, since the fragments unite more promptly and certainly when the impaction remains, and its continuance in no way damages the usefulness of the limb.

Treatment of Longitudinal Fractures of the Head and Neck, or of a Separation of the Greater Tubercle.—In the only instance which I have recognized as a fracture of the greater tubercle, and already referred to, the displacement was moderate, and could not be overcome, either by change of position or by pressure with extension. The patient was therefore merely laid upon his back in bed. No dressings of any kind were employed, and the fragments seemed to unite promptly, and with no increase in the displacement.

If the displacement is originally more considerable, attempts ought still to be made to reduce the fragments, by extension and abduction of the arm, with direct pressure; yet they will not generally prove completely successful, nor will it be found easy to retain them when reduced.

Mr. Mayo treated a fracture of this character, which occurred in a man sixty years of age, with a figure-of-8 bandage, and a sling, with a lathe splint on the outer side of the humerus, the upper part of which was made to bear on the fragments, by uniting the upper part of the circular arm roller to the figure-of-8 bandage. "The fracture united favorably," he says, but we presume that he does not mean to affirm that it united without any degree of displacement; a result which, probably, ought never to be expected. Mr. Mayo adds, however, that "for a long time the patient had some difficulty in carrying the arm backward."[1]

Treatment of Fractures of the Surgical Neck, including Separations at the Epiphysis.—I see no reason to suppose that the indications of treatment can essentially vary in separations at the epiphysis, from those in true fractures through any part of the surgical neck, since the relative action of the muscles remains the same, and the direction of the displacement is generally the same. My remarks, therefore, upon this point may be considered as equally applicable to fractures and epiphysary separations.

In a considerable proportion of these cases not much displacement of either fragment takes place, and consequently we have only to apply such moderate retentive means as will insure quiet. Indeed, under such circumstances we might not hesitate to adopt the posture treatment practised by Dupuytren in two cases, both of which terminated favorably. The treatment consisted in placing the arm, semi-flexed, on a pillow, the pillow being arranged so as to form a pyramid, the summit of which was lodged in the axilla, while the elbow was secured to the side of the body by a bandage.[2]

Unhappily, however, as we have seen, this condition is not always present; the most frequent form of displacement being that in which the lower fragment is drawn upwards and inwards, or toward the coracoid process.

In such cases it will require, often, no little perseverance and skill to effect reduction, if it is not found to be actually impossible, and still more to retain the bones in place when once reduced. Indeed, it is proper to say that a complete reduction is seldom accomplished and permanently maintained, owing, probably, to the advantageous action of the muscles which tend to produce the displacement, and in part also to the difficulty of applying any apparatus or dressing which shall act efficiently upon the fragments.

Sir Astley Cooper recommends for this accident a couple of splints, to be placed one in front of and one behind the shoulder, an axillary pad, a clavicular bandage, and a sling; the sling being made to suspend only the wrist and not the elbow, since he had observed that when the

[1] B. Cooper's edition of Sir A. Cooper on Dislocations, &c., American edition, p. 385.
[2] Dupuytren on Bones, Sydenham edition, p. 99.

elbow was lifted the upper end of the shaft was inclined to fall forwards.

Mr. Tyrrell informed Mr. Cooper that in a similar case he had found the bone best maintained in its natural position by its being raised and supported at right angles with the side, by a rectangular splint, a part of which rested against the side, while the arm reposed upon the other part; and until he had made use of this plan, he could not succeed in removing the deformity, or in keeping the bone in its place.

Mr. Erichsen has found a very convenient apparatus to consist of "a leather splint about two feet long by six inches broad, bent upon itself in the middle, so that one half of it may be applied lengthwise to the chest, and the other half to the inside of the injured arm, the angle formed by the bend, which should be somewhat obtuse, being well pressed up into the axilla."

The following is the plan which I would, however, generally recommend:—

The fragments having been reduced as completely as possible, a broad and firm gutta-percha splint should be moulded to the outside of the arm and shoulder. When it has become sufficiently hard and firm, it may be secured in place by a roller carried from the elbow to the axilla. If the splint covers well the top of the shoulder, and is sufficiently wide, it is not apt to become displaced; and by resting against the point of the acromion process, it enables the upper turns of the bandage to draw the broken end of the lower fragment outwards; at least, as effectually as any other dressing is capable of doing, and renders an axillary pad unnecessary. The sling may then be applied as recommended by Sir Astley Cooper, or the arm may be permitted to hang perpendicularly beside the body. The clavicular bandage also recommended by Sir Astley complicates the dressing very much, and does not seem to me to answer any useful purpose; while the axillary pad exposes the brachial plexus to painful if not injurious pressure.

Fig. 58.

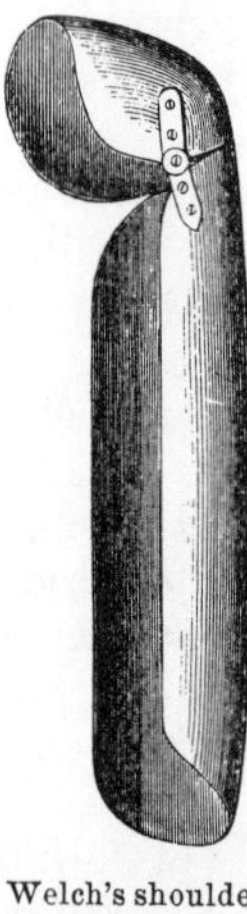

Welch's shoulder splint.

As a substitute for gutta percha, a firm sheet of felt may be employed, or a carved wooden splint, or the very complete shoulder and arm splint of Welch, but in either case the upper portion of the splint ought always to rest upon the shoulder, so as to prevent its sliding downwards.

Dr. Waters read before the Æsculapian Society of the University of New York, a remarkable case of compound and comminuted fracture of the shaft and surgical neck of the humerus, in which the constant protrusion of the upper end of the middle fragment in the region of the axilla finally rendered resection of the head and neck necessary. This operation was made by Dr. Waters, on the eighteenth day; and four months after, the patient was so far recovered as to be able to write a letter with the limb upon which the operation had been made.[1] It may be regarded, therefore, as a signal triumph of conservative surgery, since the alternative presented was only between amputation and resection. In a similar case, Dr. W. H. Van Buren, of New York, was compelled to amputate at the shoulder-joint, after which the patient made a good recovery.[2]

§ 5. Shaft, below the Surgical Neck and above the Base of the Condyles.

Causes.—In a record of seventeen cases in which the cause of the fracture is stated, I find this portion of the shaft broken from direct blows ten times; from indirect blows, the concussion being received upon the elbow, twice; once it was a consequence of tertiary lues, once it occurred during birth, and three times in the same patient it has been broken from muscular action alone, each consecutive fracture occurring at a different point. The records of surgery furnish many examples of fracture of the shaft of the humerus from muscular action, as in throwing a stone, or a snowball; but the most singular examples are those in which the bone has been broken in a trial of strength between two persons, by grasping the hands palm to palm, with the elbows resting upon a table, and twisting, when the humerus has suddenly given way a little above the condyles. I have seen one case of this kind, which was under the care of Dr. Winne, of this city, and Malgaigne has collected five other similar cases, two of which were reported by Lonsdale.

The example of fracture during birth, to which I have referred, occurred in a healthy female child, whose parents were also healthy. The mother was in labor six or eight hours, but the labor was not severe. She was attended by a midwife, and does not know whether violence was employed or not. Dr. Lockwood, of Buffalo, was called on the third day, and found the arm broken a little below its middle, and moving as freely as it did at the elbow-joint; he applied lateral splints, with bandages, &c. I saw the child on the seventeenth day after its birth, with Dr. Lockwood. There was then a perfect ferule of ensheathing callus surrounding the fragments, and which, owing to the softness of the flesh, could be easily detected and defined. The fragments were firm, and had been at least three or four days. Nearly a year after, I again examined the arm, and could not discover any traces of the accident.

Dr. Löwenhardt has also reported a case in which the evidence was conclusive that the fracture was caused solely by the contractions of the uterus, which forced the arm against the pubes; the arm being heard distinctly to snap when it was passing this point, and while the hands of the accoucheur were not aiding in the delivery. In this case the humerus was broken in its upper third.[3]

[1] Waters, New York Journal of Medicine, May, 1847, p. 318, vol. viii. First Series.

[2] Van Buren, Ibid., January, 1854, p. 152, vol. xii. Second Series.

[3] Löwenhardt, American Journal of Medical Sciences, January, 1841, p. 250, from Medicin Zeit., Mai 6, 1840.

Seat and Direction of the Fracture.—The seat of the fracture is more often below than above the middle of the bone; thus I have found the fracture thirteen times near the middle, and the same number of times below the middle third, but only six times above the middle third. The observations of Norris, who found four fractures of the shaft above the middle, and nine below, correspond with my own;[1] but M. Guèretin, in the same number of fractures, found nine above the middle and four below.[2]

Fig. 59.

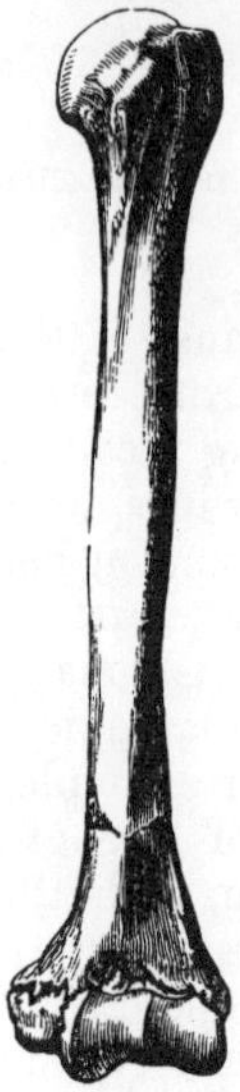

The line of fracture is generally oblique, but more often transverse than in fractures of the clavicle, femur, or tibia.

Displacement.—The direction of the displacement depends, no doubt, sometimes upon the precise point of the fracture and upon the action of the muscles operating upon the two fragments; thus, if the fracture takes place just above the insertion of the deltoid, the lower fragment is liable to be drawn upwards and outwards, in the direction of its fibres, while the upper fragment is carried toward the origin of the pectoralis major, &c.; but, in a great majority of cases, the influence of these muscles is more than counterbalanced by the direction of the force and by the direction of the fracture. Practically, therefore, it is seldom of much importance to determine the exact point of fracture, as to whether it is just above or below the insertion of a particular muscle; nor, indeed, is it generally very easy to ascertain this point with much precision.

The amount of displacement varies considerably in different persons, and in fractures at different points, but it will average about three-quarters of an inch. When the fracture is produced by muscular action alone it is generally transverse, and displacement seldom occurs. Such was the fact in every instance where my own patient broke the arm three times consecutively at different points; and union was speedily accomplished, and with no deformity. Dupuytren, however, saw a case which constituted an exception to this general rule. The fragments became completely separated, and were so movable that union could not be effected, and he was compelled, after three months, to resort to resection.

Results.—In twenty-three examples, the average shortening is about one-quarter of an inch; but of these, thirteen are not shortened at all, so that the average of shortening in the remaining ten is three-quarters of an inch; the amount of overlapping varying from one-quarter of an inch to one inch and a quarter.

In twenty-eight examples, I have twice seen the humerus refuse to unite; once when the fracture was in the lower third of the shaft. This was an oblique, compound fracture, and no union had taken place at the end of five months. The man was intemperate, but in pretty good

[1] Norris, Am. Journ. of Med. Sci., January, 1842, vol. xxix. p. 28.
[2] Guèretin, Presse Médicale, vol. i. p. 45.

health.[1] In the second case, the fracture had occurred a little below the middle of the bone, and it was simple. Five months after the accident this patient consulted me, when I found the elbow anchylosed, the forearm being fixed at right angles with the arm.[2] Neither of these patients had been under my care previously, but I learned that an intelligent Canadian surgeon had treated one of them, and the other had been seen and treated by several surgeons.

In two other cases, the elbow remained somewhat stiff a long time after the splints were removed; in one case, complete freedom of motion was not restored at the end of fifteen years.

Generally, however, the motions of the elbow-joint have been very soon restored after the removal of the splints and sling.

I ought to mention that, not unfrequently, fractures of the shaft of the humerus, and especially where they are occasioned by direct blows, are followed by great swelling, and sometimes by abscesses. In one instance the fracture having taken place within the insertion of the deltoid muscle, the sharp extremity of the lower fragment was made to penetrate the flesh, causing an abscess, and finally tetanus, of which my patient soon died. A medical gentleman, and a friend of the family, suggested that the bone had not been properly "set," for which omission I ought to be held responsible. But, fortunately for my reputation, the friends had more intelligence than the doctor, and were able to appreciate the difficulty of "setting" a very oblique fracture.

The following remarks of Malgaigne are too pertinent to be omitted in this connection: "When there is great obliquity, with overlapping, or a fracture with splintering, or a multiple fracture, a certain amount of deformity is inevitable, and the formation of callus demands one or two weeks more. With the inflammation comes also the danger of suppuration, and later, a rigidity of the articulations difficult to dissipate. In short, we must not forget that of all fractures, those of the humerus are most liable to fail of consolidation."

On the other hand, we shall find, in the case of this bone, as in all others, some remarkable exceptions, where, although the fracture may be compound, and badly comminuted, yet the limb has been saved and made useful. Ayres, of New York, reports a case of this kind, in which he removed a portion of the shaft, and although the brachial artery was probably obliterated, a good union took place;[3] and Walker, of Boston, has noticed two or three similar examples.[4]

For an account of two remarkable cases of compound fracture of the shaft of the humerus, illustrating the powers of Nature in childhood, in the restoration of broken and comminuted bones, the reader may consult, in the *New York Journal of Medicine* for November, 1849, a paper entitled "Amputations and Compound Fractures," by John O. Stone, Surgeon to Bellevue Hospital. The accidents occurred in children, one of whom was four, and the other six years of age, both of whom recovered with useful arms.

[1] Report on Deformities, &c., Case 33. [2] Ibid., Case 21.

[3] Ayres, New York Journal of Medicine, January, 1857, p. 24, 3d series, vol. xi.

[4] Walker: Essay on Compound Fractures, &c., by William J. Walker, of Boston, published in London in 1845.

Treatment.—In the treatment of fractures of that portion of the shaft of the humerus now under consideration, I have preferred generally a broad and thick splint of gutta percha—felt may answer nearly as well—sufficiently long to extend from the neck to the wrist, moulded accurately, and applied to the outside of the shoulder and arm, while the limb is flexed to a right angle, and while extension is being made upon the humerus. This being properly padded, and secured in place by rollers, I place the arm in a sling beside the body. The sling must, however, be so arranged, by being looped under the wrists, and not under the elbow, as that the weight of the elbow and lower part of the arm may aid in making extension. Welch's splint will answer the same purpose; or three narrow splints of different lengths may be used, but I do not find them so convenient as Welch's, or gutta percha applied as I have directed above.

Fig. 60.

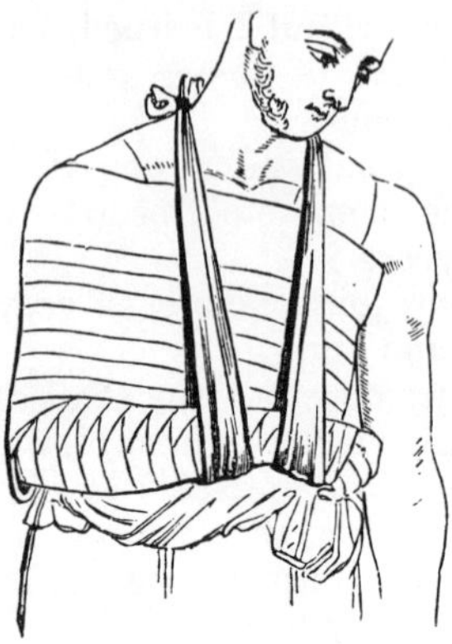

Other surgeons have sought to make permanent extension in these and certain other fractures of the humerus, by various contrivances. Mr. Lonsdale constructed an instrument which might be lengthened or shortened to suit the case; it was made of steel, and was worked with a screw operating upon cogs in a sliding bar; resembling, in some respects, the arm portion of Jarvis's adjuster. In the second London edition of a series of plates illustrating the action of the muscles in producing displacement in fractures, by S. W. Hind, is a drawing of an apparatus invented by the author for the same purpose, which is very simple, and in some respects more complete than Lonsdale's, and which may be easily adapted to almost any form of arm-splint. Indeed, nothing more is necessary than to attach to the ordinary long splint a movable crutch.

Fig. 61.

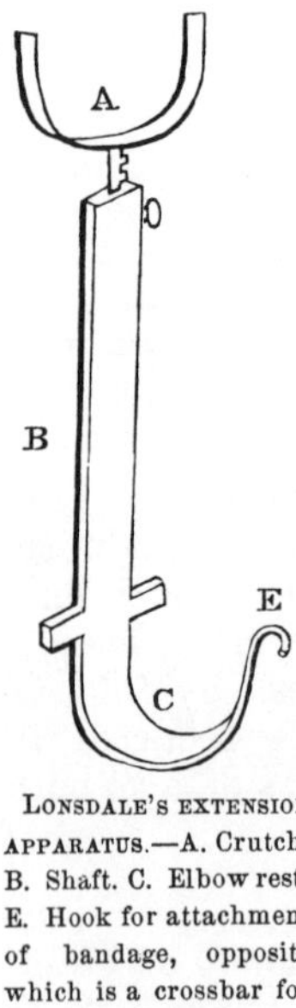

LONSDALE'S EXTENSION APPARATUS.—A. Crutch. B. Shaft. C. Elbow rest E. Hook for attachment of bandage, opposite which is a crossbar for the same purpose.

I believe that all these contrivances may prove occasionally useful, but the common experience of surgeons has shown how difficult it is to accomplish much extension by means of pressure in the axilla; a mode, too, which I think must be wholly inadmissible when the fracture approaches the upper end, since the pressure by the crutch-head upon the pectoralis major and latissimus dorsi, which constitute the margins of the axilla, must tend to displace the fragments upon which they act, inwardly, and which seldom can be applied with much force to fractures near the condyles, on account of the probable existence of inflammation and swelling about the joint.

Malgaigne, when speaking of the apparatus of

Lonsdale, remarks: "But the surgeon should never lose sight of the fact that permanent extension is a resource always dangerous, often useless, and which demands in its application much caution and watchfulness."

The following example will illustrate the practical difficulty of employing permanent extension in fractures of the humerus:—

A laborer, aged thirty, was admitted into the Buffalo Hospital of the Sisters of Charity, on the second day of October, 1853, with a simple oblique fracture of the humerus, which had occurred three days before. The fracture was situated within the insertion of the deltoid, and having been produced by the rolling of a log upon the arm, the whole limb was much swollen. The night following his admission, in a fit of delirium tremens, he removed all of the dressings. When I visited the wards in the morning, I found the fragments displaced and the muscles contracting violently. The ordinary dressings were applied, and continued until the fifth day, when, as the delirium had not ceased, and the muscles continued to contract with great violence, it was determined to attempt permanent extension. For this purpose we lifted the elbow upwards and outwards, to relax the deltoid, and then, having made extension with the forearm placed at a right angle with the arm, we fitted carefully a large gutta-percha splint to the forearm, arm, axilla, and side, in such a manner that when the splint was secured to these several parts, the arm could not fall to the side of the body completely, and in proportion as it did fall downward, it would make extension upon the arm. This splint was well padded, and secured in place with rollers.

On the sixth day the delirium had ceased, and never returned. The dressings were well in place, and seemed to accomplish the indication we had in view; but, on the seventh day, although he had kept very quiet, everything was disarranged, and the whole had to be readjusted. On the eighth and ninth, the same thing occurred. During this time we had varied the dressings, position, &c., each day, to meet, if possible, the difficulties, but it was at length deemed unwise to pursue the attempt any further, and we returned to the use of the ordinary splints, laying the arm against the side of the body. The union was finally completed without either overlapping or angular displacement.

Something may always be accomplished when the patient is walking about, by allowing the elbow to escape from the sling, so that its weight shall make constant traction upon the lower fragment; and the plan which I suggested some years since, of treating certain cases of delayed union of the humerus, namely, extending the arm at full length by the side of the body, so that the lower fragment shall receive the whole weight of the forearm and hand, might occasionally prove valuable in recent fractures where the tendency to override was very great. In two instances, I have already put this plan sufficiently to the test to determine its safety and utility.

The precise plan, and my reasons for its adoption in certain cases of delayed union, were set forth in the following paper, read before the Buffalo City Medical Association, and published in the *Buffalo Medical Journal* for August, 1854.

"I have observed that non-union results more frequently after fractures of the shaft of the humerus, than after fractures of the shaft of any other bone.

"Comparing the humerus with the femur, between which, above all others, the circumstances of form, situation, &c., are most nearly parallel, and in both of which non-union is said to be relatively frequent, I find that of forty-nine fractures of the humerus, four occurred through the surgical neck, twelve through the condyles, and twenty-nine through the shaft. In one of the twenty-nine, the patient survived the accident only a few days. In four of the remaining twenty-eight, union had not occurred after the lapse of six months, and in many more it was delayed beyond the usual time. Two of the four were simple fractures, and occurred near the middle of the humerus; the third was compound, and occurred near the middle also; the fourth was compound, and occurred near the condyles.

"This analysis supplies us, therefore, with four cases of non-union, from a table of twenty-eight cases of fractures through the shaft.

"Of eighty-seven fractures of the femur, twenty occurred through the neck, one through the trochanter major, and one through the condyles. The remaining sixty-five occurred through the shaft, and generally near the middle, and not in one case was the union delayed beyond six months.

"To make the comparison more complete, I must add that of the twenty-eight fractures of the shaft of the humerus, six were compound; and of the sixty-five fractures of the shaft of the femur, six were either compound, comminuted, or both compound and comminuted. The six compound fractures of the shaft of the humerus furnished two cases of non-union. The six cases of either compound or comminuted, or compound and comminuted fractures of the femur, furnished no case of non-union.

"I beg to suggest to the Society what seems to me to be the true explanation of these facts.

"It is the universal practice, so far as I know, in dressing fractures of the humerus, to place the forearm at a right angle with the arm. Within a few days, and, generally, I think, within a few hours, after the arm and forearm are placed in this position, a rigidity of the muscles and other structures has ensued, and to such a degree that if the splints and sling are completely removed, the elbow will remain flexed and firm; nor will it be easy to straighten it. A temporary false anchylosis has occurred, and instead of motion at the elbow-joint, when the forearm is attempted to be straightened upon the arm, there is only motion at the seat of fracture. It will thus happen that every upward and downward movement of the forearm will inflict motion upon the fracture; and inasmuch as the elbow has become the pivot, the motion at the upper end of the lower fragment will be the greater in proportion to the distance of the fracture from the elbow-joint.

"No doubt it is intended that the dressings shall prevent all motion of the forearm upon the arm; but I fear that they cannot always be made to do this. I believe it is never done when the dressing is made without angular splints, nor is it by any means certain that it will be accomplished when such splints are used. The weight of the forearm is such, when placed at a right angle with the arm, and encumbered with splints and bandages, that even when supported by a sling, it settles heavily forwards, and compels the arm-dressings to loosen themselves from the arm in front of the point of fracture, and to indent themselves in the skin and flesh behind. By these means the upper end of the lower fragment is tilted forwards. If the forearm should continue to drag upon the sling, nothing but a permanent forward displacement would probably result. The bones might unite, yet with a deformity.

But the weight of the forearm under these circumstances is not uniform, nor do I see how it can be made so. It is to the sling that we must trust mainly to accomplish this important indication. But you have all noticed that the tension or relaxation of the sling depends upon the attitude of the body, whether standing or sitting; upon the erection or inclination of the head; upon the motions of the shoulders; and in no inconsiderable degree upon the actions of respiration. Nor does the patient himself cease to add to these conditions by lifting the forearm with his opposite hand whenever provoked to it by a sense of fatigue.

This difficulty of maintaining quiet apposition of the fragments while the arm is in this position, at whatever point it may be broken, becomes more and more serious as we depart from the elbow-joint, and would be at its maximum at the upper end of the humerus, were it not that here a mass of muscles, investing and adhering to the bone, in some measure obviates the difficulty. Its true maximum is, therefore, near the middle, where there is less muscular investment, and where, on the one hand, the fracture is sufficiently remote from the pivot or fulcrum to have the motion of the upper end of the lower fragment multiplied through a long arm, while, on the other hand, it is sufficiently near the armpit and shoulder to prevent the upper portion of the splint and arm-dressings from obtaining a secure grasp upon the lower end of the upper fragment.

It must not be overlooked that the motion of which we speak belongs exclusively to the lower fragment, and that it is always in the same plane forwards and backwards, but especially that it is not a motion upon the fracture as upon a pivot, but a motion of one fragment to and from its fellow. This circumstance I regard as important to a right appreciation of the difficulty. Motion alone, I am fully convinced, does not so often prevent union as surgeons have generally believed. It is exceedingly rare to see a case of non-union of the clavicle. Of forty-seven cases of fracture of the clavicle which have come under my observation, and in by far the greater proportion of which considerable overlapping and consequent deformity ensued, only one has resulted in non-union, and in this instance no treatment whatever was practised, but from the time of the accident the patient continued to labor in the fields and hold the plough as if nothing had occurred. I have, therefore, seen no case of non-union of the clavicle where a surgeon has treated the accident. Indeed, what is most pertinent and remarkable, its union is more speedy usually than that of any other bone in the body of the same size. Yet to prevent motion of the fragments in a case of fractured clavicle with complete separation and displacement, except where the fracture is near one of the extremities of the bone, I have always found wholly impracticable. Whatever bandages or apparatus has been applied, I have still seen always that the fragments would move freely upon each other at each act of inspiration and expiration, and at almost every motion of the head, body, or upper extremities. It is probable, gentlemen, that you have made the same observation.

From this and many similar facts I have been led to suspect, for a long time, that motion has had less to do with non-union than was generally believed.

I find, however, no difficulty in reconciling this suspicion with my doctrine in reference to the case in question; and it is precisely because, as I have already explained, the motion, in case of a fractured humerus, dressed in the usual manner, is peculiar.

In a fracture of the clavicle through its middle third (its usual situation), the motion is upon the point of the fracture as upon a pivot; although, therefore, the motion is almost incessant, it does not essentially, if at all, disturb the adhesive process. The same is true in nearly all other fractures. The fragments move only upon themselves, and not to and from each other. I know of no complete exception but in the case now under consideration.

Aside from any speculation, the facts are easily verified by a personal examination of the patients during the first or second week of treatment, or at any time before union has occurred, both in fractures of the humerus and clavicle. The latter is always sufficiently exposed to permit you to see what occurs, and as soon as the swelling has a little subsided in the former case you will have no difficulty in feeling the motion outside of the dressings, or, perhaps, in introducing the finger under the dressings sufficiently far to reach the point of fracture. I believe you will not fail to recognize the difference in the motion between the two cases. Such, gentlemen, is the explanation which I wish to offer for the relative frequency of this very serious accident—non-union of the humerus.

I know of no other circumstance or condition in which this bone is peculiar, and which, therefore, might be invoked as an explanation. Overlapping of the bones, the cause assigned by some writers, is not sufficient, since it is not peculiar. The same occurs much oftener, and to a much greater extent, in fractures of the femur, and equally as often in fractures of the clavicle, yet in neither case are these results so frequent. Nor can it be due to the action of the deltoid muscle, or of any other particular muscles about the arm, whether the fracture be below or above their insertions, since similar muscles, with similar attachments, on the femur and on the clavicle, tending always powerfully to the separation of the fragments, occasion deformity, but they seldom prevent union.

If I am correct in my views, we shall be able sometimes to consummate union of a fractured humerus where it is delayed, by straightening the forearm upon the arm, and confining them to this position. A straight splint, extending from the top of the shoulder to the hand, constructed from some firm material, and made fast with rollers, will secure the requisite immobility to the fracture. The weight of the forearm and hand will only tend to keep the fragments in place, and if the splint and bandages are sufficiently tight, the motion occasioned by swinging the hand and forearm will be conveyed almost entirely to the shoulder-joint. Very little motion, indeed, can in this posture be communicated to the fragments, and what little is thus communicated, is a motion which experience has elsewhere shown not disturbing or pernicious, but a motion only upon the ends of the fragments, as upon a pivot.

I do not fail to notice that this position has serious objections, and that it is liable to inconveniences which must always, probably, prevent its being adopted as the usual plan of treatment for fractured arms. It is more inconvenient to get up and lie down, or even to sit down, in this position of the arm, and the hand is liable to swell. But I shall not be surprised to learn that experience will prove these objections to have less weight than we are now disposed to give them. Remember, the practice is yet untried—if I except the case which I am about to relate, and in which case, I am free to say, these objections scarcely existed. The swelling of the hand was trivial, and only continued through the first fortnight, and the patient never spoke of the inconvenience of getting up or sitting down, or even of lying down.

The following is the case to which I have just referred: "Michael Mahar, laborer, æt. 35, broke his left humerus just below its middle, Dec. 14th, 1853. The arm was dressed by a surgeon in Canada West, and who is well known to me as exceedingly 'clever.' After a few days from the time of the accident, 'the starch bandage was put on as tight as it could be borne, and brought down on the forearm, so as to confine the motions of the elbow-joint.' Six weeks after the injury, Jan. 29th, 1854, Mahar applied to me at the Hospital. No union had occurred. The motion between the fragments was very free, so that they passed each other with an audible click. There was little or no swelling or soreness. In short, everything indicated that union was not likely to occur without operative interference. The elbow was completely anchylosed. I explained to my students what seemed to me to be the cause of the delayed union, and declared to them that I did not intend to attempt to establish adhesive action until I had straightened the arm. They had just witnessed the failure of a precisely similar case, in which I had made the attempt to bring about union without previously straightening the arm.

"On the 6th of Feb., 1854, we had succeeded in making the arm nearly straight. I now punctured the upper end of the lower fragment with a small steel instrument, and, as well as I was able, thrust it between the fragments. Assisted by Dr. Boardman, I then applied a gutta-percha splint from the top of the shoulder to the fingers, moulding it carefully to the whole of the back and sides of the limb, and securing it firmly with a paste roller. March 4th (not quite four weeks after the application of the splint) we opened the dressings for the second time, and carefully renewed them. A slight motion was yet perceptible between the fragments. March 18th, we opened the dressings for the third time, and found the union complete. This was within less than forty days. The patient was now dismissed. On the 29th of April following, the bone was re-fractured. Mahar had been assisting to load the 'tender' to a locomotive. As the train was just getting in motion, he was hanging to the tender by his sound arm, while another laborer seized upon his broken arm to keep himself upon the car, and with a violent and sudden pull wrenched him from the tender and reproduced the fracture. The next morning I applied the dressings as before, and did not remove them during three weeks; at the end of which time the union was again complete. The splint was, however, reapplied, and has been continued to this time—a period of about six weeks."[1]

Since the date of the above paper, I have twice had opportunities to test the value of this mode of treatment in cases of somewhat delayed union of the humerus, and in each case with the same favorable result.

§ 6. Base of the Condyles. (*Fractures de l'extrêmité inférieure de l'humerus.*—Dupuytren. *Fractures sus-condyliennes de l'humerus.*—Malgaigne.)

Causes.—Of thirteen fractures at this point, nine occurred in children under ten years of age, the youngest being two years old.

In nine cases, the fracture had been produced by a fall, and it is presumed that the blow was received upon the elbow; in the remain-

Fig. 62.

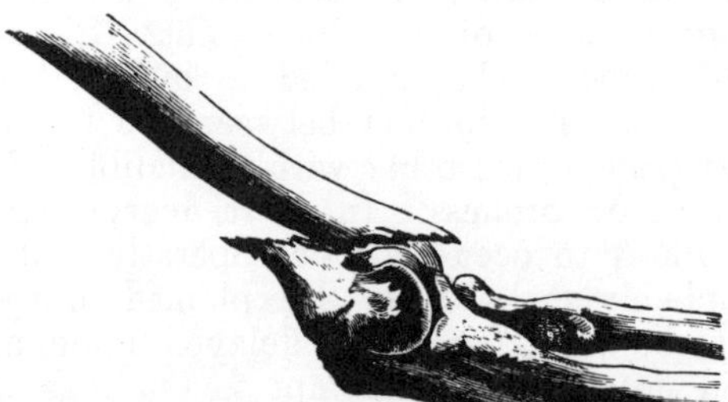

Fracture at the base of the condyles.

ing four cases the cause is not stated. I believe, therefore, that this fracture is generally the result of an indirect blow inflicted upon the extremity of the elbow; in a few examples, it has been produced by a blow received directly upon the point of fracture, as by the kick of a horse, &c., but I have never been able to trace it to a fall upon the hand. Recently, however, an "eclectic" physician in Cincinnati claimed that he had met with this fracture in a lad fourteen years old, produced

[1] Buffalo Med. Journ., vol. x. pp. 14-147.

by a fall upon the palm of the hand. Subsequently the parents of the lad sued the doctor for damages, claiming that the accident was a dislocation of the radius and ulna backwards, as it is, indeed, quite probable that it was; and alleging that his arm has been maimed by the long-continued, too tight and unnecessary bandaging.

Direction of the Fracture, Displacement, and Symptoms.—I think this fracture is generally oblique, and its line of direction upwards and backwards; in seven of the nine cases where this point was determined, such has been its apparent direction, and the lower fragment has been found drawn up behind the upper. Once I have found the lower fragment in front, and once on the outside of the upper.

Three of the thirteen were compound, comminuted fractures, this being a larger proportion of serious complications than I have found in almost any other fracture of a long bone.

I have never met with what I supposed to be a separation of the lower epiphysis, but surgical writers have occasionally spoken of this accident, and Dr. Watson, of New York, believes that he has seen one example in an infant not quite two years old. The limb had been violently wrenched by the mother, in attempting to lift her. She was not seen by Dr. Watson until the fourth day, at which time the swelling was such that the diagnosis could not be easily made out; but on the ninth day "it was apparent that the shaft of the humerus had been separated from its cartilaginous expansion at the condyles, near the elbow." By the use of angular pasteboard splints, the reduction was maintained, and the fragments became united after about four or six weeks.[1]

The diagnosis of this fracture is attended with peculiar difficulties, and it has occasionally been mistaken for a dislocation of the radius and ulna backwards. Dupuytren says: "There is nothing so common as to see a fracture of the lower end of the humerus, immediately above the elbow-joint, mistaken for a dislocation backward;" and he mentions three cases which have come under his own observation. I have found an opposite error, however, by far the most frequent, namely—a dislocation of both bones backwards has been supposed to be a fracture.

The sources of this embarrassment are found in the proximity of the fracture to the joint, in the rapidity with which swelling occurs, and in the striking similarity of the symptoms which characterize the two accidents.

It will be necessary, therefore, to establish with care the differential diagnosis. The following are the signs of fracture:—

1. Preternatural mobility, which, owing to the rapidity of the swelling and the contraction of the muscles whose tendons are stretched over the projecting ends of the bones, is often soon lost, being succeeded, sometimes after a few hours, by a rigidity equal to that which is usually present in dislocations, or even greater. It is especially difficult to flex the arm, owing to the pressure by the upper fragment into the bend of the elbow.

[1] Watson, New York Journ. Med., Nov. 1853, p. 430, second series, vol. xi.

2. Crepitus. This can usually be detected at any period if the arm is sufficiently extended, so as to bring the broken surfaces again into apposition.

3. When the extension is sufficient, reduction is easily effected, and the natural length of the arm is restored, but the limb immediately shortens when the extension is discontinued—especially if at the same moment the elbow is bent. This is a very important means of diagnosis.

4. A careful measurement, made from the point of the internal condyle to the acromion process, declares a positive shortening of the humerus.

5. By flexing and extending the forearm upon the arm, while the fingers are placed upon the lower portion of the humerus, the projecting fragments can be felt. Generally, the upper fragment being in front of the lower, and pressing down into the bend of the elbow, its end cannot be so easily recognized; but the upper end of the lower fragment can easily be made out when the forearm is considerably flexed. The lower end of the upper fragment feels more rough, and is less wide, than in dislocations.

6. The whole of the lower fragment is carried backwards, and with it the radius and ulna, producing a striking prominence of the elbow and olecranon process. Efforts to straighten the forearm upon the arm, when no extension is used, increase rather than diminish this projection.

7. The forearm is slightly flexed upon the arm; the angle made at the elbow being about 25 or 30 deg.

8. The hand and forearm are proned.

9. The relations of the olecranon process with the two condyles remain unchanged.

Signs of a dislocation of the radius and ulna backwards.

1. Preternatural rigidity.

2. Absence of crepitus. It is in this joint especially that surgeons have been deceived by the chafing of the dislocated bones upon the inflamed joint surfaces, and have supposed that they discovered crepitus when no fracture existed. The rapidity with which inflammation develops itself after dislocations of the elbow joint, and the consequent abundant effusion of lymph, afford the probable explanation of this frequent error.

3. When reduced, the bones are not generally disposed to become again displaced, even though the elbow should be flexed.

4. The humerus is not shortened, but the olecranon process approaches the acromion process.

5. There are no sharp projecting points of bone. The lower end of the humerus may not always be felt in the bend of the elbow; but when it is felt, it is found to be relatively smooth, broad and round.

6. A remarkable prominence of the elbow and olecranon process, which prominence is sensibly diminished when an effort is made to straighten the forearm on the arm.

7. Forearm flexed upon the arm to about the same degree as in fracture.

8. Hand and forearm proned, precisely as in fracture.

9. Relations of the olecranon process to the condyles changed very greatly.

The most constant diagnostic signs are, then, in the case of a fracture—crepitus, shortening of the humerus, projection of the sharp ends of the fragments, and an increase of the projection of the elbow when an attempt is made to straighten the arm; and in the case of a dislocation, the absence of crepitus, humerus not shortened, while the olecranon approaches the acromion process; the smooth, round head of the humerus lost, or indistinctly felt in the bend of the elbow and the projection of the point of the elbow diminished when an attempt is made to straighten the forearm on the arm.

It is proper, also, to repeat here what we have already said in relation to the causes of this fracture. A fracture at this point is produced almost always by a fall upon the elbow, but a dislocation of the radius and ulna backwards can never be. On the other hand, a dislocation is produced in almost every instance by a fall upon the palm of the hand, but I have never known a fracture above the condyles to be thus produced.

Results.—Eight times have I found the arm shortened from half an inch to one inch, or a little more.

Muscular anchylosis is almost always present when the apparatus is first removed, and it is seldom completely dissipated until after several months; but I have found more or less anchylosis at seven and nine months; and twice after the lapse of three years the motions of the joint have been very limited. A few years since, I examined the arm of a gentleman who was then twenty-seven years old, and who informed me that when he was four years old he broke the humerus just above the condyles. There still remained a sensible deformity at the point of fracture—he could not completely supine the arm. The whole arm was weak, and the ulnar nerve remarkably sensitive. The ulnar side of the forearm, and also the ring and little fingers, were numb, and have been in this condition ever since the accident. I know the surgeon very well who had charge of this case, and I have no doubt that the treatment was carefully and skilfully applied.

In June, of 1850, I operated upon a lad, nine years old, by sawing off the projecting end of the upper fragment, whose arm had been broken nine months before. This fragment was lying in front of the lower, and the skin covering its sharp point was very thin and tender. There was no anchylosis at the elbow-joint, but the hand was flexed forcibly upon the wrist, the first phalanx of all the fingers extended, and the second and third flexed. Supination and pronation of the forearm were lost. The forearm and hand were almost completely paralyzed, but very painful at times. The median nerve could be felt lying across the end of the bone.

In the hope that some favorable change might result to the hand by relieving the pressure upon the nerve, yet with not much expectation of success, I exposed the bone and removed the projecting fragment. The nerve had to be lifted and laid aside. About one year from this time I found the arm in the same condition as before the operation.

Non-union is a result not so frequent in fractures at this point as higher up; but Stephen Smith, of the Bellevue Hospital, New York, reports a case of non-union in a young man of twenty-three years. He was admitted to the hospital on the seventh day after the accident. The fracture was simple and transverse, yet at the end of four months he was dismissed "with perfectly free motion at the point of fracture."[1] The failure to unite was attributed to a syphilitic taint.

A case was recently tried in the Supreme Court at Brooklyn, N. Y., in which, after a simple fracture at this point, the arm being dressed with splints and bandages, the little finger sloughed off, in a condition of dry gangrene, and the adjacent parts of the hand were attacked with humid mortification. Drs. Parker and Prince believed that this serious accident was the result of bandages applied too tightly and suffered to remain too long, while Drs. Valentine Mott, Rogers, Wood, Ayres, Dixon, and others, believed that the gangrene might have been due to other causes over which the surgeon had no control.[2]

A few years ago, a similar case occurred in the town of Spencer, Tioga Co., N. Y.; a boy, six years old, having broken his humerus just above the condyles. The fracture was oblique. The surgeon who was called to treat the case was an old and highly respectable practitioner. I am not informed of the plan of treatment any farther than that a roller was applied. On the eighth day, a second surgeon was employed, who, finding the hand cold and insensible, removed all of the dressings; after which the thumb and forefinger sloughed, with other portions of the skin and flesh of the hand and arm. The surgeon who was first in attendance was prosecuted, and the case was tried in the Supreme Court of that county, but the jury found no cause of action. Dr. Hawley, of Ithaca, and the late Dr. Webster, of Geneva Medical College, testified that, in their opinion, the death of the fingers was owing to the pressure of the fragment upon the brachial artery, and not to the tightness of the bandages.

Dr. Gross has also informed us of still another case of the same character, which occurred in Warren Co., Ky. A boy, ten years old, had broken his arm above the condyles, and his parents having employed a surgeon residing at some distance, the dressings were applied, and directions given to send for the surgeon whenever it became necessary. The parents saw the arm swell excessively, and knew that the boy was suffering very much, but did not notify the surgeon until the tenth day, when the hand was found to be in a condition of mortification, and at length amputation became necessary.

Long afterward, in the year 1851, when the boy became of age, he prosecuted his surgeon, but with no result to either party beyond the payment of their respective costs.

While I would not deny that in all of these cases the sloughing might have been solely due to the tightness of the bandages, against

[1] S. Smith, New York Journal of Medicine, May, 1857, p. 386, third series, vol. ii.

[2] New York Medical Gazette, vol. xii. pp. 46, 80, 111.

which cruel and mischievous practice we cannot too loudly declaim, a knowledge of the anatomy of these parts, and the opinions of the very distinguished gentlemen who testified in defence of these surgeons, must compel us to admit the possibility of such accidents where the treatment has been skilful and faultless.

Treatment.—The splints generally employed in this country, in fractures about the elbow-joint, are simple angular side splints, without joints, such as those recommended by Physick.[1]

Fig. 63.

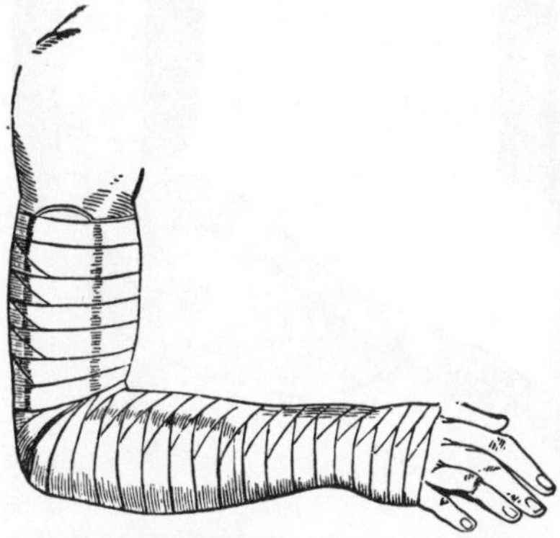

Fergusson's dressing for lower part of arm.

Fig. 64.

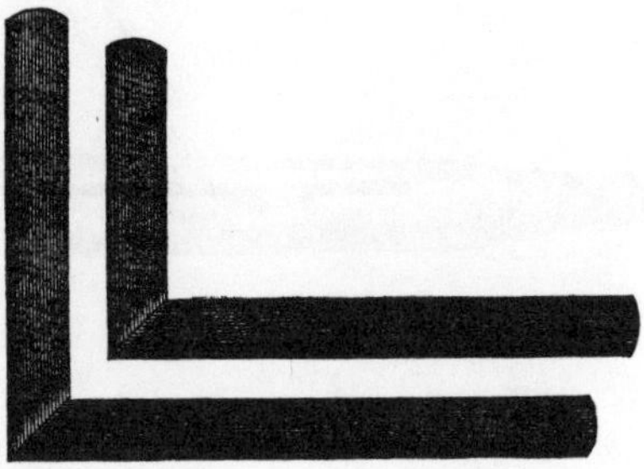

Physick's elbow splints.

Angular pasteboard splints, felt, gutta percha, &c., or angular splints with a hinge, such as Kirkbride's,[2] Thomas Hewson's, Day's, or Rose's, or the more perfect and elegant angular splint of Welch.

Fig. 65.

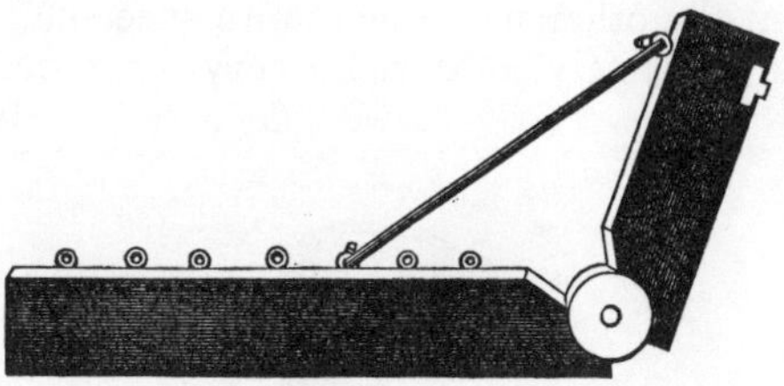

Kirkbride's elbow splint.

Fig. 66.

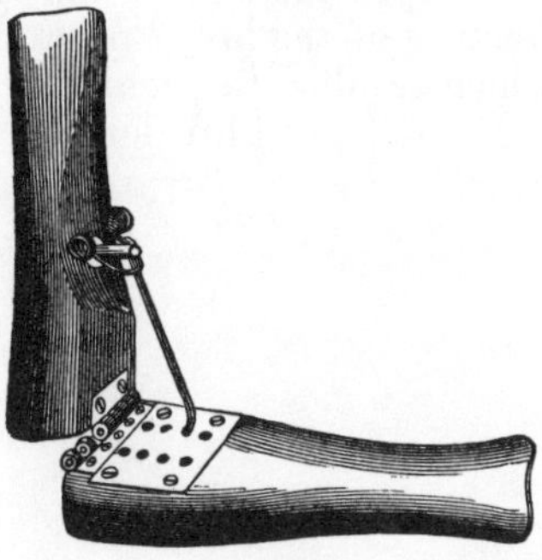

Day's splint.

Kirkbride's splint, which has been used in the Pennsylvania Hospital in several instances, is composed of two pieces of board, connected together by a circular joint, and having eyes on the inner edge, two inches apart, and holes through the splint at graduated distances be-

[1] Elements of Surgery, by John Syng Dorsey, Philadelphia edition, vol. i. p. 145.
[2] American Journal of the Medical Sciences, vol. xvi. p. 315.

tween them. There is also a swivel eye, passing through the upper part of the splint, and riveted below. A wire is fastened to the swivel, and bent at right angles at its other extremity, of a size to fit

Fig. 67.

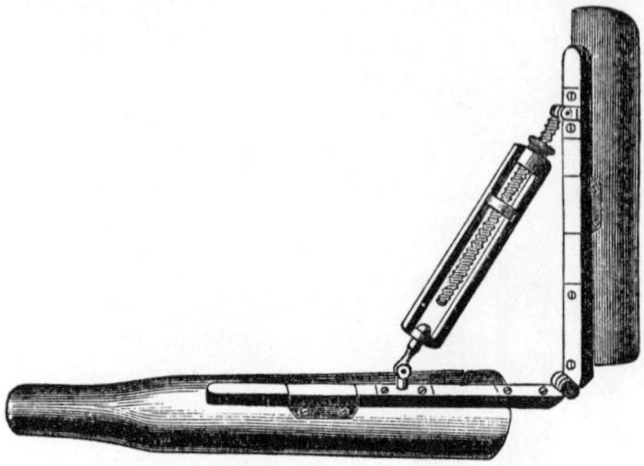

Rose's splint.

Fig. 68.

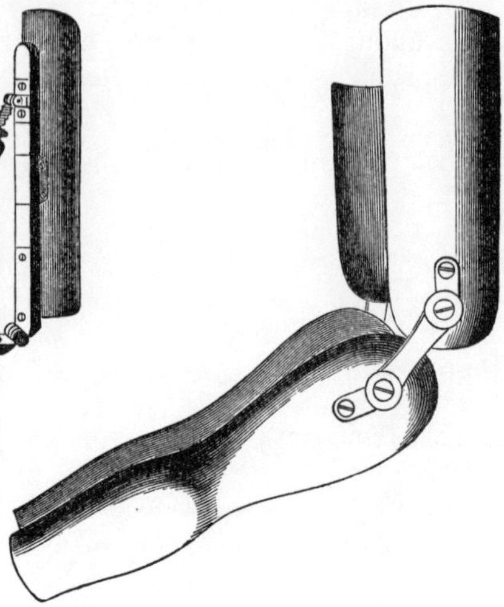

Welch's splint. The hinges may be transferred to splints of different sizes.

the eyes and holes in the splint. This splint, properly supported by pads, is to be placed either upon the outside or inside of the arm, and secured by rollers. When the angle is to be changed, the wire is unhooked and removed to another eye, or to some of the intermediate holes upon the side of the splint. Dr. Kirkbride reports two cases of fracture of the lower part of the humerus treated by this plan, one of which resulted in anchylosis, but the other was much more successful.

H. Bond, of Philadelphia, has also lately contrived a very ingenious

Fig. 69.

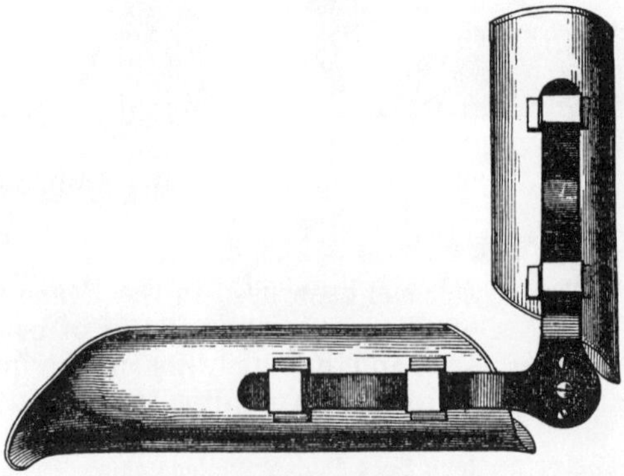

Bond's elbow splint.

splint for the elbow-joint, and which is designed also to afford a complete support to the forearm.

For myself, I generally prefer gutta percha, moulded and applied accurately to the limb, in the same manner as I have already directed in fractures of the surgical neck and shaft of the humerus, except that it shall be extended beyond the elbow to the wrist; so as to support the whole length of the arm, elbow, and forearm. Some experience in the use of wooden angular splints has convinced me that they cannot be very well fitted to the many inequalities of the limb; and neither pasteboard nor binder's board have sufficient firmness, especially in that portion which covers the joint. Angular splints, furnished with a movable joint, possess the advantage of enabling us to change the angle of the limb at pleasure, and of keeping up some degree of motion in the articulation without disturbing the fracture or removing the dressings; but the cross-bars of Days' and Rose's splints render them complicated, and are in the way of a nice application of the rollers; while they are all equally liable to the objection stated against angular wooden splints without joints, viz., that they seldom can be made to fit accurately the many irregularities of the arm, elbow, and forearm. Welch's splints, made of a material possessing a slight amount of flexibility, approach more nearly the accomplishment of these indications than any other manufactured splint with which I am acquainted, but the number of cases in practice to which they are applicable will be found to be limited, while gutta percha has no limit in its application.

Fig. 70.

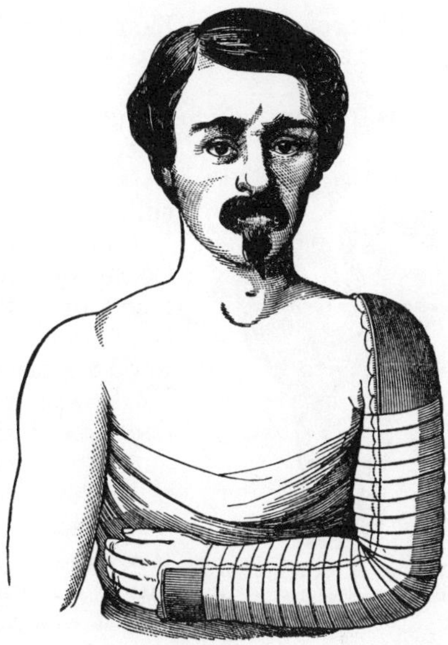

The author's elbow splint.

Whatever material is employed, a pretty large pledget of fine cotton batting ought to be laid in front of the elbow-joint, to prevent the roller from excoriating the delicate and inflamed skin, and great care should be taken to protect the bony eminences about the joint, or, rather, to relieve them from pressure, by increasing the thickness of the pads above and below these eminences.

At a very early day, so early, indeed, as the seventh or eighth day, the splint should be removed, and, while the fragments are steadied, gentle, passive motion should be inflicted upon the joint. This practice should be repeated as often as every second or third day, in order to prevent, as far as possible, anchylosis. If much swelling follows the injury, it is my custom to open the dressings, without removing the splints, on the second or third day after the accident, or at any time when the symptoms admonish us of its necessity. Occasionally it is well to change the angle of the splint before reapplying it. If the angular splint with a movable joint is used, slight changes may be made while the splint is on the arm; but if the angle is much changed without removing the rollers, they become unequally tightened over the arm, and may do mischief.

When anchylosis has actually taken place, we may more or less overcome the contraction of the muscles and of the ligaments by passive motion, or by directing the patient to swing a dumb-bell or some heavy weight in his hands, as first recommended by Hildanus.

§ 7. Fracture at the Base of the Condyles, complicated with Fracture between the Condyles, extending into the Joint.

This fracture, which is but a variety or complication of the preceding fracture, is even more difficult of diagnosis; and its signs, results, and proper treatment differ sufficiently to demand a separate consideration.

Fig. 71.

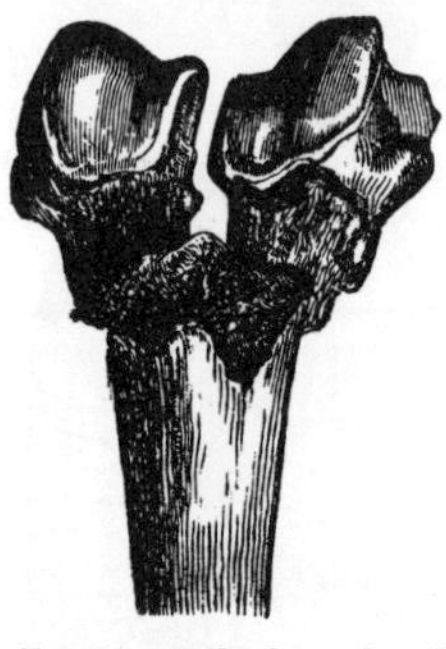

Fracture at the base of, and between the condyles.

I have recognized the accident four times. Confined to no period of life, it seems to be the result of a severe blow inflicted directly upon the lower and back part of the humerus, or upon the olecranon process. Dr. Parker, of New York, was inclined to regard an obscure accident about the elbow-joint, which he saw in a lad sixteen years old, as a longitudinal fracture of the humerus, with separation of one condyle, but which had been occasioned by a fall upon the hand.[1] For myself, I should regard this latter circumstance as presumptive evidence that it was not a fracture of this character, yet I do not mean to deny the possibility of its occurrence in this way.

Its characteristic symptoms are, increased breadth of the lower end of the humerus, occasioned by a separation of the condyles; displacement upwards and backwards of the radius and ulna; crepitus and mobility at the base of the condyles, with crepitus also between the condyles, developed by pressing the condyles together; or, when the radius and ulna are drawn up, by restoring these bones first to place by extension, and then pressing upon the opposite condyles; shortening of the humerus.

Its consequences are, generally, great inflammation about the joint, permanent deformity and bony anchylosis. An opposite result must be regarded as fortunate, and as an exception to the rule.

Of the treatment, we can only say that it must be chiefly directed to the prevention and reduction of inflammation, at least during the first few days. Nor is this inconsistent with an early reduction of the frag-

[1] Parker, New York Journal of Medicine, Nov. 1856, p. 391, 3d series, vol. i.

ments, and moderate efforts, by splints and bandages, such as we have directed in case of a simple fracture at the base of the condyles, to keep the fragments in place. No surgeon would be justified in refusing altogether to make suitable attempts to accomplish these important indications; but he must always regard them as secondary when compared with the importance of controlling the inflammation.

When splints are employed, the same rules will be applicable both as to their form and mode of application, as in cases of simple fracture above the condyles.

The following examples will more completely illustrate the character, history, and proper treatment of these cases, than any remarks or rules which we can at present make:—

A woman, living in this city, æt. 44, fell upon the sidewalk in January, 1850, striking upon her right elbow. I saw her a few minutes after the accident, but the parts about the joint were already considerably swollen, and it was not without difficulty that the diagnosis was made out. The forearm was slightly flexed upon the arm, and proned. On seizing the elbow firmly, a distinct motion was perceived above the condyles, and a crepitus. I could also feel, indistinctly, the point of the upper fragment. While moderate extension was made upon the arm, the condyles were pressed together, when it was apparent that they had been separated. On removing the extension, they again separated, and the olecranon drew up. She was in a condition of extreme exhaustion, and the bones were easily placed in position.

An angular splint was secured to the limb, and every care used to support the fragments completely, but gently.

From this date until the conclusion of the treatment, the dressings were removed often, and the elbow moved as much as it was possible to move it.

Seven months after the accident, the elbow was almost completely anchylosed at a right angle. The fingers and wrist also were quite rigid. Six years later, the anchylosis had nearly disappeared; she could now flex and extend the arm almost as much as the other; the wrist-joint was free, and the fingers could be flexed, but not sufficiently to touch the palm of the hand. The line of fracture through the base could be traced easily, but the humerus was not shortened. There was, moreover, much tenderness over the point of fracture through the base, and at other points. Occasionally, a slight grating was noticed in the radio-humeral articulation. She experienced frequent pains in the arm, and especially along the back and radial border of the ring finger. During the first year or two after the accident, the arm perished very much, but although the hand remained weak, the muscles were now well developed.

A gentleman was struck with the tongue of a carriage with which a couple of horses were running. The blow was received directly upon the back of the left elbow. Dr. Sprague and myself removed some small fragments of bone, and while opening the wound for this purpose, we could see distinctly the line of fracture extending into the joint as well as across the bone. The condyles were not separated.

The subsequent treatment consisted only in the use of such means as would best support the limb, and most successfully combat inflammation. The arm and forearm were laid upon a broad and well cushioned angular splint, covered with oil-cloth, to which they were fastened by a few light turns of a roller.

Twelve years after, I found the humerus shortened one inch and a half. During the first year, he says, there was no motion in the elbow-joint, but he can now flex and extend the forearm through about 45°; when flexed to a right angle, it seems to strike a solid body like bone. Rotation of the forearm is completely lost, the hand being in a position midway between supination and pronation. He suffers no pain, and his arm is quite strong and useful. No means have been employed to restore the functions of the limb but passive motion at first, and subsequently constant, active use of the hand and arm.

The late Dr. Thomas Spencer, of Geneva, used to relate a case in which a surgeon was called to what he supposed to be a fracture of the lower end of the humerus, and which he treated accordingly, with splints, &c. On the second or third day, another surgeon was called, who removed the splints and bandages, and pronounced it a dislocation of the radius and ulna backward; but he was unable to reduce it.

After some time, the first surgeon was prosecuted for having treated as a fracture what proved to be a dislocation. Dr. Spencer, who had examined the arm carefully, gave his testimony last, and at a time when, from the evidence, it seemed almost certain that the surgeon must be mulcted in heavy damages; but he declared his belief that both surgeons were right, since, on measuring the breadth of the humerus through its two condyles, he found that the humerus of the injured arm was three-quarters of an inch wider than the opposite. His conclusion, therefore, was that the condyles had been split asunder and were now separated; that the first surgeon properly reduced this fracture, but that when, on the second or third day, the second surgeon removed the splints and the dressings, a contraction of the muscles had taken place and the dislocation occurred, the bones of the forearm being drawn up between the fragments. Dr. Spencer believed this was an example of the variety of fracture now under consideration, but it is not quite certain that there was anything more than an oblique fracture extending into the joint, followed by a dislocation. In either case, the first surgeon was entitled to an acquittal, and so the jury promptly declared by their verdict.

In a case of compound comminuted fracture of the character now under consideration, Dr. Stone, of the Bellevue Hospital, New York, removed the condyles and sawed off the sharp end of the humerus. The woman was twenty-six years old and intemperate. The operation was made as a substitute for amputation. No serious complications followed. On the ninety-sixth day, the wounds were completely healed, and she could bend the forearm to a right angle with the arm, the action of the muscles having drawn up the radius and ulna against the lower end of the shaft of the humerus, so that the motions were natural and free.[1] The practice, as the result sufficiently shows, was

[1] Stone, New York Journ. of Med., May, 1851, p. 302, vol. vi. 2d series.

eminently judicious; and its practicability ought always to be well considered before resorting to the serious mutilation of amputation. The great principle upon which the success of resection is here based is the shortening of the bone, whereby the reduction may be accomplished without painful tension to the muscles; a principle which will demand of us hereafter a more careful consideration and a wider application.

Fractures of the Condyles.

Chaussier describes that portion of the lower end of the humerus which articulates with the ulna as the trochlea, and that portion which articulates with the radius as the condyle; naming the apophyses which arise from them, respectively, epitrochlea and epicondyle. Some of the French writers have adopted this nomenclature, but I prefer, as being more familiar to my own countrymen, the terms external and internal condyle, to which it will be convenient to add the terms external epicondyle and internal epicondyle, as indicating the extreme lateral projections, which are formed from separate points of ossification, and which do not become united to the trochlea until about the seventh year of life, and sometimes much later.

When, therefore, we speak of a fracture of the epicondyle, we refer only to a separation of the epiphysis, such as it is in early life; or to its true fracture, when, at a later period, it has become an apophysis.

§ 8. Fractures of the Internal Epicondyle (*Epitrochlea.* Chaussier.)

This is the fracture which Granger first described in the *Edinburgh Medical and Surgical Journal*,[1] and which he ascribed solely to muscular action. "A distinguishing circumstance attending this fracture is that of its being occasioned by sudden and violent muscular exertion; and it will be recollected that from the inner condyle those powerful muscles which constitute the bulk of the fleshy substance of the ulnar aspect of the forearm have their principal origin. The way in which the muscles of the inner condyle are involuntarily thrown into such sudden and excessive action I take to be this: the endeavor to prevent a fall by stretching out the arm, and thus receiving the percussion from the weight of the body on the hand."[2]

Fig. 72.

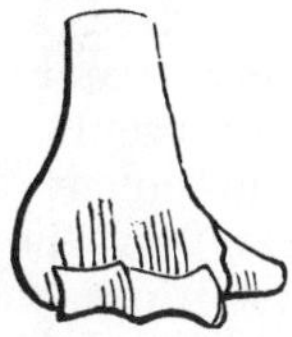

It is a fact, perhaps of some significance in this connection, that most of these fractures occur in children, before the union of the epiphysis is completed, when muscular contraction might more often prove adequate to its separation, and when the epicondyle is less prominent, and, therefore, less exposed to direct blows than in adult life; thus, of five fractures which I have distinctly recognized as frac-

[1] "On a Particular Fracture of the Inner Condyle of the Humerus," by Benjamin Granger, Surgeon, Burton-upon-Trent. Op. cit., vol. xiv. pp. 196–201, April, 1818.

[2] Ibid., p. 196.

tures of the epicondyle, all, except one, occurred between the ages of two and fifteen years. But then it is equally true that a large majority of all the fractures of the internal condyle, including those which enter the articulation, as well as those which do not, belong to childhood and youth. I have seen but one exception in fourteen cases. Since, then, direct blows generally produce those fractures which penetrate the joint, no good reason can be shown why they should not produce fractures of the epicondyle. The exception to which I have referred as not having occurred in early life, is sufficiently rare to entitle it to especial notice.

On the 16th of May, 1856, a laborer, thirty-four years of age, fell from an awning upon the side-walk, dislocating the radius and ulna backwards; the dislocation was immediately reduced by a woman who came to his assistance, but when he called on me, soon after, I found a small fragment of the inner condyle, probably the epicondyle alone, broken off and quite movable under the finger. It was slightly displaced in the direction of the hand.

I could not learn positively whether in falling he struck the elbow or the hand, but there was presumptive evidence that he struck the hand; if so, then probably the fracture was the result of muscular action, which is the more extraordinary as having taken place in a man of his age.

It is pretty certain, however, that the theory of causation adopted by Granger is too exclusive. A lad was brought to me in October, 1848, aged eleven, who had just fallen upon his elbow, the blow having been received, as he affirmed, and as the ecchymosis showed pretty conclusively, directly upon the inner condyle. The fragment was quite loose, and crepitus was distinct. He could flex and extend the arm, and rotate the forearm, without pain or inconvenience. I am quite sure the fracture did not extend into the joint; the result seemed also to confirm this opinion, for in three months from the time of the accident the motions of the elbow-joint were almost completely restored.

Indeed, Mr. Granger has failed to establish, by any particular proofs, that in more than one or two of his cases the fracture was the result of muscular action; but, on the contrary, I am disposed to infer, from the violent inflammation which generally ensued in his cases, from the frequency of ecchymosis, and especially from the injury done to the ulnar nerve in at least three instances, that most of them were produced by direct blows inflicted from below in the fall upon the ground. Fractures produced by muscular action are seldom accompanied with much inflammation or effusion of blood, and it is much more probable that the ulnar nerve should have been maimed by the direct blow which caused the fracture, than by the displacement of the apophysis, which is, as we shall presently show, almost always carried downwards, and oftener slightly forwards than backwards. It is only when the fragment is forced directly backwards that the ulnar nerve could be made to suffer; a direction which, it does not seem to me, it could ever take from muscular action alone.

Direction of Displacement, Symptoms, &c.—I have seen this fragment displaced in the direction of the hand, or downwards, very manifestly, twice, and in two other examples a careful measurement showed a slight displacement in the same direction. The greatest displacement occurred in a boy fifteen years old, who was brought to me from St. Catherines, Canada West. He had fallen upon his arm in wrestling, and his surgeon found a dislocation of the bones of the elbow-joint, which he immediately reduced. The fracture was not at that time detected, the arm being greatly swollen. No splints were applied. It was three months after the accident when I saw him, at which time I found the internal epicondyle broken off and removed downwards toward the hand one inch and a quarter; and at this point it had become immovably fixed. Partial anchylosis existed at the elbow-joint, but pronation and supination were perfect.

In one instance I believed the fragment to be carried about three lines upwards and two backwards toward the olecranon; in each of the other examples the fragment has not seemed to suffer any sensible displacement.

Granger found, also, in the five examples which came under his notice, the epicondyle carried toward the hand, with more or less variation in its lateral position, so that while in some instances it touched the olecranon, in others it was removed an inch or more in the opposite direction.

It is probable that, except where controlled by the force and direction of the blow, or by some complications in the accident, the fragment, if displaced at all, always moves downwards toward the hand, or downwards and a little forwards in the direction of the action of the principal muscles which arise from this apophysis; and when the fracture or separation is the result of muscular action alone, this form of displacement seems to me to be inevitable. In addition to the mobility, crepitus, and generally slight displacement of the fragment, which are the principal signs of this fracture, it may be noticed that there is usually some embarrassment in the motions of the elbow-joint, which may be due in part to the swelling, and in part to the detachment of the point of bone from and around which most of the pronators and flexors of the forearm have their rise. In one instance, already quoted, that of the lad aged eleven years, who broke the epicondyle from a direct blow, the motions of pronation, with flexion, were not at all impaired, neither immediately nor at any subsequent period, but the fragment was never sensibly, or only very slightly displaced.

Granger has recorded another class of symptoms, to which I have already alluded, his explanation of which, however, I am not prepared to admit. One of these cases he describes as follows: A boy, eight years old, fell with violence, and broke off completely the whole of the inner epicondyle of the right humerus. The lad said he had fallen on his hand. The fragment was displaced toward the hand. Severe inflammation followed, but he recovered the free and entire use of the elbow-joint in less than three months after the accident. No splints or bandages were ever employed.

From the moment of the accident, the little finger, the inner side of the ring finger, and the skin on the ulnar side of the hand, lost all sensation. The abductor minimi digiti and two contiguous muscles of the little finger were also paralyzed. This condition lasted eight or ten years, after which sensation and motion were gradually restored to these parts. As a consequence of this paralyzed condition of the ulnar nerve, also, successive crops of vesications, about the size of a split horse-bean, commenced to form on the little finger and ulnar edge of the hand some weeks after the accident, leaving troublesome excoriations. This eruption did not entirely cease for two or three months.

In two other cases, Mr. Granger remarks that he has found "the same paralysis of the small muscles of the little finger, the same loss of feeling in the integuments, and the same succession of crops of vesicles on the affected parts of the hand, as is described to have occurred in the preceding case."

Without intending to intimate a doubt of the accuracy of Mr. Granger's statement, that such phenomena have followed in three cases out of the five which he has seen, I must express my belief that it was only a remarkable concurrence of circumstances, since the same phenomena have never been seen by myself, nor do I know that they have been observed by any other surgeon.

Results.—As in all other accidents about the elbow-joint, a temporary rigidity is almost inevitable. The mere confinement of the arm in a flexed position is sufficient to determine this result without the interposition of a fracture; but when inflammation occurs, more or less contraction of the tendons, muscles, &c., about the joint must ensue. To this circumstance, therefore, added to the confinement, rather than to the fracture, will be due the anchylosis. If the fragment is not displaced, the fracture cannot certainly be responsible for the loss of motion, since it does not in any way involve the joint; and if displacement exists, its ultimate effect in diminishing the power of the muscles which arise from the apophysis must be only trivial and scarcely appreciable. We might, therefore reasonably conclude that where the accident has been properly treated, permanent anchylosis would be the exception and not the rule. This view of the matter seems also to be sustained by the recorded results. In Granger's cases, the full range of flexion and extension of the forearm has been finally restored, or with so trifling an exception as not to be observable without close attention, in every instance; except in the one already mentioned, which was originally complicated with dislocation; and even in this case the ultimate maiming was inconsiderable. Malgaigne, who says "it ought to be understood that in this accident articular rigidity is almost inevitable," seems nevertheless to admit the justness of Granger's observations as to the final result, if the proper means are employed to prevent it. I have myself found only once any considerable impairment of the motions of the joint after the lapse of a few years.

Treatment.—This accident does not constitute an exception to the rule which experience has established, that apophyseal projections when once displaced can seldom be restored completely to position or maintained in position, until a bony union is consummated. Granger remarks: "I have purposely avoided saying one word about replacing the detached condyle (epicondyle), and for these reasons: during the state of tumefaction of the limb, no means could be adopted for confining the retracted condyle in its place, beyond that of the relaxation of the muscles; and both before the tumefaction has commenced, and after it has subsided, all endeavors to replace the condyle, or even to change the position of it, have failed." He even proceeds so far as to declare that, while attention ought to be given to the reduction of the inflammation by appropriate means, we ought, nevertheless, to instruct the patient to flex and extend the arm daily from the moment the accident occurs until the cure is completed, and without any regard to the consolidation of the fragment; "the exercise of the joint in this manner must constitute the principal occupation of the patient for several weeks; and should it be remitted during the formation and consolidation of the callus, much of the benefit which may have been derived from this practice will be lost, and will with difficulty be regained."

With only slight qualifications I would adopt the advice of Mr. Granger. The limb ought always, at first, to be placed in a position of demiflexion, so that if anchylosis should unfortunately ensue, it should be in the condition which would render it most serviceable, and also because in this position the muscles which tend to displace the fragment would be most completely relaxed. While thus placed an attempt ought to be made, by seizing the apophysis, to restore it to position; and if the effort succeeds, as it certainly is not very likely to do, a compress and roller ought to be so applied as to maintain it in position; provided, always, that it shall not be found necessary to apply the roller so tight as to endanger the limb, or increase the inflammation. An angular splint would be an almost indispensable part of the appareil, at least with children, where this indication is in view. In no case, however, ought more than seven or fourteen days to elapse before all bandaging and splinting should be abandoned, and careful, but frequent flexion and extension be substituted.

§ 9. Fractures of the External Epicondyle. (*Epicondyle,* Chaussier.)

I have only mentioned this supposed fracture, of which some writers have spoken as a fact, in order that I may declare my conviction that its existence has never been made out. If we admit the possibility, that, while in a state of epiphysis, it might, like the corresponding internal epiphysis, be separated by muscular action, we must yet deny its probability, since it is so exceedingly small; and we must, for the same reason, be permitted to doubt whether the fact of its separation could be recognized in the living subject. Moreover, if a true fracture occurs at this point as the result of external violence, it is sufficiently plain, from an examination of the anatomical structure, that it must more or less extend into the joint and involve the condyle itself.

§ 10. Fractures of the Internal Condyle. (*Trochlea*, Chaussier.)

B. Cooper, South, Sir Astley Cooper and others, speak of fracture of the internal condyle as very common, and more so than fracture of the external condyle; while Malgaigne, who admits its existence, has never met with a single living example, and regards its occurrence as exceedingly rare. In a record of fourteen fractures I have found no difficulty in recognizing four as fractures of the inner condyle; five, I have already said, were fractures of the epicondyle, and the remaining five were undetermined, while my records furnish fourteen examples of undoubted fractures of the external condyle. It is probable that Sir Astley did not intend to make any distinction between fractures of the condyle and epicondyle, and this might explain somewhat his opinion of the relative frequency of these accidents; but even rejecting this important distinction, it has happened to me to see just as many examples of fracture of the outer condyle as of the inner.

Fig. 73.

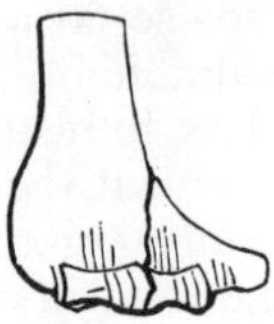

Causes.—It has already been stated that fractures of the internal condyle, as well as fractures of the epicondyle, belong almost exclusively to infancy and childhood, no instance having come under my notice after the eighteenth year of life, except in the person of a man thirty-four years old, whose case I have mentioned when speaking of fracture of the epicondyle.

I have seen no instance which could be traced to any other cause than a direct blow, such as a fall upon the elbow, the force of the concussion being received directly upon the condyle.

Lonsdale speaks of fractures of the condyles occasioned by falls upon the hands: but without intending to question their possibility, I will state frankly that they seem to me not to have been satisfactorily proven.

Line of Fracture, Displacement, Symptoms.—The direction of the line of fracture is tolerably uniform, namely, commencing about one quarter or half an inch above the epicondyle, it extends obliquely outwards through the olecranon and coronoid fossæ, and enters the joint through the centre of the trochlea.

Displacement of the lower fragment can take place only in a direction upwards, backwards, forwards and inwards (to the ulnar side). The fragment cannot be carried downwards, in the direction of the hand, nor outwards, in the direction of the radius, unless the radius also is broken or dislocated.

The most common form of displacement is upwards and backwards, and perhaps at the same time a little inwards; the ulna remaining attached to the lower fragment, and following its movements. I have seen one instance in which the fragment was carried directly downwards toward the hand, but this accident was originally complicated with a dislocation of the radius backwards. The dislocation was immediately reduced. Five years after, when the young man was twenty-three years old, I found the condyle displaced downwards and forwards about half an inch, so that when the forearm was extended it became strikingly deflected to the radial side.

The symptoms which characterize this fracture are crepitus, almost always easily detected; mobility of the fragment, discovered especially by seizing upon the epicondyle, or by flexing and extending the arm; displacement of the smaller fragment and a projection of the olecranon process, this latter being very marked when the forearm is extended upon the arm, but almost completely disappearing when the elbow is bent; projection of the lower end of the humerus in front when the arm is extended; the humerus shortened when measured along its ulnar side, from the internal epicondyle; the breadth of the humerus, through its condyles, generally increased slightly, sometimes half an inch or more; if the lesser fragment is carried upwards it will also be found that when the limb is extended, the forearm will be deflected to the ulnar side.

Sir Astley Cooper remarks that it is frequently mistaken for a dislocation; and Thomas M. Markoe, of New York, has shown that it is, in fact, frequently complicated with a dislocation of the head of the radius backwards; indeed, he expresses a belief that this dislocation of the radius seldom or never occurs without a fracture of the internal condyle.[1] I shall refer to his views again when considering dislocations of the head of the radius.

Results.—It is probable that in a majority of cases no permanent displacement exists; although the irregularity of the bony deposits around the base of the condyle, which generally may be easily felt, would lead to a contrary opinion. The fact that the lower fragment usually follows the motions of the olecranon, renders its replacement and retention comparatively easy, unless some complication exists. It is not from displacement, therefore, so much as from permanent muscular, and especially bony anchylosis, that serious maimings so often result. Under any treatment bony anchylosis will very often ensue, and under improper treatment it is almost inevitable.

Treatment.—The arm must be immediately flexed to nearly or quite a right angle, when, without much manipulation, the fragments will be made to resume their place. A gutta-percha, right-angled splint, such as I have already directed for fractures occurring just above the condyles, well and carefully cushioned, must now be applied, and secured by rollers. Suitable pads must also aid the splint and roller, in keeping the fragments in place. Markoe prefers keeping the forearm in a position about ten degrees short of a right angle, believing that in this position the ulna itself will act as a splint, and by its support on the uninjured portion of the trochlea, hold in its place the broken condyle. Very properly, also, he prefers to lay the angular splint, made of tin and fitted to the arm and forearm, upon the back of the limb instead of upon the front or sides. If it is upon the inside, it covers the broken condyle, and we are unable to know so well its position; if upon either side, it is apt to press injuriously upon the

[1] Markoe, New York Journal of Medicine, May, 1855, p. 382, second series, vol. xiv.

epicondyles; and if it is in front, the fragments cannot be so well adjusted or supported. Upon this point, however, surgeons are not very well agreed, and no doubt more will depend upon the care with which the splint is applied than upon the surface against which it is laid.

Considerable swelling is almost certain to follow, and no surgeon ought to hazard the chances of vesications, ulcerations, &c., by neglecting to open or completely remove the dressings every day. Within seven days, and perhaps earlier, passive motion must be commenced, and perseveringly employed from day to day until the cure is accomplished; indeed, in a majority of cases it is better not to resume the use of splints after this period: for although at this time no bony union has taken place, yet the effusions have somewhat steadied the fragments, and the danger of displacement is lessened, while the prevention of anchylosis demands very early and continued motion.

When the fracture is compound, or otherwise complicated, these simple rules will seldom be found applicable; indeed, fractures attended with no such complications will occasionally be found difficult to reduce, or to maintain in position after reduction.

§ 11. Fractures of the External Condyle.

Causes.—All of the fractures (14) which I have seen of the external condyle occurred in children under thirteen years of age, except one; in which instance a woman, eighty-eight years of age, fell upon her elbow while intoxicated, breaking off the outer condyle. Two months after the accident I found the fragment displaced half an inch upwards, and firmly united.

In a large majority of these cases the patients themselves have affirmed, and the surface of the skin has furnished conclusive evidence, that the fracture was produced by a direct blow, generally by a fall upon the elbow.

Line of Fracture, Displacement, and Symptoms.—The direction of the fracture is generally such that, commencing always above and without the capsule, it descends obliquely and enters the joint either just within or through the "small head" or articulating surface upon which the radius is received; or else it penetrates more deeply in its progress, and passing through the olecranon fossa, it enters the joint through the middle of the trochlea.

In the first of these classes of examples, which I think also is the most common, the condyle alone is broken off, and it is liable only to become displaced backwards, forwards, or outwards; generally, I have found it displaced a little outwards, sufficiently to increase manifestly the breadth of the condyles; or it has been carried backwards; once slightly forwards; it is also, in some cases, carried upwards in a small degree, although the action of the supinators and extensors would seem to render a downward displacement more common. These displacements are usually not considerable, and in a few cases there is none at all. Whatever may be the direction or degree in which the fragment is moved, however, the head of the radius is found almost always to accompany it. In the case which I am about to relate, the head of the radius became completely separated from the condyle.

Frederick Keaffer, æt. 11, fell from a load of hay, and he is confident that he struck the ground with the back of his elbow. Six hours after the accident, he was brought to me by the physician who was first called to him. The arm was much swollen, and the external condyle could not be distinctly felt, but when pressure was made directly upon it, crepitus and motion became manifest. The head of the radius was at the same time dislocated backwards, and separated entirely from the condyle; its smooth button-like head being very prominent. It is difficult to conceive how a blow from behind should leave the head of the radius dislocated backwards, or how the radius could have separated from the broken condyle; but as the examination was repeated several times, and while the patient was under the influence of ether, I have no doubt of the fact. Several other surgeons who were present concurred with me in opinion fully.

While prosecuting the examination, I reduced the dislocation of the radius, but it would not remain in place a moment when pressure or support was removed. The lad recovered with a very useful arm, the motions of flexion and extension, with pronation and supination, after the lapse of a year, being nearly as complete as before the accident. The radius remains unreduced.

Sometimes it will be noticed that while the portion of the condyle which is attached to the radius falls backwards, its upper and broken extremity pitches forwards; and this attitude it is especially prone to assume when the forearm is extended.

It is even possible, when the fracture traverses the trochlea, for the ulna also to become displaced backwards along with the radius and the lesser fragment.

Crepitus, which is usually very distinct, is most easily obtained by rotating the radius, or by seizing upon the condyle with the thumb and fingers, and moving it backwards and forwards.

Results.—Ordinarily, this fragment unites promptly and by the interposition of a bony callus; but in a few cases, I have noticed that either no union has occurred, or the union has been accomplished only through the medium of fibrous structure, and the fragment continued afterward to move with the radius.

As a consequence, probably, of the displacement of the lesser fragment upwards, the forearm, when straightened, is occasionally found deflected to the radial side. The surgeon must not, however, confound the deflection which is natural, and which is greater in some persons than in others, with the unnatural radial inclination which is occasioned sometimes by this accident. I have met with this phenomenon three times in children under three years of age, in one of which I could not discover that the condyle was carried toward the shoulder, but only outwards; in each of the other cases the fragment had united by ligament. The following is one of the examples referred to:—

A girl, æt. 3, fell and broke the external condyle of the left humerus; fracture extending freely into the joint; crepitus distinct; forearm slightly flexed; prone. Lesser fragment displaced outwards and a little backwards, carrying with it the radius. On the second day I was dismissed on account of the unfavorable prognosis which I gave, or rather because I refused to guarantee a perfect limb, and an empiric was employed, who readily gave the requisite guarantee, namely, his word of honor.

July 2, 1857, several months after the accident, the father brought her to me for examination. There was no anchylosis, but the lesser fragment had never united, unless by ligament, moving freely with the head of the radius. When the forearm was straightened upon the arm it fell strongly to the radial side, but resumed its natural relation again when the elbow was flexed.

The two other examples are reported at length in the second part of my *Report on Deformities after Fractures* as Cases 57 and 59 of fractures of the humerus.

In one other example, however, mentioned also in my report as Case 56, the deflection was to the opposite side. I examined the lad one year after the accident, he being then five years old, and I found the external condyle very prominent and firmly united, but not apparently displaced in any direction except outwards. The radius and ulna had evidently suffered a diastasis at their upper ends, but all of the motions of the joint were free and perfect.

Dorsey[1] speaks of this lateral inclination as being always to the ulnar side, but does not indicate to what particular fracture of the elbow it belongs. He has also described a splint, contrived by Dr. Physick, intended to remedy the deformity in question.

Chelius also speaks of the same deformity as occurring after fractures of the internal, but does not mention it in connection with fractures of the external condyle, that is, an inclination of the forearm to the ulnar side.

In more than half of the cases of fracture of this condyle some degree of anchylosis has resulted, lasting at least several months. I have seen it remaining after a lapse of from one to twenty years, but generally it gradually diminishes, and, in a majority of cases, completely disappears after a few years.

Treatment.—I do not know that I need add much to what has already been said in relation to the treatment of fractures of the opposite condyle, and at the base of the condyles, since the measures applicable to the one are, in general, applicable to the other.

Generally, the forearm ought to be flexed upon the arm, especially with a view to overcome the usual tendency in the upper end of the lower fragment to pitch forwards, and which form of displacement is greatly increased by straightening the arm. A remarkable exception to this rule, and the only one I have seen, must be mentioned.

James Cronyn, aged six, was brought to me in March, 1857, having, a few minutes before, fallen from a height of four or five feet to the ground. His father said the elbow had been broken at the same point two years before, and from that time had remained stiff and crooked. I found the external condyle broken off, and, with the head of the

[1] Elements of Surgery, by Philip Syng Dorsey, Phila. ed., 1813, vol. i. p. 146.

radius, carried backwards. This was the position which it occupied constantly, though it was easily restored and maintained in position when the arm was straight, but not by any possible means when the elbow was flexed. I dressed the arm, therefore, in an extended position, with a long felt splint, and the fragments remained well in place until a cure was accomplished.

In certain examples, I have no doubt also that advantage might be derived from the use of Physick's splint, intended to obviate the outward or inward inclination of the forearm.

Fig. 74.

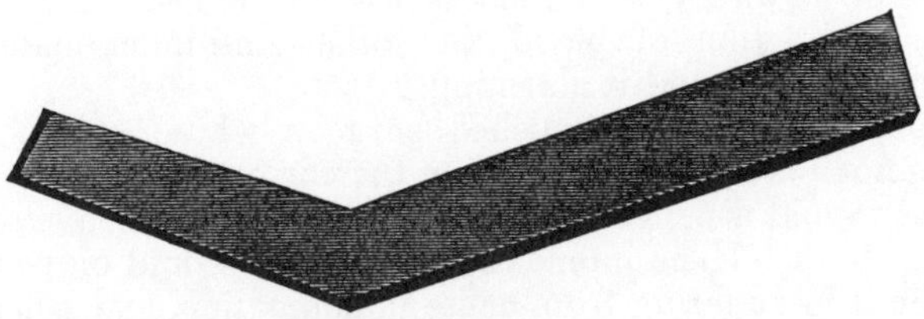

Physick's splint.

It is especially deserving of notice that, in the three cases in which I have observed bony union to fail, and the fragments to continue movable, the motions of the elbow-joint have, in a very short time, been completely restored. If it does not prove that Granger was correct in his views as applied to fractures of the internal epicondyle, namely, that it was of little or no consequence whether the fragment united or not, and that the elbow-joint ought to be submitted to free motion from the beginning to the end of the treatment—if it does not absolutely prove, I say, the correctness of his views, it at least must abate our apprehensions of the supposed evil results of non-union in the case of the fracture now under consideration.

I shall take the liberty of quoting also, with a qualified approval, the opinion of Dr. John C. Warren, of Boston, as stated by Dr. Norris in his *Report on Surgery*, made to the American Medical Association in 1848.

"In the treatment of fractures of the condyles of the os humeri, a course is usually recommended which he believes to be hurtful, inasmuch as it favors the worst consequences of the injury, namely, loss of motion in the joint. By this mode of treatment, the fractured piece becomes sufficiently fixed to create partial anchylosis; and there is so much pain afterwards in the proposed passive movements as to cause the omission of these measures until permanent stiffness takes place. The proper course in the management of these accidents he conceives to be, 1st. To apply no splints, but in the earlier days to make use of the proper means to prevent inflammation. 2d. To accustom the patient to early and daily movements of flexion and extension. 3d. When the action of the joint becomes limited, to overcome the resistance by force, and repeat it daily, until the tendency of the joint to stiffen ceases.

"The accomplishment of this process, he adds, is so very painful that few patients have courage to submit to it, and few surgeons firmness to prosecute it. The consequence has been that in a great number of cases the use of the articulation to a greater or less extent has been lost. The introduction of etherization, by preventing the pain, gives us, in the opinion of Dr. Warren, the means of overcoming the resistance. By its aid he has restored the motion of a considerable number of anchylosed elbows, and has successfully applied the same measures to other joints, particularly to the shoulder and knee. This has now become his settled practice, with the results of which he is entirely satisfied. The inflammation consequent upon the forced movements of an anchylosed joint is not to be lost sight of. By a reasonable abstraction of blood, and other anti-inflammatory treatment, he has never found it alarming."[1]

My respect for the distinguished surgeon whose opinion is here given does not permit me to question the correctness of his practice; but I cannot avoid a belief that his language does not convey a precise idea of his views. If he intends to say that he would move the joint freely when it is suffering from acute inflammation, and when motion occasions great pain, I must protest against the practice as likely to do vastly more harm than good in any case; but if he would move the joint from the first when the inflammation and swelling are trivial, and when it occasions only an endurable amount of pain, then his views are just and his practice worthy of imitation.

CHAPTER XXI.

FRACTURES OF THE RADIUS.

Of sixty-one fractures of the radius which have come under my observation, three belonged to the upper third, two to the middle third, and fifty-six to the lower third. Two were compound, and fifty-nine simple. Thirty-nine are recorded of males, and twenty one of females; twenty-seven as having occurred in the left arm, and sixteen in the right.

Fracture of the neck of the radius, as a simple accident, uncomplicated with any other fracture or dislocation, is exceedingly rare; yet, owing to the depth of the superincumbent mass of muscles, and the difficulty of determining, where so many bones and processes approach each other, precisely from what point the crepitus, if any is found, proceeds, surgeons have often been deceived, and they believed that they were the fortunate possessors of this rare pathological treasure,

[1] Transactions of the American Medical Association, vol. i. p. 174.

when the autopsy has too soon disclosed their error. Both B. Cooper and Robert Smith have alluded to this difficulty, and the case reported by Dr. Markoe to the New York Pathological Society, and published in the April number of the *American Medical Monthly*, will serve to illustrate the same point; in which case the signs of a fracture of the radius at its neck were such as to deceive that experienced surgeon, yet the autopsy disclosed the fact that it was a dislocation of the head of the radius forwards, with a fracture of the ulna. Indeed, its existence as a form of fracture was doubted by Sir Astley Cooper, and by others has been actually denied. I have seen no specimen obtained from the cadaver, except the doubtful one contained in Dr. Watts' cabinet, and of which I have furnished an account, accompanied with a drawing, in my report to the American Medical Association,[1] and the specimen owned by Dr. Mütter, of Philadelphia, of which he has kindly furnished me the following description: "History unknown. The line of fracture seems to have passed through the neck of the left radius, just at the upper extremity of the bicipital protuberance. Union with deformity has resulted. Owing to the fracture having taken place within the insertion of the biceps, that muscle appears to have drawn forward and upward the lower end of the short upper fragment. In consequence of this movement, the articulating facet of the head of the radius is tilted backwards, so as no longer to be in contact with the humerus. As a secondary consequence, the anterior edge of the head of the radius rests permanently against the articulating surface of the humerus. At this new point of contact a new surface of articulation is seen to have been formed, while the original articulating facet is directed backwards, and lies at right angles to the one of more recent formation. At the inner edge of the new articulation of the head of the radius with the humerus, contact with the ulna has developed another surface of articulation. The upper and lower fragments are united at an angle, and the radius does not appear to have lost in length."

Fig. 75.

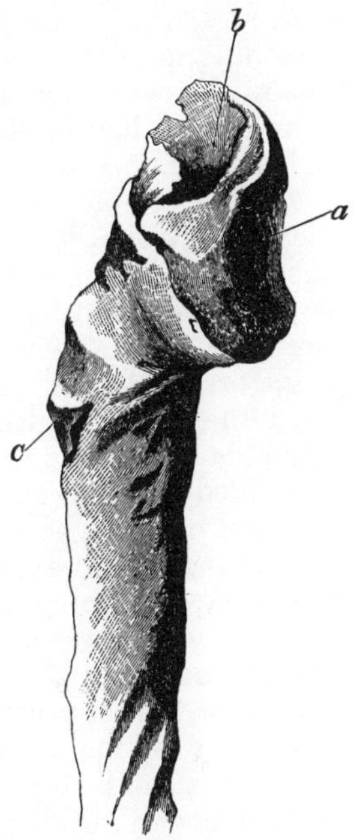

Fracture of neck of radius. (Mütter's cabinet.) *a*. Original articulating facet. *b, b*. New articulating facets. *c*. Projecting fragments.

Velpeau has once demonstrated the existence of this fracture in a dissection, but the fracture was accompanied with a fracture also of the coronoid process; and Bérard obtained possession of a similar specimen. I do not remember to have seen a notice of any others. Malgaigne affirms, with his usual frankness, that although he has occasionally believed that he had met with it, the autopsy, whenever it has

[1] Transactions, vol. ix. pp. 157 and 229.

been obtained, has shown that it was rather a subluxation than a fracture. On the other hand, Mr. South calls it a "not unfrequent accident," but in confirmation of this declaration he cites no examples.

While, therefore, the presence of what appear to be the rational diagnostic signs has compelled me to record one case as an uncomplicated fracture of the neck of the radius, and two others as fractures at this point accompanied either with a fracture of the humerus or a dislocation of the ulna, I am prepared to admit that some doubt remains in my own mind as to whether in either case the fact was clearly ascertained; nor do I think, speaking only of the simple fracture, that it will ever be safe to declare positively that we have before us this accident, lest, as has happened many times before, in the final appeal to that court whose judgment waits until after death, our decisions should be reversed.

Nothing, perhaps, could more fully illustrate the difficulty of diagnosis in the case of injuries received in the neighborhood of the head of the radius than the testimony given in the case of Noyes *vs.* Allen, tried in the Supreme Court at Cambridge, January, 1856, before Judge Bigelow. Mr. Noyes injured his elbow, January 7, 1854, and Dr. Allen, who was called immediately, believed that the ligaments of the joint had been torn, but that no bones were broken or displaced. On the following morning he was dismissed, and Mr. Noyes went home. Three weeks later it was seen by Dr. Dow, who also thought there was no fracture. About eight weeks after the accident a physician examined the arm, and declared the neck of the radius broken and the fragments displaced; and when the case was finally brought to trial, he testified still that such was certainly the fact: and five other physicians, not one of whom, however, we are told, was a member of the State Medical Society, testified positively that the radius was broken at its neck, producing a bony protuberance; that such an injury only could account for the symptoms manifested at the time of the accident, and that no other fractures or injuries of the joint could explain so well the present appearances of the arm. While, on the part of the defence, six of the most intelligent medical gentlemen of the State, Drs. Kimbal and Huntington, of Lowell, and Drs. Townsend, Lewis, Clark, and Gay, of Boston, testified that the head and neck of the radius were not displaced, nor was there any evidence that this bone had ever been broken. There is every reason to believe that these latter gentlemen were correct; yet it is to be presumed that the gentlemen who first testified were not without some grounds for their opinions, so confidently expressed.

The case was given to the jury after a trial of five days, who promptly returned a verdict for the defendant.[1]

When this fracture occurs, the upper end of the lower fragment will probably be carried forwards by the action of that portion of the biceps which has its insertion into the tubercle; and the displacement in this direction must necessarily be increased in proportion as the arm is straightened. In the cabinet specimen belonging to Dr. Mütter,

[1] Amer. Med. Gazette, vol. vii. p. 299.

the line of fracture, commencing in the neck, has terminated in the tubercle; consequently the biceps, having still some attachment to the upper fragment as well as the lower, has drawn them both forwards.

The same anterior displacement I have noticed in all of the supposed living examples, but whether both fragments or only one had suffered displacement I am unable to say.

A girl, æt. 11, living in Ontario Co., N. Y., fell from a tree and injured her right arm. Her surgeon, who regarded it as a fracture of the neck of the radius, reduced the fragments, and placed the forearm at a right angle with the arm. On the twenty-eighth day, all dressings were removed, and the patient was dismissed; the fragments seemed to be in place. The parents, finding the elbow stiff, now made violent and successful efforts to straighten the arm.

Fifteen months after the accident, the child was brought to me. There was at this time a bony projection in front, opposite the neck of the radius, which I believed to be the point of fracture. The hand was forcibly proned, and she had only a limited amount of motion at the elbow-joint. The anchylosis was probably due to inflammation directly resulting from the severe contusion; but it is quite probable that the forward displacement of the fragments was alone due to the too early and too violent attempts to straighten the arm; at least, this was the explanation which I ventured to give to the parents at the time.

The second case occurred in a lad eight years old, living in Wyoming Co., N. Y. His parents brought him to me ten weeks after the injury was received, and I then found the forearm bent to a right angle with the arm, and anchylosed at the elbow-joint. The hand was also forcibly proned, and could not be supined. In front, and opposite the neck of the radius, there was a distinct bony projection, which I believed to be the point of union of the broken fragments. The external condyle seemed also to have been broken.

The third example, treated originally by Dr. Nott, of Buffalo, was seen by me six months after the accident. The upper end of the lower fragment seemed to be displaced forwards. There was very little motion at the elbow-joint, and both pronation and supination were completely lost.

I have seen, in Dr. Mütter's cabinet, two specimens of fracture of the outer half of the head of the radius. In one case, the small fragment is slightly displaced downwards in the direction of the axis of the bone; and, in the other, the fragment is thrown outwards, or to the radial side. Both are firmly united in their new positions.

In the treatment of fractures of the neck of the radius, we must not neglect to flex the forearm upon the arm, so as to relax, as completely as possible, the biceps, whose advantageous insertion into the tubercle of the radius would be certain to produce displacement, unless this position was adopted. A single dorsal splint, properly padded, should support the forearm, while the surgeon, having placed a compress over the upper end of the lower fragment, proceeds to secure the whole with a roller.

Especial care must also be taken to prevent the forearm from being extended before the bony union is fairly consummated, lest the biceps, now firmly contracted, should draw the lower fragment forwards, as it must inevitably do while the bony union is imperfect; an accident which, there is some reason to believe, occurred in one of the examples which I have already cited.

If the patient be a child, or if there is any reason to suppose that these rules will not be faithfully complied with, it would be well to secure the arm in this position with a right-angled splint.

When the fracture occurs in any portion of the radius below the insertion of the biceps and above the insertion of the pronator radii teres, Mr. Lonsdale suggests the propriety of placing the forearm in a condition of supination, at least so far as is practicable, for the purpose of securing a proper apposition of the fragments. His argument in favor of this practice is ingenious, and deserves consideration.

When the bone is broken anywhere in this portion, the action of the pronators upon the upper fragment ceases; while that of the biceps, which is a powerful supinator, continues; consequently the upper fragment becomes at once, and completely, rotated outwards or supined. Now, if the hand, to which the lower end of the radius alone remains attached, should be forcibly proned, the radius will also be rotated inwards upon its own axis; and although it might be possible in this condition to bring the broken ends into contact, and a bony union, without deformity might be consummated, yet the power of supination must be forever lost; since the union has been effected while the head and upper fragment are already in a state of complete supination, and if such is the fact it is evident that the whole bone, together with the hand, will be incapable of any further supination.

It is not, indeed, the practice with any surgeons, so far as I know, to treat this fracture with the hand placed in a position of extreme pronation; but the case has been supposed for the purpose of rendering the argument more intelligible. The usual practice is to place the forearm and hand in a position midway between supination and pronation, and then to lay it across the body at a right angle with the arm; but it is plain that the same objection, differing only in degree, will apply to this position as to that of pronation. The axes of the two fragments are not made to correspond, since, while the lower fragment is only half rotated outwards, the upper fragment is completely, and the result of the union must be the loss of one-half the power of supination in the hand.

It is only, then, by complete supination of the hand during treatment that this difficulty can be avoided, and I have no doubt that we ought to adopt this plan whenever it is practicable to do so, or whenever we are not hindered by serious obstacles; and the only obstacle which occurs to me as likely to interpose itself, is the practical one which most surgeons must have experienced in treating all injuries of the forearm, whether fractures, or only severe contusions of the muscles, &c., namely, the constant and almost uncontrollable tendency of the hand to assume the prone or semi-prone position. This is due, no doubt, to the great preponderance of the power of the pronators; and such is the resistance which they afford to supination that it is often quite impossible to lay the hand upon its back while the forearm is across the body, and if accomplished, the position generally becomes in a few hours so painful as to be unendurable. By extending the arm, however, and laying it upon a pillow, the hand will be found again to rest easily upon its back, because in this way we avail ourselves of the outward rotation of the humerus at the shoulder-joint.

It has already been stated that of the whole number of fractures of this bone seen by me, amounting in all to just sixty, only two belonged to the middle third. An observation which is in striking contrast with the remark of Chelius, that it is broken most frequently in its middle.

Generally the fragments incline toward the ulna, but they may also be carried either forwards or backwards, according to the direction and force of the blow, or the seat of the fracture.

A laboring man, æt. 35, broke the radius near the lower end of the middle third. On the same day I replaced the fragments as well as I could in the midst of the swelling which had already occurred, and applied two broad and well-padded splints, one to the palmar and one to the dorsal surface of the forearm.

Fig. 76.

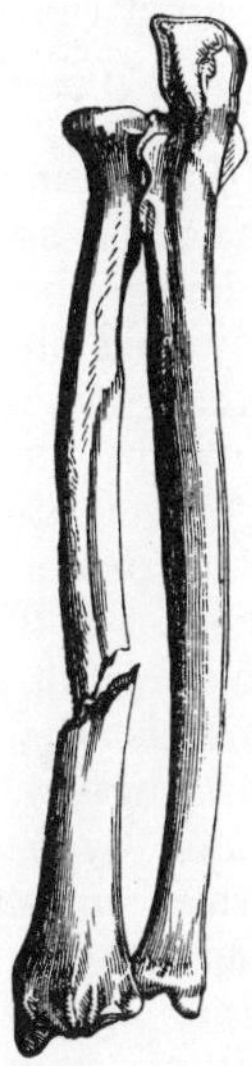

Fracture of the shaft of the radius.

On the twenty-eighth day I first discovered that the fragments were projecting in front, and I at once proposed to thrust them back by force, but the patient declined allowing me to do so. I then applied a compress near the summit of the projection, but not exactly upon it, lest it should produce ulceration, and secured over this a firm splint. At first, this seemed to produce a change in the fragments, but after a couple of weeks I found there was no improvement, and it was discontinued. About six months after the fracture occurred, this man had the same arm terribly lacerated in a railroad accident, and I was obliged to amputate near the shoulder-joint; and I thus obtained the broken radius. The bone was firmly united, but with an angle, salient forwards, of about ten degrees. There was no inclination toward the ulna.

My impression is that these fragments were never completely replaced, a point which I could not well determine at first on account of the rapid effusion. If they had been, I think they could have been retained in place with the appliances used. Almost every day the limb was examined, and as often as every fourth or fifth day the dressings were removed and carefully reapplied. And only once did they become so loose as not to afford the requisite support, and this at a period too late to have occasioned the deformity.

We ought not to be deceived, therefore, and promise too confidently a perfect limb, even when but the middle of the radius is broken, since we may not always be certain that the ends are well replaced, or perhaps they may become displaced subsequently, and in either case we are not likely to discover the deformity until the swelling has subsided, and it is too late to apply the remedy.

In the treatment of fractures of the middle third, the same rules, with only slight modifications, will be applicable, as in fractures of both bones. Two straight, long, and broad splints must be applied after being carefully padded; and especial attention should be paid to the tendency of the fragments to become displaced forwards and toward the ulna through the action of both the biceps and the pronator radii teres; a tendency which may in some measure be provided against by flexion of the arm, but which must be overcome chiefly by steady and well-adjusted pressure, near, but not upon, the ends of the fragments.

Fractures of the lower third, occurring above the line of Colles' fracture, are almost as rare as fractures of the middle or upper thirds. I have met with five; one of which it will be proper to relate as a representative example.

Geo. Vogel, æt. 30, was admitted to the Buffalo Hospital of the Sisters of Charity, Nov. 2, 1852, with a fracture of the right radius about three and a half inches above its lower end. The hand was proned, and inclined to the radial side; while the broken ends of the radius fell against the ulna, from which it was found difficult to separate them. The lower end of the ulna was prominent, and projecting upon the ulnar margin of the hand.

I was unable completely to separate the fragments of the radius from the ulna, by either pressure with my fingers between the bones, or by seizing upon them with my thumb and fingers. Having, however, adjusted them as well as possible, I flexed the arm, and applied a broad and well-padded splint to the palmar surface of the forearm, securing it in place with a paste bandage. These dressings were finally removed at the end of four weeks, when I found scarcely any displacement or deformity remaining.

Most of these fractures, when properly treated, result in perfect limbs. In a certain proportion, however, it will be found impossible effectually to resist the action of the pronator radii teres and of the quadratus, and the fragments will unite at an angle resting against the ulna, and sometimes, by the interposition of intermediate callus, they will become firmly united to the ulna. Occasionally also, especially where the fracture has been produced by a fall upon the hand, and the radio-ulnar ligaments of the wrist have been torn or stretched, the lower end of the ulna will be found to project permanently, and the hand to fall more or less to the radial side.

Of the fifty-six fractures belonging to the lower third of the radius, forty-eight traversed the bone completely and were near the lower end, or within from half an inch to one inch and a half from the articular surface; all being included in those fractures called "Colles' fractures," most of which were no doubt true fractures, and probably a small proportion separations of the epiphysis.

Colles described this fracture as occurring always about one inch and a half above the carpal end of the bone; but Robert Smith, who has carefully examined all of the cabinet specimens he could find, about twenty-three in number, has never seen the line of fracture removed farther than one inch from the lower end of the bone, and in several specimens it was within one-quarter of an inch of this extremity. Dupuytren has also described the fracture as occurring from three to twelve lines above the joint. I think I have found the fracture generally as low as these latter surgeons have placed it, but occasionally as high as it was placed by Colles.

Fig. 77.

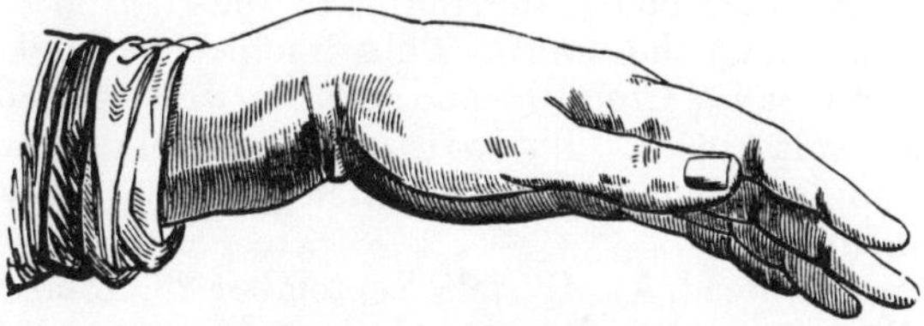

Fracture of radius near its lower end.

Case. A woman, æt. 40, fell upon the side-walk, striking upon the palm of her left hand. She was brought immediately to my office, and I found the radius was broken about one inch and a half above the wrist. The lower fragment was tilted back considerably. Hand proned.

Placing my thumb against the back of the lower fragment, it was easily restored to position, and with only a slight crepitus. When my thumb was removed it manifested no tendency to displacement. The arm was dressed with a curved palmar splint, secured in place with a roller applied moderately tight. On the seventh day a straight splint was substituted for the curved. The arm was examined almost every day, and the dressings occasionally renewed until the twenty-sixth day, when the splint was finally removed. The wrist was at this time only slightly anchylosed, and there seemed to be no deformity or imperfection remaining. Passive motion, which had been practised at each removal of the dressings, was directed to be continued.

Case. A boy, æt. 11, was brought to me having just fallen from a pair of stilts. His right radius was broken transversely, three-quarters of an inch above the wrist, and the lower fragment was much tilted back; the lower end of the ulna was prominent, and the hand fell to the radial side.

Pushing from behind, the lower fragment was made to resume its place, and the deformity immediately disappeared. It was noticed, however, that it required unusual force to accomplish this, but it was not found necessary to use extension. There was also, accompanying the reduction, a slight crepitus.

The treatment was the same as in the first case, except that the curved splint was employed throughout. Little or no deformity existed when the dressings were removed.

Case. George Lofinch, æt. 42, fell upon an icy side-walk, striking upon the palm of his left hand. Fracture three-quarters of an inch above the lower end. Fragment displaced backwards. A friend had partially replaced the fragment by pushing upon it, before he came to me. Within half an hour after the accident he was at my office, and I restored the lower end of the bone very easily to place by pushing from behind with my thumb. No extension was necessary. It would not, however, remain in place unless the forearm was proned so that the weight of the hand could aid in the retention.

I applied my own palmar splint. The recovery was rapid and complete.

CASE. Lewis Brittin, æt. 60, fell from a fourth story window, breaking, among other bones, the radius of the right arm three-quarters of an inch above the joint. This fracture was not discovered until the fourth day. Crepitus and motion were then distinct, but there was no displacement. The wrist was considerably swollen. No splints were applied; and the bone united promptly, leaving no deformity or anchylosis.

CASE. Margaret Read, æt. 48, fell, September 23, 1855, striking on the palm of the left hand, and breaking the radius about one inch from its lower end. One week after, she came under my care at the hospital. The arm had been previously dressed carefully by one of my colleagues, with curved, dorsal, and palmar splints; but, on examination, we found the fragments a good deal displaced. It was found necessary now to use both extension and pressure from behind to restore the lower fragment to position. This we finally succeeded in doing, and immediately splints were again snugly applied. Two days after, on opening the dressings, the lower fragment was a second time found displaced backwards. It was again reduced, but only by using great force. Fifteen days later, we were pleased to find the bone firm and without deformity.

Margaret left the hospital on the 4th of November, with her hand and wrist still swollen, and with a good deal of stiffness at the elbow and wrist joints.

CASE. Charles Stratton, a healthy and temperate laborer, æt. 36, fell forwards from a wagon, Nov. 22, 1854, striking upon the palm of his hand, and breaking the radius a little more than one inch above the joint. I found the lower fragment displaced backwards, and it was easily reduced by pressure in the opposite direction. The fore part of the wrist being quite tender to pressure, the splint was applied to the dorsal surface of the forearm. The splint was pistol-shaped, and the surface which was applied to the arm was padded with care; it was secured in place by a few light turns of a roller, and laid across the body in a sling.

The arm was seen by me on each of the succeeding seven days, and on the third, fifth, and seventh days, the splint was removed completely; but on this last day an erysipelatous inflammation had commenced in the neighborhood of the wrist. The splint and roller were therefore not reapplied, but the limb was laid upon a broad board, cushioned and covered with oiled silk, and cool water irrigations were directed. The inflammation soon subsided, but the splint was never resumed, as the fragments were found to stay in place perfectly without its aid. At the end of five weeks, union seemed to be consummated; and one year later the bone was found to be perfectly straight, yet the wrist-joint and the finger-joints remained stiff, so much so that he was unable to perform any labor. The stiffness was, however, gradually disappearing; while all swelling and tenderness had long ceased.

The observations of M. Vollemier also have shown that, instead of being oblique, as has generally been supposed, the fracture is almost uniformly transverse from the palmar to the dorsal surfaces of the bone, and only occasionally slightly oblique in its other diameter, or from the radial to the ulnar side. I have seen, however, in the museum of the College of Physicians of Philadelphia, a specimen of this fracture in which the line of fracture is transverse, from side to side, but very oblique from before backwards, and from below upwards. There is also a line of incomplete fracture extending into the joint. It is united by bone, with the usual displacement backwards.

The observations of both R. Smith and Vollemier have shown, moreover, that the displacement of the lower fragment is seldom sufficient to enable it to escape completely from the upper; and that where, in extremely rare instances, and in consequence of extraordinary violence, such complete separation does occur, a disruption of those ligaments which attach the lower fragment to the ulna occurs also, and the deformity becomes at once very great, so that it no longer presents the peculiar features of Colles' fracture, but resembles a dislocation.

In the so-called Colles' fracture, the lower and outer border of the radius, or its styloid apophysis, is swung around or tilted, as it were, upon the ulna; the lower and inner border of the same fragment being retained in place by the radio-ulnar ligaments, which do not usually suffer a complete disruption, but only a stretching or partial laceration. The upper or broken margin of the lower fragment, and also the ulnar margin, undergo very little displacement; while the lower or articular surface, and the radial margin, are carried backwards, upwards, and outwards.

Surgeons have spoken of a falling in of the upper end of the lower fragment toward the ulna, as an almost inevitable result of the action of the pronator quadratus, and against which tendency they have sought carefully to provide; but there is much reason to believe that any considerable degree of displacement in this direction is a rare event, and that, when it does exist, it is in consequence mostly of the direction of the force which has produced the fracture, rather than of the action of this muscle, only a few of the fibres of which are usually attached to the lower fragment, and, in some instances, when the fracture is within a half or a quarter of an inch of the articulation, not any. Besides, there is actually in these latter cases, no interosseous space into which the fragment may fall, and its displacement toward the ulna becomes, therefore, impossible.

Still, however, if one were disposed to speculate upon the condition of these parts after the fracture, it might perhaps be easy to persuade ourselves that the action of the pronator quadratus upon the upper fragment, whose broken extremity was not completely or at all disengaged from the lower, would carry both fragments together toward the ulna. But whatever might be the result of our speculations, still the fact, as proved by specimens, is not generally so; and this is not the first time that facts and theories have disagreed.

The truth is, that it is unusual to find in any of the museums specimens of this fracture having thus united. But they may be found constantly tilted back in the manner I have described, occasionally tilted forwards, and, still more rarely, slightly displaced upon their broken surfaces antero-posteriorly.

The general absence of this internal displacement may find its explanation in the direction of the force which generally produces this fracture, in the occurrence of the fracture sometimes at a point so low as to render its displacement in this direction impossible, and in the breadth of the bone, at the seat of the fracture, which does not permit it to fall laterally without actually increasing its length; a circumstance which its secure ligamentous attachment to the ulna at its opposite extremities, and its complete apposition to the wrist and elbow-joint, do not allow.

The mistake of those surgeons who have attempted to describe this fracture, has originated in the appearance presented in nearly all recent fractures occurring at this point. The hand falls to the radial side, and seems to carry the lower end of the lower fragment with it, while the lower end of the ulna becomes unnaturally prominent in front and to the ulnar side; a condition of things which has naturally enough been ascribed to the displacement of the upper end of the lower fragment in the direction of the interosseous space.

But this same radial inclination of the hand, and prominence of the ulna, are present frequently when the radius is broken at its lower end and no displacement in any direction has taken place; and I have even observed it in simple sprains of the wrist, and in the hands of old or feeble persons where all the ligaments have become relaxed. It is seen, however, in a more marked degree when the bone is actually both broken and displaced backwards in its usual direction. In short, the deformity in question is due, in a large majority of instances, to the relaxation, stretching, or more or less disruption of the radio-ulnar ligaments, which permits the hand to fall to the radial side by a simple rotatory movement over its articular surface. For this reason, also, because these ligaments once lengthened or broken can never, or only after a lapse of many years, be completely restored, this deformity may be expected to continue, however exact and perfect may be the bony union.

It must be added, however, that, so long as the tilting remains, the articular surface is actually presenting somewhat to the radial side. While in the normal condition it presents downwards, forwards, and inwards, it now presents, when the displacement is considerable, downwards, backwards, and outwards.

Diday maintained that there existed usually in this fracture an overlapping or shortening of the bone in its entire diameter, and Vollemier thought that the specimens which he had examined proved that an impaction was almost universal.

Both of these opinions it seems to me, have been successfully combated by Robert Smith; the shortening observed by Diday being found only on that side of the bone to which the hand inclines, and being the result of the motion of the lower fragment already described; and the appearance of impaction being due to the ensheathing callus which is deposited usually, if the displacement is allowed to continue, in the retiring angle, opposite the seat of fracture.

These are questions, however, requiring for their decision a very careful study of specimens, and in relation to which further observations may be necessary.

Meanwhile there is no doubt that occasional examples may be found illustrating one or more of all these varieties of displacement, and that to the impaction is sometimes added a comminution of the lower fragment, the lines of the fracture extending freely into the joint. One of the most curious examples of which has been reported by Dr. Bigelow, of Boston. The patient had fallen, and being otherwise seriously injured, ultimately died in the Massachusetts Hospital. At first he had only complained of lameness at the wrist, as if it had been severely sprained; but at the end of several days the joint became swollen, and from the persistence of the swelling Dr. Bigelow was led to diagnosticate a stellate crack in the articulating extremity of the radius, he having met with a similar case two years before, when a patient with the same symptoms had died of other injuries, and exhibited a crack in the same place, but less extensive than in this case. There was found in this last example, a star-shaped fissure on the articulating surface, without displacement. These fissures penetrated the shaft for an inch or more. Dr. Bigelow thought that the bones of the wrist acted as a wedge to spread the corresponding hollow of the articulating extremity; and that this specimen would explain the persistence of some cases of sprained wrist.[1]

Fig. 78.

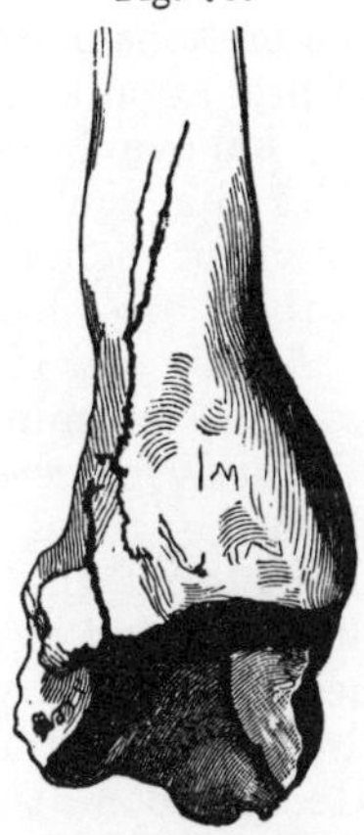

Bigelow's case of comminuted fracture of the lower end of the radius.

Robert Smith has described a fracture occurring at the same point, and probably possessing the same characters as Colles' fractures; in which the lower fragment is thrown forwards instead of backwards, and which has generally been the result of a fall upon the back of the hand. There is no such specimen, however, in any of the pathological collections in Dublin, nor has Mr. Smith ever seen a specimen obtained from the cadaver, although he reports a case which fell under his observation in practice.

I have myself seen one such case,[2] but I regret to say that my examination of the condition of the arm was not such as to enable me to add anything to the information already possessed upon this subject; indeed, until we shall have an opportunity of studying it in the cadaver, we cannot speak very definitely of its anatomical characters.

[1] Boston Med. and Surg. Journ., vol. lviii. p. 99.
[2] Trans. Am. Med. Assoc., vol. ix. p. 145.

Nélaton observes that all the varieties of this fracture which he has seen are often accompanied with fracture of the styloid apophysis of the ulna, and with a tearing of the triangular ligament. I am not aware that any other writer has made the same observation in relation to the frequent occurrence of a fracture of the styloid apophysis of the ulna, and I think the accident is not so common as the remark of Nélaton would lead us to suppose.

Dr. Butler, House Surgeon to the Brooklyn Hospital, reports a case of fracture of the right radius at the junction of the middle and lower thirds, accompanied with a fracture also of the styloid apophysis in the same bone. The accident occurred in a lad fourteen years old, who had fallen from a height of thirty feet upon the pavement. The lower fracture commenced at the base of the styloid process of the radius, and extended down obliquely into the wrist-joint, breaking off about one-fifth of the articular surface. The process was drawn up on the posterior surface of the radius, about one inch and a half, by the supinator radii longus muscle. It was movable, but in consequence of the contusion and swelling, could not be returned to its place. The hand occupied the same position that it does in Colles' fracture.

On the eighth day an attempt was made to force down the process with a compress secured by adhesive plaster straps; but it could not be done. The hand and arm were confined also to a pistol shaped splint; ulcerations ensued from the pressure of the compress, and the process was laid bare, but, it finally became united in its abnormal position; the motions of the wrist, however, were not impaired, and the power of pronation and supination soon returned.[1]

I believe I have seen two examples of a fracture commencing on the radial side of the bone and terminating in the joint, the separated fragment including considerable more than the apophysis; but neither of these cases has been verified by an autopsy.

A boy, æt. 18, fell twelve feet, striking upon the right hand and wrist. I examined him at the hospital soon after, and thought I could distinctly feel the line of fracture extending very obliquely downwards, from the radial side into the joint, and without traversing the entire diameter of the bone. The fragment thus separated fell backwards, and the hand inclined to the radial side. Reduction was immediately accomplished by pushing the fragment forwards, and the arm was dressed with straight palmar and dorsal splints, with compresses, &c. He was soon dismissed.

Five months after I found the bones united without displacement, and the motions of the joint were perfect.

A man, æt. 38, fell upon the palm of his left hand. On the same day he was admitted to the Buffalo Hospital of the Sisters of Charity, and the diagnosis was confirmed by Drs. Lay and Lemon. The symptoms were the same as in the first case, and we adopted the same treatment. On the thirty-first day, it was noted in the hospital record, that "the splints have been for some time removed, but the wrist remains swollen and stiff. The lower end of the ulna is prominent, but the fragments of the radius seem to be in exact line."

[1] New York Journ. of Med., 1857.

In the first volume of the *Philadelphia Medical Examiner* (1838) will be found a description by J. Rhea Barton, of Philadelphia, of a form of fracture occurring through the lower end of the radius, which is probably much less common than Colles' fracture, and which had hitherto escaped the notice of surgeons. Its peculiarity consists in the line of fracture extending very obliquely from the articulation, upwards and backwards, separating and displacing the whole, or only a portion, as the case may be, of the posterior margin of the articulating surface. I have not recognized this fracture in any instance which has come under my own observation, nor have I been able to find a cabinet specimen in any pathological collection. Dr. Barton was not able to prove the correctness of his diagnosis by an autopsy, and the only well-authenticated example which I can find upon record is that to which Malgaigne has alluded, as having been seen by M. Lenoir, and of which an account was published in the *Archives Générale de Médecine* in 1839. M. Lenoir believed it to be a simple luxation of the hand backwards, but the patient having died, he was able to correct his diagnosis by an autopsy. A considerable fragment had been broken from the posterior lip of the articular surface, the line of fracture being from below upwards, and from before backwards. This fragment had become displaced upwards and backwards, carrying with it the carpal bones, and producing thus the appearance of a simple dislocation.[1] I believe that the accident so carefully described by Barton was either a Colles' fracture, or a fracture simply of the radial margin, of which I have given two supposed examples, with the usual signs of which his account so exactly coincides, and that it was not a fracture of the posterior lip of the articulating surface, as he believed.

Fifty examples of simple fracture near the lower end of the radius have furnished no cases of non-union, nor indeed do I remember ever to have seen the union delayed; yet only sixteen are positively known to have left no perceptible deformity or stiffness about the joint: it is probable, however, that the number of perfect results might be extended to twenty. In one example, the case of a man whose arm was broken in Germany, when he was only ten years old, the fragments of the radius were driven into each other, or overlapped one inch, and the ulna had been displaced downwards toward the fingers the same distance. This was examined twelve years after the accident, and he had then a very useful arm. Twice I have found the wrist and finger-joints quite stiff after a lapse of one year; in one case I have found the same condition after two years; in one case after three years, and in two cases after five years.

If we confine our remarks to Colles' fracture, the deformity which has been observed most often, and, indeed, with only rare exceptions, being found in some degree more or less in several of those cases which I have marked as perfect, consists in a projection of the lower end of the ulna inwards and generally a little forwards. In a large majority of cases this is accompanied with a perceptible falling of the hand to the radial side, while in a few it is not. After this, in point

[1] Malgaigne, Traité des Frac., etc., tom. ii. p. 700.

of frequency, I have met with the backward inclination of the lower fragment. Robert Smith found this displacement almost constant in the cabinet specimens examined by him; and it is very probable that nearly all of the examples examined by myself would present more or less of the same deviation upon the naked bone; but in the living examples a slight deviation would be concealed by the numerous tendons which cover this part of the arm, and perhaps by some permanent effusions, of which I shall speak more particularly presently.

There remains for a long time, in a majority of cases, a broad, firm, uniform swelling on the palmar surface of the forearm, commencing near the upper margin of the annular ligament and extending upwards two inches or more. This swelling continues much longer in old and feeble persons than in the young and vigorous. It is pretty generally proportioned to the amount of anchylosis existing at the wrist and finger-joints, and it disappears usually, *pari passû*, with these conditions. There can be no doubt that this phenomenon is due to an effusion, first serous, and subsequently fibrinous, along the sheaths of the tendons; and it is as often present after sprains and other severe injuries about this part, as in fractures. In many cases, however, its prolonged continuance and its firmness have led to a suspicion that the bones were displaced, a suspicion which only a moderate degree of care in the examination ought easily to dispel. A similar effusion, but in less amount, is frequently seen also on the back of the hand, below the annular ligament. When both exist simultaneously the appearances of deformity and of displacement are greatly increased. Here, then, we shall find a partial explanation of the anchylosis in the wrist and finger-joints, which, often for a time almost complete, continues occasionally many months, or even years, if, indeed, it is not perpetual. An anchylosis produced, not, as has generally been affirmed, by extension of the inflammation to these joints, but by the inflammatory effusion and consequent adhesions along the thecæ and serous sheaths, through which the tendons all pass in their course to the hands and fingers; and by simple contraction of the articular ligaments as a consequence of disuse. The fingers are quite as often thus anchylosed as the wrist-joint itself, a circumstance which is wholly inexplicable on the doctrine that the anchylosis is due to an inflammation in the joints. Indeed, I have seen the fingers rigid after many months, when, having observed the case throughout myself, I was certain that no inflammatory action had ever reached them.

Nor is it any more difficult to show, I think, that the anchylosis of the wrist-joint is not due to a malposition of its articular surfaces, as has often been asserted in the written treatises; for, if the anchylosis of the fingers in all these cases is known to be the result of inflammation of the tendinous sheaths and of contraction of the articular ligaments, why shall we refuse to accept the same explanations for anchylosis of the wrist?

The most superficial examination of the mechanism of this joint ought to satisfy us that any moderate or even considerable malposition of the lower fragment after a fracture of the radius is not sufficient in itself to occasion anchylosis. It is true that the direction of the articular surface of the radius is changed also, and that, while it was directed downwards, forwards, and to the ulnar side, it is now, perhaps, directed downwards, backwards, and to the radial side. But of what consequence is this so long as the carpal bones, with which alone this bone is articulated, preserve their relations to the radius unchanged?

I suspect it will be found very difficult for any one, however ingenious, to offer even a plausible argument in defence of this doctrine of anchylosis, as applied to this fracture, so long and so positively affirmed that to-day it is thought to be established.

But if any other evidence than such as I have furnished be demanded, it may be supplied by the experience of most surgeons in examples of anchylosis without displacement; in examples of displacement without anchylosis, but in which the anchylosis has yielded gradually to the lapse of time, while the displacement has continued. Examples, also, of all these results, so incompatible with the supposition named, have frequently come under my own notice, some of which I have already mentioned in this chapter, and many more of which may be found in my report On Deformities after Fractures.

To what I have said as to the prognosis in these accidents, I may be permitted to add the opinion of our distinguished countryman, Dr. Mott, given in a clinical lecture before his class in the University of New York.

"Fractures of the radius within two inches of the wrist, where treated by the most eminent surgeons, are of very difficult management so as to avoid all deformity; indeed, more or less deformity may occur under the treatment of the most eminent surgeons, and more or less imperfection in the motion of the wrist or radius is very apt to follow for a longer or shorter time. Even when the fracture is well cured, an anterior prominence at the wrist, or near it, will sometimes result from swelling of the soft parts."

To which the reporter, himself a surgeon in the city of New York, adds:—

"As the above opinion of Professor Mott coincides with my own observations, both in Europe and in this city, as well as with many of our most distinguished surgical authorities, I venture to hope that it may assist in removing some of the groundless and ill-merited aspersions which are occasionally thrown on the members of our profession by the ignorant or designing."[1]

Of gangrene as an occasional result of this fracture, I shall speak presently, in connection with the subject of treatment.

The peculiar character of the displacement which characterizes Colles' fracture, and the constant difficulty experienced by surgeons in obviating deformity, have led to much speculation and ingenious invention; and modern surgeons, especially, have thought it necessary to introduce here an essential modification of the usual apparel for broken forearms. This modification consists in employing a pistol-shaped splint, instead of a straight splint, by means of which the hand may be thrown more or less strongly to the ulnar side.

[1] Boston Med. and Surg. Journ., vol. xxv. p. 289.

Heister[1] speaks of inclining the hand toward the ulna, while reducing a fracture of the radius, but when the reduction has been effected he recommends a straight splint.

Among the first to advocate the permanent confinement of the hand in this position, were Mr. Cline, of London,[2] and M. Dupuytren, of Paris.[3] Mr. Cline, and after him Bransby Cooper,[4] and Mr. South,[5] recommend the ordinary straight splints for the forearm, but the rollers by which the splints are secured in place are not permitted to extend lower than the wrist; so that when the forearm is suspended in a sling, in a state of semi-pronation, the hand shall fall by its own weight to the ulnar side.

Dupuytren, and, after him, Chelius, adopt, in addition to the palmar and dorsal splints, the "attelle cubitale," or ulnar splint; which is a gutter, composed of steel, iron, tin, or some other metal, and made to fit the ulnar margin of the forearm and hand, when the hand is drawn forcibly to the ulnar side. Blandin,[6] Nélaton,[7] and Goyraud,[8] also, under certain contingencies employ the same. An instrument similar to this, but constructed of wood and gutta percha, and much less curved, has been invented by Welch.

Fig. 79.

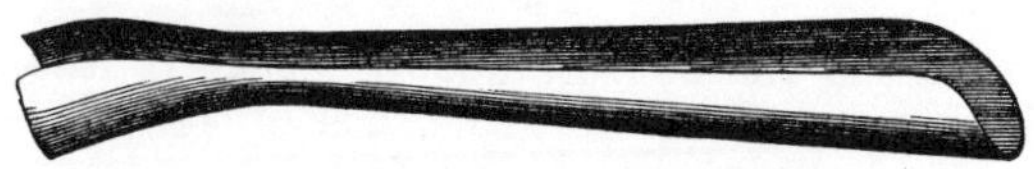

Welch's "ulnar splint" for fracture of the radius.

Most surgeons, however, employ either a palmar or a dorsal splint; or both palmar and dorsal splints, constructed with a knee, or pistol-shaped, and they thus avoid the necessity of the ulnar splint. Thus,

Fig. 80.

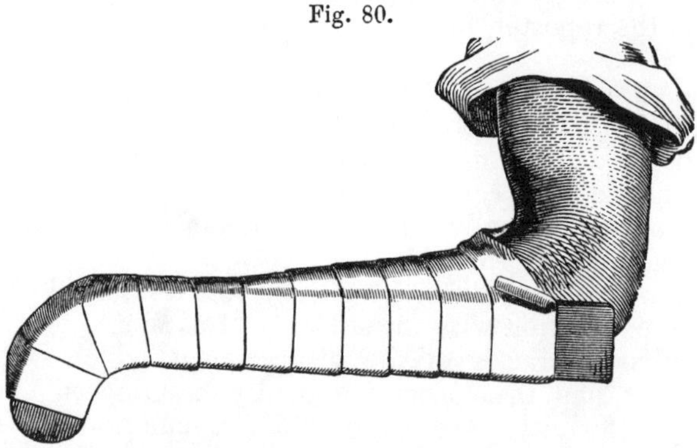

Nélaton's splint for fracture of the radius.

[1] De Lavrentii Heisteri, Institutiones Chirurgicæ, pars prima, p. 202, Amsterdam ed., 1739.
[2] Malgaigne, Traité de Frac., etc., tom. i. p. 614, Paris ed.
[3] Dupuytren, on Bones, London ed., p. 140.
[4] B. Cooper, Lectures on Surg., p. 232, Amer. ed.
[5] Chelius's Surg., vol. i. p. 613.
[6] Malgaigne, op. cit., tom i. p. 614.
[7] Nélaton, Elém. de Path. Chir., tom. i. p. 747.
[8] Ibid., p. 746.

Nélaton,[1] Robert Smith,[2] and Erichsen,[3] recommend this peculiar form only in the dorsal splint; while Bond,[4] Hays,[5] E. P. Smith,[6] and others, especially among the Americans, place the pistol-shaped splint against

Fig. 81.

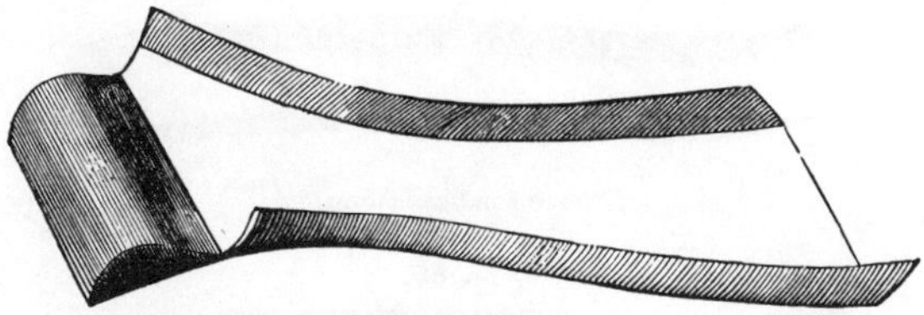

Bond's splint.

Fig. 82.

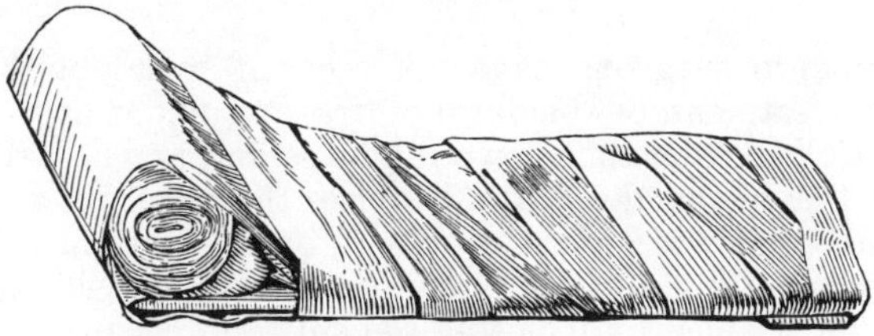

Hays' splint.

Fig. 83.

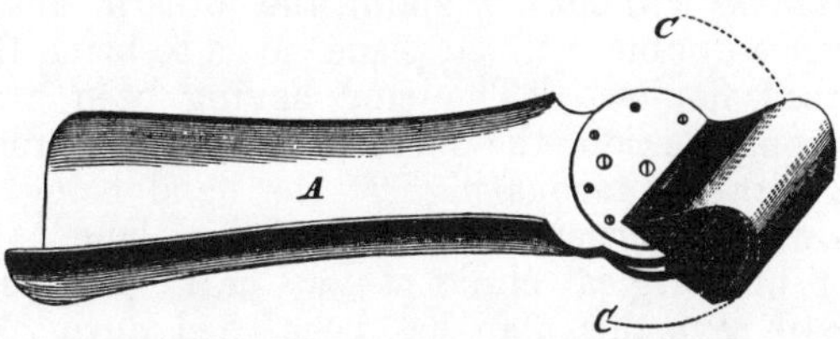

E. P. Smith's splint. Surface applied to forearm. *A*. Forearm piece, made of felt, with incurvated margins.

Fig. 84.

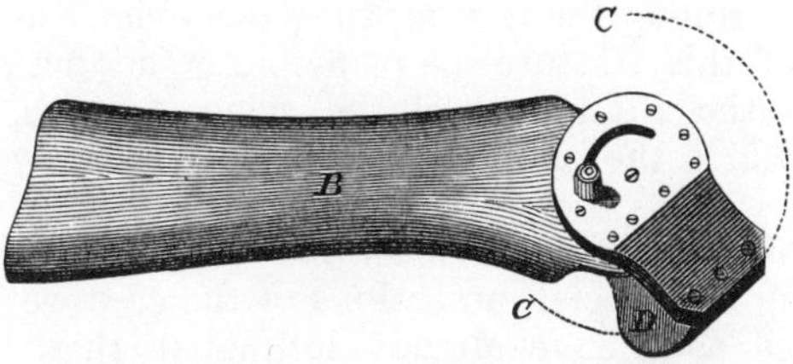

E. P. Smith's splint. *B*. Opposite surface. *D*, the hand-block, is connected with the forearm piece by two circular brass plates, which move upon each other, in order that the hand-block may assume any desired angle with the arm. In this way it may be adapted to either the right or left arm. It is fixed by a nut seen on the brass plate. The letters *C C* indicate the extent of motion allowed to the hand-block.

[1] Nélaton, op. cit., p. 747.
[2] R. Smith, op. cit., p. 168.
[3] Erichsen, Surgery, p. 215.
[4] Bond, Amer. Journ. Med. Sci., April, 1852.
[5] Ibid., Jan., 1853.
E. P. Smith, Buffalo Med. Journ., vol. ix. p. 225.

the palmar surface of the forearm and hand. Welch has manufactured, also, as a substitute for his single ulnar splint, a palmar and a dorsal splint, made of gutta percha and wood.

Fig. 85.

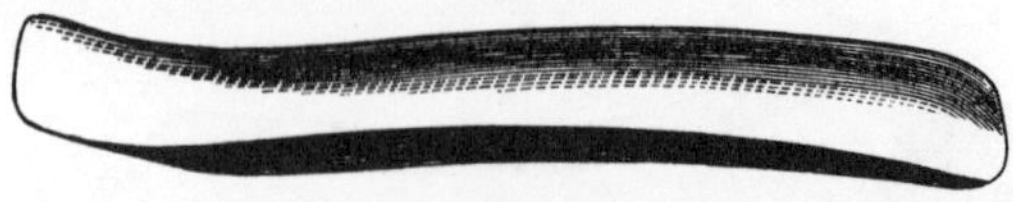

Welch's palmar splint.

Fig. 86.

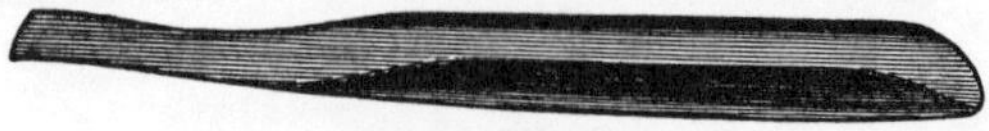

Welch's dorsal splint.

A few modern surgeons have not seen fit to adopt this peculiar principle of treatment, or this form of dressing under any of its modifications. Colles[1] recommends a straight palmar and dorsal splint, and does not incline the hand. Barton[2] advises the same, and Skey, having declared his preference for a couple of broad, straight splints, adds: "Great care should be taken to prevent the hand falling, and this object will be attained by inclosing the entire forearm and hand in a well-applied sling."[3]

Professor Fauger, of Copenhagen, has undertaken to treat this fracture in some sense without any splint, the forearm and hand being simply laid over a double inclined plane, so as to bring the wrist into a state of forced flexion. "The hand having been brought into a position of strong flexion, the forearm is placed, pronated, on an oblique plane, with the carpus highest, the hand being permitted to hang freely down the perpendicular end of the plane."[4] M. Velpeau, in a report of his surgical clinic at La Charité for the year ending September, 1846, says this plan has been tried during the year, and "the result has not been very satisfactory. The experiment, however, has not been decisive upon this mode of treatment."[5]

Notwithstanding these exceptions, the practice seems to be pretty well established among the leading surgeons everywhere to employ in the treatment of this fracture the principle of adduction of the hand, and always to the attainment of the same purpose, namely, rotary extension, by which they hope to retain more securely the lower fragment in place.

We come now to consider how far this peculiar treatment is capable of answering the special indications of the case we are studying.

It is assumed, as I have already intimated, that, by bearing the hand strongly to the ulnar side, the fragments of the radius are brought more exactly into apposition, and more easily and effectually retained; an assumption which supposes two things to have been

[1] Colles, Lectures on Surgery, p. 325.
[2] Barton, Phil. Med. Exam., 1838.
[3] Skey, Operative Surgery, p. 161.
[4] Fauger, London Lancet, May 8, 1847.
[5] Velpeau, Boston Med. Journ., vol. xxxv. p. 213.

determined; first, that there exists an overlapping of the fragments, either through the whole extent of their broken surfaces or especially toward the radial side, or that the upper end of the lower fragment is inclined to fall against the ulna, or that all of these several conditions coexist; and, secondly, that if such displacements do exist, they can be remedied by this manœuvre.

The first of these suppositions seems to have been sufficiently considered and fully controverted by all those gentlemen who have particularly examined the specimens contained in the various pathological collections, and to whose careful investigations I have already frequently adverted. My own observation confirms also their statements. With rare exceptions, none of these displacements have been found to exist, although, as has been observed, a casual inspection of the arm when recently broken would often lead to an opposite conclusion.

In regard to the second supposition, namely, that where such displacements do exist, a forced adduction will aid in the retention of the fragments, I shall have to speak more cautiously, because, so far as I know, my opinions have received as yet no public and authoritative indorsement. In order that adduction may prove effective, there must be some point upon which to act as a fulcrum. It is of no use that we rotate the hand for the purpose of making extension unless there can be found a resistance or limit to the rotary motion. Such a limit exists, no doubt, but to determine its availability we must ascertain its character and position.

It is not in the lower end of the ulna, for the ulna has no point of contact with the carpal bones, and when, in the natural state of these parts, the hand is inclined to the ulnar side, the lower end of the ulna rides freely downwards upon the wrist until arrested by the ligaments which unite it with the carpus, and by the capacity of the joint to move in this direction. When the lower end of the radius is broken, and the ligaments of the joint more or less torn, the ulna, although thrust downwards much further than it could ever descend in its normal state, still fails to find a support, and spreading wider and wider from the radius as it is thrust further upon the hand, no limit can be given to its progress in this direction. It was thus that, in one example already mentioned, I found the ulna carried downwards one inch or more.

If the fragments overlap each other in their entire diameter, it is very certain then that a fulcrum could not be obtained upon any point of their broken surfaces; and if the fracture is transverse in its antero-posterior diameter, and transverse, or only slightly oblique, in its lateral diameter, when once replaced, the surfaces must of necessity support themselves, and the indication in question cannot be present. If, again, the direction of the fracture is from before backwards and oblique, and reduction has been effected, no chance still remains to prevent the sliding off of the radial edge, if it is disposed to happen, by making use of the ulnar extremity of the broken surface as a fulcrum. If the radial side is inclined to fall off, what shall prevent the ulnar from doing the same? And how then can it, the ulnar side, be used as a fulcrum? It only remains to suppose an impaction of the radial margin of the broken radius without similar impaction of the ulnar margin, or a fracture extending very obliquely from the radial margin into the joint, as the sole examples in which the lower fragment can find a sufficient fulcrum upon which the rotary extension may operate. The first of these examples I have supposed without being aware of the proof of its existence, and the second is probably rare.

I have not spoken of the ligaments which bind the lower fragment to the lower end of the ulna, and the ulna to the carpal bones, viz: the radio-ulnar, and the internal lateral ligaments, which in the normal state of the parts constitute the centre upon which forced adduction expends its power, and which still continue to be the point of resistance when the radius is broken. And this brings me to the point and purpose of my inquiry. How feeble and uncertain must be a resistance which depends solely on these broken ligaments! And how painful to the patient must be an extension sufficient to overcome the action of nearly all the muscles of the wrist, which is borne entirely by a few lacerated and inflamed fibres! even in health this position, when forced, cannot be endured beyond a few seconds, and it must be difficult to estimate the sufferings which the same position must occasion when the ligaments are torn and inflamed.

I am not to be told that surgeons have not intended to teach this extreme practice; that they have never recommended forced adduction, but only a moderate and easy lateral inclination, such as can be comfortably borne. If they have not, then they should not have spoken of making extension by this means. An easy lateral inclination has no power to do good so far as extension is concerned, any more than it has power to do harm. But the fact is, while a majority of surgeons have no doubt used less force than was hurtful, some have used more than was useful or safe; indeed, the sharpness of the curve given to the splints figured and recommended by Dupuytren, Nélaton, and others, sufficiently indicate that their distinguished inventors intended to accomplish by these means a forced and violent adduction.

Malgaigne, speaking of other means of extension applied to the forearm, suggested by Godin, Diday, and Velpeau, intended to operate only in a straight line, and alluding especially to the modes devised by Huguier and Velpeau, remarks: "Without discussing here, the comparative value of the two appareils, I believe that they could scarcely be endured by the patients; and M. Diday tells us that in the trials which he has made, the pain produced by the extension was so great that he was compelled to renounce it." Which observations cannot but apply equally to this plan of extension by adduction, or to any other which might be adopted.

After all, it must not be inferred that I have concluded to reject this mode of dressing in all of its modifications; for although I am far from being persuaded of its utility as a means of extension and retention in any case, yet I am not prepared to deny to it some very considerable value in another point of view; and when judiciously employed it can certainly do no harm. It is, I repeat, for another reason altogether than the one heretofore assigned, that I would recommend its continuance, a reason which I cannot so well explain, or hope to render intelligible, except to the practical surgeon. This position throws the whole lower end of both radius and ulna outwards toward the radial margin of the splints, and by keeping the radius more completely in view, it enables the surgeon better to judge of the accuracy of the reduction, and to recognize more readily the condition and situation of the compresses, etc. This alone I have always considered a sufficient ground for retaining the angular splint; although I have treated a number of arms satisfactorily with the straight splints alone.

Finally, while surgeons have been seeking to accomplish an indication, the existence of which is at least rendered doubtful, and by means which appear to me totally inadequate, if it did exist, they have probably too often overlooked or regarded indifferently an indication which is almost uniformly present, namely, to press forwards the tilted fragment by a force applied upon the wrist from behind, and to retain it in place by suitable compresses. And I cannot help thinking that if they had regarded this as the sole indication, an indication generally so easily accomplished, they would have made fewer crooked arms, and have saved their patients much suffering and themselves much trouble.

It only remains for us to determine the precise form of splint which ought to be preferred, and to describe its mode of application.

The narrow "attelle cubitale" of Dupuytren, is inconvenient; nor can I give the preference to the curved dorsal splint recommended by Nélaton, and employed by Robert Smith, Erichsen, and others. It is not to me a matter of entire indifference, in case only one curved splint is employed, whether this be applied to the palmar or dorsal surfaces of the forearm. Foreign surgeons, so far as I know, have applied this splint to the dorsal surface, and the straight splint to the palmar; while American surgeons have adopted almost as uniformly the opposite rule—to whose practice, in this respect, I acknowledge myself also partial. It is to the curved splint rather than to the straight, that we mainly trust; not simply, or at all, perhaps, because of its form, but because the curved splint is also the long splint. This is the splint, therefore, which ought to be the most steady and immovable in its position. Now, the very irregularities of surface upon the palmar aspect of the forearm and hand, instead of constituting an embarrassment, enable us, when the splint is suitably prepared and adjusted, to fix it more securely. Moreover, upon it alone, after a few days, the surgeon may see fit to rely, and in that case it ought to be applied to that surface of the arm which is most tolerant of continued pressure. The palmar surface, as being more muscular, and as having been more accustomed to friction and to pressure, must necessarily have the advantage in this respect. The palmar splint terminating also at the metacarpo-phalangeal articulations, instead of at the wrist, as the short straight splint must do when the hand is adducted, enables the hand to be flexed upon its extremity over a hand-block, or pad of proper size. Such are the not insignificant advantages which we claim for this mode, over that pursued by our transatlantic brethren.

The block suggested first by Bond, of Philadelphia, is a valuable addition; since the flexed position is always more easy for the fingers, and in case of anchylosis this position renders the whole hand more useful.

For myself, I am in the habit of preparing extemporaneously a splint from a wooden shingle, which I first cut into the requisite shape and length; the length being obtained by measuring from the front of the elbow joint, when the arm is flexed to a right angle, to the metacarpo-phalangeal articulations. It ought, indeed, to fall half an inch short of the bend of the elbow, to render it certain that it shall make no uncomfortable pressure at this point; and the direction to measure with the arm flexed, is of sufficient importance to warrant a repetition. The breadth of the splint should be in all its extent just equal to the breadth of the forearm in its widest part, so that there shall be no lateral pressure upon the bones. If the splint is of unequal breadth, the roller cannot be so neatly applied, and it is more likely to become disarranged.

Fig. 87.

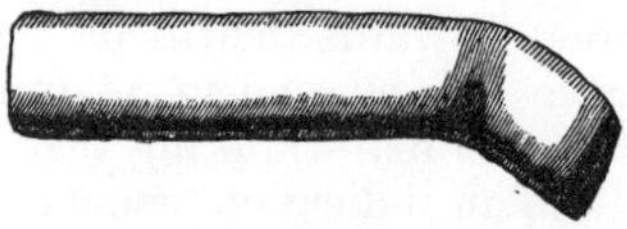

The author's splint.

Thus constructed it is to be covered with a sack of cotton cloth, made to fit tightly, with the seam along its back; and afterwards stuffed with cotton batting or with curled hair. These materials may be passed in and easily adjusted, wherever they are most needed, from the open extremities of the sack. While preparing, the splint must be occasionally applied to the arm until it fits accurately every part of the forearm and hand, only that the stuffing must be rather more firm a little above the lower end of the upper fragment. The open ends of the sack are then to be neatly stitched over the ends of the splint. This splint is now to be laid directly upon the skin without any intermediate compresses or rollers.

The advantages of this form of splint are easily comprehended. They consist in facility and cheapness of construction, accuracy of adaptation, neatness, permanency and fitness to the ends proposed.

The extemporaneous splint recommended by Dr. Isaac Hays, of Philadelphia, is very similar, but it lacks the neatness and permanency of that which I have now described.

In all cases it is better to employ, also, at least during the first fortnight, a straight dorsal splint, of the same breadth as the palmar splint, and of sufficient length to extend from the elbow to the middle of the metacarpus. This should be covered and stuffed in the same manner as the palmar splint, except that here the thickest and firmest part of the splint must be opposite the carpus and the lower end of the lower fragment. It will answer the indications also a little more completely if, at this point, the padding is thicker on the radial than on the ulnar side.

Having restored the fragments to place, in case of Colles' fracture, by pressing forcibly upon the back of the lower fragment, the force being applied near the styloid apophysis of the radius, the arm is to be flexed upon the body and placed in a position of semi-pronation; when the splints are to be applied and secured with a sufficient number of turns of the roller, taking especial care not to include the thumb, the forcible confinement of which is always painful and never useful.

Fig. 88.

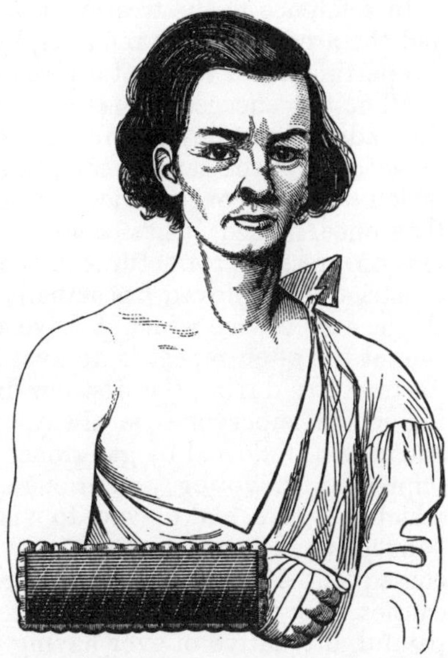

The author's dressing complete. The curved palmar splint is not in view, only the dorsal. The dotted lines represent the roller. The sling is omitted for the purpose of bringing the other dressings into view.

I cannot too severely reprobate the practice of violent extension of the wrist in the efforts at reduction, and that, whether this extension be applied in a straight line, or with the hand adducted. It has been shown that in a great majority of cases no indication in this direction is to be accomplished, and to pull violently upon the wrist is not only useless but hurtful. It is adding to the fracture, and to the other injuries already received, the graver pathological lesion of a stretching, a sprain, of all the ligaments connected with the joint. I am persuaded that to this violence, added to the unequal and too firm pressure of the splints, are, in a great measure, to be attributed the subsequent inflammation and anchylosis, in very many cases.

The first application of the bandages ought to be only moderately tight, and as the inflammation and swelling develop in these structures with rapidity, they should be attentively watched and loosened as soon as they become painful. It must be constantly borne in mind that, to prevent and control inflammation, in this fracture, is the most difficult and by far the most important object to be accomplished, while to retain the fragments in place when once reduced, is comparatively easy and unimportant.

During the first seven or ten days, therefore, these cases demand the most assiduous attention; and we had much better dispense with the splints entirely than to retain them at the risk of increasing the inflammatory action. Indeed, I have no doubt that very many cases would come to a successful termination without splints, if only the hand and arm were kept perfectly still in a suitable position until bony union was effected.

I must also enter my protest against many or all of those carved splints which are manufactured, hawked about the country and sold by mechanics, who are not surgeons; with a fossa for each styloid process, a ridge to press between the bones, and various other curious provisions for supposed necessities, but which never find in any arm their exact counterparts, and only deceive the inexperienced surgeon into neglect of the proper means for making a suitable adaptation. They are the fruitful sources of excoriations, ulcerations, inflammations and deformities.

In reference to the treatment of these fractures, the following cases and the accompanying remarks, by that great surgeon Dupuytren, are too pertinent not to merit a place in every treatise of this character.

"The two succeeding cases are not only interesting as fractures of the radius, but they are further deserving of attentive consideration on account of the serious complications which accompanied them, and which were the consequence of forgetting an important precept. More than once, indeed, it has occurred that the surgeons have been so intent on preserving fractures in their proper position, that the extreme constriction employed has actually caused destruction of the soft parts. A piece of advice which I have very frequently given, and which I cannot too often repeat is, to avoid tightening too much the apparatus for fractures during the first few days of its being worn; for the swelling which supervenes is always accompanied by considerable pain, and may be followed by gangrene. It cannot therefore be too urgently impressed on young practitioners, to pay attention to the complaints which patients make; and to visit them twice daily, and relax the bandages and straps as need may be, in order to obviate the frightful consequences which may spring from not heeding this necessary precaution: by carefully attending to this point I have been saved the painful alternative of ever having to sacrifice a limb for complications which its neglect may entail.

"Antoine Rilard, æt. 44, fractured his right radius whilst going down into a cellar, in Feb. 1828, and went at once to the Hospital of La Charité. When the fracture was reduced (it was near the base of the bone) an apparatus was applied, but fastened too tightly; and, notwithstanding the great swelling, and the acute pain which the patient endured, it was not removed until the fourth day, when the hand was cold and œdematous, and the forearm red, painful, and covered with vesications. Leeches, poultices, and fomentations were applied, and followed by some alleviation of the local symptoms, though there was much constitutional disturbance. At the close of a fortnight from the accident, the palmar surface of the forearm presented a point where fluctuation was supposed to exist; but when a bistoury was plunged into it no matter followed. Portions of the flexor muscles subsequently sloughed, and the skin subsequently mortified. The only resource was amputation, which was performed above the elbow, six weeks after his admission; and he afterwards recovered without the occurrence of any further untoward symptoms.

"R., æt. 36, was at work boring an artesian well in 1832, when he was struck by a part of the machinery on the right forearm; he was instantly knocked down and thrown violently on the right thigh. A surgeon who was sent for detected a fracture of the radius, and applied the usual apparatus, consisting of pads and splints, confined by a roller extending from the extremities of the fingers to the elbow, which compressed the arm so tightly as to give rise to very great suffering. The fingers, hand, and forearm were numbed almost to insensibility, and yet the surgeon in attendance did not think proper to loosen the apparatus. Such was the condition of the patient until he came to the Hôtel Dieu, four days after the accident; the fingers were then black, cold, and insensible, and when I removed the splints I found the hand likewise black, especially on its palmar surface. The lower part of the forearm was a shade less livid, but equally cold and insensible; and several vesicles filled with pink-colored serum were apparent on both its surfaces where the splints had pressed; the upper part of the forearm was inflamed, swollen, and very painful. He was bled and leeches were applied to the inflamed part of the arm; camphorated spirit was applied to the fingers.

"On the following day heat was restored as low as the wrist, but the hand remained for the most part livid and cold, and the radial artery did not pulsate. Seventy leeches were applied to the forearm, and the local application was continued." On the second day after admission thirty more leeches were applied. On the fourth day the hand looked a little better, so as to "encourage some hope of its being saved; but this was again blighted on the sixth day, by the entire loss of heat and sensibility in the part, and increased pain and swelling in the forearm, to which the gangrene subsequently extended. On the twelfth day amputation was performed at the elbow-joint; but the patient did not survive the operation more than ten days, the immediate cause of death being acute pleurisy. There was a considerable quantity of purulent serosity poured out on the right side of the chest; and abscesses were found in the lungs and liver. On examining the arm, there was found to be a simple fracture of the radius about its centre.

"The above case presents a painful illustration of the neglect to which I have alluded. In nearly every instance the swelling of the limb requires that careful attention should be paid to the bandage or straps, by which the apparatus is confined. Similar accidents are likely to result from the employment of an immovable apparatus, of which an example occurred in the practice of M. Thiéry, one of my pupils. He was summoned to visit a young girl, on whom such an apparatus had been applied for supposed fracture of the radius. After suffering excruciating torment, the forearm mortified, and amputation was the only resource; on examining the limb no trace of fracture could be discovered. Had a simple apparatus been here employed, and properly watched, this patient's limb would not have been sacrificed."[1]

Robert Smith, mentions also the case of a boy, æt. 18, who had a fracture of the lower extremity of the radius, through the line of the junction of the epiphysis with the diaphysis, caused by being thrown from a horse. A surgeon applied within an hour, a narrow roller tightly around the wrist. On the following day the limb was intensely painful, cold and discolored; still the roller was not removed, nor even slackened. On the fourth day he was admitted into the Richmond Hospital, when the gangrene had reached the forearm. Spon-

[1] Dupuytren, Injuries and Diseases of Bones, Syd. ed., London, 1847, pp. 145–7.

taneous separation of the soft parts finally occurred, and the bones were sawn through twenty-four days after the fracture was produced, from which time "everything proceeded favorably."[1]

Nov. 21, 1851, a boy ten years old, living in the town of Andover, Mass., had his left hand drawn into the picker of a woollen mill, producing several severe wounds of the hand and a fracture of the radius near its middle. One of the wounds was situated directly over the point of fracture, but whether it communicated with the bone or not was not ascertained. A surgeon was called, who closed the wounds, covered the forearm with a bandage from the hand to above the elbow, and applied compresses and splints. This lad made no complaint, his appetite remaining good and his sleep continuing undisturbed, until the third day, when he began to speak of a pain in his shoulder; on the same day also it was noticed that his hand was rather insensible to the prick of a pin. Early on the morning of the fourth day his surgeon being summoned, found him suffering more pain and quite restless; and on removing the dressings, the arm was discovered to be insensible and actually mortified from the shoulder downwards.

Opiates and cordials were immediately given to sustain the patient, and fomentations ordered.

On the sixth day a line of demarcation commenced across the shoulder, and on the twenty-first day, the father himself removed the arm from the body by merely separating the dead tissues with a feather. Subsequently a surgeon found the head of the humerus remaining in the socket, and removed it, the epiphysis having become separated from the diaphysis. The boy now rapidly got well.

In the year 1853, this case became the subject of a legal investigation, in the course of which Dr. Pilsbury, of Lowell, Mass., declared that in his opinion this unfortunate result had been caused by too tight bandaging, and by neglecting to examine the arm during four days.

On the other hand, Drs. Hayward, Bigelow, Townsend, and Ainsworth, of Boston, with Kimball, of Lowell, Drs. Loring, and Pierce, of Salem, believed that the death of the limb was due to some injury done to the artery near the shoulder-joint; and in no other way could they explain the total absence of pain during the first two days; nor could they regard this condition as consistent with the supposition that the bandage occasioned the death of the limb.[2]

I cannot but think, however, that these gentlemen were mistaken, and that the gangrene was alone due to the bandages. In a similar case which came under my own observation, and in which both the radius and ulna were broken, the roller extended no higher than just above the elbow, and the patient complained of no pain until the bandages were unloosed, yet the arm separated at the shoulder-joint. I shall refer again to this example in the chapter on fractures of the radius and ulna; and I shall take occasion then also to speak more fully of the causes of these terrible accidents.

Norris mentions another case of compound fracture of the lower

[1] R. Smith, Treatise on Fractures, &c., Dublin, 1854, p. 170.

[2] Bost. Med. and Surg. Journ., vol. xlviii. p. 281.

end of the radius which came under his notice at the Pennsylvania Hospital, in August, 1837, the arm having been dressed by a country surgeon within half an hour after the accident, with bandages and splints. When these bandages were removed at the hospital, on the fifth day, "the soft parts around the fracture were found to have sloughed, an abscess extended up to the elbow-joint, and sloughs existed over the condyles. Severe constitutional symptoms arose, making amputation of the arm necessary."[1]

A lady, æt. 50, was also seen by Thiérry, who, having broken the radius near its lower end, lost her fingers by the sloughing consequent upon a tight bandage.[2]

The remarks which have now been made in relation to the treatment of Colles' fracture, are applicable, with only such slight modifications as would naturally be suggested, to fractures of the lower end of the radius commencing upon the radial side of the bone and extending obliquely downwards into the joint; and it is to this form of fracture especially, that the pistol-shaped splint must be found applicable. If the fracture actually extends into the joint, it is even the more necessary that, in order to the prevention of anchylosis, the wrist should be early subjected to passive motion.

The following example of a compound, comminuted fracture of the radius, may serve to illustrate the value of a somewhat novel mode of treatment under certain circumstances:—

William Croak, of Buffalo, æt. 30. Jan. 29, 1856, a large piece of iron casting fell upon his arm, crushing and lacerating the wrist, and comminuting the lower part of the radius; he was immediately taken to the Hospital of the Sisters of Charity. I found the whole of the soft parts torn away in front of the joint, and the fragments of the radius projected into the flesh in every direction. The hope of saving the hand seemed to be scarcely sufficient to warrant the attempt; at least by the ordinary mode of procedure. I, however, stated to the gentlemen present, among whom were Dr. Rochester, my colleague, and the house surgeon, Dr. Lemon, that I believed it could be saved if, having removed the fragments of the radius, we practised resection of the lower end of the ulna, and allowed the muscles to become completely relaxed. Accordingly, after placing my patient under the influence of chloroform, I enlarged the wounds so as to enable me to remove six or seven fragments of the radius, leaving others which were broken off but not much displaced. I then removed with the saw one inch and a half of the lower end of the ulna. The hand was immediately drawn up by the contraction of the remaining muscles, but their tension was completely relieved.

The wounds were closed and dressed lightly, and the whole limb was placed on a broad and well-padded splint covered with oiled cloth. The hand, which was very pale and exsanguine, was covered with warm cotton batting.

The subsequent treatment was changed from time to time to suit

[1] Norris, note to Liston's Surgery, p. 54.

[2] Amer. Journ. Med. Sci., vol. xxv. p. 461, from L'Expérience for 1838.

the indications; but his recovery was rapid and complete, nor was there at any time excessive inflammation in any part of the limb.

I have seen this man frequently since he left the hospital, and while he has recovered only a little motion in the wrist-joint, his hand and fingers are nearly as useful as before the accident. He is able to perform all ordinary kinds of labor with almost as much ease as most other men; and what is always gratifying to the humane surgeon, he does not fail to appreciate fully the service which has been conferred upon him by the preservation of his somewhat mutilated hand.

CHAPTER XXII.

FRACTURES OF THE ULNA.

§ 1. Shaft of the Ulna.

Causes.—The shaft of the ulna is generally broken by a direct blow. I have never seen an exception to this rule; but Voisin has related in the *Gazette Médicale* for 1833, a single example in which it was said to have been broken by a fall upon the palm of the hand. Malgaigne thinks it is most often broken when one seeks to ward off a blow with the arm; but it has happened most often to me to see it broken by a fall upon the side of the arm.

Fig. 89.

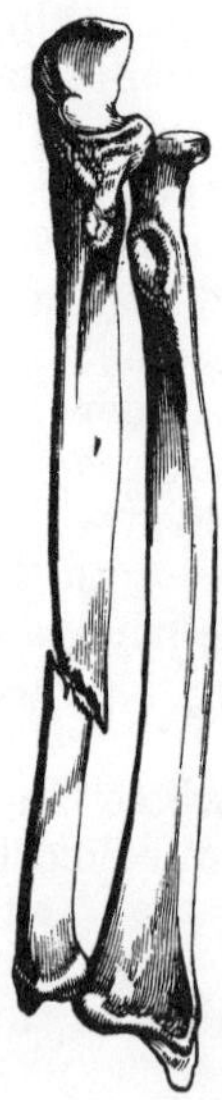

Fracture of the shaft of the ulna.

Point of Fracture, Direction of Displacement, &c.—In an analysis of twenty-three cases, I find the shaft has been broken seven times in its upper third, eight times in its middle third, and eight times in its lower third. All portions seem, therefore, to be about equally liable to fracture. I think, also, the fractures have generally been oblique.

Contrary to what has been observed by other writers, I have noticed that no law prevailed as to the direction in which the fragments have become displaced; the broken ends being found directed forwards, backwards, inwards, or outwards, according to the direction of the blow which has occasioned the fracture; and this is in accordance with the general rule in other fractures occasioned by direct blows. No doubt, however, other things being equal, the tendency of the lower fragment would be toward the interosseous space, in consequence of the action of the pronator quadratus in this direction, and if the fracture is above the middle, the pronator radii teres also will increase this tendency; while the upper fragment, owing to its broad and firm articulation at the elbow-joint, can only be displaced forwards or backwards, at least to any great extent.

Complications.—In no case of the shaft of a long bone have I found serious complications so frequent as in fractures of the shaft of the ulna. Three have been compound; seven complicated with a forward dislocation of the head of the radius; one with a partial dislocation of the lower end of the radius backwards, and one with a dislocation of both radius and ulna backwards at the elbow-joint. It will be seen, therefore, that twelve, or more than one-half of the whole number, have been seriously complicated.

Symptoms.—Occasionally this fracture is found to exist without sensible displacement. In such cases the diagnosis is sometimes difficult, and can only be determined by the crepitus and mobility. If, however, the ulna is firmly seized above and below the point which has suffered contusion, and pressed in opposite directions, these signs will generally be sufficiently manifest, and will render the diagnosis certain.

But in cases where there is considerable displacement, the inner surface of the bone is so superficial as to enable us to detect its deviations with the eye alone, or, when swelling has already occurred, by the fingers carried firmly and slowly along this margin.

If the head of the radius is dislocated also, the displacement of the broken ends of the ulna must always be considerable, and the consequent deformity palpable. I have known one instance, however, in which a surgeon living in the neighboring Province of Upper Canada, recognized and reduced a dislocation of the radius and ulna backwards, but did not detect a fracture of the ulna two inches above its lower end. Six months after, in the month of March, 1856, the patient called upon me with a marked deformity near the wrist, occasioned by the backward projection of the broken ulna, and with a complete loss of the power of supination. It will not surprise us that this fracture was overlooked when we learn that the man had fallen fifty-five feet.

Prognosis.—In simple fractures the prognosis is generally favorable, since no overlapping can occur, and the lateral displacements are not usually sufficient to produce a marked deformity, or to interfere materially with the functions of the arm; yet it is not unfrequent to find the fragments inclining slightly forwards or backwards, inwards or outwards. If the fragments fall toward the radius, I have noticed in three or four instances a slight projection of the lower end or styloid process of the ulna to the ulnar side; but not interfering in any degree with the motions of the wrist-joint.

I have seen the radius left unreduced three times after a fracture of the ulna, and in each example the forearm was shortened. A boy, æt. 17, was struck by a locomotive, and severely injured in various parts of his body, June 5, 1855. I saw him with two very intelligent country practitioners, a few hours after the accident. The whole left arm was then greatly swollen. Crepitus was distinct, and we easily recognized the fracture of the ulna about three inches below its upper end, with which an open wound was in direct communication. We suspected, also, a dislocation of the head of the radius forwards, but as we could not make ourselves certain, and finding that the arm was in such a condition as to preclude any farther manipulation without greatly diminishing the chance of saving the limb, we made no attempt at reduction, but laid the arm upon a pillow and directed cool water lotions.

At no subsequent period, in the opinion of the medical gentleman who was left in charge, did a favorable opportunity occur to reduce the radius; and at the end of two months I found the ulna united, with the fragments bent forwards and outwards toward the radius, while the head of the radius lay in front of the humerus. The forearm was shortened three-quarters of an inch. He could flex his arm freely to a right angle and a little beyond; and he could straighten it perfectly. Hand slightly proned, with partial loss of supination. Whole arm nearly as strong and as useful as before the accident. Above the olecranon process, on the back of the humerus, I observed a remarkable fulness occasioned by the shortening of the triceps muscle.

The second case occurred in the person of a man æt. 26, residing about twenty miles from town, and was occasioned by the kick of a horse. This was also a compound fracture. It does not appear that his surgeon discovered the dislocation of the radius, but supposed that it was a fracture of both bones. On the ninth day the patient became dissatisfied and dismissed his surgeon, but employed no other.

Oct. 1, 1849, eleven weeks after the accident, he called upon me at Buffalo. I found the ulna united with a manifest displacement, but I could not discover that there had been any fracture of the radius. The head of the radius was in front of the external condyle, and a depression existed where it formerly articulated. When the arm was flexed, the head did not strike the humerus so as to arrest the flexion, but it glided upwards and outwards along the inclined base of the external condyle. He had already begun to use his arm considerably in labor. The forearm was shortened one inch.

The third example was in the person of John Lewis, of Pa., æt. 25, who told me, in Sept. 1851, that his left ulna had been broken two years before, and at several points. He was attended by two surgeons living at Montrose, Pa.

I found the ulna much bent forwards a little below its middle, the head of the radius displaced forwards, and the forearm shortened one inch.

Three times I have noticed after the lapse of several years that the forearm could not be perfectly supined; but pronation was never permanently impaired. I think, also, that the motions of flexion and extension have always, except where the radius has remained dislocated, been completely restored soon after the splints were removed; and even in these latter cases, it is only extreme flexion which has been hindered.

Treatment.—In simple fracture we must look carefully to the lateral deviation of the fragments, and if they are found to be salient forwards or backwards, pressure made directly upon or near their extremities, restores them to place, but it often requires considerable force to accomplish this. A gentleman fell and broke the right ulna near its middle. He came immediately to me, and I found the fragments displaced backwards. Pressing strongly with my fingers, they sprung forwards with a distinct crepitus, and I thought they were now in exact line. A broad and well-padded splint was applied to the forearm, and I took especial pains with compresses nicely adjusted, from day to day, to keep everything in place. The arm was placed in a sling. Eight months after the accident this gentleman died of cholera, and I was permitted to dissect the arm. I found the fragments well united, but with a very palpable projection of the fragments backwards, in the direction in which they were at first.

If the displacement is in the direction of the radius, it is more difficult to overcome, but its necessity is much more urgent, since if the fragments fall completely against the radius, a bony union may take place, occasioning a complete loss of the power of pronation and of supination.

While moderate extension is being made, and the hand is firmly supined, the fingers of the surgeon should be pressed firmly, and in spite sometimes of the complaints of the patient, between the radius and ulna, and the fragments of the broken ulna fairly pushed out from the radius.

The forearm may now be laid in the usual position against the front of the chest, midway between supination and pronation, and the same splints applied and in the manner which we shall hereafter describe for fractures of the shaft of both bones.

We ought, however, especially to bear in mind the danger of thrusting the fragments against the ulna, by allowing the sling or the bandages to rest against the middle of the ulnar side of the bone. To prevent this, the sling ought to support the arm by passing only under the hand and wrist, or the forearm may be laid in a firm gutter which will touch the forearm only at the elbow and wrist, or it may be laid upon its back as suggested and practised by Fleury, who, according to Malgaigne, had a case which had been treated in the position of semi-pronation, and which remained not only displaced but refused to unite; but when the arm was supined, the fragments came at once into contact and bony union speedily took place. This position may be adopted whenever it is found to be practicable; but the position of demi-pronation is generally much more comfortable to the patient, at least when the forearm is laid across the chest, and very few patients will submit to a position of complete supination.

In fractures accompanied with dislocation of the head of the radius forwards or backwards, nothing should prevent the immediate reduction of the dislocation but a demonstration of its impossibility, or a condition of the limb which would render manipulation hazardous. It can be reduced, generally, by pushing forcibly upon the head of the bone in the direction of the socket, while the arm is moderately flexed so as to relax the biceps, and while extension is being made at the forearm by an assistant. In making the counter-extension, care should be taken to seize the lower end of the humerus by the condyles, rather than by its anterior aspect, by which precaution we shall avoid pressing upon and rendering tense the tendon of the biceps.

July 29, 1845, a lad, æt. 9, fell from his bed, breaking the ulna and dislocating the head of the radius. Dr. Austin Flint was called on the following morning, and at his request I was invited to see the patient with him. We found the ulna broken obliquely near its middle, and the head of the radius dislocated forwards. While Dr. Flint seized the elbow in front of the condyles, I made extension from the hand, the forearm being slightly flexed upon the arm, and at the same moment I pushed forcibly the head of the radius back to its socket. The reduction was accomplished easily and completely.

We then dressed the arm with Rose's angular splints, constructed with a joint opposite the elbow. This was laid upon the palmar surface, and the whole was nicely padded, especially in front of the head of the radius. In two weeks pasteboard was substituted for the angular splint. At the end of six weeks I was permitted to examine the arm and found the head of the radius perfectly in place, but the points of fracture slightly salient. All of the motions of the arm were fully restored.

June 2, 1845. C. C., æt. 9, fell upon his arm, breaking the ulna obliquely near its middle, and dislocating the head of the radius forwards. Dr. J. P. White being called, requested me to visit the patient also with him. We found one of the broken fragments protruding through the skin, on the inside of the arm.

With great ease, and by simply pressing with considerable force upon the head of the radius, it was made to slide into its socket. The case was left in charge of Dr. White.

Five weeks after, I found all of the motions of the forearm completely restored, except that he could not extend it perfectly. The head of the radius was also a little more prominent in front than in the opposite arm.

Four or five years afterwards, the projection of the head of the radius had disappeared, and the functions of the arm were perfect.

The following example of compound and comminuted fracture of the ulna will illustrate how much may be accomplished by conservative surgery:—

A German lad, æt. 10, was run over by a railroad car, Sept. 4, 1857. Drs. C. F. Gay and Austin Flint, Jr., were summoned immediately; but the limb presented such a discouraging appearance as induced them to send for me also.

We found the ulna very much broken near its lower end, and about two inches of it entirely gone. The radius was sound. The skin and muscles were extensively lacerated and torn off in shreds.

After a careful examination, finding that the radial and ulnar arteries continued to pulsate, upon consultation together, we agreed to attempt to save the limb. It was accordingly laid upon a board covered with a soft and nicely adjusted cushion; such vessels as were bleeding were tied; the skin was loosely stitched together, and the whole covered with a cotton cloth smeared with simple cerate. Cool water dressings were directed, and the boy was left in charge of Drs. Gay and Flint. The skin subsequently sloughed extensively, and also more or less of the muscular tissue; but on the 1st of May, 1858, about eight months from the time of the accident, it had nearly or quite closed over, and although his arm was very much deformed and maimed, it was still very useful; indeed, to one who must earn his living by his hands alone, its value is beyond estimate.

§ 2. Coronoid Process of the Ulna.

Dissections have established the possibility of this fracture as a simple accident in the living subject; but I have not myself seen any example of which I can speak positively. In the two following cases, the existence of such a fracture was at first suspected, but I have now very little doubt but that my diagnosis was incorrect. I shall relate them, however, as examples of those accidents which are likely to be mistaken for fracture of this process.

A laboring man aged about twenty-five years, had been seen and treated by another surgeon, for what was supposed to be a simple dislocation of the radius and ulna backwards. The surgeon thought he had reduced the dislocation very soon after the accident. On the following day he found the dislocation reproduced, and he requested me to see the patient with him. The arm was then much swollen, but the character of the dislocation was apparent. By moderate extension, applied while the arm was slightly flexed, and continued for a few seconds, reduction was again effected; the bones returning to their places with a distinct sensation; but on releasing the arm the dislocation was immediately reproduced. These attempts to reduce and retain in place the dislocated bones were repeated several times during

Fig. 90.

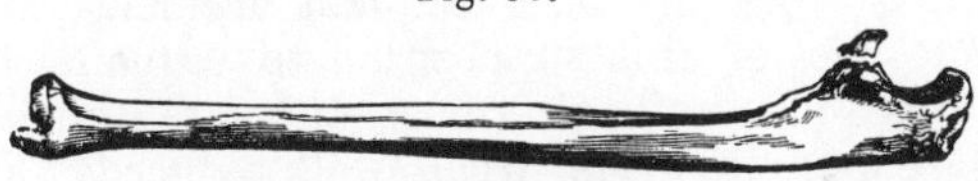

Fracture of the coronoid process.

this day, and on subsequent days, but to no purpose, and the patient was dismissed after about two weeks with the bones unreduced.

The impossibility of retaining the bones in place, and the existence of an occasional crepitus during the manipulation, inclined me to believe at the time that the dislocation was accompanied with a fracture of the coronoid process.

Another similar case has since presented itself in a child nine years old, and in which the subsequent examinations not only demonstrated the non-existence of a fracture, but also rendered doubtful the justness of the conclusions which I had drawn in the case just related.

This lad fell, Nov. 4, 1855, and his parents immediately brought him to me; but as he lived many miles from town, I did not see him until eighteen hours after the injury was received. I found the arm much swollen, slightly flexed and proned. Flexion and extension of the arm were very painful; the pain being referred chiefly to the front of the joint, near the situation of the coronoid process; and at this point also there was a discoloration of the size of a twenty-five cent piece. Flexing the forearm moderately upon the arm and making extension, the bones came readily into place, but without sensation of any kind, either a snap or a crepitus. That the bones had now resumed their position, however, I made certain by a very careful examination with the hand and by measurement; yet they would not remain in place one moment when the extension was discontinued. The reduction was made several times, and constantly with the same result. We then applied a right-angled splint to the arm, having first reduced the bones, and thus were able to retain them in position. I believed that the coronoid process was broken, and so informed the surgeon to whose care the boy was returned.

Five months after, he was brought again to me, and I then found that the radius and ulna had been kept in place; the motions of the joint were perfect, and if the coronoid process had ever been broken it was now again in its natural position, and with every structure about it in a condition as complete as it was before the accident. For myself, I do not believe that so perfect a union of this process can happen—at least in a case where, as must have been the fact in this example, the separation and displacement of the process are such that it no longer offers an obstacle to the dislocation of the ulna backwards and upwards.

Malgaigne thinks that the fracture is more frequent than the small number of reported examples would lead us to suppose, especially because he has noticed how often the summit of the process is broken off, when dislocation of the radius and ulna backwards are produced artificially on the dead subject. In three or four cases, also, of dislocations of these bones backwards and inwards, which had come under his notice, he was unable to feel this process, and he therefore thought it probable that it was broken off. Other surgeons have thought, also, that it was a not infrequent accident; and they have constantly made use of this supposition to explain those cases in which, the radius and ulna having been dislocated backwards, would not afterward remain in place when well reduced. Fergusson has indeed made the extraordinary statement in relation to dislocations of the radius and ulna backwards generally, that in these cases "the coronoid process will probably be broken."

But in my opinion, these fractures are exceedingly rare; and I think these gentleman need to have furnished some more conclusive evidence of the correctness of their opinions, than can be found in their writings, or in the writings of any other surgeons, which I have seen.

Malgaigne mentions three reported examples, namely: one published by Combes Brassard, an Italian surgeon, in 1811, which Brassard saw only after a lapse of three months; one seen by Penneck, and published in the *Lancet* in 1828, the patient then being sixty years old and the accident having occurred while he was a young man; the third was seen by Sir Astley Cooper, several months after the accident, and is reported by himself in his excellent treatise on Fractures and Dislocations. Says Mr. Cooper: "It was thought, at the consultation which was held about him in London, that the coronoid process was detached from the ulna." This was the only living example seen by Mr. Cooper in his long and immensely varied surgical practice; and even here we cannot fail to notice the apparent reserve with which he expresses his opinion—"It was thought at the consultation."

To these examples our own researches have added a few others.

Dorsey says that Dr. Physick once saw a fracture of the coronoid process. The symptoms resembled a luxation of the forearm backwards, "except that when the reduction was effected, the dislocation was repeated, and by careful examination, crepitation was discovered. The forearm was kept flexed at a right angle with the humerus. The tendency of the brachieus internus to draw up the superior fragment, was counteracted in some measure by the pressure of the roller above the elbow. A perfect cure was readily obtained."[1] In 1830, Dr. Wm. M. Fahnestock reported a case occurring in a boy, who, having fallen from a haymow, received the whole weight of his body "on the back part of the palm of the left hand," while the arm was extended forwards. It seemed to be a dislocation of the forearm backwards, but when reduced it was again immediately displaced, with an evident crepitus. The arm was secured in the angular splint of Dr. Physick, and "recovered very speedily."[2] Dr. Couper, of the Glasgow Infirmary, also has reported a dislocation of the forearm backwards and outwards occurring in a young man aged seventeen, and which he thinks was accompanied with this fracture. The dislocation was easily reduced, but returned again immediately on ceasing the extension. The fragment was not felt, nor does he speak of crepitus; the existence of the fracture being inferred from the fact that the bones would not remain in place without help. The forearm was placed across the chest, with the fingers pointing toward the opposite shoulder, and secured in this position with splints and a bandage. At the end of four weeks union had taken place, with only slight deformity, although with some stiffness of the joint.

In relation to this example, the editor remarks that the symptoms were not to his mind conclusive in determining the existence of a fracture of the coronoid process, and he inclines to the belief that it was rather an oblique fracture of the lower extremity of the humerus. "In cases like these," he adds, "where very rare accidents are suspected, we think that unless the diagnosis is clear, the leaning should always be the other way: we mean, that, *cæteris paribus*, the symptoms should rather be referred to the common than the extraordinary injury. The contrary practice introduces a dangerous laxity in diagnosis."[3]

In the *American Medical Monthly* for October, 1855, also, I find the report of a trial for malpractice, in which a lad nine years old received some injury about the elbow-joint which resulted in a maiming. The defendant claimed that there had been a dislocation of the forearm backwards, accompanied either with a fracture of the trochlea of the humerus, or of the coronoid process of the ulna.

Dr. Crosby, of Dartmouth College, testified that he had never met with a fracture of this process, yet he would not say that it did not exist in this case. He was not able to decide positively. Dr. Peaslee,

[1] Dorsey, Elements of Surgery, vol. i. p. 152. Philadelphia, 1813.
[2] Fahnestock, Amer. Journ. Med. Sci., vol. vi. p. 267.
[3] Couper, Lond. Med.-Chir. Rev., new ser, vol. xi. p. 509.

of the same college, thought it altogether probable that it had been broken, and Dr. Spaulding was of the opinion fully that it had been broken.

The jury did not agree, and a non-suit was finally allowed by the court.

The defendant, in his report of the trial, seems to me to have justly complained that Mr. Fergusson has said, that in a dislocation of the forearm backwards "the coronoid process will probably be broken." This was urged in the trial by the plaintiff's counsel as contradicting the medical testimony, and as evidence of a conspiracy on the part of the surgeons to defeat the ends of justice; since they constantly affirmed that the accident was so rare as not to have been reasonably expected, and that a failure to look for or to discover it did not imply a lack of ordinary skill or care.[1]

Says Mr. Liston: "The coronoid process is occasionally pulled or pushed off from the shaft, more especially in young subjects. I saw a case of it lately, in which the injury arose in consequence of the patient, a boy of eight years, having hung for a long time from the top of a wall by one hand, afraid to drop down;"[2] after whom, Miller, Erichsen, Skey, Lonsdale, and most of the Scotch and English surgeons have repeated the assertion that this process may be broken in this manner by the action of the brachialis anticus alone, yet no one of them has to this day seen another example.

The explanation of the accident in the case of the boy, given by Liston, implies two anatomical errors: first, that the coronoid process is an epiphysis during childhood; and second, that the brachialis anticus is inserted upon its summit. The coronoid process is never an epiphysis, but is formed from a common point of ossification with the shaft; the olecranon process and the lower extremity of the ulna having also separate points of ossification. Moreover, the brachialis anticus has its insertion at the base of the process and partly upon the body of the ulna, but in no part upon its summit; indeed, the process seems rather to be intended as a pulley over which the brachialis anticus may play; resembling also, somewhat, in its function, the patella; serving to protect the joint and perhaps the muscle itself from becoming compressed in the motions of the joint. Certainly it could never have been broken by the action of this muscle, and the case mentioned by Mr. Liston must find some other explanation. It may have been a rupture of the brachialis anticus itself, or of the biceps, or possibly a forward luxation of the head of the radius. Either of these suppositions is more rational than the statement made by Mr. Liston, because either one of them is possible, while his supposition is impossible.

These, if I except my own, constitute all of the supposed examples seen in the living subject, of which I find any record; eight in all.

The first two were not entirely satisfactory to Malgaigne; the third is spoken of cautiously by Sir Astley Cooper, as if it needed, in addition to his own great name, the indorsement of the "London council."

[1] Op. cit., vol. iv. p. 339.

[2] Liston, Practical Surgery, p. 55.

Dorsey reports his case upon hearsay, and the result is quite too satisfactory to give it much claim to credibility. Fahnestock's case is to our mind far from being fully proven. Couper's case is doubted by Dr. Johnson; and the New Hampshire case was not made out satisfactorily to either the jury or the medical men. Liston's case was simply impossible.

Certainly it is not upon such testimony as this that we can rely to sustain Mr. Fergusson's opinion that it is likely to occur in all dislocations of the forearm backwards, or of Malgaigne's conjecture that it is of more frequent occurrence than the published cases would seem to show. Nor will it be regarded as conclusive, that the beak of the process is often found broken after luxations made upon the subject; since between luxations thus produced and luxations occurring in the living subject there exists this important difference: that in the case of the latter, muscular action is the principal agent in the production of the dislocation, while in the former it is the external force alone which drives the bone from its socket.

The fact, therefore, that so few cases have ever been reported, and that most of these are far from having been clearly made out, remains presumptive evidence that the actual cases are exceedingly rare; but if to this we add such negative evidence as is furnished by actual dissections, and by examinations of the pathological cabinets of the world, we think the testimony is almost conclusive.

Only four specimens have been mentioned by any of the surgical writers known to me. Sir Astley Cooper says that a person was brought to the dissecting room at St. Thomas's Hospital, who had been the subject of this accident. "The coronoid process, which had been broken off within the joint, had united by a ligament only, so as to move readily upon the ulna, and thus alter the sigmoid cavity of the ulna so much as to allow in extension that bone to glide backwards upon the condyles of the humerus."[1] Mr. Bransby Cooper adds in a note that the external condyle of the humerus was also broken and united by ligament.

Samuel Cooper describes, rather obscurely, a specimen contained in the University College Museum, "in which the ulna is broken at the elbow, the posterior fragment being displaced backwards by the action of the triceps; the coronoid process is broken off; the upper head of the radius is also dislocated from the lesser sigmoid cavity of the ulna, and drawn upwards by the action of the biceps. In this complicated accident, the ulna is broken in two places."

Malgaigne says that Velpeau has also established by an autopsy the existence of a fracture of the coronoid apophysis, but without having given any further particulars in relation to the case.

In addition to these examples, Charles Gibson, of Richmond, Va., has stated to me by letter that he has in his possession a specimen of this fracture, evidently belonging to an adult. The process was broken transversely near its extremity, and has united again quite closely and without any displacement, and without ensheathing callus.

[1] A. Cooper, Dislocations and Fractures, p. 411.

We must subject these specimens to analysis also. The first two were complicated with other fractures, and the second, especially, seems to have been a general crushing of all the bones concerned in the formation of the elbow-joint: neither of them could have been occasioned by contractions of the brachialis anticus, while only that one described by Sir Astley Cooper could have been the result of a dislocation of the forearm backwards. Of the specimen said to have been seen by Velpeau, I am unable to speak without more circumstantial knowledge of its condition. Nor can I speak very confidently of that belonging to my distinguished friend, Dr. Gibson, of Virginia. Notwithstanding the respect which I entertain for his opinion, I cannot avoid a suspicion that the bone was never broken at all, since I find it more easy to believe that he is deceived by certain appearances, than that it should have united by bone again, and so perfectly as not to leave any line of separation or degree of displacement. Certainly the fracture was too high to have been produced by the action of the muscle, if such a thing were ever possible; and if broken by a dislocation, which must have forced it violently from its position, as the ulna was driven upwards, it is to me incredible that it should ever be made to unite again so perfectly.

We are therefore left as before with no evidence that the coronoid process was ever broken by the action of a muscle, and with only one example in which it is probable that a fracture occurred as a consequence of a dislocation of the radius and ulna backwards. If then it does happen that in this dislocation it is pretty often found difficult or impossible to retain the bones in place without aid, it will be the part of prudence to ascribe this troublesome circumstance to some more common accident than a fracture of the coronoid process: perhaps to a fracture of some portion of the lower end of the humerus, or to a disruption, more or less complete, of the tendons of the biceps and brachialis anticus, together with the ligaments which surround the joint.

Causes.—It is probable that this process will be sometimes broken in a fall upon the palm of the hand; the force of the blow being received directly upon the lower end of the radius, and through its numerous muscles and ligamentous attachments being indirectly conveyed to the ulna, producing a violent concussion of the coronoid process against the trochlea of the humerus, and resulting finally in a fracture of this process and a dislocation of both bones of the forearm backwards. The gentleman seen by Sir Astley had fallen upon his extended hand while in the act of running. Brassard's patient had fallen also upon his hand with his arm extended in front. Penneck's patient, an old man of sixty years, had fallen upon the palm of his hand, and Fahnestock's fell upon the "back of the palm." In no other case is the point upon which the blow was received particularly mentioned. In two of the examples mentioned by Malgaigne there was a luxation of the forearm backwards; such was also the fact in the case seen by Fahnestock; in Couper's case it was dislocated backwards and outwards, and in Sir Astley's case I infer that there was only a subluxation of the ulna backwards.

We know of no other causes, therefore, than such as equally tend to produce dislocations at the elbow-joint, unless we except direct crushing blows, which of course may break the bones at any point upon which the force happens to be applied.

Symptoms.—Partial or complete displacement of the ulna, or of the radius and ulna backwards, accompanied with the usual signs of these luxations; to which may be possibly added crepitus; and it is fair to presume that in some examples the fragment carried forwards by being driven against the trochlea, may be felt displaced and movable in the bend of the elbow. Brassard affirms that it was so with the patient whom he saw. If only the summit is broken off, the brachialis anticus could have no influence upon it, but if it were broken fairly through the base, it might be displaced slightly in the direction of the action of this muscle.

The symptoms, however, which have been regarded as most diagnostic are the disposition to re-luxation manifested in most of these examples when the extension has been discontinued; and especially the fact that the olecranon was particularly prominent when the arm was extended, but that it resumed its natural position when the arm was flexed to a right angle. But I am unable to understand how either of these circumstances can be better explained upon the supposition of a fracture of this apophysis, than without such a supposition. If the reduction of both bones is once effected, even though the support of the coronoid process is completely lost, the head of the radius ought to prevent a re-luxation unless the arm is disturbed again; nor can I understand why, when the elbow is bent, the re-luxation is less likely to occur; since, although in this position the humerus bears less directly upon the process, the difference in this respect must be very little, for in whatever position the arm is placed, so long as the radius retains its position the ulna cannot be drawn very forcibly against the humerus; while, on the other hand, by flexing the arm the power of the biceps, and of such fibres of the brachialis as remain attached to the ulna, to aid in the maintenance of reduction is completely lost; and at the same moment the resistance, and consequent power of the triceps to produce the luxation, are greatly increased.

In short, we must confess that we are here, also, notwithstanding the confidence with which writers have spoken of the signs of this accident, very much in doubt; nor do we see how these doubts can be removed until we have in detail the symptoms of at least one example, the indubitable existence of which has been subsequently verified by dissection.

Prognosis.—In the case of Cooper's patient, seen several months after the accident, the ulna projected backwards while the arm was extended, but it was without much difficulty drawn forwards and bent, and then the deformity disappeared. He thought that during extension the ulna slipped back behind the inner condyle of the humerus. Brassard's patient, seen after three months, retained the power of pronation and supination, with also extension, but flexion was completely impossible, the forearm being arrested in this direction by the small, slightly movable fragment of bone in front of the elbow-joint, and which was supposed to be the process itself. Penneck's old man, who had met with the accident in boyhood, had still the radius luxated forwards and outwards, and the olecranon more salient backwards than in the sound arm. Extension and flexion were nearly but not quite complete. Fahnestock informs us that his patient "recovered completely," but whether without deformity or maiming we are not told. Couper says the bone was united in four weeks, and that only a slight deformity and a little stiffness remained. Physick's patient made a perfect recovery.

Let us come again to the dissections. Rejecting the doubtful specimen belonging to Dr. Gibson, we have an exact account of only two, and, indeed, Sir Astley Cooper alone has described the mode of union. Samuel Cooper says that in the case of the University College specimen the radius is dislocated forwards and upwards, and the olecranon is displaced backwards, but he does not say whether the coronoid process has united, nor describe its position; but Sir Astley informs us that in the example seen and dissected by him the process was united by ligament, which was sufficiently long and flexible to allow the fragment to move upwards and downwards in the motions of flexion and extension.

In the absence of any other testimony, we may be allowed to express an opinion that when the fracture has taken place across the summit or above the insertion of the brachialis anticus, nothing but a ligamentous union can be regarded as possible, since the fragment can only derive nourishment from a few untorn fibres of the capsule and perhaps of the internal lateral ligaments; and although it may not be displaced, it cannot have the advantage of impaction, upon which alone, I suspect, a fracture of the neck of the femur within the capsule must rely for a bony union, if it ever does so unite. If, however, the fracture has taken place at the base, and fortunately it has not become much displaced by the force of the concussion against the humerus, it does not seem to me so impossible that under favorable circumstances a bony union might now and then occur. It will be remembered that a good portion of the attachment of the brachialis anticus is still below the fracture, and the remaining fibres are not therefore very likely to displace the fragment, especially when the arm is sufficiently flexed, so as to properly relax this muscle.

It will be of small importance, however, whether the union is bony or ligamentous, provided only there is not great displacement.

Treatment.—Whatever view we take of the pathology of this accident, the rational mode of treatment would seem to consist in flexing the arm at a right angle, and retaining it a sufficient length of time in that position; not forgetting, however, the danger of anchylosis from long-continued confinement in one position.

An angular splint may be useful in preventing motion at first, but I think it ought not to be continued beyond seven or ten days at the most. After this, a simple sling is all that can be necessary, since from this period some motion must be given to the joint if we would take the proper precautions to prevent stiffness. Sir Astley Cooper thought the limb ought to be kept immovable three weeks, and Velpeau preferred four; but I cannot agree with them, believing that the question of the future mobility of the elbow-joint is vastly more important than the question of a bony or ligamentous union between the fragments. Couper says that he adopted in the treatment of the case reported by him, extreme flexion, but both Physick and Fahnestock placed the arm at right angles, and Sir Astley Cooper has recommended the same position. The latter position has always the advantage in case permanent anchylosis occurs, and the former cannot add much to the chance of complete replacement of the fragment.

Bandages are only serviceable to retain the splint in place, and they may be thrown aside as soon as the splint is removed.

While these pages are going to press, I have met with the following two additional reported examples of fracture of the coronoid process:—

Thomas Jenkins, admitted to the New York City Hospital, Feb. 5, 1850, having fallen, a few hours before admission, from the roof of a building to the ground, a height of thirty feet. Both bones of the right forearm were dislocated backwards at the elbow; the right radius had also sustained a comminuted fracture of its head and of its lower extremity, the head being completely detached from the articular surface of the os brachii. Besides this injury, there was a fracture of the coronoid process of the right ulna, a comminuted fracture of the left radius, fracture of the left ulna, compound fracture of the right patella, and compound fracture of the skull at its base and above it, with laceration of the dura mater and brain; under which injuries the patient soon expired.[1]

Terrance O'Brian, æt. 16, was admitted to the Brooklyn Hospital, Aug. 13, 1856. In attempting to pass his hand over a pulley connected with some machinery, his arm was caught, and he was drawn over the shaft, producing a compound dislocation at the elbow joint, a fracture of the inner condyle of the humerus, and a fracture of the coronoid process of the ulna. The lower end of the humerus protruded through the skin in front of the joint, two inches. The dislocation was reduced, the arm placed upon an angular splint, and cold water dressings applied. At the end of about seven weeks, the wounds were granulating nicely, and the surgeon felt assured that the limb would be saved, and he hoped also that some motion in the joint would be obtained.[2]

The first of these examples does not appear to have been proven by a dissection, although the man died.

The second example lacks also this same important testimony; and indeed the report is too brief and loose to inspire full confidence in its accuracy. In neither case does the surgeon seem to have regarded the fracture of this process as an unusual circumstance, or as an accident of difficult diagnosis, and to substantiate which he would be expected to say more than simply that it had occurred. It must be noticed also, that if we admit these two as well-proven examples of this fracture, they are neither of them examples of simple, uncomplicated fractures.

[1] Lente's Hospital Reports. N. Y. Journ. Med., &c., N. S., vol. v. p. 25, July, 1850.

[2] Enos's Brooklyn Hospital Reports. N. Y. Journ. Med., &c., Third Ser., vol. ii. p. 98, Jan. 1857.

§ 3. Fractures of the Olecranon Process.

Causes.—So far as I have been able to ascertain, all of the fractures of this process which I have seen were occasioned by falls upon the elbow, or by blows inflicted directly upon the part. Malgaigne has, however, been able to collect accounts of six examples of fracture of the olecranon, produced, as is affirmed, by the violent action of the triceps; as in pushing with the arm slightly flexed, in throwing a ball, in plunging into the water with the arms extended, etc.; but only four of these reported examples does he think are sufficiently authenticated to entitle them to be received as facts; nor do I think it possible to affirm positively that in any instance, where the whole process is broken off, the triceps alone has occasioned the separation. For example, Capiomont reports the case of a cavalier, who, being intoxicated, was thrown head foremost from his horse, and striking probably upon his hand, was found to have broken the olecranon process. We do not, in this example, see evidence alone of a forcible contraction of the triceps, but also of violent pressure against the hand and in the direction of the axis of the forearm toward the elbow-joint, by which the olecranon process might have been so thrown forwards against the fossa of the humerus as to cause its separation. The same explanation might apply to several of the other examples.

Point and Direction of Fracture; Displacement, etc.—The process may be broken at its summit, at its base, or intermediate between these two extremes, the last of which is the most common.

It is probable that when the action of the triceps alone has produced the fracture, it will be found that only the summit, or that portion which receives the insertion of the triceps, has been broken off. Malgaigne, who had been able to find upon record only two cases of a fracture of the extreme end of the process, declares that they were both occasioned by muscular action.

Fractures of the middle are generally transverse, or only slightly oblique, occurring in the line of the junction of the epiphysis with the diaphysis. We think, also, we have reasons for believing that these only occur as a consequence of a fall upon the elbow, or of a blow upon the extreme point of the elbow, when the forearm is considerably flexed upon the arm; the direction of the obliquity, when any is found to exist, being generally from above downwards and from behind forwards, indicating that the direction of the force was also from behind.

Fig. 91.

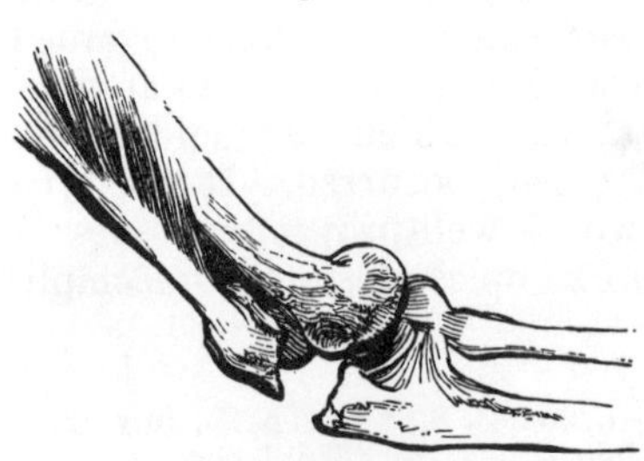

Fracture at the base.

Fractures through the base are generally quite oblique, the line of fracture extending from before downwards and backwards, so that not only the whole of the process, but a portion of the back of the shaft, is carried away; and this accident can scarcely happen, except by a blow received upon the lower end of the humerus, directly in front of the process; or, what would amount to the same thing, by a blow from behind, received upon the ulna just below the olecranon process, or by wrenching the forearm violently back, while the humerus is fixed.

The only displacement to which the upper fragment seems to be liable, is in the direction of the triceps; and the degree of this displacement does not depend so much upon the point at which the fracture has taken place as upon the violence which has occasioned it, the extent of the disruption of the ligaments, aponeurosis of the triceps and of the capsule, and upon whether, since the accident, the arm has been flexed or kept extended.

In two instances, I have found distinct crepitus immediately after the fracture had occurred, produced by only moving the fragment laterally, showing plainly that little or no displacement had taken place. The following example will show also that this displacement does not always happen even after the lapse of several days, and where no surgical treatment has been adopted.

Samuel Duckett, æt. 14, fell upon the point of the elbow, and two days after was admitted to the Buffalo Hospital of the Sisters of Charity. The elbow was then much swollen, but no crepitus could be detected, and he could nearly straighten his arm by the action of the triceps. On the sixth day, the swelling having sufficiently subsided, a distinct crepitus was discovered when the olecranon process was seized between the fingers, and moved laterally. We extended the arm immediately, and applied a long gutta-percha splint to the whole front of the arm and forearm, securing it in place with a roller. On the eleventh day, five days after the first dressing, the splint was taken off, and its angle at the elbow-joint slightly changed; and this was repeated every day until the twenty-second from the time of the accident. The splint was then finally removed, when the fragment was found to be united without any perceptible displacement, and the motions of the joint were unimpaired.

It must not be inferred, however, that it is always prudent to leave this fracture thus unsupported, since it has occasionally happened that the displacement, which did not exist at first, has taken place to the extent of half an inch or more, after the lapse of several days. Mr. Earle mentions a case in which the separation did not take place until the sixth day, when it was occasioned by the patient's attempting to tie his neck-cloth.

Symptoms.—The usual signs of a fracture of the olecranon process, are, when the fragments are not separated, crepitus discovered especially by seizing the process, and moving it laterally; or, when displacement has actually taken place the crepitus may be discovered sometimes by extending the forearm, and pressing the fragment downwards until it is made to touch the lower fragment; the existence of a palpable depression between the fragments, partial flexion of the forearm, and total inability, on the part of the patient, to straighten it completely, or even to flex the arm in some cases. If the fragments do not separate, gentle flexion and extension of the arm, while the finger rests upon the process, may enable us to detect the fracture.

It will sometimes happen that, owing to the rapid occurrence of tumefaction, the evidences of a fracture will be quite equivocal; but, in all cases where a severe injury has been inflicted upon the point of the elbow, it will be well to suspend judgment until, by repeated examinations, made on successive days, the question is determined. Meanwhile, the arm ought to be kept constantly in an extended position, as if a fracture was known to exist.

Prognosis.—In a large majority of cases, this process becomes reunited to the shaft by ligament, which may vary in length from a line to an inch or more, and which is more or less perfect in different cases. Sometimes it is composed of two separate bands, with an intermediate space, or the ligament may have several holes in it; at other times it is composed in part of bone and in part of fibrous tissue; but most frequently it is a single, firm, fibrous cord, whose breadth and thickness are less than that of the process to which it is attached.

If the fragments are maintained in perfect apposition, a bony union is likely to occur, yet it is not invariably found to have taken place, even under these circumstances. Malgaigne thinks, also, he has seen one case in which there was neither bone nor fibrous tissue deposited between the fragments. This was an ancient fracture at the base of the olecranon; the superior fragment remained immovable during the flexion and extension of the arm, yet it could be moved easily from side to side.

Fig. 92.

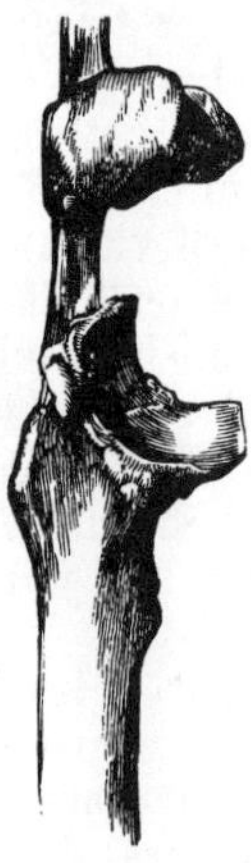

Union by ligament.

In my own cases, I have three times found the fragments united without any appreciable separation, and have presumed that the union was bony. One of these examples I have already mentioned; the second, was in the person of a lady aged about forty years, who, having fallen down a flight of steps on the 8th of September, 1857, sent for me immediately. I found a large bloody tumor covering the elbow-joint, but there was no difficulty in detecting a fracture of the olecranon process. It was easily moved from side to side, and this motion was accompanied with a distinct crepitus. During the first week, the arm was only laid upon a pillow, but as it was found to become gradually more flexed, and the swelling having in a great measure subsided, the arm was nearly, but not quite, straightened, and a long gutta-percha splint applied to the palmar surface of the forearm and arm. The fragments united in about twenty or twenty-five days, and without separation, so far as could be discovered in a very careful examination.

The third example to which I have referred, occurred in a boy fourteen years old, and was treated by Dr. Benjamin Smith, of Berkshire, Massachusetts. Sixty-nine years after, he being then eighty-three years old, I found the olecranon process united apparently by

rapidly acquire a tolerance, which soon dissipates all feeling of fatigue, and that, after a few hours, or days at most, the patients express themselves as being more comfortable in this position than in the flexed.

Finally, the advocates of complete extension claim that in this position alone, is the triceps most perfectly relaxed, and consequently the most important indication, namely, the descent of the olecranon, most fully accomplished. In this opinion we also concur; and regarding all other considerations, in the early days of the treatment, as secondary to this one, we unhesitatingly declare our preference for what has been called the "position of complete extension."

It only remains for us to determine by what means the limb can be best maintained in the extended position, and the olecranon process most easily and effectually secured in place.

For this purpose a variety of ingenious plans have been devised; such as the compress and "figure-of-8" bandage of Duverney, without

Fig. 93.

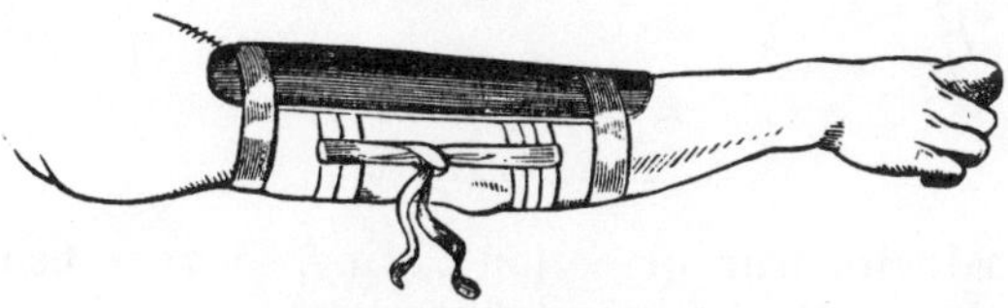

Sir Astley Cooper's method.

splints; or a similar bandage employed by Desault, with the addition of a long splint in front; the circular and transverse bandages of Sir Astley Cooper, with lateral tapes to draw them together, to which also a splint was added; and many other modes not varying essentially from those already described, but nearly all of which are liable to one serious objection, namely, that if they are applied with sufficient firmness to hold upon the fragment, and Boyer says they "ought to be drawn very tight," they ligate the limb so completely as to interrupt its circulation, and expose the limb greatly to the hazards of swelling, ulceration, and even gangrene. How else is it possible to make the bandage effective upon a small fragment of bone, scarcely larger than the tendon which envelops its upper end, and with no salient points against which the compress or the roller can make advantageous pressure? If, then, these accidents, swelling, ulceration, and gangrene, are not of frequent occurrence, it is only because the bandage has not been generally applied "very tight," and while it has done no harm, it has as plainly done no good.

The dangers to which I allude may be easily avoided, without relaxing the security afforded by the compress and bandage, by a method which is very simple, and the value of which I have already sufficiently determined by my own practice.

The surgeon will prepare, extemporaneously always, for no single pattern will fit two arms, a splint, from a long and sound wooden shingle, or from any piece of thin, light board. This must be long enough to reach from near the wrist-joint, to within three or four inches of the shoulder, and of a width equal to the widest part of the limb. Its width must be uniform throughout, except that, at a point corresponding to a point three inches, or thereabouts, below the top of the olecranon process, there shall be a notch on each side, or a slight narrowing of the splint. One surface of the splint is now to be

Fig. 94.

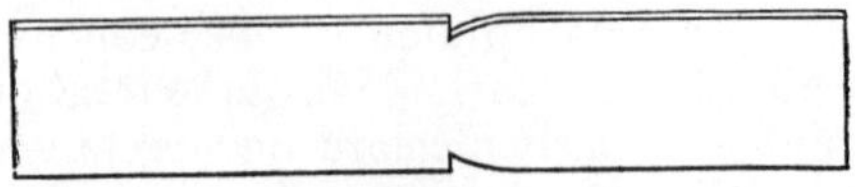

Fig. 95.

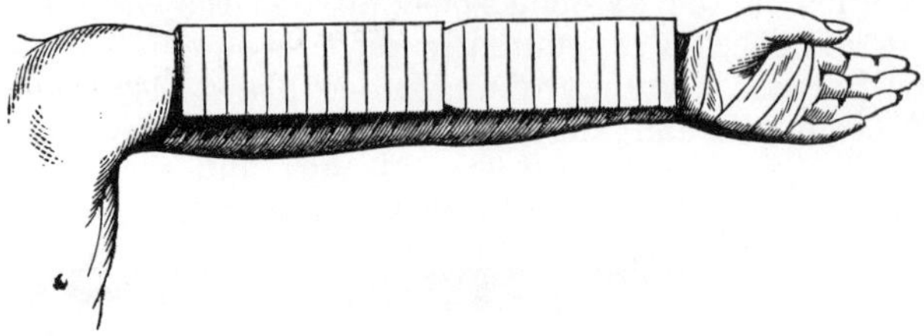

The author's method.

thickly padded with hair or cotton-batting, so as to fit all of the inequalities of the arm, forearm, and elbow, and the whole covered neatly with a piece of cotton cloth, stitched together upon the back of the splint. Thus prepared, it is to be laid upon the palmar surface of the limb, and a roller is to be applied, commencing at the hand and covering the splint, by successive circular turns, until the notch is reached, from which point the roller is to pass upwards and backwards behind the olecranon process and down again to the same point on the opposite side of the splint; after making a second oblique turn above the olecranon, to render it more secure, the roller may begin gradually to descend, each turn being less oblique, and passing through the same notch, until the whole of the back of the elbow-joint is covered. This completes the adjustment of the fragments, and it only remains to carry the roller again upwards, by circular turns, until the whole arm is covered as high as the top of the splint.

The advantage of this mode of dressing must be apparent. It leaves, on each side of the splint, a space upon which neither the splint nor bandage can make pressure, and the circulation of the limb is, therefore, unembarrassed, while it is equally effective in retaining the olecranon in place, and much less liable to become disarranged.

Before the bandage is applied about the elbow-joint, the olecranon must be drawn down, as well as it can be, by pressure with the fingers, and a compress of folded linen, wetted to prevent its sliding, must be placed partly above and partly upon the process; at the same time, also, care must be taken that the skin is not folded in between the fragments.

This dressing ought, no doubt, to be applied immediately, since, if we wait, as Boyer seems to advise, until the swelling has subsided, it will be found much more difficult to straighten the arm completely than it would have been at first, and the olecranon process will be more drawn up and fixed in its abnormal position. Something will be gained by these means, adopted early, even if the bandage cannot be applied tightly, and moderate bandaging will not in any way interfere with the proper and successful treatment of the inflammation. We must always keep in mind, however, the fact that the fracture being usually the result of a direct blow, considerable inflammation and swelling about the joint are about to follow rapidly; and on each successive day, or oftener if necessary, the bandages must be examined carefully, and promptly loosened whenever it seems to be necessary. For this purpose it is better not to unroll the bandages, but to cut them with a pair of scissors, along the face of the splint, cutting only a small portion at a time, and as they draw back, stitch them together again lightly; and thus proceed until the whole has been rendered sufficiently loose.

As soon as the inflammation has subsided, and as early sometimes as the fifth or seventh day, the dressings ought to be removed completely; and while the fingers of the surgeon, resting upon a compress, sustain the process, the elbow ought to be gently and slightly flexed and extended two or three times. From this time forward, until the union is consummated, this practice should be continued daily, only increasing the flexion each time, as the inflammation and pain may permit. If it is thought best, at length, to change the angle of the arm, and to flex it more and more, it may be done easily by substituting a very thick sheet of gutta percha for the board.

Dieffenbach has several times, in old fractures of both the olecranon and patella, where the fragments were dragged far apart, divided the tendons, so as to be able to bring the two portions together, and, by friction of them one upon the other, has endeavored to excite such action as might end in the formation of a shorter and a firmer bond of union. In some instances, it is said, considerable benefit was obtained, after all other means had failed; in others, the result was negative. One example of an old ununited fracture of the olecranon is mentioned, in which he divided the tendon of the triceps, secured the upper fragment in place, and every fourteen days rubbed it well against the lower one; in three months "the union was firm."[1]

The practice, not without its hazards, needs further observations to determine its value.

[1] Dieffenbach, American Journal of Medical Science, vol. xxix. p. 478; from Casper's Wochenschrift, Oct. 2d, 1841.

CHAPTER XXIII.

FRACTURES OF THE RADIUS AND ULNA.

Causes.—In a large majority of the examples of this fracture seen by me, which have been of such a character as to warrant an attempt to save the limb, the accident has been occasioned by a fall upon the palm of the hand while the arm was extended in front of the body. Yet this cause is not so constant as in fractures of the radius alone, since a considerable number have been occasioned by direct blows; and if we were to add to this estimate all of those bad compound fractures which have demanded immediate amputation, the proportion of fractures occasioned by direct and indirect blows might be found to be pretty nearly balanced.

Point of Fracture, Character, Direction of Displacement, &c.—In a record of fifty-three fractures of both bones, I have noticed but two examples in the upper third; while I have found that twenty-one happened in the middle third, twenty-eight in the lower third; and

Fig. 96.

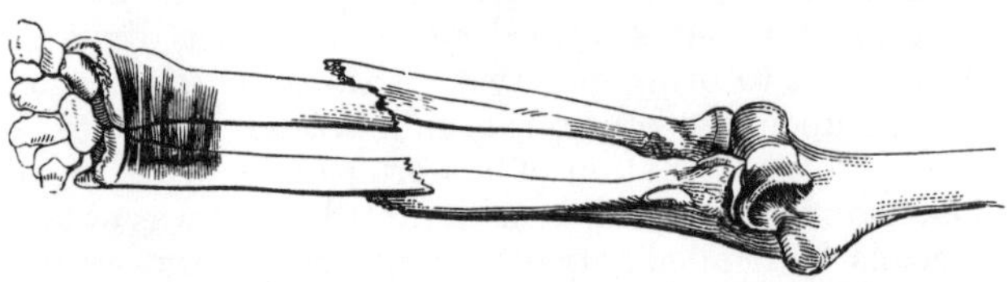

Fracture in the middle third.

Fig. 97.

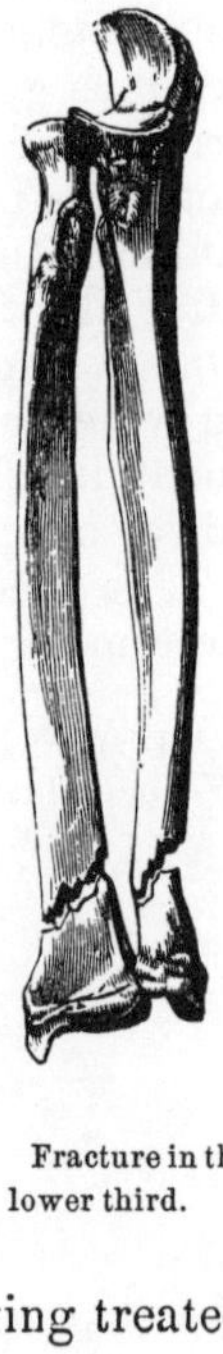

Fracture in the lower third.

in one case the radius was broken three-quarters of an inch above its lower end, and the ulna about one inch below the coronoid process. Three of the fractures belonging to the lower third were probably epiphyseal separations.

Forty-four were in males, and nine in females. Nineteen are known to have occurred in the right arm and thirteen in the left.

Forty-one were simple, seven compound, one was comminuted, three both compound and comminuted, one complicated with a fracture of the humerus, and one with a partial luxation of the lower end of the radius. With three exceptions, all of these more serious accidents were arranged among fractures of the lower third, and generally the bones had been broken near the wrist.

Partial fractures have been frequently observed, but having treated of these fractures fully in another chapter, I shall not think it necessary to make any further allusion to them in this place.

Prognosis.—Generally these bones unite in from twenty to thirty days; but I have seen the union occasionally delayed considerably beyond this time, and this delay has occurred especially in the case of the radius. Thus, in three cases of compound and comminuted fracture, the ulna united within four or five weeks, while the radius did not unite until the ninth or tenth week. Twice in simple fractures the ulna has united in the usual time, but the radius not until the sixteenth week. Once the ulna has united promptly and the radius remained ununited at the end of two years, at which time I practised resection of the broken ends of the radius, and union was speedily established.

On the other hand I have once seen the union delayed four months in the case of the ulna, when the radius had united in the usual time; and in one example of compound fracture both bones refused to unite until after the fifth month.

Fig. 98.

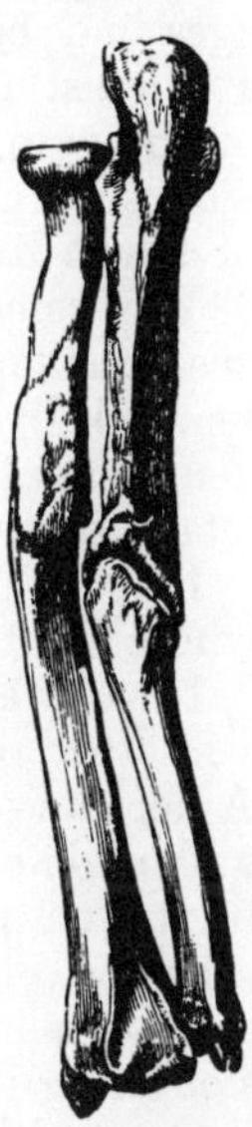

Union with slight lateral displacement.

Thirty-two of the whole number have united without any appreciable deformity, and twelve are known to have left some marked defect, while two have resulted finally in the loss of the arm.

I have seen the fragments deviate slightly in almost every direction, but most often it has been noticed that the deviation was to the radial or ulnar sides. Thus, in three examples, two of which had been compound fractures, the bones have united in such a position as that from the point of fracture downwards the forearm has been deflected to the ulnar side, and a marked projection has been left at the seat of fracture on the radial side; while in two examples, both of which were simple fractures, exactly the opposite condition has obtained, the lower part of the forearm being deflected to the radial side.

In a majority of cases the hand has been left with some tendency to pronation; in many instances this tendency was very slight and scarcely appreciable, but in others it has been quite marked, so that the patients have been wholly unable to supine the forearm except by a motion of the humerus in its socket.

From what has been said it must be seen that the prognosis in these accidents takes the widest range: for while a larger proportion than in the case of almost any other of the long bones, unite without any appreciable deformity, a considerable number delay to unite or do not unite at all, and some, even where the fracture is most simple, result in the complete loss of the limb. I am not now speaking of those more severe accidents in which the limb is at once condemned to amputation, and which, in the case of the arm, are numerous; but as I have already mentioned, our observations here apply only to cases which came under treatment with a view especially to the fracture.

I shall state the facts more fully, and then perhaps we shall think it proper to inquire why, when, as a rule, the treatment is found to be so simple and successful, occasionally, and pretty often indeed, it results so disastrously.

A boy, aged about ten years, fell from a tree, April 22, 1856, fracturing the right forearm near the lower end of the middle third. It was evident that he had fallen upon the palm of his hand, as the lower fragments were inclined backwards, and one of the bones had been thrust through the skin on the front of the arm.

It was at first dressed carefully by Dr. Wilcox, but the father of the lad on the following day placed him under the care of an empiric.

Six days after the fracture occurred, I was called to see him, with several other gentlemen. He was then suffering under a severe attack of tetanus which had commenced the night before. His arm was much swollen and very painful. He died the same evening.

I was unable to learn very particularly what had been the treatment since the patient was seen by Dr. Wilcox, except that the bandages had been most of the time very tight, and that the doctor had applied stimulating liniments, the boy constantly complaining greatly of the pain. I found the arm done up in a most slovenly manner with several narrow splints, underlaid with loose and knotty fragments of cotton batting.

We removed all of these immediately, and laid the arm upon a cushion supported by a board, to both of which the arm was lightly secured by a few turns of a bandage; cool water lotions were diligently applied and chloroform administered by inhalation; but the fatal event was delayed only a few hours.

I shall not stop to inquire the cause of a result so unfortunate, where the treatment has been so palpably unskilful.

I have already mentioned one case of gangrene of the hand, after a fracture of the lower part of the humerus; Norris, in a note to the American edition of *Liston's Surgery*, mentions a case which came under his observation in the Pennsylvania Hospital, the fracture having taken place just above the condyles, and still another has been related to me lately. I have brought together also no less than five cases of sloughing of the arm, after fracture of the radius, and one of sloughing from tight bandaging, where the radius was supposed to be broken, although the dissection proved that it was not.

Robert Smith says, that similar cases have been recorded in the *Gazette Médicale*. To these I shall now add two examples of sloughing after fracture of both radius and ulna; making a total of eleven cases in the upper extremities, in addition to those reported in the *Gazette Médicale*, an exact account of which I have not seen.

John McGrath, æt. 9, fell, July 2, 1847, from a ladder, about thirty feet to the ground, breaking the right radius and ulna in their middle thirds. A surgeon, residing in this city, was in attendance about four or five hours after the accident occurred. He then reduced the fractures and applied two broad splints, one on the palmar and one on the dorsal surface of the forearm. Whether a roller was first applied to the arm, or not, I am unable to say. The splints were secured in place by a roller and the arm laid in a sling.

The third day was our national holiday, and the patient was not visited. Nor was he seen on the fourth day, not being found at home. On the fifth day the surgeon removed the bandages and found the arm gangrenous; and within an hour afterwards I was requested to see it also.

I found him lying in a miserable apartment, with his right arm resting upon a pillow. The arm, forearm, and hand were gangrenous through their whole extent; and the skin of the right side, on the front of the chest, had assumed a dusky color, the extreme margin of which was indicated by an abrupt crescentic line. The thumb and fingers were black. His countenance was bright and cheerful, and his mind intelligent; pulse 75, and soft; tongue clean. He had slept undisturbed the night before, and he had all along felt perfectly well, except that he had a slight diarrhœa. I was assured by the surgeon and by all of the family, that the bandages had not been applied tightly; but we were told that on the third day of the accident, having been locked into the house by his mother, who was a pedler, he climbed out of the window, and that during all of that, and most of the following day he was running about the streets firing crackers, during most of which time his arm was removed from his sling and hanging by his side. On the morning of the fourth day, his mother noticed that his fingers were black, but she thought they were stained with powder.

We ordered him to take one-quarter of a grain of opium every four hours, and applied a yeast poultice to the arm. On the seventh day the gangrene was still extending, and the pulse was 124; yet he continued to feel well and to eat as usual. On the tenth day, the line of demarcation had commenced opposite the shoulder-joint; and the crescentic discoloration on the breast, which had at first spread rapidly until it covered nearly the whole upper half of the chest, was quite faint, in some parts almost lost.

In a few days more he was removed to the county almshouse, the separation continuing rapidly to take place until the arm fell off at the shoulder-joint; after which he made a good recovery.

A child two years and three months old, had fallen from a chair upon the floor, a distance of about two feet. A German physician being called, found, as he believes, a fracture of both bones of the left arm. The fracture was near the middle. He immediately applied a roller from the fingers to the elbow, and over this three narrow splints made of the wood of a cigar box. One of these was laid upon the palmar, one upon the dorsal, and one upon the radial side of the forearm, and the whole were bound together by another roller. From this time until the tenth day the child continued to play about on the floor. Ten days after the accident occurred the doctor noticed that the ulnar side of the little finger was blue. The bandages were immediately removed, and were never again applied tightly.

Three or four days after I was requested to see the arm with the attending physician. The gangrene had continued to extend, involving now the whole of the little finger and most of the thumb. There were also gangrenous spots over the hand and forearm, extending to within one inch from the elbow-joint; these spots were more numerous in front and on the back of the forearm, and seemed to correspond to the pressure of the splints. The hand was much swollen, and also the arm above the line of the gangrene. The sloughs had already commenced to be thrown off, and the gangrene was only extending in a few points. The child appeared well and rather playful, except when the arm was being dressed.

I ordered a yeast poultice, and a nourishing diet.

I have since learned that the arm and a large portion of the hand were finally saved.

South also says that he has seen one or two instances of mortification produced by splints applied too tightly, and previous to the accession of the swelling after fracture, and which have not been loosened as the swelling increased.[1]

How shall we explain the frequency of these accidents after fracture, especially of the forearm?

Malgaigne, speaking of fractures of both bones of the forearm, remarks that "when the displacement is considerable, or more especially when the outward violence has been excessive, we frequently see follow a very intense inflammatory swelling, and there is no fracture which complicates itself so easily with gangrene under the pressure of apparatus."[2]

Says Nélaton: "If we make choice of the apparatus of J. L. Petit, it is necessary that it shall not be applied too tightly, for, as Professor Roux has long since remarked, fractures of the forearm are those which furnish most of the examples of gangrene in consequence of an arrest of the circulation. This is easily understood, if we consider on the one hand the superficial position of the two principal arteries of the forearm, and on the other the disposition of the appareil, which must almost infallibly compress the arteries to a great extent."[3]

I do not think that this accident is due always to the negligence of the surgeon. It may be due many times to the carelessness of the parents or of the patient himself; as in the case of the boy who came under my own observation, and who lost his arm at the shoulder-joint. Sometimes also it may be due rather to the severity of the original injury, which, the experience of every surgeon will prove, is occasionally competent to the production of such bad results. A number of unfortunate circumstances may have concurred, such as a severe injury, especially where the skin has remained unbroken and the effused blood has had no opportunity to escape—the broken bone may have rested against the trunk of a main artery causing an arrest of its circulation—the constitution may be impaired by previous illness, or it may be suffering under the shock of the injury; yet that it may be and too often is the result of maltreatment, on the part of the surgeon, is undeniable. It is proper, however, to discriminate between

[1] South, note to Chelius's Surg., vol. i. p. 69.
[2] Malgaigne, Frac. et Disloc., tom. i. p. 589.
[3] Nélaton, Pathologie Chirurgicale, p. 735.

the responsibility which attaches to the surgeon as the true exponent of the state of his art, and that which attaches to the art itself as taught by the masters.

The old surgeons applied first a roller to the hand and forearm, and over this their various splints. J. L. Petit thought he had made a valuable improvement upon this simple plan in laying over the roller a compress, supported by a splint, designed to press between the bones, and to antagonize thus the action of the roller in drawing the fragments toward each other. Duverney believed that this object would be best accomplished by placing the pad against the skin, and under a circular compress; while Desault declares all of these modes inefficient, and announces a method which he regards as accomplishing at once and completely all of the indications; the sole peculiarity of which method consists in placing the graduated pads against the skin, and securing them in place by a roller. Boyer adopts the same method without any modifications, and Mr. Hind, in his illustrations of fractures already referred to, has seen fit to recommend the same, at least in fractures of the radius.

It is quite obvious that between these various methods there remains very little if anything to choose, the differences being too trifling and unessential to claim serious consideration. Each alike is inadequate to accomplish any amount of useful pressure between the fragments; each alike is calculated to bind the bones one against the other, and each alike exposes to the danger of ligation and of gangrene.

Says M. Dupuytren: "The practice of rolling the arm before the splints are applied, whether internal or external to the pads and compresses, is eminently mischievous; and instead of fulfilling, directly counteracts, the indications which it is most important to keep in view in the treatment of fractures of the forearm."

And notwithstanding the same sentiment has been reiterated by Velpeau, Malgaigne, Nélaton, Samuel Cooper, Bransby Cooper, Erichsen, Amesbury, Gibson and others, yet we find to-day the great surgeon of Heidelburgh, Chelius, recommending the roller to be applied under the splints, after the manner of Desault: while Liston, Syme, and Fergusson, who perhaps represent the Edinburgh school, use only pasteboard splints above the compresses, over which is immediately applied the roller; a practice which differs very little from that recommended by Desault, and is equally obnoxious to criticism.

Among the American surgeons, I believe, the advice and practice of Dupuytren have received almost universal assent, only that we have always employed splints much wider than those recommended by this distinguished surgeon. I cannot therefore agree with my accomplished countryman, Dr. Reynell Coates, if in the following paragraph he means to imply that American surgeons generally adopt Desault's treatment. Such at least is not my experience. "It would be wrong," says Dr. Coates, "not to bear testimony, on every possible occasion, against the folly so universally prevalent, that induces surgeons to apply a bandage directly to the forearm before applying splints in injuries of this character. We have often asked for a rational explanation of this practice, without effect. It is directly at war with the acknowledged indications in the coaptation of the fragments, and when the object of the whole apparatus is to thrust asunder their extremities, it commences by binding them together. Few plans in surgery are more generally followed; none can be more absurd."

Of the estimate placed upon the roller by M. Mayor, the reader will judge by a reference to the passage which I shall quote further on, when I shall speak of the value of the interosseous compresses.

Amesbury and Bransby Cooper use no rollers at all—not even to secure the splints in place, they being made fast to the forearm by straps or tapes; a practice which, I am happy to say, has found hitherto, except perhaps among the English, very few followers.

Mr. Amesbury and Mr. South also endeavor to give to their splints an appropriate shape, by having them constructed with more or less convexity. It must be noticed, however, that the practice of these two gentlemen is very dissimilar, for while Mr. South applies the convex surface of his splint to the interosseous space, Mr. Amesbury reverses this plan, and applies the concave surface directly to the skin.

As to the width of the splints, surgeons are also very generally agreed, at the present day, that they ought to be at least wider than the arm, so as to prevent the roller or the tapes from resting against its sides.

I do not intend to deny peremptorily, and without qualification, the value of the graduated compresses, which, as we have seen, are usually laid along the interosseous space to press the fragments asunder. It is necessary, however, to caution the surgeon against their injudicious use. M. Nélaton has well remarked of the apparel employed by J. L. Petit, that it must inevitably compress, to a great extent, the arteries of the forearm; and the remark is applicable, in only a less degree, to all of those other plans in which the compress is employed. And I suspect that to this portion of the dressing, quite as much as to any other cause, are due those frightful accidents of which we have already spoken. The arteries are not only exposed, from their superficial position, to pressure from a compress, but, in addition to this, it will be noticed that the two principal arteries, the radial and the ulnar, are situated upon a broad and flat surface of bone, along which this pressure must operate most advantageously. So early as the year 1833, M. Lenoir, in his inaugural thesis, at Paris, called attention to this danger, and from time to time surgeons have continued to advert to it, but they have seldom given to its consideration that prominence which its importance deserves.

I have observed another fact in this connection: when this compress is extended low down on the palmar surface, within an inch or two of the wrist-joint, it soon becomes excessively painful, and sometimes even wholly insupportable, in consequence of the pressure made upon the median nerve; and I find myself always obliged to exercise great care in the adaptation of the pads at this point. For this reason alone I believe, in case of a fracture near the base of the radius, the lower fragment, if it were thrown toward the ulna, could not be retained in its place by graduated compresses.

In short, finding that broad splints, properly covered and padded, answer very well to crowd the muscles into the interosseous space, so far as it is proper to do so, and believing that this mode is less painful and less dangerous, I seldom resort to graduated compresses, nor can I appreciate their necessity, or, indeed, their utility. Mr. Lonsdale also concurs with me in attaching very little value to this part of the accustomed apparel.

But listen to the surgeon of Lausanne, M. Mayor: " What signify graduated compresses placed between the bones of the forearm for the purpose of separating them from each other? These bones will not have that constant tendency to approach each other which has been supposed, provided, first, that they have been well reduced; second, that for the purpose of maintaining them in position we do not make use of a preliminary circular bandage, whose action is an absurdity; and in short, provided we make the retentive means act chiefly upon the palmar and dorsal surfaces of the forearm."[1]

M. Mayor proceeds to declare these convictions to be the result of his own experience, both in the treatment of simple and compound fractures of the forearm, and he intimates that in the use of the circular bandage with compresses, surgeons seem to have rolled the arm into a cylinder and drawn the bones together, in order that they might tax their ingenuity to discover some means to again separate them.

Surgeons have generally, after the splints have been applied, placed the forearm in a position of semi-pronation, or midway between supination and pronation, so that the radius should be uppermost; it being assumed that in this position the two bones are most nearly parallel, and least inclined to displacement. Such, indeed, was the practice of Hippocrates, Paulus Ægineta, Celsus, Albucasis, and of most surgeons down to this day; but Lonsdale, Robert Smith, Nélaton and South have lately called in question the correctness of this mode of dressing, at least when it is adopted as a universal rule.

I have before mentioned, when treating of fractures of the ulna, that M. Fleury had, in one instance, been unable to bring the fragments into apposition except by forced supination of the forearm; and in certain fractures we have seen the same position recommended by Lonsdale.

Says Mr. South, in a note to Chelius: "In fractures of both bones the forearm is best laid supine;" and Nélaton declares that in fractures of the radius and ulna at any point of their upper thirds it will be necessary to supine the arm, both in the reduction and during the subsequent treatment; but that in fractures of the inferior two-thirds we may place the limb in a condition of semi-pronation.

It seems very probable, however, that both of these gentlemen have received their suggestions from Mr. Lonsdale, who, as we have already seen, has treated the question very much at length, and who has finally declared his decided preference for the supine position in the treatment

[1] Bandages et Appareils à Pansements, ou Nouveau Système de Déligation Chirurgicale, par M. Mathias Mayor, Chirurg. en Chef de l'Hôpital de Lausanne, Switzerland. Paris ed. 1 38, p. 345.

of all fractures of the forearm. His arguments are certainly very ingenious, and as applied to fractures of the radius above the insertion of the pronator radii teres, they seem altogether conclusive; and, indeed, they commend themselves very strongly to our judgment, as applied to all fractures of the forearm. They are sustained also by the results of his own experience, and I see no good reason why they should not be more thoroughly examined and tested by other surgeons. The advantages which he claims for this method are more perfect coaptation of the broken ends, less liability of the fragments to encroach upon the interosseous space, and consequently less danger of anchylosis between the bones, and of non-union of the fragments, more complete restoration of the power of supination, and less tendency to lateral distortion, or of falling off to the ulnar or radial sides.

My own cases, treated by the usual method, have shown that while supination is frequently impaired, and sometimes entirely lost, pronation is rarely affected; and that lateral displacements are much more common than displacements forwards or backwards. How this position, semi-pronation, may tend to the production of a permanent pronation, I have fully explained when speaking of fractures of the head of the radius; and the influence of the same position, the forearm resting upon its ulnar margin in the sling, in the production of a lateral deviation is also easily understood. If the arm rests upon the sling so that its weight bears more upon the point of fracture than upon the extremities of the bones, then the ulna, or both ulna and radius, will incline gradually to the radial side, and the hand will fall off to the ulnar side; or if the sling rests under the wrist or hand chiefly, the hand will ascend to the radial side, and the broken ends of the two bones will project to the ulnar side.

If this plan is adopted, viz: laying the hand and forearm upon its back, instead of upon its ulnar margin, the elbow should remain at the side, the humerus falling perpendicularly from its socket; and the forearm should rest in the sling directed forwards from the body. Or, if it is found impossible or inconvenient, owing to the resistance of the pronator muscles, to supine the arm while it is suspended in a sling, it will be best to keep the patient in the recumbent posture with the arm extended upon a pillow.

Finally, whatever may be the mode of dressing, let me repeat the injunction to examine the arm frequently. No surgeon can do justice to himself, or to his patient, who does not look at the arm at least once in twenty-four hours during the first ten or fourteen days, and in some cases the patient ought to be seen twice daily.

When the fracture is compound, it is often quite impossible to retain the forearm in the half-proned position; since, when thus placed, and only slightly supported, as it must necessarily be, it inevitably falls over upon its palmar surface.

There can be no doubt that in such a case we ought from the first, if it is found practicable, to place it upon its back, in a position of complete, or nearly complete supination. For this purpose, a single broad splint, carefully cushioned and covered with oiled cloth, is the most suitable. Upon this the forearm is to be laid and secured gently with a few turns of the roller. If the patient is able to do so, and wishes to walk about, the board may be suspended to the neck, as recommended by M. Mayor.

I have said that we ought in case of a compound fracture to lay the forearm upon its back if practicable. I am sure, however, that the surgeon will find very many patients who cannot endure this position, and he may be compelled therefore to lay the limb upon its palmar surface, or to leave it to assume any other position in which it may be the most at ease.

CHAPTER XXIV.

FRACTURES OF THE CARPAL BONES.

THE few cases of fracture of the carpal bones which have come under my observation were, without exception, compound and complicated, and have resulted in the complete loss of the hand, or in some less serious, but never inconsiderable mutilation or maiming.

In no case has a treatment been adopted which might be regarded as having reference to the fracture, or the purpose of which was to insure apposition and union of the fragments.

It may be proper to assume, in a matter so easily comprehended, what actual and recorded experience has not proven, namely, that simple fractures of these bones will demand very little surgical interference, and that they will unite generally without much displacement, and without any considerable maiming. It is, indeed, quite probable that some degree of anchylosis between their adjacent surfaces will occur, yet even in the normal condition they enjoy so little motion as to render it doubtful whether its complete loss would be very sensibly felt.

In cases of comminuted, compound, and otherwise complicated fractures of the carpal bones, which accidents are sufficiently common, the surgeon has only, I conceive, to follow carefully those general or special indications which may happen to be present, the precise character of which it would be difficult to anticipate, and for the treatment of which it would be unsafe to attempt in a written treatise to provide.

CHAPTER XXV.

FRACTURES OF THE METACARPAL BONES.

Causes.—These bones, also, are generally broken by direct blows; and in that case the injury is often of such a character as to demand amputation, and does not therefore belong to that class of accidents of which it is the purpose of this volume to treat. Not an inconsiderable number, however, are the results of indirect blows, and especially of blows upon the knuckles received in pugilistic encounters. Thus, in a record of ten fractures, I find this cause assigned in three; in one other instance it was occasioned by falling upon the clenched fist, and in one by striking a board; so that the fracture has resulted from a blow upon the ends of the bones in five of the ten examples.

Dorsey, in his *Elements of Surgery*, mentions also that he has known the metacarpal bones to be fractured in pugilistic contests.

Point of Fracture; Direction of Displacement; Symptoms.—Once the fracture has occurred in the metacarpal bone of the thumb; four times in the metacarpal bone of the index finger; three times in the ring finger, and twice in the metacarpal bone of the little finger. Two of those belonging to the ring finger, and the two occurring in the little finger, were produced by blows with the clenched fist, and in each instance the fracture was in the lower or distal third of the bone. One of the fractures of the metacarpal bone of the index finger was produced also in the same way; but the fracture was near the middle of the bone. Of the whole number, six were broken through the lower third, two through the middle, and two through the upper third.

In every instance where the bone is known to have been broken by a blow upon the knuckles, the lower end of the lower fragment was thrown toward the palm, and the bone was salient backwards at the point of fracture.

In the following case the bone was probably separated at the epiphysis.

Thomas Rose, æt. 8, fell down a flight of steps, Sept. 11, 1855, breaking the metacarpal bone of the index finger of the right hand near its lower extremity, and apparently at the junction of the epiphysis with the diaphysis.

I saw the lad about sixteen hours after the accident. The lower fragment, projecting abruptly into the palm of the hand, could be easily replaced, or with only moderate effort, yet immediately when the support was removed it would become displaced. There was no crepitus.

It was dressed very carefully with a splint and compress; but notwithstanding our continued efforts to keep the fragments in place, the epiphysis united considerably depressed toward the palm.

In one instance, also, I think the bone was rather bent, or partially fractured, than broken completely. This was the case of fracture of the metacarpal bone of the ring finger, produced in a gymnasium by striking with the clenched fist against a board, and to which I have already alluded. I did not see the young man until four weeks after the accident, when I found the lower end of the bone depressed toward the palm and the angle made at the point of fracture was rather rounded and quite smooth; it was also tender at this point, but the bone was firm and unyielding. Four years after I was permitted to examine it again, and I found the same slight deformity still continuing.

A partial explanation of the fact that the joint end of the lower fragment is generally displaced toward the palm, may be found in the natural curve of these bones, which is such that when the fracture has been produced by a counter-stroke, the distal end would almost necessarily be driven in this direction; and a further explanation has been suggested by Mr. B. Cooper, namely, the action of the interossei.

Results.—Generally, when the fracture is simple, and the displacement is not considerable, the nature of the accident is overlooked, and some deformity must inevitably ensue. In a majority of the cases which have come under my observation this has been the fact, and the bone has remained slightly bent at the seat of fracture, but without affecting in any degree the value of the hand.

The following example has furnished the most serious result of any case of simple fracture of these bones which has come under my notice.

Louis Mooney, æt. 25, struck a man with his clenched fist, Nov. 4, 1856, breaking the metacarpal bone of the index finger of the right hand, near its middle. He was under the care of a surgeon residing in this city. Great swelling and suppuration followed the injury.

February 21, 1857, nearly four months after the injury was received, he consulted me. There existed at this time a complete anchylosis at the wrist-joint, and partial anchylosis in the fingers. The hand was deflected forcibly to the radial side. At the point of fracture the fragments were salient backwards and quite prominent, but firmly united.

Even when the existence of the fracture is recognized, it is not always easy to retain the fragments in place, as the case of epiphyseal separation already mentioned, and the following case, will illustrate.

Miss E., of Erie Co., N. Y., æt. 18, fell, Aug. 7, 1853, striking upon her right hand with her fingers forcibly bent into the palm of the hand. On the following day she consulted me at my office, and I found the metacarpal bone of the ring finger broken about three-quarters of an inch from its lower end, and the distal extremity of the fragment depressed toward the palm. A feeble crepitus, with distinct motion, completed the diagnosis. The young lady was very anxious to have a perfect hand, and I was determined if possible to accomplish it. Finding that the lower fragment was constantly disposed to fall toward the palm, I constructed a gutta-percha splint for the hand and fingers, and after placing a pad directly underneath this fragment, I secured it firmly with a roller. From this time until the end of four weeks she remained under my care, visiting me as often as once or twice a week; and at each dressing I found the lower fragment slightly displaced in the same direction as at first, nor was I able ever to make it resume completely its position.

Ordinarily, however, no such difficulty is experienced, and the bone, supported by such simple means as we shall presently direct, unites quickly and without deformity.

An engineer, residing in this city, was struck by a piece of iron in such a way as to break his right forearm and the second metacarpal bone of the same hand. The fracture of the metacarpal bone was compound and about three-quarters of an inch from its proximal extremity. When he called upon me, which was immediately after the injury was received, I found the proximal fragment projecting directly backwards, its sharp point rising above the skin; into which position it was evidently drawn by the action of the extensor carpi radialis longior muscle. By pressure alone it could be replaced, but it was much more easily reduced when the hand was forcibly carried backwards on the forearm. I therefore secured the hand in this position with appropriate splints, and it was maintained in this posture during most of the subsequent treatment. Union finally took place, but not without some backward displacement. Four months after the accident occurred, on the 31st of Dec. 1858, I examined the hand, and found the skin healed over completely, the end of the fragment having become rounded and smooth so as not to give him any degree of annoyance. His wrist was as flexible and as strong as before. No doubt the projection of the fragment might have been prevented entirely by cutting at the point of its attachment the tendon of the extensor muscle, but this would have sensibly weakened the wrist-joint, and I preferred the alternative of a projection of the fragment.

Treatment.—With moderate extension made upon the finger corresponding to the broken bone, while the fragments are forced home by firm pressure, the bone may generally be brought at once into line, and we may now proceed to adapt a gutta-percha, felt, or thick pasteboard splint, to either the whole surface of the back or palm of the hand and fingers, while they are held in a position of easy flexion. It is not very material to which of these surfaces the splint is applied; or rather, I may say, it ought to be applied to the one or the other according as circumstances seem to indicate. It should be well padded, and especially at certain points, in order to the more effectual support of the fragments. It is then to be secured in place with several turns of a roller. When either of the metacarpal bones, except those of the great or ring finger, is broken, the splint must be wide enough to secure the sides of the hand against the pressure of the roller.

Thus dressed, the hand may be laid in a sling beside the chest, or while sitting it may rest upon a table.

The apparel must be examined daily, and readjusted as often as it shall become disarranged, or as a doubt shall arise as to the condition of the parts.

When the fracture is followed by much inflammation, or occurs near, and especially if it actually involves a joint, the same precautions must be adopted to prevent anchylosis as in the case of similar fractures in other bones.

CHAPTER XXVI.

FRACTURES OF THE FINGERS.

Causes.—I do not remember to have seen a fracture of one of the phalanges produced by a counter-stroke; I am aware, however, that they are occasionally produced in this way, as by falling upon the ends of the fingers, and especially by the stroke of a ball in the game of base.

The fact, however, that they are generally the consequence of a direct blow, and that the finger bones are small and only protected by a thin covering of skin and tendons, renders them peculiarly liable to comminution and to other serious complications. Thus, in a record of thirty fractures, only eighteen were sufficiently simple to warrant an attempt to save them; and only five are recorded as simple fractures without complications.

The majority of those fingers which were saved were broken through the first phalanx.

Twice the fracture has seemed to be a mere separation of the epiphysis. The first was in the person of a boy twelve years old, the separation having taken place, in consequence of a crushing injury, at the distal end of the first phalanx of the second or large finger. A peculiar crepitus, with motion, was easily detected, but there was no displacement. A splint was applied and union occurred in a few days, and without any deformity.

The second was in a lad four years old, who was admitted to the Hospital of the Sisters of Charity, Dec. 24, 1849, with a simple fracture of the first phalanx of the ring finger of the left hand; the fracture being at the proximal end of the bone, and at the junction of the epiphysis with the shaft.

The finger was so much swollen at first, that no dressings were applied until the fifth day, at which time a gutta-percha splint was moulded to it carefully. It resulted in a perfect cure.

I have never seen the fragments much overlapped, except in one instance. Frequently there has been no perceptible displacement whatever; but generally there will be found a slight displacement in the direction of the diameter of the bone.

The case to which I refer as presenting an extraordinary overlapping, was that of an Irish laboring woman, aged about thirty-five years, who, having fallen down a flight of steps, broke the first phalanx of the thumb, below its middle. Dr. Congar, of this city, was first called on the day following the accident, but was unable to reduce the fracture, and on the same day invited me to see the patient with him. The distal fragment was displaced backwards, overlapping the proximal fragment a little more than one-quarter of an inch. We made repeated efforts, by pulling upon the thumb with a sliding noose, and with all the strength of our four hands, but to no purpose. The fragments could not be reduced for one moment; and we left the patient as we had found her, only somewhat the worse for our violent and repeated extensions and manipulations. The finger was already considerably swollen when we began our efforts, and we cannot therefore say what might have been accomplished at an earlier moment, but I confess that our defeat was unexpected, and does not seem to me to be satisfactorily explained.

Results.—At least ten have left no appreciable lameness or deformity, and possibly several more. It is therefore probably true that these consequences may be avoided with proper care in one-half of the examples in which we attempt to save the finger; and perhaps it will occasion surprise that a perfect result may not be claimed in a larger proportion; but when we consider how frequently the accident is compound, and that even when it is not, the blow having generally been received directly upon the point of fracture, how promptly swelling ensues, it will be easily understood that it will be often found difficult to determine whether the bone is exactly in line or not, or to maintain it in this position after absolute coaptation has been once secured.

I have seen the finger in two or three cases deviate laterally, or become permanently deflected to one side or the other; and once I have found it united, but rotated on its own axis. This latter case is not without instruction.

A girl, æt. 6, had her little finger caught by a door violently shut, breaking one of the phalanges, and nearly severing the finger. I closed the wound and dressed the finger with a moulded pasteboard splint. My dressings were repeated often, and applied carefully; nor did I detect the rotation which the lower fragment had made upon its own axis until the union was consummated. I then found the extremity of the finger turned so that its palmar surface presented diagonally toward the ring finger.

If the surgeon believes that this ought to have been prevented, and that the result evinces a lack of skill or of care, its record may still serve one of the purposes for which it was designed, and secure to the patient sometimes hereafter more faithful and assiduous attention.

Treatment.—Boyer, and after him Bransby Cooper, have taught that when the extreme phalanx is broken, from the small size of the bone, and from its having attached to it the nail and its matrix, it is better, in all cases, to amputate at once, as the process of reparation is in such case extremely slow and uncertain.

Whether in any of the cases treated by myself, or which have been seen by me, the fracture involved the last phalanx, I am not now able to say, but my impression is that such cases have come under my notice which have been successfully treated, and I cannot but regard the rule established by these gentlemen as much too stringent. Examples must, no doubt, sometimes occur, in which the fracture is so simple in its character as to render prompt reunion pretty certain; and even though the restoration should prove tedious, this ought scarcely to be regarded as a sufficient justification for so serious a mutilation as these surgeons propose, since the loss of even an extreme phalanx is not only a deformity, but must prove in many occupations a troublesome maiming.

The rule ought still to be held inviolate, which surgeons have so often repeated in reference to injuries inflicted upon the hand and fingers, namely, that we should save always as much as possible.

It is remarkable, too, how much nature, assisted by art, can do toward the accomplishment of this purpose. If the bone of a finger is not only severed completely, but also all of its soft coverings, save only a narrow band of integument, are torn asunder, a chance remains for its restoration. And it is especially interesting to observe what recuperative powers are possessed by the articular surfaces of these smaller joints, so that although they may be broken into, or sawn through, or comminuted, and although small fragments be entirely removed, a complete restoration of their functions is sometimes permitted. I have seen and reported some such examples. It is true, however, that such fortunate results are rare, and they are rather to be hoped for than anticipated.

Since, in the case of these delicate bones, the slightest deviation from the natural form or position determines in the end an ugly deformity, it becomes exceedingly necessary, especially with females, that we should open and examine the fingers carefully from day to day, so that, as the swelling subsides, we may discover and correct any displacement which may happen to exist.

As a splint, I have found nothing so convenient as gutta percha, or felt, moulded accurately to either the dorsal or palmar aspect of the finger; and the form of which I have found it generally necessary to change slightly every third or fourth day, until consolidation is nearly, or quite completed.

If the fracture is near, or extends into a joint, the finger ought to be a little flexed so as to place it in the most useful position in the event that anchylosis should occur; and as early as the end of the second week the joint surfaces should be slightly moved upon each other in order to the prevention of fibrous or bony adhesions. Nor is there much danger of preventing the union of the bone by moving the joints at this early day. Union occurs between these fragments very speedily, and I have never met with a case of non-union of the phalanges, nor do I remember to have seen a case reported.

It is the lateral inclination of the distal end of the finger which, according to my experience, it will be found most difficult to obviate, and which may, perhaps, in some cases be most successfully combated by laying the two adjoining sound fingers against the broken finger, and then applying a moulded splint to the palmar surface of the whole. In other cases it will be more convenient to apply the splint only to the broken finger.

Rotation of the lower fragment on its own axis is especially to be guarded against, as the deformity which it occasions is more unseemly, and the impairment of utility more decided, than that occasioned by a lateral deviation.

It may be well also to remind the surgeon of the convenience of extending the splint beyond the end of the last phalanx, and moulding it to this extremity, in order that the finger may be protected against injuries, and that when, from time to time, the splint is removed, it may be reapplied with accuracy.

In all cases the splint should be lined with two or three folds of cotton cloth, or soft flannel, or patent lint, and secured in place with narrow and neatly cut cotton rollers. Bandages of this width should never be torn, but carefully cut with scissors.

CHAPTER XXVII.

FRACTURES OF THE PELVIS, AND TRAUMATIC SEPARATIONS OF ITS SYMPHYSES.

§ 1. PUBES.

LENTE, in his reports from the New York Hospital, mentions the case of a young man, æt. 18, who was crushed between a couple of cars, in consequence of which he died two days after. The autopsy disclosed a separation at the symphysis pubis, unaccompanied with any other fracture. The right side was displaced backwards about half an inch, so that the fingers could be passed between the bones. There was also a wound in the top of the bladder large enough to admit the thumb.[1] Similar accidents have been several times met with by surgeons. Hall reports a case in the *Provincial Medical and Surgical Journal*, May 1, 1844, in which the pubes thus separated, was actually thrust into the bladder; but in this example the ilium was broken also. I need scarcely add that this patient died;[2] but Sir Astley Cooper has furnished us with an example of a simple fracture or traumatic separation at the symphysis, from which the patient after a long time almost completely recovered. The following is Sir Astley's account of the case:—

[1] Lente, New York Journ. Med., 2d ser., vol. iv. p. 286.
[2] Hall, Amer. Journ. Med. Sci., vol. xxxiv. p. 248.

"Case 79. Richard White, æt. 22, was admitted into Guy's Hospital on the 30th of July, 1832, having sustained a severe injury in consequence of a large quantity of gravel having fallen upon his back while in the act of stooping. It knocked him down; and on rising, which he did with considerable difficulty, he attempted to walk; this produced violent pain in the region of the bladder, extending upwards in the course of the ureters to the kidneys. Upon inquiry, he stated that the urine he had voided since the accident was bloody and passed with difficulty.

"On examination, a fissure was found at the symphysis pubis, producing a separation of about two fingers' breadth. On pressure being made upon any part of the ilium, he complained of increased pain in the region of the pubes, and of numbness down the left thigh.

"A catheter was immediately passed, and the urine which was drawn off was clear and healthy. Leeches were applied over the pubes, and a broad belt was firmly buckled around the pelvis, sufficiently tight to bring the separated pubes nearly in contact, and the patient ordered to be kept perfectly quiet in the recumbent posture, on low diet. The leech-bites ulcerated, and some slight degree of fever resulted, which, however, readily yielded to the usual treatment.

"He remained in the hospital for three months without any check to the progress of his cure; the length of time it required being accounted for by the difficulty of reparation in an amphiarthrodial articulation; and when he left there was some slight separation of the pubes remaining; nor were the two lower extremities, or the anterior and superior spinous processes of the ilia, perfectly symmetrical, although he could walk very well."[1]

Malgaigne has collected four cases of simple separations at the symphysis pubis occasioned by external violence, and in three of the four cases, it was occasioned by pressing out the thighs with great force; the separation being directly due, therefore, to muscular action.

Two of these patients succumbed to the accidents. The same author has brought together, also, seventeen cases of separations of this symphysis occurring in childbirth, of which only seven survived.

It is much more common, however, to find the pubes broken through its horizontal or ascending ramus; and Clark, of the Massachusetts General Hospital, has described a case of simultaneous fracture of the pubes and ischium in three places. The man, æt. 29, had been caught between two heavy timbers, and on the following day, May 7, 1852, he was brought to the hospital.

No crepitus could be detected, but he was unable to lie upon the right side, and the right limb was nearly paralyzed. It was evident that the bladder or urethra had been ruptured, and on the third day Dr. Clark opened the bladder through the perineum, evacuating a large amount of blood and urine, and affording to the patient very sensible relief. on the first of June, however, he died, having survived the accident twenty five days.

[1] Sir Astley Cooper, Frac. and Disloc., Amer. ed., p. 144.

The autopsy disclosed several fractures, all of which belonged to the right os innominatum. First, a fracture of the pubes, near the symphysis; second, a fracture near the junction of the pubes and ilium; third, a fracture through the ramus of the ischium anterior to the tuberosity.[1]

Fig. 99.

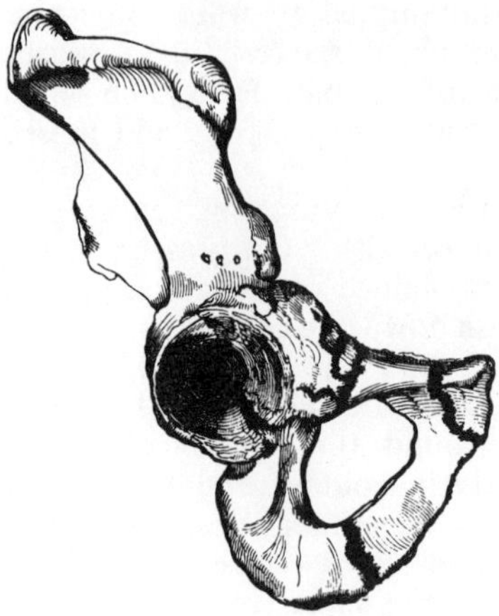

Clark's case of fracture of the pelvis.

Sir Astley mentions a case (Case 83) of fracture of the "ramus of the pubes," unaccompanied with injury to the bladder or urethra, which resulted in a complete recovery; and in another case (Case 84) the patient recovered in eight weeks, and was able to walk nearly as well as before: but he soon after died of disease of the chest. The os pubis was found, at the autopsy, to have been broken in three places; there was also a fracture extending in two directions through the acetabulum, with an extensive comminuted fracture of the ilium accompanied with great displacement.

Maret has even found it necessary after a fracture to remove nearly the whole of the body of the pubes by incision, in a girl of 18 years, and who not only recovered completely, but having subsequently married, she gave birth to two children in easy and natural labors.[2]

Cappelletti relates that a man, æt. 54, jumped from a carriage, the horses having run away, and alighted with his feet to the ground, but with one limb in the greatest possible degree of abduction. A surgeon, who saw him immediately, found an enormous swelling at the superior part of the thigh, accompanied with very acute pain. When seen by Cappelletti, at Trieste, six months after, there still remained a slight swelling near the ramus of the ischium and pubes, under which a careful examination detected a fragment of bone two and a half inches long and of the "size of the finger." The patient was able to walk, but not without pain and limping. Cappelletti soon began to suspect that this fragment of bone consisted of a part of the ramus of the ischium and pubes detached by muscular contraction. On examining it anteriorly he found this part of the pelvis defective, and the loose portion of bone had all of the anatomical characters of the defective part. He felt distinctly the circular projection indicating the point where the ascending branch of the ischium unites with the descending branch of the pubes.[3]

Whitaker, of Lewiston, N.Y., saw the body of the left os pubis broken in a female while in the seventh month of pregnancy. She

[1] Clark, Boston Med. and Surg. Journ., vol. liii. p. 185.

[2] Maret, from Malgaigne, op. cit., p. 646.

[3] Cappelletti, Ranking's Abstract, No. viii. p. 83; from Giornale per servire al Progressi della Patologie della Teraputica, 1847.

had fallen down a pair of stairs, striking astride the edge of an open, upright barrel. The fracture was oblique, and with but little displacement, yet she complained of excruciating pain in the left pubic region on the least motion. The accident was followed by no positive attempt at miscarriage.[1]

The danger in these accidents consists not so much in the fracture, as in the injury done to the bladder, and other pelvic viscera. If the bladder is opened into the peritoneal cavity, death is almost inevitable, and even when the bladder or urethra has suffered laceration lower down or at any point above the deep perineal fascia, extensive urinary infiltrations, followed by abscesses and gangrene, generally expose these patients to the most imminent hazards.

The practice pursued at Guy's Hospital in the case of separation at the symphysis pubis, commends itself both by its simplicity and by its success. Antiphlogistic remedies steadily pursued, rest in the recumbent posture, the use of the catheter when necessary, and in certain cases the girding the pelvis with a firm belt or band, are measures which seem to meet all of the important indications.

If the fracture is accompanied with displacement, it will be proper to attempt to restore the fragments, but except in the case of separation at the symphysis very little aid can be expected from a band or any similar means, in retaining them in place. It will be sufficient, generally, in such examples to place the patient quietly upon his back, with his thighs flexed upon his body, and to treat the accident in all other respects as a case of inflammation.

If the urine has become extravasated underneath the pelvic fascia, no time ought to be lost in opening freely through the perineum, and in extending the incisions, if necessary, into the urethra and bladder.

§ 2. Ischium.

When speaking of fractures of the pubes we have already noticed some examples of fractures of the ischium also; indeed, it is seldom that one of the bones of the innominata is broken without a coincident fracture of one or both of the others. The records of surgery furnish several other examples, produced generally by a fall upon the tuberosities; but perhaps the most remarkable instance is that mentioned by Maret as having occurred in a female during labor.

The following summary of a case of fracture of the ischium, reported by Sir Astley Cooper, will serve to illustrate one of the most fortunate terminations of these accidents when accompanied with a rupture of the urethra:—

A young man who was driving a cart, was thrown down and a wheel passed over him. On the following morning he was found to have a fracture of the left leg and a contusion of the inner side of the left thigh. There was also great swelling and ecchymosis of the scrotum, with a slight appearance of injury over the pubes and left

[1] Whittaker, Amer. Journ. Med. Sci., July, 1857, p. 283.

hypochondrium. No fracture of the pelvis was at that time discovered. The patient was suffering great pain, and was cold and exhausted. Bloody urine escaped from the bladder. On the eighth day an abscess had pointed on the left side of the perineum, which, being opened, discharged a great quantity of pus having the odor of urine; extensive sloughing occurred, and the patient sank very low. On introducing the finger into the wound, the ascending ramus of the ischium could be distinctly felt, and the fracture traced in an oblique course, the upper fragment being slightly displaced forwards. When the catheter was introduced into the urethra it was found to enter this wound, and could be felt resting against the naked bone. From this time until the twenty-sixth day, the urine continued to escape freely through the wound. In about six weeks more the fistulous opening had entirely closed, and after several months his recovery was complete.[1]

The signs of this accident are generally even more obscure than those of fracture of the pubes, but in a case of doubt the bones ought not only to be carefully examined from without, but the finger should be introduced freely into the rectum and the anterior surface explored; or the tuber ischii may be grasped between the thumb and finger and moved laterally in order to determine the existence of motion or crepitus. If the patient is a female, this exploration can be best made through the vagina. By flexing and extending the thigh, also, crepitus may sometimes be discovered. The examination will generally be made while the patient lies upon his back, but if turning is not found too painful, it will be well to lay him upon his face that the tuberosities of the ischium may be more plainly brought into view.

A considerable proportion of the fractures of both the pubes and the ischium are accompanied with lesions of the bladder or of the urethra, either of which circumstances will render the prognosis very unfavorable; but in simple fractures recoveries may generally be expected, yet only after a tedious confinement.

It is not usual except in cases which must almost necessarily prove fatal, to find much displacement of the fragments; nor is it probable that by any manœuvres the slight displacements which are found to exist can be entirely overcome. Instances may occur, however, in which careful pressure from without, or the introduction of a finger into the rectum or vagina may aid in the restoration.

The posture best suited to these cases will be indicated usually by the sensations of the patient himself. Ordinarily he will prefer to lie upon his back with his thighs flexed and supported by pillows; and his hips slightly elevated by a firm cushion laid under the upper part of the sacrum. His knees ought also to be gently bound together; but if the patient finds this position painful or excessively irksome, as sometimes he will, he may be permitted to occupy any position which he finds most comfortable.

[1] A. Cooper, by Bransby Cooper, Amer. ed., p. 140.

§ 3. Ilium.

Fractures of the ilium are much more common than fractures of either the ischium or pubes, and they assume a great variety of forms, directions, and degrees of complications.

In the two following examples the anterior superior spinous process alone was broken off:—

John Kelly, æt. 36, admitted to the Hospital of the Sisters of Charity Dec. 28, 1852, having just fallen and broken the anterior superior spinous process of the ilium. The fragment was displaced downwards about one-quarter of an inch. Motion and crepitus distinct. Slight ecchymosis over the point of fracture, and other signs of contusion about the hip. He was intoxicated at the time of the accident, and could not tell how or where he fell.

He was laid upon his back in bed, with his thighs flexed upon his body; and in this position we attempted to reduce the fragment and retain it in place with a bandage, but finding this impossible, we left him with only instructions to remain quietly in bed. In about two weeks the fragment was firmly fixed in its new position, and he was allowed to get up and walk about, which he was able to do without inconvenience.

July 13, 1853, Matthias Morrison was caught under a bank of falling earth, and on the following day Dr. Mixer, his attending surgeon, requested me to see the case with him. He was unable to stand upon his feet. There was a lacerated wound and an extensive bruise on his left hip; but the thigh was not shortened nor everted, and he could flex it slightly upon his body. Noticing a swelling and discoloration in the region of the anterior superior spinous process of the ilium, I pressed upon it and felt it recede with a distinct crepitus; the fragment, however, immediately resumed its place when the pressure was removed. I was able also, by a careful manipulation, to trace the line of fracture, and to determine that it included a small portion of the anterior extremity and wing of the pelvis.

We directed the patient to remain quietly upon his bed with his legs drawn up. He soon recovered, but I am unable to say what is the present position of the fragment.

More frequently, however, the fracture involves a still larger portion of the crest, as in the following examples:—

Joseph Joquoy, æt. 40, was caught by the bumpers between two cars, Feb. 10, 1854, breaking obliquely the anterior superior portion of the ilium. I saw him within an hour, and found him greatly prostrated; the fragment of the pelvis broken off was quite movable, and crepitus was easily detected. His abdomen was very tender and slightly bloated.

He was laid upon his back with his legs drawn up, and hot fomentations of hops and vinegar were directed to be applied to his belly. He took also one grain of morphine. The broken ala did not seem disposed to become displaced. With no other treatment, his recovery was rapid; and the bones seemed to have united without displacement.

James Roche, æt. 41, fell, March 7, 1854, from a height of fourteen feet, breaking off the anterior superior portion of the right ala of the pelvis. On the following day, I found him at the Hospital of the Sisters of Charity. The fragment, which was quite large, was movable, and occasionally a crepitus could be detected. It was displaced downwards and forwards about three-quarters of an inch.

He was laid upon his back, with his thighs and legs moderately flexed. At the end of two weeks he found himself able to walk without much difficulty, and he immediately left the hospital. At this time the fragment was displaced in the same manner and direction as at first, but I cannot say whether it had united or not.

I have once seen a fracture of the posterior superior spinous process, and I do not know of any other example.

Miss B., æt. 16, was thrown from her horse backwards, striking with her back upon the ground. She was at first attended by Dr. Coan, of Ovid, N. Y.; and she did not come under my care until two weeks after the accident.

I found a small fragment broken from the posterior superior spinous process of the ilium, and displaced backwards in the direction of the spine about half an inch. It was movable, and by pressure it could be partially restored to place, but it would immediately return to its abnormal position when the pressure was removed. The injured hip was painful, and occasionally it felt numb. She had previously sufferred from spinal irritation.

I laid a compress behind the fragment, and secured it in place with a roller, enjoining perfect rest. She recovered from her lameness in a few weeks, but I believe the fragment remains displaced.

Extensive comminuted fractures of the ilium are generally accompanied with so much injury of the pelvic viscera as to prove rapidly fatal; but the following example will show that this rule admits of exceptions.

June 5, 1854, Bernard Duffie, æt. 32, was crushed under a very heavy stone which fell upon his back. I found the left ala of the pelvis broken into several fragments, between the different portions of which motion and crepitus were distinct. The fractures were near the superior part of the bone, commencing about two inches back of the anterior superior spinous process, and extending backwards irregularly. There was a narrow wound communicating with the fracture, from which I removed a loose fragment of bone. The right leg was also broken.

Four months after, he was still confined to his bed, and a fistulous opening continued opposite the point of fracture; there existed also a large and irregular mass of ossific matter or callus around the fragments. He soon after left the hospital.

Dr. Sargent, of the Massachusetts General Hospital, has reported a case in which a man received a compound fracture of the left ilium, and several small fragments were removed. He was discharged at the end of three months with a fistulous opening still remaining, but in other respects he was quite well.[1]

The two following cases illustrate the more fatal injuries of this character.

A man was injured by a steam boiler explosion in this city on the 11th of February, 1857, and died in about two hours. I found the anterior half of the crest of the ilium broken off, and the fragments driven into the belly. There was no other serious injury which I could discover.

John O'Keaf was crushed under a heavy stone Oct. 23, 1851, breaking and comminuting the alæ of the pelvis on both sides, and wounding also the iliac vein. He was taken to the Hospital of the Sisters of Charity, and died in a few hours, partly from the shock to his system and partly from the hemorrhage.

Lente, of the New York Hospital, has reported a case of dislocation of the hip, which was accompanied with a fracture also of the ala of the pelvis upon the same side. The dislocation was reduced on the third day, and the patient soon after died. The autopsy disclosed what had not been suspected during life, namely, that the left ilium was broken horizontally about through its middle, and vertically through the crest; and also that there was a fracture extending through the sacro-iliac synchondrosis, accompanied with considerable comminution of the articular surfaces. It was also found that a portion of the small intestine was ruptured, and probably by one of the sharp fragments of the broken pelvis.[2]

It is seldom, I think, that the fragments become much displaced; such, at least, has been my experience; and I have noticed in Dr. Neill's cabinet three specimens of fracture of the crest of the ilium, all of which had united without any appreciable displacement. Dr. Neill also called my attention to the fact that in two of these specimens the ensheathing callus was confined to the outer surface of the bone, an observation which this gentleman assures me he has had frequent occasion to make before where the fracture belonged to a flat bone.

The same cabinet contains a specimen of gunshot fracture of the ilium, the ala being perforated by a smooth, round hole, about one inch below the crest.

If any displacement exists, the upper or loose fragment is generally carried slightly inwards; occasionally, however, it is found displaced upwards, outwards, or downwards.

Treatment.—In a large majority of cases the fragments, if displaced, cannot be replaced. Occasionally, however, as where the anterior superior spinous process is broken off with only a small portion of the crest, the fragment may be seized with the fingers and carried outwards or upwards, or in whatever direction may be necessary; but to retain it in this position is generally quite impossible. The bandage or broad belt which we have recommended in certain fractures of the pubes would be in these cases not only useless, but absolutely mis-

[1] Sargent, Boston Med. and Surg. Journ., vol. liii. p. 121.
[2] Lente, New York Journ. of Med., Jan. 1851, p. 29.

chievous, since its effect must be to press inwards the fragments, and thus to create a displacement which might not otherwise exist.

The surgeon ought to determine by a careful examination the extent and direction of the fracture, and, having done what was in his power to replace the fragments, he should lay his patient upon his back with the thighs drawn up and supported. This is the position which will generally be found most comfortable; but, as in other fractures of the pelvis, it may be well always to try the effect of other positions, and especially to determine their influence upon the fragments, and finally to adopt that precise posture which accomplishes the indications best.

If the fracture is compound, and the fragments have penetrated the belly, the wound should be enlarged, and, as far as possible, every piece of bone should be removed; but if the fragments cannot be found, the external opening should be allowed to remain so as to favor their escape when suppuration shall have taken place.

§ 4. Acetabulum.

Although, strictly speaking, fractures of the acetabulum belong always to one or all of those bones of the pelvis whose lesions have already been described, yet the peculiar relations of this cavity to the femur render it necessary that they should be considered as a separate class of accidents.

Fractures of the acetabulum divide themselves naturally into two varieties.

First, Fractures of the base of the cavity, with or without displacement.

Second, Fractures of the rim, with or without displacement.

In fractures of the base of the cavity, not accompanied with displacement, nothing but crepitus can be present as a sign of the accident; and this will scarcely be sufficient, in itself, to enable the surgeon to distinguish it from a fracture of the neck of the femur within the capsule without displacement.

It is probable, therefore, that its existence will only be determined by dissection. Nor is it of much importance that the diagnosis should be made out; since in either case neither splints nor any other surgical appliances could be of service. An injury so severe as to fracture the acetabulum will necessarily so much bruise the body, and concuss the viscera of the pelvis as to compel the patient to remain quiet for a number of days, and this is all that would be thought necessary if the nature of the accident was exactly determined.

Dr. Neill's cabinet contains a specimen of this kind, in which the fracture, commencing near the centre, extends in three directions across the cotyloid margins; and in which perfect bony union has occurred without displacement.

M. Bouvier related to the Academy the case of a man, æt. 71, who, in consequence of a fall from his bed, remained for three weeks unable to walk, and never was able afterwards to walk without crutches. No fracture could be discovered during life, but after his death, which occurred some months subsequent to the accident, a fracture was found extending from the ilio-pectineal eminence to the spine of the ischium, and traversing the centre of the acetabulum. The fragments were not displaced, but remained slightly movable.[1]

The following case was reported by Mr. Earle to the London Medico-Chirurgical Society, and will be found in the nineteenth volume of its *Transactions*. It is also referred to by Sir Astley, in his *Treatise on Fractures and Dislocations*.

In the month of October, 1829, a man, æt. 40, was admitted into St. Bartholomew's Hospital, with a severe injury caused by having fallen from a height of thirty-one feet and striking upon the left side. The left leg was powerless, and shortened. The foot was everted. Any attempt to rotate the limb caused great pain, and was accompanied with a sensible crepitus. The left trochanter was very much depressed, and when it was pressed upon the patient complained of deep-seated pain in the hip-joint.

He recovered in eight weeks, and was able to walk nearly as well as before; but he soon after died of disease in the chest.

On dissection, a fracture was found extending in two directions through the acetabulum; there was an extensive comminuted fracture of the ilium, with great displacement, and the os pubis was broken in three places.

The repair was very complete, and Mr. Earle remarked how nature had guarded against any considerable deposit of new bone within the articulation, which might have interfered with the functions of the joint, while there was an abundant deposit of callus around the other parts of the fractured bone.

Fractures of the base of the acetabulum, with displacement of the femur into the pelvic cavity, constitute a much more formidable, and unfortunately a more common form of accident.

Like the preceding variety of acetabular fractures, they are produced generally by falls upon the trochanter major, but the force of the concussion has been greater.

Even here, it is not often that the diagnosis has been clearly made out during life; and indeed, generally, the true character of the accident has not even been suspected, the surgeons believing that they had to do with a fracture of the neck of the femur, or with a dislocation. In two examples (Cases 71 and 72) mentioned by Sir Astley Cooper as having been presented at St. Thomas's Hospital, the thigh was thought to be dislocated backwards.

In the following example, reported by Lendrick, of Dublin, the patient was supposed to have a fracture of the neck of the femur:—

An old man, well known as the "Wandering Piper," was admitted into the Mercer Hospital in January, 1839, suffering under phthisis pulmonalis and acute inflammation of the hip-joint. Some years before, he had received a severe injury by the upsetting of a coach, and was under treatment several months for what was supposed to be

[1] Bouvier, Amer. Journ. Med. Sci., vol. xxiii. p. 486; from Bullét. de l'Acad. Roy. de Méd., August 15, 1838.

a fracture of the neck of the femur. Since that time he had been lame, but still able to take a great deal of exercise on foot both in Great Britain and in America. The acute disease of the joint commenced about two months before his admission, and he was at first under the care of Sir Philip Crampton, who remarked that the thigh was only shortened about half an inch, and expressed his surprise at this fact.

This man died on the 17th of February, and the dissection showed that there had been no fracture of the femur, but its head and neck were affected with "morbus coxæ senilis." The head was also thrust through a rent in the acetabulum into the cavity of the pelvis; but the head had again been covered by a bony case, complete, except in a small portion about the size of a shilling piece, and at this point the covering was ligamentous.

The os pubis had also been broken at the same time, and it had united so much overlapped that the space between the inferior anterior spinous process and the symphysis pubis was shortened nearly an inch. A portion of intestine was found protruding through an opening in the pelvis and adherent to the bone, in which situation it seemed to have been caught by the broken fragments and retained.[1]

Morel-Lavallée, in his thesis upon complicated luxations, mentions a case which had come under his observation, and which had been treated as a fracture of the neck of the femur. The patient survived the accident many years; during a part of which time he suffered such pain in the hip-joint as to induce a belief that it was itself diseased. At his death he was found to have had a multiple fracture of the bones of the pelvis, and the head of the femur had penetrated more than an inch into the cavity of the pelvis, pressing upon the obturator nerve to such a degree as to have, no doubt, caused the severe pain from which he had suffered, and which had been ascribed to coxalgia.[2]

In the two cases mentioned by Sir Astley, as having been received into St. Thomas's Hospital, the toes were turned in. In the example mentioned by the same author as having been presented at St. Bartholomew's Hospital, the toes were everted; the two persons seen by Lendrick and Morel-Lavallée were supposed before death to have had a fracture of the neck; it is probable, therefore, that in both of these cases the toes were also everted. While Moore has dissected a subject whose pelvis was broken into many fragments—the left os innominatum was divided into three portions, corresponding to the three bones of which it was composed in infancy; the head of the femur had completely penetrated the basin—the limb was shortened two inches, and in a position of slight flexion and adduction, but neither rotated outwards nor inwards.[3]

There seems, therefore, to be no certain rule in relation to the position of the limb; but it is found to take the one position or the other, probably according to the direction of the force which has inflicted the

[1] Lendrick, Amer. Journ. Med. Sci., vol. xxiv. p. 481, August, 1839; from London Med. Gazette, March, 1839.

[2] Morel-Lavallée, from Malgaigne, op. cit., vol. ii. p. 881.

[3] Moore, Med.-Chir. Trans., vol. xxxiv. p. 107, 1851.

injury, and perhaps in obedience to circumstances not always easily explained.

The shortening has been observed to vary from half an inch to two inches or more; the trochanter is also usually driven in toward the pelvis. Pressure upon the trochanter occasions a deep seated pain. If the limb is drawn down to the same length with the other, it immediately resumes its position when the extension is discontinued. Crepitus is more uniformly present than in fractures of the neck of the femur, and it is especially felt while the limb is being extended or while it is again shortening, and not so much in flexion or rotation.

If, in addition to all of these phenomena, we learn that the accident has occurred from a severe blow, or a fall from a great height upon the trochanter; and that the viscera of the pelvis, and especially the bladder, seem to have suffered considerable injury; or if we detect at the same time a fracture of some other portion of the pelvis, we may reasonably conclude that the head of the femur has penetrated the acetabulum. Yet it must be confessed that no one of these symptoms is positively distinctive of this accident, and that they are seldom found sufficiently grouped to render the diagnosis certain.

The old "Piper" mentioned by Lendrick, and the man dissected by Morel-Lavallée, lived many years, and managed to walk about, but not without considerable pain; the other three, to whom I have alluded, died soon after the injuries were received.

Some have thought of treating these cases by extension and counter-extension; the latter being accomplished through the aid of a perineal band; but it is not probable that after an injury of this character, any patient will be able to endure the requisite pressure about the perineum or groins. It will be better to lay the patient upon Daniel's invalid bed, or some bed similarly constructed, so that it may be converted into a double-inclined plane; allowing the knees to be suspended over the angle of the thigh and leg-piece, in order that the weight of the body may have some effect to draw away the pelvis from the femur.

Fractures of the rim of the acetabulum have frequently been discovered in dissections, and the records of surgery abound with cases of unreduced dislocations of the femur, in which the failure to reduce or to retain the bone in place has been ascribed, not always with sufficient reason, perhaps, to this fracture.

Dr. M'Tyer, of the Glasgow Royal Infirmary, published in the *Glasgow Medical Journal*, for February, 1830, four cases of this fracture.

The first was that of a man, æt. 27, on whose back a number of bricks had fallen while he had his right knee placed on the bank of a trench. His right leg was found shortened about one inch and a half, bent, and the toes turned a little outwards. The limb could be moved without much difficulty, but every motion gave him pain; motion was also attended with crepitus. On making extension, the limb was easily brought to the same length with the other, but it became shortened again immediately when the extension was discontinued.

These symptoms, differing but little, if at all, from those which are usually present in a case of fracture of the neck of the femur, led to the supposition that this was actually the nature of the accident. Subsequently, the toes became slightly turned in, but this circumstance was not regarded as sufficiently distinctive to warrant a change in the diagnosis.

Having succumbed to the injuries after a few days, the autopsy revealed a fracture extending through the bottom of the right acetabulum, and about one inch and a half of the rim at its upper and posterior margin completely detached, except as it was held in place by a portion of the capsular ligament. The head of the bone could be easily pushed upwards and backwards upon the dorsum, the fragment of the acetabular margin being moved aside and swinging upon its fibrous attachment as upon a hinge, but resuming its place again perfectly when the head of the femur was restored to the socket. The femur was not broken.

In the second case the limb was found shortened, the knee slightly bent, and turned a little forwards and inwards, and the toes pointing to the tarsus of the other foot. It was thought to be a fracture also of the neck of the femur, but the autopsy disclosed only a fracture of the upper margin of the rim of the acetabulum.

In the third case, seen only after death, the limb was not shortened much, but the toes were stretched downwards, and turned slightly inwards. It was supposed at first to be a simple dislocation, but on dissection the posterior and inferior margin of the acetabulum was found to be broken and displaced toward the coccyx, while the head of the femur rested upon the pyriformis muscle, over the ischiatic notch.

The fourth example was found in the dissecting-room, and the history of the case is not known. A fragment of the superior and posterior margin of the acetabulum had been broken off and had reunited slightly displaced.[1]

Several other similar examples have been established by dissection, and we are able, therefore, to determine pretty accurately what are the usual phenomena and terminations of this accident, though we are far from having arrived at a satisfactory means of diagnosis; indeed, the accident has seldom been recognized before death. Its causes are generally the same with those which produce dislocations of the hip, but in most instances the violence has been greater than in the case of dislocations.

The symptoms are, first, such as indicate a dislocation, to which must be added crepitus and a difficulty, if not impossibility, of retaining the head of the femur in its place when it is reduced. The crepitus is sometimes discovered the moment we begin to move the limb, and this will aid us to distinguish it from a fracture of the neck of the femur accompanied with much displacement, since, in the latter case, crepitus is not felt usually until the extension is complete and the fragments are again brought into apposition.

The majority of these accidents, either from a failure to recognize them or from the impossibility of maintaining the head of the femur in place when once it has been reduced, have resulted in a permanent dislocation of the hip and a serious maiming. The following case was

[1] M'Tyer, Amer. Journ. Med. Sci., vol. viii. p. 517, Aug. 1831.

recognized and reduced, but it was found impossible to maintain the reduction.

February 3, 1847, a strong German laborer was crushed under a mass of iron weighing several tons. Drs. Sprague and Loomis, of this city, were called and found the left thigh dislocated upwards and backwards, and by the aid of six men they succeeded in reducing it, the reduction being attended, as the gentlemen have informed me, with a slight sensation of crepitus. The legs were then laid beside each other, and the knees tied together, the patient lying on his back; and now the two limbs appeared to be of the same length. On the second and third days the injured limb was examined by the same gentlemen and there was no displacement. On the fourth day I was invited to meet these gentlemen, the patient having had muscular spasms during the previous night, and the thigh being reluxated. I found the limb shortened one inch and a half, adducted, and the toes turned in. We immediately applied the pulleys and soon drew the trochanter down to a point apparently opposite the acetabulum, and a careful measurement showed that the two limbs were of the same length. The pulleys being removed, the leg did not draw up again, nor did the foot turn in, yet we had felt no sensation to indicate that the bone had slipped into its socket, nor had we felt crepitus. The legs and thighs were now laid over a double inclined plane and well secured. He remained in this condition three days more, during which time Dr. Sprague saw him each day and found nothing disarranged. On the night of the seventh day the spasms returned, and in the morning the thigh was displaced. The next day we again applied the pulleys, but soon found that the bone would not remain in place one minute after the pulleys were removed.

At this time, while moderate extension was being made at the foot by rotating the foot inwards, we could distinctly feel a slight crepitus. A straight splint was applied and as much extension made as he could conveniently bear, and in this condition the limb was kept several weeks. Seven years after I found the thigh still displaced upon the dorsum ilii. He limped badly, but he could walk fast and perform as much labor as before the accident.

In one case mentioned by Mr. Keate the bone had become dislocated downwards and could be felt lying against the tuber ischii, and the presence of a "distinct grating as of ruptured cartilage" led him to conclude that the cartilaginous labrum of the socket was broken off; but as the fracture was on the lower margin of the socket no difficulty was experienced in retaining the bone in position.[1]

If the diagnosis is satisfactorily made out, and upon complete reduction the femur will not remain in place, the treatment ought to be the same as for a fracture of the thigh, except that no lateral splints or bandages to the thigh will be necessary. The limb ought to be kept drawn out to its proper length, as far as this shall be found to be practicable, by extending and counter-extending apparatus. A band around the pelvis, so adjusted as to press the head of the bone into its

[1] Keate, Amer. Journ. of Med. Sci., vol. xvi. p. 225.

socket, may also be of service in preventing the tendency to displacement; and in case the bone manifests little or none of this tendency, the hip bandage will probably alone be sufficient, yet even here no harm could come of applying the long straight splint and the extending apparatus, secured moderately tight, simply as a measure of precaution.

§ 5. Sacrum.

Simple fractures of the sacrum, known to be exceedingly rare,[1] are occasioned either by such injuries as break at the same time the other bones of the pelvis, and which may act in any direction, or by blows or falls received directly upon the sacrum. It may be broken at any point, and in any direction, when the fracture is produced by the first of this class of causes; but if the fracture is the result of a direct blow upon the sacrum, it will generally be transverse, and below the sacro-iliac symphysis. The direction of the displacement is almost invariably the same, the coccygeal extremity being simply carried forwards, and this is seldom sufficient to interfere in any degree with the functions of the rectum and anus; but in one case seen by Bermond it nearly closed the rectum. Sometimes, also, there is a slight lateral deviation. There is also in the Dupuytren museum, at Paris, a specimen in which the whole of the lower fragment is displaced a little forwards.

The signs of this fracture are pain at the seat of injury, aggravated greatly in the attempts to flex or elevate the body, and especially in the efforts at defecation; swelling and discoloration of the soft parts covering the sacrum; displacement of the coccyx forwards; an angular projection at the point of fracture, with a corresponding retiring angle upon the opposite side; mobility.

Ambrose Paré declared that he had many times seen patients recover after fractures of the sacrum, but if the fracture reaches the spine, "scarcely," says he, "can the patient escape death." Later experience has shown, moreover, that where the fracture of the sacrum is accompanied with other fractures of the pelvis the patients seldom recover; and only because so extensive an injury implies usually great force in the cause which produced the fractures, and of necessity, greater lesions among the pelvic viscera. Simple fractures, from direct blows, or falls upon the sacrum, occurring below the sacro-iliac symphysis, are generally followed by speedy recoveries, although the inward displacement is not often completely overcome.

By introducing a finger into the rectum, the lower fragment can be easily pressed back to its natural position, but the difficulty consists in finding any means of retaining it there until bony union is effected. Judes succeeded to his satisfaction with a wooden plug, which he compelled the patient to wear forty-five days; removing it, however, every third day, in order to cleanse the rectum with an enema. Bermond

[1] Malgaigne has referred to eight cases; and I have not been able to find a record of any others.

introduced first a linen bag, which he immediately proceeded to fill with lint, but during the night it was forced away in an involuntary effort to empty the bowels of wind and stercoraceous matter. He now substituted a silver canula covered with a shirt, which latter he filled with lint in the same manner as before. This was retained without much inconvenience, nineteen days; having only been removed once during this time. The union now seemed to be firm, and the apparatus was removed. Plugging the rectum in this manner may be necessary whenever the inward inclination of the lower fragment is found to be considerable, but not otherwise; ordinarily, it will be sufficient to lay the patient upon his back, with a firm cushion above the point of fracture, so as to prevent the bed from pressing in the lower fragment, and having emptied his rectum thoroughly by an enema of warm water, he should be placed under the influence of an opiate sufficiently to restrain the action of the bowels for several days, or for as long a time as may be consistent with health or comfort. To the same end, also, the diet ought to be light and dry; nothing should be allowed which might prove laxative. By constipating the bowels, two ends may be gained. We shall prevent that frequent action of the sphincters, which might tend to disturb the union; and the hardened feces, by their accumulation in the rectum may serve to press back the lower fragment of the sacrum, in a manner much more natural and quite as effective as any apparatus which can be contrived.

I have already mentioned a case of separation of the bones at the sacro-iliac symphysis, reported by Lente (p. 339), but which was accompanied also with a fracture of the ilium and a dislocation of the hip. Several other similar examples have been reported, in some of which both of the sacro-iliac symphyses have been separated, or displaced. Such accidents are the results only of great violence, and the subjects of them seldom recover. In a few instances, however, this articulation has been known to give way during labor, while the symphysis pubis has suffered little or no diastasis; and in these cases recovery has generally taken place.

§ 6. Coccyx.

Cloquet mentions two cases as having come under his notice, one produced by a kick, and the other by a fall. In the latter case one thigh and both legs were also broken, and the coccyx having become carious in consequence of the fracture was gradually exfoliated.[1]

The symptoms, mode of diagnosis and the treatment in case of a fracture of the coccyx will scarcely demand of us consideration after having treated fully of these points in their relation to fractures of the sacrum.

It is more common, however, to meet with examples of separations of the coccyx from the sacrum, which may be regarded in some cases as veritable fractures, and in others as a species of luxation.

[1] Cloquet, art. Bassin, of Dict. en trente vol.

Due to the same causes which produce fractures of the coccyx itself, its symptoms differ only in the increased length of the movable fragment, and its consequent greater projection in the direction of its displacement. If it is thrown forwards, as it usually is, the rectum may be almost or completely blocked up by its presence; or, if it is carried backwards, its pointed extremity presses almost through the skin.

Its mode of reduction and retention are the same as in fractures of the coccyx and sacrum.

CHAPTER XXVIII.

FRACTURES OF THE FEMUR.

Division.—Of 115 fractures of the femur which have come under my observation, 43 belong to the upper third, 50 to the middle third, and 21 to the lower third; or, if we confine our analysis to the shaft alone, 18 belong to the upper third, 50 to the middle, and 21 to the lower.

The femur constitutes, therefore, a striking exception to the rule which my observations have established, that in the case of the long bones the lower third is most often the seat of fracture. The femur is most often broken in its middle third.

§ 1. NECK OF THE FEMUR.

Twenty-four of the whole number were fractures of the neck; either intra or extra-capsular. The youngest of these patients was thirty-nine years, the oldest eighty-four, and the average age was about sixty. Thirteen were males and eleven females. Nine occurred in the right femur and twelve in the left. All were simple. Six were believed to be without the capsule, and nine were believed to be within; the remainder were undetermined.

Surgeons have differed in their opinions as to the relative frequency of fractures of the neck of the femur within or without the capsule. This has arisen, no doubt, in part from the difficulty and probable inaccuracy of many of the diagnoses. Malgaigne, who has adopted a mode of deciding this question which, it must be conceded, is much less liable to error than simple clinical observation, namely, an examination of cabinet specimens, finds in four large collections sixty-one intra-capsular fractures, and only forty-two extra-capsular. So that, according to his observations, they stand in the proportion of about three to two; the intra-capsular being the most common. On the contrary, Nélaton believes that extra-capsular fractures are much the most common, and Bonnet, of Lyons, affirms that they constitute the immense majority. Bonnet made four dissections, and in each case he found the fracture extra-capsular. This testimony, so far as it goes, is positive, but the number is not sufficient to establish anything more than a probability in favor of the greater frequency of extra-capsular fractures.

Clinical observations are too uncertain to be made available in so nice a question. Cabinet specimens may have been collected for a special purpose, and this is well known to have been the fact with the celebrated Dupuytren collection, the specimens in which constitute nearly one-third of the whole number referred to by Malgaigne. I allude to the effort which was made while the controversy was pending between Dupuytren and Sir Astley Cooper as to the probability of bony union in intra-capsular fractures, to accumulate cabinet specimens of this fracture; and which effort extended itself, no doubt, both to London and Dublin, from which sources alone Malgaigne has gathered the balance of his figures. In Dr. Mütter's collection, at Philadelphia, I think there are only three examples of intra-capsular fracture, to seven extra-capsular.

Dr. Reuben D. Mussey, of Cincinnati, has in his cabinet twelve examples of fractures of the neck of the femur without the capsule, and only ten within.

We ought, therefore, to regard the question of relative frequency as still undetermined.

(a.) *Neck of the Femur within the Capsule.*

Causes.—In no other fracture do the predisposing causes play so important a part as in fractures of the neck of the femur, and this whether within or without the capsule; indeed, experience has shown that without the concurrence of those pathological changes which usually accompany old age, these fractures can scarcely occur. Sir Astley Cooper thought that the majority of fractures of the neck after the fiftieth year were intra-capsular; but Robert Smith has given us the ages of sixty persons having fractures of the neck of the femur, and the average age of thirty-two in whom the fractures were within the capsule, is sixty-two years, while the average age of twenty-eight in whom the fractures were extra-capsular, is sixty-eight years. Malgaigne has referred to this testimony in proof of the inaccuracy of the opinion held by Sir Astley Cooper; but I trust it will not be regarded impertinent or hypercritical for us to inquire how Mr. Smith

Fig. 100.

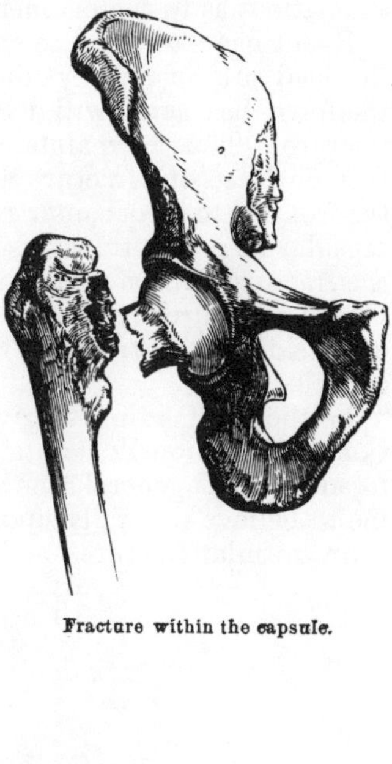

Fracture within the capsule.

became possessed of the ages of all these persons from whom these specimens were obtained; for more than half of the whole number, that is, just thirty-two, have their ages set down in round decimals, such as 50, 60, 70, &c., and it would be easy to show by the inevitable law of chances that this could not possibly be a true statement. If Mr. Smith does not pretend to have given the ages with accuracy, but only to have arrived as near to the truth as his sources of information would permit, then I protest that these tables do not constitute proper evidence in relation to this point; and until better evidence is furnished I shall continue to think, with Sir Astley Cooper, that fractures within the capsule belong generally to an older class of subjects than fractures without the capsule. This opinion, confirmed by my own experience, does not, however, as Malgaigne seems to think, imply that fractures within the capsule may not occasionally occur in persons much younger than the average limit, namely, under fifty years.

It is also believed that intra-capsular fractures are more frequent in women than in men.

The position of the neck of the femur and the great thickness of its muscular coverings render its fracture from a direct blow a very rare circumstance; indeed, it can only happen as the result of gunshot accidents, or other similar penetrating injuries.

It is broken therefore usually by indirect blows, such as a fall upon the bottom of the foot, upon the knee, or upon the trochanter major; or by muscular action alone, as has sometimes happened with very old people, who, in walking across the floor, have tripped upon the carpet, breaking the bone in the effort to sustain themselves. We must not always infer, however, because the patient has tripped, that the bone was broken by muscular action; since it is quite as likely that the fall, consequent upon the tripping, has occasioned the fracture; and we ought to make a careful examination of the hip over the trochanter to ascertain whether it has been bruised, and to interrogate the patient as to the manner of the fall.

Rodet has attempted to show by a series of experiments made upon the dead subject, and by other observations, that the direction in which the force has acted will determine the situation and direction of the fracture. Thus he maintains that when the person has fallen upon the foot or knee, the fracture will be intra-capsular and oblique; that if the front of the trochanter receives the blow, the fracture will be intra-capsular also, but transverse; if the back of the trochanter is struck, the fracture will be partly intra and partly extra-capsular; and if the person falls directly upon the side or receives the blow fairly upon the outer side of the trochanter, the fracture will be entirely without the capsule.[1]

Without intending to give my unqualified assent to these propositions so ingeniously maintained by Rodet, I am nevertheless prepared to admit their general accuracy; and especially has my experience led me to believe that falls upon the feet or knees in most cases produce intra-capsular fractures, and that falls upon the outside of the hip, or

[1] L'Experience, March 14, 1844.

upon the trochanter, generally produce extra-capsular fractures. I have seen also the intra-capsular fracture produced by so slight a cause as stepping down unexpectedly two or three inches upon an irregular surface.

Pathology.—I have already, when speaking of partial fractures, expressed my conviction of the possibility of a partial fracture, or a fissure of the neck of the femur, and I have referred to the case reported by Dr. J. B. S. Jackson, of Boston, as having determined this question beyond all possibility of a doubt; yet its occurrence must be regarded as an exceedingly rare, and, we may say, improbable event.

It is much more common to meet with examples of complete fracture of the neck both within and without the capsule, unaccompanied with a rupture of either the periosteum or the reflected capsule. Such was the fact in eight cases examined by Colles: in three of which, however, he believed the fracture not to have been complete, but Robert Smith thinks they were all of them examples of complete fracture.[1] Stanley has also related a case of complete separation of the bone unaccompanied with laceration or injury of either the periosteum or capsular ligament. This was in the person of a man aged sixty years, who had been knocked down in the street. On being admitted into St. Bartholomew's Hospital, shortly after the injury, he complained of pain in the hip, but there was neither shortening nor eversion of the limb, and its several motions could be executed with freedom and power. A fracture was not suspected; but five weeks after this he died of inflammation of the bowels. The dissection showed a fracture extending through the neck accompanied with a slight bloody effusion, but no displacement of the fragments or laceration of the soft parts.[2]

In other examples the bone is not only broken but displaced to such an extent that the capsule is completely torn in two.

But in a large majority of cases both the capsule and the periosteum are only partially torn asunder.

The fracture is generally somewhat oblique, and its direction is usually from above downwards and from within outwards. Sometimes its direction is such as to include a portion of the head; occasionally it is quite transverse. In one example of an old fracture I have seen the ends dove-tailed upon each other, the fracture having a double obliquity, and not admitting of displacement.

There may occur also a species of impaction, the lower portion of the neck entering the cancellous structure of the head, while its upper portion rides upon the articular surface, a circumstance which is well illustrated by the annexed woodcut (Fig. 101), copied by Mr. Smith from a specimen in the Dupuytren Museum at Paris; or the impaction may occur without any degree of either upward or lateral displacement.

Mr. Liston says: "Even in children separation of the head of the bone may, on good grounds, be supposed occasionally to take place;"[3] by which we understand him to mean that a separation of the epiphy-

[1] Colles, Dublin Hosp. Reports, vol. ii. p. 339.
[2] Stanley, Med.-Chir. Trans., vol. xiii.
[3] Liston, Elements of Surgery, Phila. ed., 1837, p. 480.

sis which completes the head of the femur, may occur. Mr. South relates a case in a boy ten years of age, who had fallen out of a first floor window upon his left hip. The limb was slightly turned out, but scarcely at all shortened. The thigh could be readily moved in any direction without much pain, but on bending the limb and rotating it outwards, a very distinct dummy sensation was frequently felt, apparently within the joint, as if one articular surface had slipped off another. This was regarded by both Mr. South and Mr. Green as an example of epiphyseal separation, and he was placed upon a double inclined plane, but he felt so little inconvenience from it that he several times left his bed and walked about. We have no information as to the result or as to the farther progress of the case.[1]

Fig. 101.

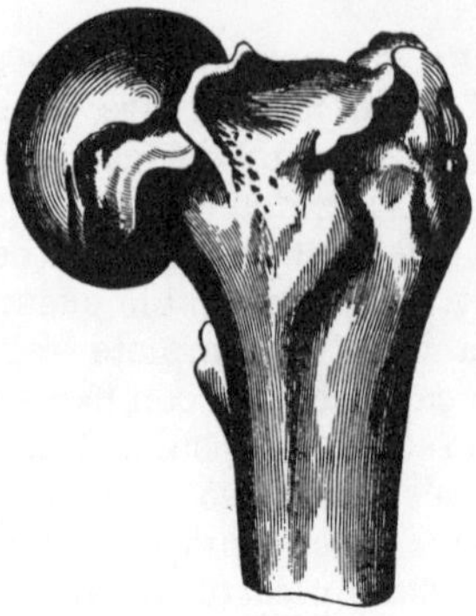

Impacted fracture within the capsule.

A girl, æt. 18, was brought before Dr. Parker, of New York, at his surgical clinic, Nov., 1850, who had been injured by a fall upon a curb-stone, when eleven years old. The accident was followed by suppuration and a fistulous discharge, from which, however, she finally recovered, but with the foot everted, and a shortening of one inch and a half. "Flexion and rotation of the joint occasioned no inconvenience." Dr. Parker thought this circumstance alone sufficient to distinguish it from hip disease in which anchylosis is the termination.[2]

At a meeting of the Kappa Lambda Society, held in New York, March 25, 1840, Dr. Post mentioned a case which he had seen in a girl sixteen years old, who, in taking a slight step with a child in her arms, made a false movement, and feeling something give way, she was obliged to lean against a wall. Dr. Post saw her the next day, when he found the affected limb one inch shorter than the opposite one, movable, the toes turned outwards, no swelling, some slight pain at the upper part of the thigh. The trochanter major moved with the shaft. There was also crepitus. From the age of the patient and the slight amount of violence by which the injury was produced, Dr. Post thought a separation of the epiphysis of the head had taken place. The extending apparatus was applied, but the limb remains from a quarter to half an inch shorter than its fellow.[3]

These three constitute the only examples of this accident which I find reported, and although there may be much reason to suppose that the diagnosis was correct in each instance, I cannot regard any one of them as actually proven; nor can I admit the accident as fairly established, or the diagnostic signs as being properly made out until these important points have received the confirmation of at least one dissection.

Symptoms.—Whether the limb will be shortened or not must depend

[1] South, Note to Chelius's Surgery, vol. i. p. 619.
[2] Parker, Amer. Med. Gazette, vol. i. p. 342, Nov. 30, 1850.
[3] Post, New York Journ. Med., vol. iii. p. 190, July, 1840.

upon whether the fragments have become displaced in the direction of the axis of the shaft of the femur. It is well established that in this fracture the broken ends frequently remain in contact for several hours or days, or until the gradual contraction of the muscles or the weight of the body upon the limb occasions a separation, and that consequently there is often at first no appreciable or actual shortening of the limb. To determine, however, its existence, it is not sufficient to lay the patient upon his back and place the limbs beside each other; we ought also to measure carefully with a tape line from the pelvis to the leg or foot, and from various other points, until we have placed this question beyond a doubt.

If shortening occurs, it may vary from one-quarter of an inch to two inches, or even more; but this extreme shortening is not reached usually, except after the lapse of several weeks or months, when the ligaments have gradually given way under the weight of the body in walking, or not until the neck has undergone a partial or almost complete absorption.

Sir Astley Cooper has stated that a shortening to this degree may occur at once; but Boyer, Earle, and others, doubt the accuracy of this opinion, and Robert Smith declares that he does not think the capsule would admit of such an amount of immediate displacement, unless it were extensively torn, an occurrence which he thinks very rare indeed.

With this qualification, the opinion of Mr. Smith does not differ from that entertained by Sir Astley, who only admits its possibility as a rare event; in a large majority of cases the shortening does not exceed one inch.

Crepitus, unlike shortening, is generally absent when the displacement of the fragments is complete; but under no circumstance is it easily developed. When the fragments remain in apposition and the femur is rotated for the purpose of moving the broken surfaces upon each other, the small acetabular fragment, resting in a smooth cup-like socket, and holding upon the opposite fragment by denticulations or by the untorn periosteum or capsule, glides about in obedience to the motions of this latter, and no crepitus can be produced. Nor is the difficulty rendered less by pressing firmly upon the trochanter, as some surgeons have recommended, since, while this pressure tends, no doubt, to fasten the upper fragment in the acetabulum, it tends much more to fasten the broken ends together, and thus defeats the purpose in view. When, on the other hand, the fragments have become completely separated, it is almost impossible to bring them again into contact. The limb may, perhaps, be easily brought down to the same length with the other, but it must by no means be inferred that, consequently, the broken ends are in apposition. It is almost certain, indeed, that in its progress downwards the trochanteric fragment has caught upon the acetabular fragment and pushed its floating and broken extremity downwards before it. Under these circumstances, the discovery of a crepitus must be accidental, and scarcely to be looked for. Sometimes, however, we may recognize a sound not unlike crepitus, but less harsh, produced by the friction of the trochanteric fragment against the rim of the acetabulum or dorsum of the ilium.

One thing we ought never to forget, namely, that by extraordinary efforts to obtain a crepitus we may lacerate the capsule or produce a displacement of the fragments which we never can remedy, and which, without such unwarrantable manipulation, might never have occurred.

Eversion of the foot is almost uniformly present in some degree, taking place immediately or more gradually, in proportion as the fragments become displaced, and the external rotators contract. The opposite condition or an inversion of the foot is occasionally present, and sometimes also the foot is neither turned in or out, but the toes point directly forwards. In sixty cases of fracture of the neck seen by Cloquet the foot was never turned in, and Boyer never met with such an example in all of his immense experience; but Langstaff, Guthrie, Stanley, and Cruveilhier have each seen one example, and Robert Smith has seen two.[1]

The explanation of the fact that the foot is usually turned out is simple. It is owing in part, no doubt, to the natural position and form of the foot and leg, which incline them to fall outwards by their own weight, but mainly to the powerful action of the external rotators, which are so feebly antagonized upon the opposite side. But those rare examples of fracture of the neck of the femur both within and without the capsule, accompanied with a permanent or a temporary inversion of the foot, are of more difficult explanation; and, indeed, a complete solution of this phenomenon does not seem to have been yet satisfactorily reached.

Fracture of the neck of the femur within the capsule is not usually attended with much pain when the patient is at rest, but any attempt to move the limb produces intense suffering, and especially when an attempt is made to rotate the limb inwards, or to carry it upwards and inwards.

Occasionally, also, during the first few days or hours after the fracture, a spasmodic action of the muscles compels the patient to cry out from the severity of the pain which it produces. At first, the sufferer is unable to indicate clearly the seat of this pain, or, perhaps, it is diffused and uncertain in its position, but after a time he is able to refer it chiefly to the region of the groin, opposite the neck of the bone, or to near the point of attachment of the psoas magnus and iliacus internus. There is also usually in this region a great degree of tenderness and an unusual fulness.

If now the limb be seized, and extension gradually but firmly applied, it will soon be made of the same length with the opposite thigh; but, the moment the extension is discontinued, the shortening and eversion will recur, accompanied with pain, and perhaps crepitus.

The trochanter major is less prominent than upon the opposite side, and if eversion of the limb exists, the trochanter may be felt indistinctly upwards and backwards from its usual position. The patient having been placed under the influence of an anæsthetic, we may

[1] Robert Smith, op. cit., p. 25. A. Cooper by B. Cooper, op. cit., p. 151, note.

prosecute the investigation still further, and by rotating the limb inwards and outwards as far as it will admit, we shall notice that the trochanter describes the arc of a smaller circle than in the opposite limb, or that the length of its radius has been shortened.

The patient is generally unable to move his limb, or to bear the least weight upon it; but many examples are on record of persons who walked some distance after the fracture had taken place, the capsule, and perhaps, also, the periosteum not being torn, and, consequently, the fragments not being displaced; or, possibly, it was at first an impacted fracture.

Finally, after having examined the patient as well as we are able to do, in the recumbent posture, if any doubt remains, and it is found practicable for the patient to be elevated upon his sound foot, this should be done. The broken limb can now be examined thoroughly on all sides, and a more accurate opinion formed of the amount of shortening and eversion. It will be especially noticed that if the weight of the body is allowed to rest upon the limb in the slightest degree it produces insupportable pain.

Prognosis.—The question of bony union after a complete fracture of the neck of the femur within the capsule, has occupied the attention of the ablest surgeons and pathologists for a long period; and while great differences of opinion have been expressed as to the probability of the occurrence, and as to the value of the testimony on the one side or the other, very few have ventured to deny its possibility.

Among these latter are found, however, the distinguished names of Cruveilhier, Colles, Lonsdale, and Bransby Cooper. It has been affirmed, also, that Sir Astley Cooper taught the same doctrine, but with how much show of reason, the following paragraphs from his own pen will determine:—

"In the examinations which I have made of transverse fractures of the cervix femoris, entirely within the capsular ligament, I have only met with one in which a bony union had taken place, or which did not admit of a motion of one bone upon the other. To deny the possibility of this union, and to maintain that no exception to the general rule can take place, would be presumptuous, especially when we consider the varieties of direction in which a fracture may occur, and the degree of violence by which it may have been produced. For example, when the fracture is through the head of the bone, with no separation of the fractured ends; when the bone is broken without its periosteum being torn; or, when it is broken obliquely, partly within and partly externally to the capsular ligament, I believe that bony union may take place, although at the same time I am of opinion that such a favorable combination of circumstances is of very rare occurrence. Much trouble has been taken to impress the minds of the public with the false idea that I have denied the possibility of union of the fracture of the neck of the thigh-bone; and therefore I beg at once to be understood to contend for the principle only, that I believe the reason that fractures of the neck of the thigh-bone do not unite, is that the ligamentous sheath and periosteum of the neck of the bone are torn through, that the bones are consequently drawn asunder by the muscles, and that there is a want of nourishment of the head of the bone; but I can readily believe that if a fracture should happen without the reflected ligament being torn, that as the nutrition would continue, the bone might unite; but the character of the accident would differ; the nature of the injury could scarcely be discerned, and the patient's bone would unite with little attention on the part of the surgeon.

"In proof of the correctness of my opinion, I enumerated, in the early editions of this work, forty-three specimens of this fracture, in different collections in London, which had not united by bone. At the present day these might be multiplied, were it necessary.

"Such has been the accumulated evidence of the want of power of the neck of the femur to unite by bone, in my practice of forty years, during which period I have seen but two or three cases which militate against this opinion, for many of the preparations which have been brought for my inspection, as specimens of united fractures of this part, have proved to be nothing more than the result of the changes concomitant with old age; and in many of them the two thigh-bones of the same subject had undergone the same alteration in texture and in form."[1]

The following passages from a communication made by Sir Astley to the *London Medical Gazette*, for the 25th of April, 1834, are equally pertinent.

"I find in a report of the Baron Dupuytren's lecture that he attributes to me the opinion that fractures of the neck of the thigh-bone, within the capsular ligament, not only 'never unite, but that it is impossible that they should unite by bone.'

"It is quite true that, as a general principle, I believe that those fractures unite by ligament, and not by bone, as do those of the patella and olecranon. But I deny that I have ever stated the impossibility of their ossific union; on the contrary, I have given the reason why they may occasionally unite by bone.

"The following are my words: 'To deny the possibility of their union, and to maintain that no exception to this general rule may take place, would be presumptuous,'" &c. &c.

In conclusion, Sir Astley remarks: "I should not have given you this trouble, nor should I have taken it myself, but for the respect I bear my friend, the Baron Dupuytren; for although I have already submitted myself to be misrepresented by many individuals, yet I should be sorry to be misunderstood by so excellent a surgeon, and so valuable a friend, as Le Baron Dupuytren."[2]

What apology now can be found for a writer who, in a lecture before the Royal College of Surgeons, delivered so late as the year 1858, uses the following language:—

"It is well known that Sir Astley Cooper always taught the doctrine that fractures of the neck of the thigh-bone were incapable of being repaired by osseous matter, and that in the whole course of his

[1] Sir Astley Cooper, on Dislocations and Fractures of the Joints, edited by Bransby Cooper, Amer. ed., p. 156.

[2] See also Sir Astley's letter to Prof. Cox, written in 1835, and published in the Prov. Med. and Surg. Journ. for July 12, 1848, and New York Journ. Med. for Sept. 1848.

practice he had never met with a single instance, nor could he meet with any one who had seen a case where such an occurrence had happened; and that union within the capsular ligament (when any such union takes place) is always by membrane. However, it appears that he had no sooner published the last edition of his work *On Fractures and Dislocations*, than Mr. Swan forwarded to him a specimen of the thigh-bone, in which the fracture of the neck had become reunited by osseous matter. Sir Astley retained the specimen until his death, and it appears that he never had the courage or policy to promulgate the discovery of the error of that doctrine which had so pervaded his mind, and which had misled the profession during a period of forty years."[1]

What pusillanimity is apparent in this repetition of a slander which had been refuted a hundred times by Sir Astley, but who, being now dead, might be assailed with impunity! Do not the surgeons of the Royal College who listened to these ungenerous insinuations, know full well their falsity? or is it possible that they derived a secret pleasure in hearing these insults cast upon one who, although he had done more than any other man to exalt the fame of English surgery, had, nevertheless, been only lately their rival, and from the shadow of whose colossal form they were just beginning to emerge into light. Sir Astley, so far from denying, frankly admitted its possibility, and explained the circumstances under which he believed it might occur. The true point in dispute was, whether certain cabinet specimens were actually examples of complete fractures, wholly within the capsule, united by bone. Some of them Sir Astley thought were only examples of chronic rheumatic arthritis, or of interstitial and progressive absorption. Some were partial rather than complete fractures; others were partly within and partly without the capsule; and for this he was accused of wilful blindness or stupidity, chiefly by those who themselves being the owners of these rare pathological treasures, might possibly have felt somewhat annoyed at seeing their value thus depreciated, and who, no doubt, would be quite as apt to fall into blindness and partisanship as Sir Astley himself. The truth is, however, that although the claim has been set up and stoutly maintained for more than thirty cabinet specimens, in one part of the world or another, a majority of these, including several whose claims were urged upon Sir Astley, have been at length declared by all parties unsatisfactory, or absolutely fictitious, and only a fraction of the whole number continue to be mentioned by any surgical writer as probable examples.[2]

[1] Lettsomian Lectures on the Physical Constitution, Diseases and Fractures of Bones, by John Bishop, F. R. S. London, 1855, p. 55.

[2] The following European surgeons have claimed to have in their possession, each, one example: Langstaff (Med.-Chir. Trans., vol. xiii. 1827); Brulatour (Ibid., vol. xiii. 1827); Stanley (Ibid., vol. xviii.); Swan (Swan on Diseases of Nerves, p. 304); Adams (Todd's Cyclop., p. 813); Jones (Med.-Chir. Trans., vol. xxiv.); Chorley (Amesbury on Frac., p. 125); Field (Ibid., p. 128); Soemmering (Chelius's Surgery by South, vol. i. p. 621); South (Ibid., p. 621). South also mentions another example as being in the museum of St. Bartholomew's Hospital. This is probably Jones' case, which Robert Smith says is preserved in this museum, and which has already been enumerated. Bryant (Memphis Med. Rec., vol. vi. p. 108, from British Med. Journ., March 14);

Robert Smith reduces the number to seven, but Malgaigne recognizes only three, namely: Swan's case, admitted by Sir Astley himself; Stanley's case, and one specimen in the Dupuytren museum. In neither of these cases, he affirms, has the neck lost anything of its form or length by absorption, from which we are to infer that he would reject as doubtful all such specimens as had undergone these pathological changes.

Indeed, I think we are not left in doubt as to Malgaigne's opinion upon this point. Six of the nineteen cases which I have enumerated are declared by him to resemble much more rachitic alterations of the neck than true fractures; and yet Robert Smith admits three of the six as well established examples; but as to the precise grounds upon which he rejects these cases, he shall speak for himself: "And it is sufficient that we consider the beautiful drawings designed by Sir Astley Cooper, to illustrate certain varieties of the alterations, to place us on our guard against every pretended consolidation which presents itself, accompanied with a shortening and deformity of the head and neck. When fractures unite by bone they do not suffer such enormous losses of substance which it would become necessary to admit for the neck of the femur."[1]

A reference to Stanley's case, as reported by Robert Smith, will show that, contrary to Malgaigne's statement, this was also shortened and deformed, and that, consequently, according to his own rules of exclusion, it also must be rejected; after which only two remain, namely, Swan's case, admitted by Sir Astley himself, and No. 188 of the Dupuytren museum.

I should do injustice to my own convictions, moreover, were I not to refer my readers to the following judicious criticism upon Mr. Swan's case:—

"Mr. Smith's notes are as follows: 'Mrs. Powel, above eighty years of age, fell down, November 14, 1824. Sir Astley Cooper, who saw her soon after, believed that there was a fracture of the neck of the femur, although there was no appreciable shortening of the limb, and only a slight inclination of the toes outwards; crepitus could not be perceived; the patient died about five weeks after the accident; upon examination of the joint after death, the fracture was found to have been entirely within the capsular ligament, and the greater part of it was firmly united. A section was made through the fractured part, and a faint white line was seen in one portion of the union, but the rest appeared entirely of bone. The cervical ligament had not been injured.'" (*Smith*, page 59.) In this case the patient was an old lady, above eighty years of age, with the fracture not certainly made out; there was no appreciable shortening of the limb; no crepitus; and

Fawdington (Amer. Journ. Med. Sci., vol. xv. p. 534, from London, Med. Gaz., Aug. 16, 1834); Harris (Ibid., vol. xviii. p. 246, from Dublin Journ., Sept. 1835). Robert Hamilton says that Prof. Tilanus showed him three specimens in the museum of the Hospital of St. Peter, at Amsterdam (Ibid., vol. xxxi. p. 470, from Lond. Med. Gaz., Jan. 6, 1843). Malgaigne says there are three specimens in the Dupuytren museum which have been described with the same interpretation. The whole number claimed by transatlantic surgeons is therefore nineteen.

[1] Malgaigne Traité des Fractures et des Luxations, tom. i. p. 678.

only a slight inclination of the toes outwards. The strongest point in favor of there having been a fracture, was the opinion of Sir Astley Cooper, which opinion is entitled to great weight; but there are no satisfactory facts given upon which he formed that opinion. This slight eversion of the foot might be given by the patient to relieve the tension on the bruised and inflamed part. We may well query if the vessels of the ligamentum teres would not have shown evidences of having performed an increased function? Would five weeks have been sufficient time for them to furnish osseous union, and resume their original size?

"Again, the old woman died in five weeks after the receipt of the injury. Now, it seems to us quite improbable, nay, impossible, that bony union of an intra-capsular fracture of the femur in an old woman, above eighty years of age, in whom there was not left vitality enough to sustain life, should take place, in five weeks after the injury, in less time than is allowed for the ordinary union of a fracture of the shaft of the femur in a healthy person in the prime of life."[1]

On this side of the Atlantic, the number of specimens for which the honor is claimed is nearly equal to the original number in Europe; but they have not yet, all of them, been subjected to the same sifting process as their foreign congeners; and it remains to be seen how many of them will come successfully out of a similar fifty years' contest.

Three of the specimens belong to the venerable and distinguished surgeon, Reuben D. Mussey, Professor of Surgery in the Miami Medical College, at Cincinnati, Ohio, and whose many valuable contributions to the science which he has so long adorned are familiar to all American surgeons. He has also himself furnished a complete history and description of the specimens, accompanied with drawings, which is published in the April number for 1857 of the *American Journal of the Medical Sciences.*

The first patient was a Mr. S., æt. 78, a hardy yeoman from one of the hilly districts of Northern New England. When more than one hundred miles from home, his two-horse wagon was upset, and falling upon his hip he was so much injured as to be unable to rise. Dr. J. C. Dalton, of Lowell, Massachusetts, a highly distinguished gentleman, examined the limb, and pronounced it a fracture of the neck of the thigh-bone, and accordingly he applied a modified Desault's apparatus.

On the fourth or fifth day, contrary to the remonstrances of his surgeon, the man had himself, apparatus, and bed placed in a long box, and the whole being laid in a country wagon he started for home. On the eighteenth day of the accident, after reaching home, and while yet in the box and apparatus, Dr. Mussey was called to see him. On removing the bedclothes Dr. Mussey noticed that the foot and knee were turned considerably outwards. He immediately took off the splint, and moved the hip-joint; finding that it gave him no pain, he flexed the thigh to a right angle with the body, and kept it a minute or two in that position, still occasioning no pain, but on flexing it a little further

[1] An inaugural thesis on intra-capsular fractures of the cervix femoris, by John Geo. Johnson, New York, 1857, p. 23. New York Journ. Med., 3d ser., vol. ii. p. 295.

he complained that it hurt him in his groin. Pressure with the finger at this point and behind the trochanter gave him decided uneasiness. No shortening could be detected.

Fig. 102.

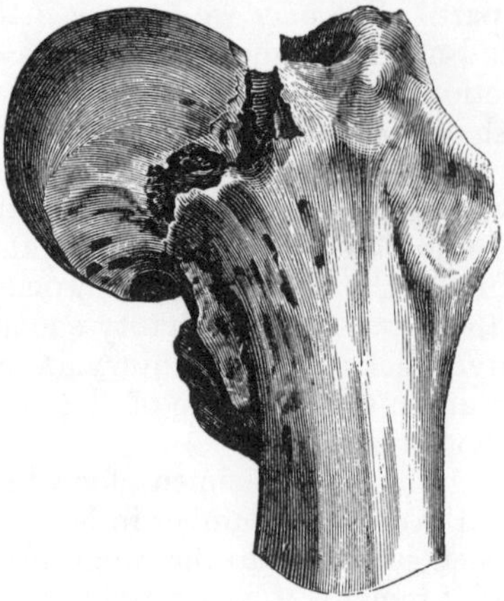

Left, or injured femur, of Mr. S.

Fig. 103.

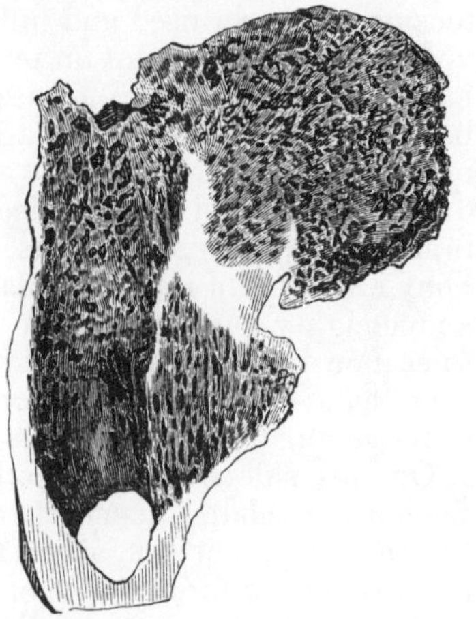

Vertical section of the same.

Dr. Mussey now felt so confident that the bone was not broken that he asked the old gentleman if he wished to get up, and upon his replying in the affirmative he was helped into a chair and sat for some time. He also bore the weight of his body for a minute or two upon his limb. From that day onward he wore no splint, and was got from his bed daily. In the course of four months the patient was able to walk with a cane, but he remained lame, and was never able again to ride on horseback as he had been accustomed to do.

Fig. 104.

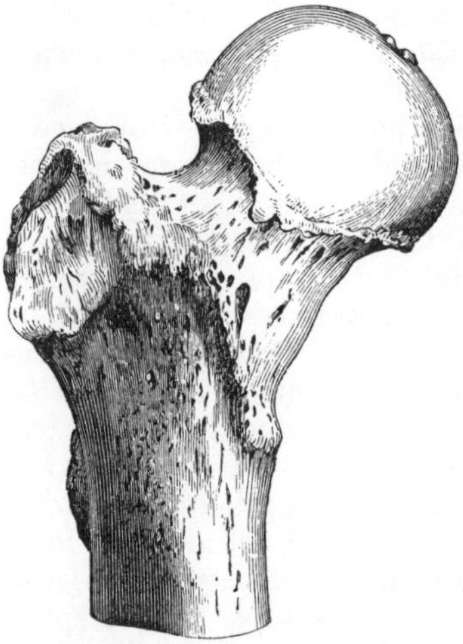

Right, or sound femur of Mr. S.

Dr. Dalton hearing of Dr. Mussey's opinion, wrote to him that on his visit to the patient he found the limb not only everted but shortened more than an inch, and that he had detected crepitus. Yet this does not seem to have changed Dr. Mussey's belief that it was not broken.

Two or three years after this the man died of an acute disease. Both thigh-bones were obtained. The right femur was sound (Fig. 104), but on being carefully cleaned the neck of the left femur was found to be shortened, so that in front it measured from the head to the intertrochanteric line one inch and three-eighths, and behind only one-third of an inch, the shaft being rotated outwards. The head was sunk below the level of the top of the trochanter major, occasioning a shortening of more than half an inch. "A vertical section" (Figs. 102, 103), says Dr. Mussey, "made by a saw, shows a consolidation of the fracture by a deposit of a mass as compact and white as ivory."

"In the year 1830," he continues, "I showed this to Messrs. Roux and Amussat, and some other professional gentlemen in Paris; they regarded it as a fair specimen of bony union of intra-capsular fracture. In London I also showed it to Mr. Lawrence, Mr. Travers, Mr. Stanley, and Dr. Hodgkin, who was then Curator of the Museum at Guy's Hospital. These gentlemen were interested with the specimen, and considered it as a satisfactory example of bony union within the capsular ligament. On my presenting it for inspection to Sir Astley Cooper, he remarked, 'This bone never was broken.' I said, 'Sir Astley, please to look at the interior of the bone.' He separated the two halves, and said, 'This does look a little more like it, to be sure; but I do not think it is wholly within the capsular ligament.' It is well known that Sir Astley, for some years, had taught the doctrine that bony union does not take place in intra-capsular fracture. His views, among the surgeons of Great Britain, were extensively admitted as correct."

At Edinburgh, Dr. Mussey also showed the specimen to John Thompson, author of the great work on inflammation, who called it an example of absorption, &c., consequent upon old age, and affirmed, "upon his truth and honor," that it had never been broken.

Dr. Mussey says, moreover, that the surgeons in this country, "who have examined these specimens, unhesitatingly pronounce this to be a case of union by bone of intra-capsular fracture."

There are one or two points in this case which give it extraordinary claims to attention. The first circumstance is the shortening discovered by Dr. Dalton, and which was absent on the eighteenth day, when the limb was examined by Dr. Mussey. One of these two gentlemen was mistaken. If it had united, the bones were never completely displaced, and it could not have been shortened when Dr. Dalton first saw it. This position I need not now attempt to defend; the testimony of all surgeons who have written upon this subject will warrant me in assuming thus much. Again, if it had been thus displaced, and Dr. Dalton had restored it to place, it seems impossible that, after a journey of one hundred miles over a rough country in a wagon, on the eighteenth day it should not have been again displaced and shortened, and especially if at this time the thigh was not only flexed to an acute angle upon the body, but the patient was permitted to stand upon it. If, however, Dr. Mussey still maintains that the limb was not shortened when he examined it, it remains for him to show how the bone was brought to position, and afterward kept in place so effectually, under such unfavorable circumstances; or if he admits that the shortening existed at that time, but was overlooked by him, then we must inquire, When (subsequently, of course) was the bone set? and how does it happen that it has united at all? There must have been a mistake somewhere in relation to this matter of shortening; and if so, with all my respect for Dr. Dalton, whose veracity and skill no man will dare to question, I am sceptical also as to the existence of crepitus. It is not entirely clear to me that he was not deceived.

In the history of the case, then, we see no reliable evidence of a fracture either within or without the capsule, nor did Dr. Mussey before the death of the patient. The bone itself, however, has convinced Dr. Mussey that it was broken within the capsule, and that it is well united by ossific matter. I have not seen it, and therefore am an incompetent judge of its value; but I must acknowledge that neither the description nor the drawing furnishes me with any positive proof that it was ever broken, and still less that the fracture was wholly within the capsule. Sir Astley Cooper doubted whether, if it was a fracture at all, it was a fracture wholly within the capsule; and I am willing to leave the question between these distinguished gentlemen as they have themselves left it, each one of whom was, in my opinion, equally earnest and sincere in his convictions, and each one of whom was equally competent to decide the point at issue.

Dr. Mussey's second specimen was obtained from a Mr. N., who, when fifty-one years old, fell, in alighting from his chaise, striking upon his left hip. He was unable to walk. Dr. Mussey saw him on the third day, and found him a corpulent man, lying with his foot everted, and the limb shortened from one inch to one inch and a third. He could extend the leg to within about one-third of an inch of its natural length, and when thus extended and rotated a distinct crepitus was produced. He applied Hartshorne's long splint, which was continued eighty-four days, the extension never being sufficient, however, to completely overcome the shortening. He ultimately walked with a cane, the shortening, which was about half an inch, being concealed by a high-heeled shoe.

Fig. 105.

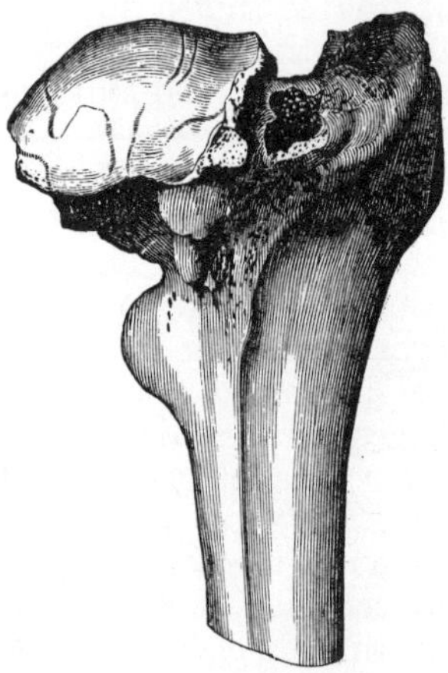

The left, or injured femur of Mr. N.

This man survived the injury twelve years, and eight years after his death Dr. Mussey obtained the specimen of injured bone (Fig. 105), together with its fellow (Fig 107). The head of the injured bone is elongated and depressed, or flattened, the neck is very much shortened, and the trochanter turned back as in the first specimen. A section (Fig. 106) shows a white, condensed tissue traversing the neck, near its junction with the head.

Mrs. Mason, æt. 73, was the subject of the third accident. She was a small, thin woman, and had fallen upon her side. Two days after, Dr. Mussey saw her in consultation with his friend, Dr. Judkins. The knee and foot were a little everted, with slight shortening and tenderness on pressure in the groin and behind the trochanter major. She was averse to the application of any kind of splint, and, being in a delicate state of health, she was allowed to remain upon her couch, with the thigh and leg somewhat flexed and supported by a pillow.

Fig. 106.

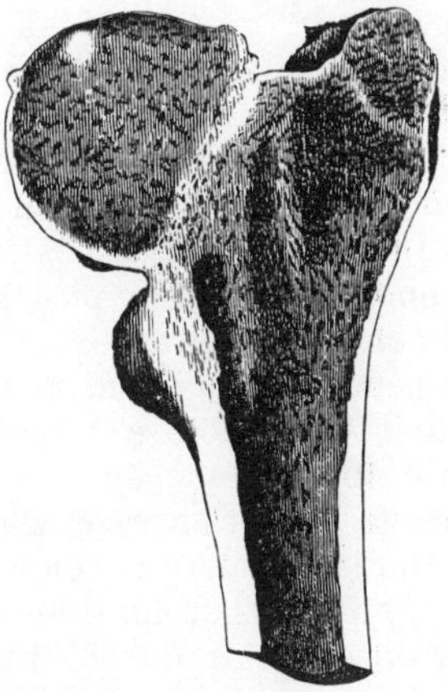

Vertical section of the injured femur of Mr. N.

Fig. 107.

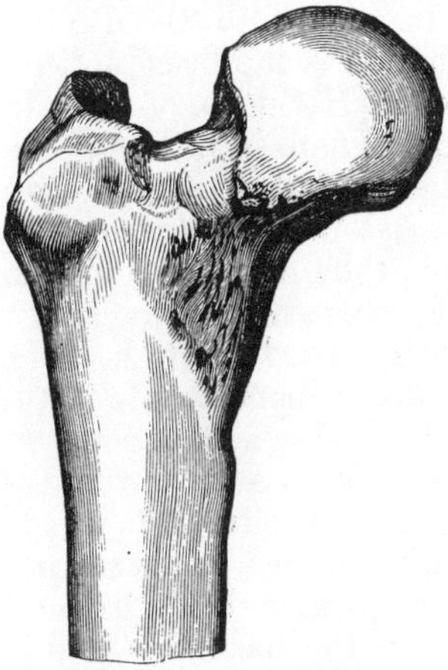

The right, or sound femur of Mr. N.

She remained in this situation about three months, after which she could move with the aid of crutches. She died in a year and a half from the accident, worn out by age and exhaustion.

Fig. 108.

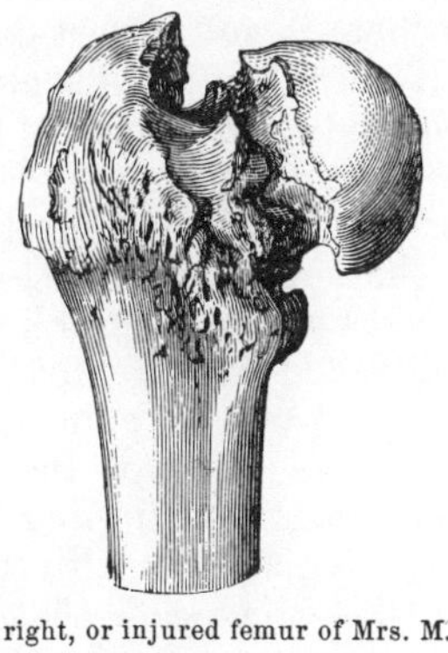

The right, or injured femur of Mrs. M.

Fig. 109.

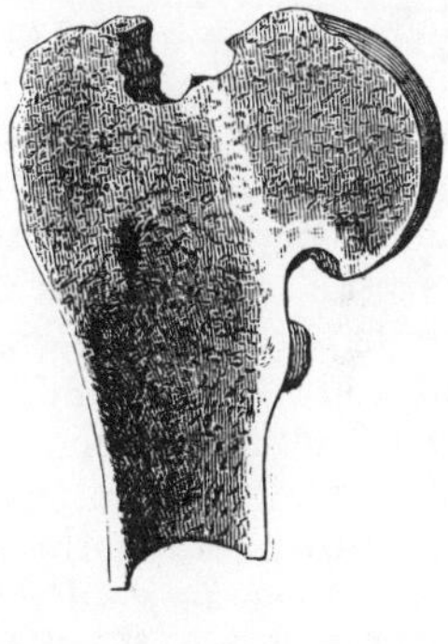

Vertical section of the injured femur of Mrs. M.

The neck of the bone (Fig. 108) is shortened to seven-eighths of an inch anteriorly, and to half an inch posteriorly. A considerable ridge runs across the anterior part of the neck, between which and the head is an irregular superficial groove. A section of the bone (Fig. 109) presents "a narrow, white, eburnated line, corresponding with the aforesaid ridge, exhibiting a firm consolidation."

I shall express no opinion of these two last described specimens further than to say that they seem to be liable to the same objections as several others of which I have already spoken, and that they do not belong to that class which has alone been accepted by Malgaigne.

It is proper, however, to say that, according to Dr. Johnson, in the paper already referred to, some of the surgeons who have examined these specimens have declared to him that they were not satisfactory.

Says Dr. Johnson, in the same paper:—

"In regard to the Philadelphia specimens, my only source of information is the brief notice of them in the new work on surgery by Prof. H. H. Smith, of Philadelphia. His statement is as follows (page 399): 'There is, in the Wistar and Horner Museum of the University of Pennsylvania, a femur, apparently of an old woman, in which the neck has been fractured near the head, yet in which complete osseous union, though with some degree of shortening, has taken place. I have, moreover, in my own cabinet a specimen in which the bone has been fractured through the neck near the head, the fragment having slid down beneath its natural position, and the fracture travelled obliquely down the neck, though still within the capsule, splitting it off in the line of the inter-trochanteric ridge. In this case, which must have produced marked shortening of the limb, there is complete osseous union.' This report is so exceedingly brief that no inference can be drawn from it; in fact, the writer does not appear to know whether the specimen is from a male or female. If this is true, then he knows nothing of the history of it. He does not give us the direction of the fracture, or a drawing of it, or even a positive statement that it is entirely within the capsule. In regard to his own specimen he is more explicit; he gives a drawing and shows that the fractured head has slipped down, and even now the line of fracture can be traced to the inter-trochanteric line. If this is so now, it is probable that the end of the fractured bone extended below the capsule in the first place, as in all cases of fracture, where there is not perfect coaptation, the rough points become absorbed. If we allow for this absorption, it would make the end of the bone below the trochanteric line a point without the capsule, thus excluding it from this class. If we adopt Prof. Smith's view, that this was entirely within, we meet with this objection. He states that the head of the bone has slipped down beneath its natural position, and the fracture has traversed it obliquely. This, of course, could not have been an impacted fracture, for in an impacted fracture we should have had the shaft of the bone driven into the cancellated portion of the head, not the head of the bone 'slipping down' along the shaft. If this was a case of slipping down of the head, we leave Prof. Smith, of Philadelphia, to controvert the position taken by Mr. Smith, of Dublin, where he says that only *impacted* intra-capsular fractures can have an osseous union."

Speaking of a specimen, also, which may be found in the Crosby-street Medical College, of New York, he says:—

"This belongs to Prof. Willard Parker, of this city. I am under obligations to Prof. Parker, for his kindness in explaining to me the various points which he considers the case presents. He loaned me the specimen to examine at my leisure, that I might become thoroughly acquainted with all the facts of the case. According to the description of the case given by Prof. Parker, in his lecture, the patient was a maiden, about sixty years of age, an inmate of the almshouse of Barnard, Vt. One morning, while going out of doors, she fell, striking upon her hip. The doctor in attendance, who did not pretend to be a surgeon, or accurate in his diagnosis, came to the conclusion that there was a fracture. He was of the opinion that he obtained crepitus, accordingly he dressed the limb with the straight splint for six weeks, and at the end of that time found half an inch shortening. The specimen afterwards came into Prof. Parker's possession. The points Prof. Parker relies on to show that this was a fracture, are: 1. The supposed crepitus. 2. A ridge of bone along the inter-trochanteric line, termed the 'callus.' 3. The neck of the bone shortened on the outer side one-third of an inch more than on the inner side, this being accounted for on the supposition that it was produced by the position the limb was allowed to retain. 4. No such changes are to be found in the femur of the opposite side, which is pronounced healthy.

"These specimens were procured four years after the injury. The capsule is entirely gone, and there is nothing to show positively where it was inserted; a line is pointed out about three lines below the so-called callus, as the line of insertion of the capsule. On examination of the interior of the specimen, there is nothing to indicate the line of fracture; no callus, such as is shown on internal examination of other fractures of long bones.

"There is one point very marked on the inner edge of the compact structure of the shaft; it is what Sir Astley Cooper terms a "buttress of bone" shooting up from the body into the neck and head, evidently as a support to the head in the new angle which it has assumed, with respect to the shaft. This buttress is formed apparently by the cancellated structure being more compact than in other points. On comparing this specimen with the femur of the well limb, a very marked difference is observable: this line or buttress is stronger, better developed, and is evidently for the purpose of giving support to the head of the bone in this new position.

"The specimen is far from being satisfactory. If this rough line extending along the inter-trochanteric line, is in reality the line of callus, then it is extremely probable that the fracture was partially *extra-capsular*. For if the capsule extended along the line which runs below this line that is pointed out as the line of fracture, then the insertion of the capsule must have been as low down as the middle of the trochanter minor, an anomaly in regard to insertion of the capsule. If this really was the line of insertion, it is extremely unfortunate that the capsule was not left to show where it was inserted.

"Again, there is no callus on the inside of the bone corresponding to this so-called external callus, but throughout the whole line corresponding to this external 'callus' the cancellated structure is perfect. If it should be admitted that crepitus was here obtained, a point which is extremely doubtful, as we have only the opinion of a doctor who practised many years ago in the small town of Barnard, Vt., a town which now numbers less than two thousand inhabitants—if it should be admitted on such authority that this was a fracture—still, it is by no means established that this was an intra-capsular fracture, for this so-called callus extends along the inter-trochanteric line. The capsule itself is gone, so that it cannot be shown positively where it was inserted, and it is probable, if there was a fracture, it was partly extracapsular.

"Again, the view which Prof. Parker takes of his specimen conflicts with that taken by Robert W. Smith, of Dublin, on fractures of this class, in his work already quoted. For if there was crepitus, then there must have been motion of one fragment on the other; and if there was motion, then the fracture was not impacted; and it is only this latter class which, Mr. Smith contends, can unite. My own impression is that there never was a fracture here at all. I think this is a case of interstitial absorption of the neck of the bone, the cause of this absorption being the contusion received by the fall. This view is sustained by analogy. Sir Astley Cooper says this is common in old people. 'As the shell becomes thin, ossific matter is deposited on the upper side of the cervix, opposite the edge of the acetabulum, and often a similar portion at its lower part, and thus the strength of the bone is in some degree preserved. This state of things may be frequently seen in very old persons.' 'When the absorption of the neck proceeds faster than the deposit on the surface, the bone breaks from the slightest cause; and this deposit wears so much the appearance of a united fracture, that it might be easily mistaken for it before the bone thus alters. We sometimes meet with a remarkable buttress shooting up from the shaft of the bone into its head, giving it additional support to that which it receives from the deposit of bone on its external surface.'

"Mr. Liston says: 'Gradual shortening of the lower extremity often ensues upon contusions of the hip in persons advanced in life, in consequence of interstitial absorption of the neck of the thigh-bone, and alteration of the angle in which it is set upon the shaft. The head of the bone undergoes a change in form; it becomes flattened and expanded, and the cotyloid cavity is made to correspond. This cause of lameness ought to be kept in view. The risk of its occurrence ought to be explained to those who have suffered injury of the hip, and, if possible, it must be prevented.'

"Mr. Gulliver, in the *Edinburgh Medical and Surgical Journal*, No. 128, July, 1836, *et seq.*, has written very fully on this subject of interstitial absorption, and has adduced cases which we would copy if our limits would allow. He shows by his specimens that the head is enlarged at its lower part; that these cases may occur in young persons; that it is not disease of the joint, from the fact that there is no anchylosis; and that the cartilages are not involved. The cases of John Lynn, J. McGath, and J. Fox, etc., are adduced, and the specimens preserved from autopsies. We have abundant evidence of interstitial absorption occurring from contusion in persons like this maiden, and Mr. Gulliver says this shortening may take place as rapidly as in five or six days. Now, Prof. Parker's specimen corresponds to the facts we have given. 1. There is a ridge formed along the lower part of the neck, as Sir Astley Cooper states occurs in these cases of interstitial absorption. 2. There is the buttress of bone shooting up from the shaft into the head as a means of support; this is clearly shown by comparing the two specimens, the one from the well limb, and the one from the contused limb. 3. There was a contusion sufficient for an exciting cause. 4. This occurs in one limb, and not in the other, as shown in the case of J. Fox, reported by Gulliver, where one limb was in every respect natural, and in the other interstitial absorption had taken place. This, we believe, is the case in Prof. Parker's specimen. If this specimen is in reality a fracture, it was most probably partly extra-capsular; if not, it was a case of interstitial absorption."[1]

Dr. Alden March, the distinguished Professor of Surgery in Albany Medical College, has permitted me to examine two specimens belonging to his collection, which he regards as examples of bony union within the capsule. He has, however, rendered it unnecessary that I should describe particularly the appearances which they present, by having himself given an account of them, accompanied with drawings, in a paper entitled "Osseous Union of Intra-Capsular Fracture of the Neck of the Femur," published in the *Transactions of the Medical Society of the State of New York*, for the year 1858. The account of the first specimen is as follows:—

"Of the two specimens here presented for examination, as examples of intra-capsular fracture of the femur united by bone, the smaller one, numbered 884, was procured in London some years since, and at that time was regarded by the curator of the old London Hospital Museum as a good specimen of fracture and bony union of the neck of the femur within the capsular ligament. I can give no history of the patient, or subject, from whom it was taken. I think it could not have belonged to an old person, and it is quite clear that he or she, as the case may be, lived long enough after the occurrence of the fracture for it to become thoroughly reunited by bony material.

"The neck of the bone is very much absorbed, which will be found to be the case in almost all instances of intra-capsular fracture, whether united by bony or ligamentous material. This specimen, with several others of various kinds of organic change, was submitted to the examination of an able professor of surgery, who has recently devoted much attention to the study of fractures, and who remarks upon it as follows: 'Specimen 884 is plainly enough a fracture, and I think there can be no doubt that on one side of the neck the fracture was within the capsule, but I have no means of determining whether it was also within the capsule on the opposite side, since the neck is almost completely absorbed.'

"On close examination," continues Dr. March, "it will be found that about all the part of the bone that can be called neck is connected with the shaft, and that the fracture appears to be nearly transverse, and close to the articulating, or cartilaginous border of the head. It strikes me that it is just as clearly altogether within the capsule as it is a fracture."

In defence of the opinion already expressed by myself in relation to this specimen, and to which Dr. March has seen fit to refer in the pas-

[1] This specimen is probably the same to which Prof. Parker has made allusion in his notes to the fourth American edition of Samuel Cooper's *First Lines of Surgery*, at page 354 of volume second.

sage above quoted, I will say, that the almost total absence of the neck posteriorly, where, in the natural condition of the parts, quite half an inch of the neck belongs outside of the capsule, renders it impossible, in my opinion, to determine whether the fracture was not in part without the capsule. This remark will apply to all similar examples, unless, indeed, the capsule itself remains to indicate precisely where this small portion of the neck belongs; but the capsule is gone from this specimen, and the neck is lost posteriorly. If it is true, then, that the line of fracture can be shown to be close to the head of the bone, it is equally true that it hugs the trochanter; we have just as much right, therefore, to interpret its proximity to the trochanter in favor of an extra-capsular fracture, as has my distinguished friend to interpret its proximity to the head in favor of an intra-capsular fracture.

Moreover, this specimen has never been sawn open, or subjected to the test of boiling, or of maceration, nor in any other way has the most important question of all been definitely settled, namely, whether the union is by bony or by fibrous tissue.

The second specimen is described by Dr. March much more at length, rendering it necessary that our own account of it should be somewhat condensed.

Fred. L. fell from a shed when ten or twelve years old, and, according to the testimony of respectable citizens, was attended by a surgeon, and treated, as they think, for a fractured thigh; but it does not appear probable that splints were used, as a woman was known to carry him up and down stairs on her shoulders during the time he was under the surgeon's care. It appears, also, that "immediately after getting about he was just about as lame, as much of a cripple, and as much distorted in his figure as he was at any time previous to his death." He is mentioned by one of the witnesses who knew him for many years after, as a "distorted cripple." Dr. March himself had known him twenty-five or thirty years, and describes him as a large framed man, with a "peculiar" gait, "a kind of *side waddle*, one limb appearing to be two or three inches shorter than the other, and with the hip of the shortened side greatly projecting laterally." He was about 58 years of age when he died.

More or less of the skeleton of this man came subsequently into the possession of Dr. March, and he describes one of the thigh-bones as follows:—

"A pretty large surface at its upper part and toward the trochanter major is a little flattened, and has the appearance of having been worn away, deprived of its cartilage, and becoming eburnated, or presenting at one point a porcelaneous polish." This change Dr. March regards as the result of interstitial and progressive absorption, aided by attrition, and as having occurred at an advanced period of life.

On the anterior superior part of the neck is a ridge of bone, to which a portion of the capsular ligament remains attached. Most of the cartilaginous covering of the head has been either entirely removed, or very much thinned, leaving at certain points a polished surface. That part occupied originally by the round ligament "seems to have been getting into a state of ulceration." The whole head is depressed and turned obliquely backwards. There is also a long spine or rib of bone extending upwards and inwards, which was imbedded in the fibres of the psoas magnus and iliacus, and "seems to have its attachment at its base, to the point where we should look for a trochanter minor."

At first Dr. March thought that the shaft of the opposite femur had also been broken three inches below the trochanter minor, and that it had united with some slight deformity. He also found the ala of the pelvis on the right side bent inwards, so that the distance from the crest to the centre of the sacrum was three-fourths of an inch less than on the opposite side. This, too, he ascribed at first to the original injury, but further investigation has satisfied him that it was due to the action of the muscles, and that the opposite limb had never been broken.

To this description, condensed from the paper alluded to, I need only add, that the whole head of the bone is very much flattened and changed in shape, and that there is scarcely anything which can be appropriately called a neck. The bone has been sawed in two, but Dr. March does not pretend that the bisection furnishes any additional evidence that it had been broken.

My objections to this case are briefly :—

It is not satisfactorily made out that there was ever a fracture, either by a reference to the original history, or by an examination of the bone. The age at which the accident occurred (10 or 12 years), is presumptive evidence against a fracture of the neck of the femur within the capsule, if not almost conclusive, unless it is claimed to be an example of epiphyseal separation with a bony union, a supposition which, so far as I can learn, no surgeon has yet ventured to make. Dupuytren says he never saw a fracture of the neck of the femur in a child. The youngest I have seen recorded is that mentioned by Sabatier, in which case the boy was fifteen years old.[1] Dupuytren has also well explained the causes of this infrequency of a fracture of the neck of the femur in early life.

On the other hand, the age at which the accident occurred was favorable to the production of disease of the hip-joint. The whole history of the patient, from that time onwards, especially his peculiar "waddle," seems to indicate that his hip-joints were both diseased. The autopsy shows that they actually were diseased, and renders it quite probable also that all of the bones of his body were in an unhealthy condition. The specimen itself is in nearly all respects a counterpart of many others to be found in the museums of this and other countries, and which are now, by almost unanimous consent, declared to be examples of chronic rheumatic arthritis.

Dr. Mütter thinks also that specimen B, 71, in his collection of bones, now lying in the Jefferson Medical College at Philadelphia, is a genuine example. It is a cleaned and dried specimen, from which the capsule, and all the soft parts, have been removed. The neck is very nearly absorbed, and the trochanter major is rotated backwards,

[1] Dupuytren on Dis. and Injuries of Bones, p. 187.

as we see in nearly all examples of interstitial absorption, so that it almost touches the head. The interior has never been exposed, to determine the line of the supposed fracture, nor is there anything upon its external surface by which this point, so essential to the question at issue, can be decided. It may be an example in point, but the proof is not before us.

Dr. Charles A. Pope, Professor of Surgery in the St. Louis University, Missouri, informs me that he has an example of "intra-capsular fracture of the neck of the femur, with concomitant fracture of the acetabulum. The union by bone is perfect, although the neck is, as it were, gone, the head being almost squarely set on the shaft of the bone. The head is much deformed, being an enlarged cone, and fitting into a similarly shaped acetabulum. The motions of the joints were well preserved."

I have never seen this specimen, and I am therefore unable to speak of it authoritatively, but I confess I do not see how it is possible to know that the fracture was wholly within the capsule when the neck is gone. If the capsule remains attached to the specimen, it may aid in the elucidation of this point; but it does not appear from Dr. Pope's communication that such is the fact. I should be gratified if this distinguished surgeon would give the profession a more complete account of the case.

From various sources, including several private letters, I have been able to gather a few of the particulars relating to a case which for some time attracted the attention of the profession in this country; but a full account of which, I regret to say, has never been published.[1]

Somewhere about the year 1832, Mrs. William Nelson, of Derby, Vt., fell, and was slightly lamed. Dr. M. F. Colby, of Stanstead, Lower Canada, being consulted, declared that she had broken the neck of the thigh-bone. She was accordingly placed in a horizontal position, and an extending apparatus applied. This treatment was continued one month, during which time she became insane; but from this condition she ultimately recovered. At the end of one month the apparatus was removed, and she was able to walk after her recovery without much halt, and the limb did not seem to be much shortened.

Subsequently the husband of Mrs. Nelson prosecuted Dr. Colby for causing insanity through unnecessary confinement, alleging that the bone was not broken; and, as evidence that it was not, testimony was presented to show that she was able to walk a few steps immediately after the injury was received; that she could draw up her legs; that she rode, sitting upon the seat of a wagon; that the extending splint was continued only four weeks, and that, although it was loosened occasionally by the friends, the limb did not shorten; and, finally, that she had a perfect, or nearly perfect, limb.

The case remained in court several years, until both parties were nearly ruined; but ten years after the accident Mrs. Nelson died, and both femurs, says Dr. Mussey, were secured by Dr. Colby. The one

[1] Boston Med. and Surg. Journ., Jan. 26, 1842; Amer. Journ. Med. Sci., April, 1857, p. 310.

believed to have been broken was then sent to several of our larger cities, and, among others, it was examined by Hayward and one of the Warrens in Boston; Dixi Crosby, of Dartmouth; Willard Parker; one of the Rogers in New York; and Robert Nelson, of Canada.

Robert Nelson and Rogers still denied that it had been broken, both of these surgeons affirming that the bone was perfect; but, on the part of the defence, it was subsequently charged that a spurious bone had been laid before these latter gentlemen. Drs. Warren[1] and Hayward thought it had been a dislocation; Drs. Parker and Crosby believed it to have been a fracture within the capsule, and that it was united by bone.

Dr. Mussey, to whom the specimen has been described, but who has never seen it himself, says that "the bone belonging to the injured limb had a ridge across the neck, while the head was so far depressed as to shorten the thigh-bone three-sixteenths of an inch."

Dr. Colby finally received a judgment in his favor for one cent costs, and a bond, signed by the prosecuting attorney, to the effect that the bone, which was now in the possession of the prosecutor, should be given up to the defendant, and remain in his possession during a period of six months, in order that he might show it to the public; but this part of the contract has been broken, and the bone seems now to be lost to science.

Whatever may be our opinion as to the probability of the fracture in this case, the absurdity and cruelty of the allegation of malpractice is too plain to admit of discussion or a doubt among intelligent medical men. If Dr. Colby thought there was a fracture—and he certainly had reasons to think so—his treatment was such as every judicious surgeon would have adopted, and for not adopting which he might justly have been held responsible.

I have in my cabinet a cast which I made nearly twenty years since, from a femur then owned by Prof. James Webster, of Rochester, late Professor of Anatomy in the University of Buffalo, and which he believed to be a case of union by bone after a fracture within the capsule. The patient from whom this specimen was obtained was a female, and had been seen by him before death. Its resemblance to the specimen owned by Dr. March, and purchased by him in London, is so perfect, that I believed it to be the same until Dr. March informed me that it was not. It is almost its exact counterpart, however, as I know by a comparison of the specimen with my own cast of Prof. Webster's. This fact will render it unnecessary that I should state my objections to it, since the same remarks will apply to it as to Dr. March's specimen.

I have also in my own cabinet a femur of no inconsiderable pretensions, belonging clearly to that class of specimens recognized by Robert Smith. Its neck is greatly shortened, and this surgeon would regard it, I think, as an impacted intra-capsular fracture, but its claim would be promptly denied by Malgaigne, on account of the absorption and distortion of its neck. Its history has been kindly furnished to me by Dr. H. H. Bissell, of this city.

[1] Dr. Mussey says "Dr. Warren decided there had been a fracture;" but I have it upon the authority of Dr. Colby that Dr. Warren had called it a dislocation, or that a witness so testified. Perhaps it was not the same Warren.

About the year 1833 Mrs. Wakelee, of Clarence, Erie County, New York, æt. 68, who was then very low with tubercular consumption, and so ill as to be scarcely able to walk across the floor, tripped upon the carpet and fell, striking upon her left side. She was unable to rise, but was laid upon a bed by her son, Dr. Wakelee, a very intelligent physician, residing in the same house, who did not suspect a fracture. Dr. Bissell saw her on the following day, and on rotating the limb outwards, he says that he discovered a crepitus. His examination was greatly facilitated by her extreme emaciation.

Mrs. W. was placed upon a double-inclined plane, with apparatus for extension, &c., and left in charge of Dr. Wakelee. On the fifth day the splint was removed, and from this time no dressings of any kind were applied. The reason for this change of treatment was, that she was likely to live but a few days, in consequence of the state of her lungs, and that such confinement would only hasten her death. Contrary, however, to all expectation, she gradually convalesced, so that after two or three years she could walk on crutches, her toes turning out and her limb becoming somewhat shortened. Four years after the accident she died, and Dr. Bissell obtained from Dr. Wakelee the specimen, of which the accompanying drawing is a faithful delineation.

Fig. 110.

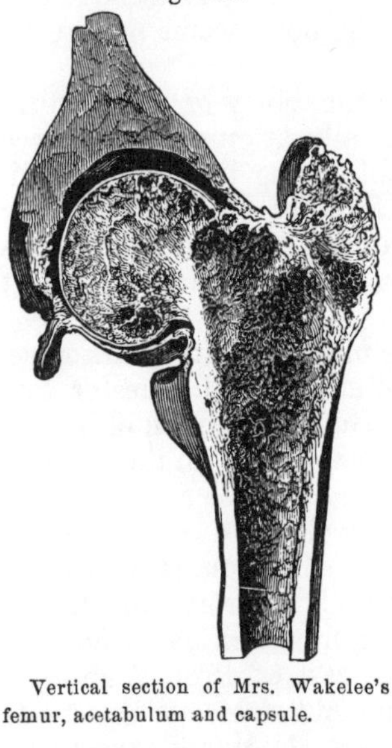

Vertical section of Mrs. Wakelee's femur, acetabulum and capsule.

I am informed, also, that there are two specimens in the Boston Museums, but the descriptions which I have received of them are too imperfect to allow me to speak of their merits.

Such is the present state of the testimony upon this interesting but difficult subject. In it all we think we see enough to warrant a belief that under certain favorable circumstances bony union may occur, but not enough to establish it beyond all doubt. There are those who feel much more assured, and who are as confident of this fact as that the shaft of the femur will unite by bone; we do not accuse them of credulity, and we invoke for ourselves the same exercise of charity toward our scepticism. We have never yet seen a specimen which, upon a careful examination, proved satisfactory; but unless our want of conviction can be shown to be the result of a wilful blindness, we shall demand protection against the assaults and insinuations which have so frequently fallen upon those who ventured to doubt the authenticity of every specimen which was laid before them.

I repeat, that it seems to me probable, that under certain favorable circumstances this union will occur; these favorable circumstances have relation to several conditions, such as age, health, degree of separation of the fragments, laceration of the periosteum and capsule, treatment, &c. Robert Smith thinks it is not likely to occur unless the fragments are impacted, but Sir Astley Cooper, as we have already seen, admitted its possibility whenever the reflected capsule and the periosteum were not torn, and at the same time the fragments were not displaced. If to these conditions we were to add moderate but not extreme age, with good health, we can see no sufficient reason why, under judicious treatment, bony union might not occasionally be expected. But such a combination of circumstances is probably exceedingly rare; and, what is more unfortunate, if they exist, the fracture is not likely to be recognized, and the surgeon will fail to avail himself of those advantageous coincidences which might, if understood and properly treated, secure a bony union. Dupuytren says, when the fragments are not displaced "its existence may be suspected, but cannot be positively asserted." There will not be wanting, however, examples in which surgeons will believe or affirm that they have recognized the fracture and wrought the cure. I have heard of many such instances, and Mr. Smith has referred to one, which is quite pertinent, as having been reported in the *Gazette des Hôpitaux*. A woman, æt. 64, was treated for an intra-capsular fracture of the neck of the femur at one of the hospitals in Paris, and "at the end of four weeks she was discharged perfectly cured, and without shortening." We fully partake of Mr. Smith's surprise at the impudence of this claim, yet we do not see in it much greater improbability than in Mr. Swan's case, received by both Mr. Smith and Sir Astley himself, where the neck was found almost wholly united by bone in five weeks, although the woman was 80 years old, and actually dying while the process was going on! Says Dupuytren, "I would lay it down as a general principle that all fractures of the neck of a cylindrical bone should be kept at rest twice as long as ordinary fractures of the same bone; and even after that period I have seen displacement take place. The term may, therefore, be lengthened to a hundred days, or even longer in aged and feeble persons, whose powers of reparation are much deteriorated."

It is not the purpose of the writer to describe particularly all of the accidents or pathological conditions with which these fractures may be confounded. It is sufficient to allude to them, and to leave to others the labor of a complete historical record; but I am tempted to devote a paragraph to what has been variously termed "morbus coxæ senilis" (*Robert Smith*); "chronic rheumatic arthritis" (*Adams*); "interstitial absorption of the neck of the thigh-bone" (*B. Bell*); and by others "interstitial and progressive absorption," but the exact nature and cause of which morbid changes are not yet fully understood. Mr. Colles does not think this partakes of the nature of rheumatism. I have myself a specimen of what has been more generally called chronic rheumatic arthritis, occurring in the knee-joint, accompanied with a flattening and eburnation of the articular surfaces, and Gulliver has shown that similar changes of form in the neck of the bone may occur in tolerably young persons.

I suspect also that it will be found to occur under a greater variety of circumstances, and to present a greater variety of forms than have yet been described; and we shall perhaps find a partial explanation of this diversity and frequency in one single circumstance, namely, the peculiar anatomical structure of the neck. The neck of the femur stands nearly at a right angle with the shaft, or at an angle so great as that the weight of the body, even in health, has the effect to gradually depress the head below the top of the trochanter major, and to diminish its length. This is seen constantly in the striking change of form which occurs between childhood and old age. Now, if from any cause whatever, such as a blow upon the trochanter or upon the foot, the neck or head are made to suffer, and inflammation, or perhaps only a slight degree of increased action in the absorbents ensues, resulting in an equally slight softening of the bony tissue, these pathological circumstances may end, sooner or later, in a striking change of form in the neck or head. But it is not necessary to suppose an external injury to explain the occurrence of this inflammation, and consequent softening of the bone; a scrofulous, or rickety, or tuberculous constitution may occasion it, and

Fig. 111.

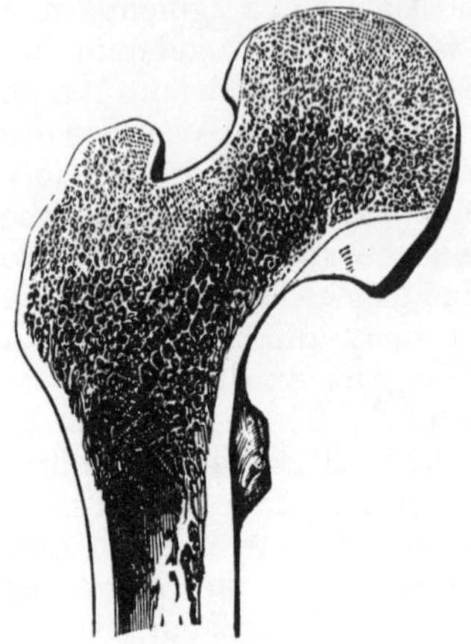

Section of the femur of an adult.

Fig. 112.

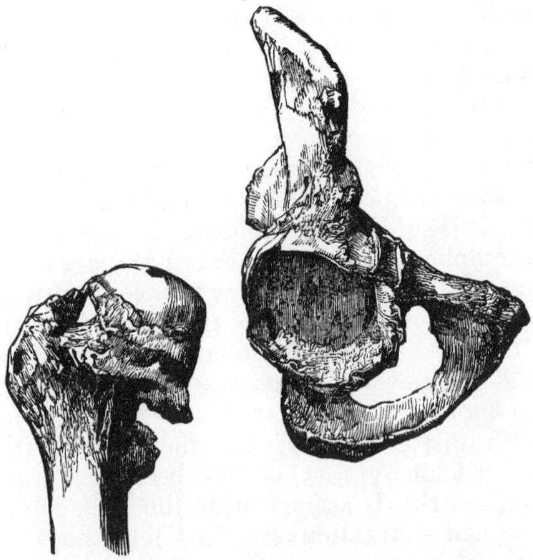

Chronic rheumatic arthritis. (Miller.)

we see no reason why these conditions are not as likely to lead to a change of form here as in the bones of the leg or of the spine. A change of form in the head may be the result of an ulceration of the cartilage, and a change of form in the neck, of ulceration of the neck. Among other causes, also, "chronic rheumatic arthritis" may operate in a large proportion of those examples which belong to advanced life. One case, reported by Gulliver, would seem to show that a deformity may occur here as a result of disease, and independently of pressure,[1] yet it is plain, from the direction which the deviation of the head and neck usually takes, that pressure performs an important part in the causation.

From these various causes, operating in these diverse ways, we shall have the different deformities enumerated and described by surgical writers. The head flattened, irregularly spread out, depressed and polished; the neck shortened and irregularly thickened and expanded; the trochanter major rotated outwards and drawn upwards; sinuous chasms traversing the neck, produced by ulceration; and finally, shortening of the neck, by a true interstitial absorption, and with little or no increase in its breadth, the trochanter major also being rotated outwards. It would be strange, moreover, if the interior of these bones did not present some changes in structure, such as have been frequently observed, namely—an irregular expansion or condensation of the cellular tissue, and which latter might easily be supposed by one who was inattentive to all of these circumstances, to indicate the line of an imaginary fracture.

The following example will illustrate the incipient stage of one class of these cases, namely—that in which the neck is not only shortened, but its surface is irregularly seamed, as if it had been broken and imperfectly united.

Wm. Clarkson, æt. 43, was admitted into the Toronto Hospital, C. W., May 5, 1858, with tubercular consumption, of which he died on the 25th of the same month.

He had been under the care of Dr. Scott, and it having been noticed that he complained of his right hip, at the time of admission, an autopsy was made on the 25th, at which I was, through the courtesy of the house surgeon, permitted to be present.

We examined both hip-joints, and found the neck of the right femur shortened, especially in its posterior aspect. At the junction of the head with the neck, posteriorly, and extending about half way around, the bone was carious, and so far absorbed as to leave a sulcus of a line or two in depth, and of about the same width. Adjacent to this, also, the bone was quite soft, yielding under the slightest pressure of the knife. There was no other appearance of disease. The opposite femur was sound.

The hospital record furnished the following account of his case, so far as the injury to his hip was concerned:—

About nine months before admission, then laboring under the malady of which he finally died, he received a blow upon his right trochanter, ever since which he had been lame, and suffered pain in the region of the hip-joint. The pain was felt especially in the groin, when the trochanter was pressed upon, or when the sole of his foot was per-

[1] Gulliver, Lond. Med.-Chir. Rev., vol. xxxix. p. 544.

cussed. The thigh was slightly flexed; the toes a little everted; and he walked with some halt.

The case of the soldier, Fox, reported by Gulliver, and who died of tuberculosis, presents a case also exactly in point, but illustrating a later stage, or the completion of the same process.

Of the precise nature of the changes in the two following examples, I cannot be certain, since they have not been determined by dissection. They will serve, however, to illustrate the usual history and progress of a considerable number of cases. They certainly were not examples of fracture.

Ephraim Brown, when twelve years old, fell from a tree and struck upon his right foot. Dr. Silas Holmes, of Stonington, Ct., was called. Of the particular symptoms at this time, I have only learned that the leg was not shortened. The doctor laid a plaster upon his hip, and left him without any further treatment. In three days he was able to walk on crutches; in three weeks he walked without crutches, and in four months was at work as usual. There was at this time no shortening or deformity of any kind.

Mr. Brown subsequently enlisted as a soldier in the war of the American Revolution, and experienced no difficulty in this hip until after a severe illness which followed upon an unusual exposure, when he was about thirty-five years old. At this period the leg began to shorten, but the shortening was unaccompanied with pain or soreness.

He consulted me, July 17, 1845, at which time he was eighty-three years old, and a remarkably strong and healthy-looking man. The shortening, which had ceased to progress some years before, amounted at this time to two and a half inches.

An officer in the United States army addressed to me the following letter, dated Nov. 13, 1849:—

"My mother-in-law, Mrs. S., of D., some three years since fell down a flight of stairs, striking on her side upon a stone, injuring the hip-joint severely; but upon examination, her physician declared that there was neither a fracture nor a dislocation, and said that she would gradually recover. Something like one year since the injured limb commenced shortening, so that she can now barely touch her toe to the floor as she walks. She can bear but little weight upon it, and is compelled to use a crutch or a cane constantly. So much time has now elapsed, and the limb is so little better, and constantly becoming shorter, I have proposed to ask your opinion," &c.

I need scarcely say that I had no hesitation in pronouncing this a case of chronic inflammation of the bone, accompanied with softening and gradual change of form, either of the neck or head, or of both.

It is proper that I should state briefly, before I leave this subject, what constitute the chief difficulties in the way of union by bone within the capsule.

The persons to whom the accident occurs are generally advanced in life, and consequently the process of repair is feeble and slow.

The head of the bone receives its supply of blood chiefly through the neck and reflected capsule, and when both are severed, the small amount furnished by the round ligament is found to be insufficient.

When the fragments are once displaced, it is difficult, as I have already explained, if not impossible, to replace them.

The direction of the fracture is generally such that the ends of the fragments do not properly support and sustain each other when they are in apposition.

The fracture is at a point where the most powerful muscles in the body, acting with great advantage, tend to displace the broken ends.

Aged persons, who are chiefly the subjects of this accident, do not bear well the necessary confinement, and especially as the union requires generally a longer time than the union of any other fracture; so that a persistence in the attempt to confine the patient the requisite time often causes death.

Whether the absence of provisional callus as a bond of union, and the interposition of synovial fluid between the ends of the fragments, constitute additional obstacles, I am not fully prepared to say. In the opinion of many surgeons these circumstances constitute very serious, if not the chief, obstacles.

It remains only to consider what is the usual result of this fracture.

The fragments, more or less displaced, undergo various changes. The acetabular fragment is generally rapidly absorbed as far as the head, and occasionally a considerable portion of this latter disappears also; while the trochanteric fragment appears rather as if it had been

Fig. 113.

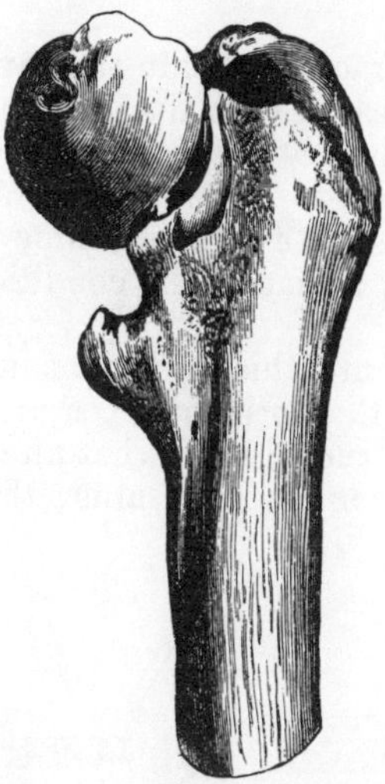

Fracture of cervix femoris within capsule. Ununited. Opposite surfaces irregularly convex and concave, and polished; moving slightly upon each other. (From a specimen in the possession of Dr. Crosby.)

Fig. 114.

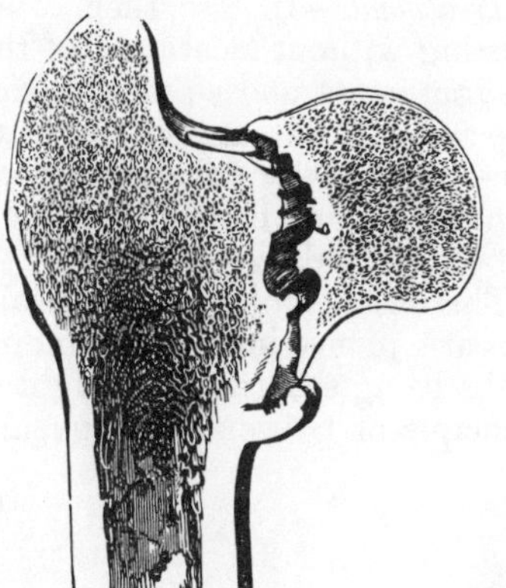

Mayo's specimen. United by ligament. Patient lived nine months after the accident. The trochanter minor arrested the descent of the head. (From Sir A. Cooper.)

flattened out by pressure and friction, it having gained as much generally in thickness as it has lost in length. To this observation, however, there will be found many exceptions. Sometimes the trochanteric fragment forms an open, shallow socket, into which the acetabular fragment is received; or its extremity may be irregularly convex and concave, to correspond with an exactly opposite condition of the acetabular fragment. (Fig. 113.)

Ordinarily the two fragments move upon each other, without the intervention of any substance; but often they become united, more or less completely, by fibrous bands (Fig. 114), which bands may be short or long, according to the amount of motion which has been maintained between the fragments while they were forming, or to the degree of separation which exists.

The capsular ligaments are usually considerably thickened and elongated in certain directions, and not unfrequently penetrated by spiculæ of bone. They are also found sometimes attached by firm bands to the acetabular fragment.

A permanent shortening, either with or without eversion of the limb, are the invariable consequences of this accident. Indeed, not a few succumb rapidly to the injury, perishing from a low, irritative fever, or from gradual exhaustion, within a month or two from the time of its occurrence. Says Robert Smith: "Our prognosis, in cases of fracture of the neck of the femur, must always be unfavorable. In many instances the injury soon proves fatal, and in all the functions of the limb are forever impaired; no matter whether the fracture has taken place within or external to the capsule—whether it has united by ligament or bone—shortening of the limb and lameness are the inevitable results."

Treatment.—In case, then, of a complete fracture within the capsule, existing without laceration of the reflected capsule, or displacement of the fragments, and equally in case of a fracture at the same point with impaction, the treatment ought to be directed to the retention of the bone in place, by suitable mechanical means, for a length of time sufficient to insure bony union, or for as long a time as the condition of the patient will warrant.

The means which are best calculated to fulfil this important indication are, in my judgment, complete rest in the horizontal posture, the limbs being secured in straight splints constructed somewhat after the principle of Gibson's improvement of Hagedorn's apparatus; that is,

Fig. 115.

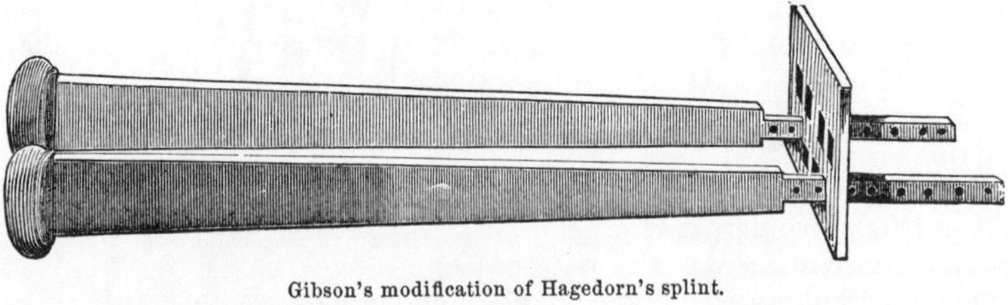

Gibson's modification of Hagedorn's splint.

the sound limb being first secured to the foot-board, and the broken limb subsequently brought down to the same point. In this way we may dispense with the perineal band as a means of counter-extension, which is so painful, indeed insupportable often, when the fracture is at the neck, the hip of the broken limb being prevented from descending by the lateral pressure of the two long splints. This apparatus possesses also this advantage, namely, that it presses the broken fragments more firmly against each other, and thus operates to prevent their displacement in the direction of the axis of the shaft.

Fig. 116.

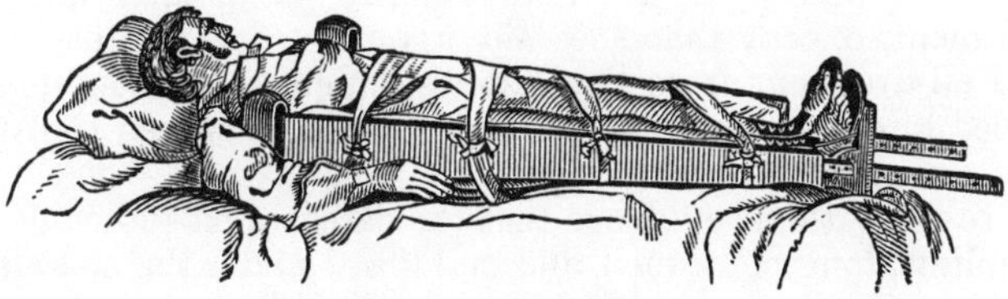

Gibson's splint applied.

In treating this fracture, supposing no displacement to exist, no extension beyond that which is necessary to insure perfect quiet can be proper, inasmuch as the fragments are not overlapped; and they need only a moderate assistance to enable them to maintain their position against the action of the muscles. Moreover, if the fragments are impacted, violent extension would disengage them and render their displacement and non-union inevitable.

Of course no side splints are necessary, but both limbs should be secured through their whole length to the long lateral splints, and properly supported by junks and pads.

I am prepared to affirm, from my own experience, that more patients will endure quietly this position for a length of time than the flexed position, whether in this latter the patient is placed upon his side or upon his back.

How long the patient will submit to this, or to any other mode of securing perfect rest, is very uncertain, and the decision of this question must rest with the individual cases and the good sense of the surgeon. Not very many old and feeble people will bear such confinement many days without presenting such palpable signs of failure as to demand their complete abandonment.

A mode of treatment similar to this was adopted in Jones' case, and also in the case reported by Fawdington, and is said to have been successful. In Brulatour's case the limb was kept extended two months; in Mussey's second case Hartshorne's straight splint for extension remained upon the limb eighty-four days; in Bryant's case a long splint was used "some weeks."

It is true, however, that other plans of treatment seem to have been equally successful. In the case reported by Adams the limb was placed over a double inclined plane, made of pillows, five weeks; and in Mussey's third example the limb remained in the same position three months. Chorley laid his patient upon the sound side, with the thighs flexed, for a space of two weeks, and then turned him upon his back, still keeping the thighs flexed. At the end of six weeks he was placed in the straight position, &c.

But in a majority of the examples reported, the existence of the fracture was either not suspected, or bony union was not anticipated or desired, consequently no treatment, having in view the confinement of the broken bone, was adopted. Yet the success was as great as that which has followed from either of the other plans. Harris' patient was simply laid on a sofa. Field's patient, who broke the neck of both femurs within the capsule at different times, was in each case left without treatment, except that she laid upon her bed. Mussey himself removed all dressings from Dr. Dalton's patient on the eighteenth day, and placed him upon his feet, and Dr. Wakelee removed the apparatus from his mother on the fifth day.

Nor are we without evidence that the careful and judicious application of splints, long continued, and employed under the most favorable circumstances, will sometimes fail. The two following cases confirm these remarks. The first occurred in the practice of Dr. James R. Wood, of the city of New York: "M. J., a young lady, æt. 16 years; of vigorous constitution; perfectly free from any constitutional taint either of scrofula, syphilis, or cancer; was caught between the wheels of two carriages, the one stationary, the other in motion. The blow was received directly on the trochanter major of the right side. The symptoms which presented themselves showed conclusively that there was a fracture. There was shortening, loss of voluntary motion, and eversion; by placing the finger on the trochanter major, and the thumb in the groin, a well-marked crepitus could be felt on extension and rotation being made. There was no laceration or other complication of the injury. She was placed on Amesbury's splint, with side splints accurately adjusted, and every precaution taken to insure a perfect union. The limb was kept on this splint without being disturbed for six weeks. At the end of that time, it was taken from the splint and examined with care. The signs of fracture still remained; the limb was replaced on the splint, and the dressings as before; everything was attended to in the general management of the case which the doctor thought would be conducive to perfect union. The patient was kept for three weeks longer on the splint, which was then removed. It was found that there was no union. Patient lived for three years, and was so lame that she was always obliged to use a crutch in walking. At the expiration of three years she died of an acute disease.

"On examination of the cervix femoris, it was found that there had been a transverse fracture of the bone just at the junction of the head and neck. The head of the bone was still attached to the acetabulum by the ligamentum teres. The process of absorption had been going on, and the head of the bone had already been absorbed below the level of the acetabulum, and what remained was soft and spongy, easily broken with the handle of the scalpel. The neck of the bone was rounded off, and covered with a fibrous deposit. This was not a case of diastasis, as has been suggested by an eminent surgeon, who judged simply from the age of the patient. She was full sixteen when the accident happened, and over nineteen when she died."

The second was in the person of a man, æt. 25 years, who was at the time of the accident robust and in good health: "He was dancing at his sister's wedding; while cutting a pigeon wing, he struck the foot upon which he was resting from under him, and fell, striking directly upon the trochanter major. He was unable to rise; a carriage was called and he was taken directly to the New York Hospital. There he came under the charge of Dr. J. Kearney Rodgers. A fracture was immediately diagnosticated, and for a few days he was kept on the double inclined plane. The straight splint was then used, and the dressings kept up for six weeks; at the end of that time they were taken off and the limb examined; there was no union. The limb was continued in the straight splints for three weeks longer, and again examined—there was still no union. The patient was again replaced in the straight splint for two weeks longer, but no union occurred. At the end of three months from his admission he was discharged; he was in good health, but so lame that he was obliged to use two crutches in walking. After his discharge the patient became very intemperate; and, in the course of a few weeks he applied for admission to Bellevue Hospital. He was much debilitated, and had an exhausting diarrhœa. Shortly after his admission, an immense abscess formed over the joint, which discharged profusely. The man died shortly after from exhaustion, and the specimen came into Dr. Van Buren's hands, the patient having been in his service. Dr. Van Buren was aware of the patient's previous history, the treatment, etc., at the New York Hospital, and a careful examination was made.

"The capsular ligament was destroyed entirely by the suppurative process; there was a formation of callus upon the trochanter major; the ligamentum teres was entirely absorbed; the head of the bone was spongy, as if worm eaten; the direction of the fracture was oblique, commencing just at the articulating surface of the head and ending just within the capsule; the upper end of the shaft of the bone showed this same appearance that was marked in the head. These points are beautifully shown in the specimen at the present time. The opinion of Charles E. Isaacs, M. D., the able Demonstrator of Anatomy of the University Medical College, is, that this fracture was entirely within the capsule."[1] The bone may be seen in the museum of Prof. Wm. H. Van Buren, of the University Medical College, New York.

Such equal results from opposite plans, and unequal results from similar plans of treatment, are not calculated to increase our faith in the testimony which most of the foregoing examples are supposed to furnish of the possibility of bony union. On the contrary, they cannot fail to suggest a doubt as to whether some of them, at least, were not inaccurately diagnosticated.

But admitting that they were not, the testimony which they furnish in relation to treatment is too inconclusive to be made available for instruction, and we are still at liberty to adopt that which seems most rational, without reference to the experience of others.

The reasons why I would prefer Hagedorn's plan, have already been

[1] Johnson, op. cit. pp. 13–15.

stated in part, to which I will now add, that if an error should occur in the diagnosis—if it should prove finally to have been a fracture without the capsule, then this treatment would be correct, and no injury would come to the patient from the error in diagnosis; but if we adopt Sir Astley Cooper's suggestion, namely, to get the patient upon crutches as soon as possible, perhaps as soon as fourteen days, an error in diagnosis might be followed by the most disastrous consequences.

I ought to add, that if this plan for any reason is found inconvenient or inapplicable, nothing which I have seen will prove so comfortable and available an alternative as the fracture bed, invented by Dr. Daniels, of New York.

(b.) *Neck of the Femur without the Capsule.*

Causes.—Like fractures within the capsule, these also occur most frequently in advanced life; age may therefore be regarded as the grand predisposing cause.

As to the immediate causes, we have already mentioned in the preceding section that fractures without the capsule seem to be the result generally of falls or of blows received directly upon the trochanter; occasionally, also, they are produced by falls upon the feet or upon the knees.

Pathology.—These fractures may occur at any point external to the capsule, but generally the line of fracture is at the base, corresponding very nearly with the anterior and posterior inter-trochanteric crests. Almost invariably the acetabular penetrates the trochanteric fragment in such a manner as to split the latter into two or more pieces. The direction of the lesions in the outer fragments preserves also a remark-

Fig. 117.

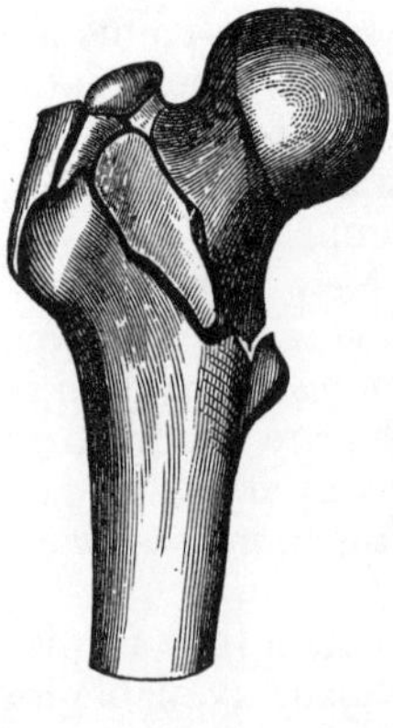

Fig. 118.

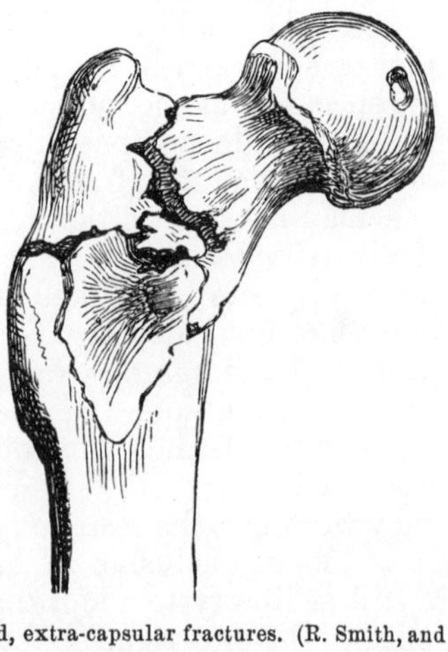

Fig. 119.

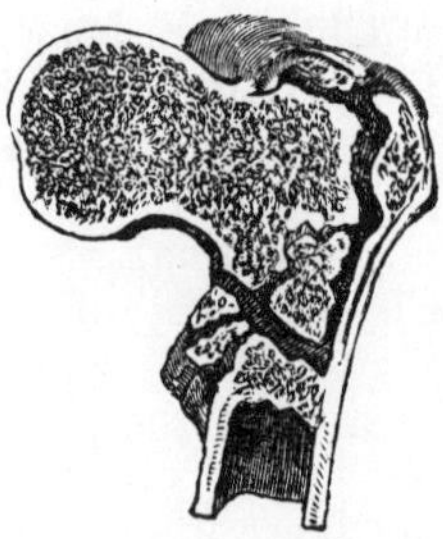

Impacted, extra-capsular fractures. (R. Smith, and Erichsen.)

able uniformity; the trochanter major being usually divided from near the centre of its summit, obliquely downwards and forwards toward its base, and the line of fracture terminating a little short of the trochanter minor, or penetrating beneath its base; while one or two lines of fracture usually traverse the trochanter major horizontally.

In an examination of more than twenty specimens, I have noticed but two or three exceptions to the general rules above stated.

In Dr. Mütter's collection, specimen marked B 115 is not accompanied with either impaction or splitting of the trochanteric fragment; but the neck having been broken close to the inter-trochanteric lines, has, apparently, slid down upon the shaft about one inch, at which point it is firmly united by bone.

Dr. Neill has also a specimen of fracture at the same point, but without union of any kind, in which no traces remain of a fracture of the trochanters. The acetabular fragment has moved up and down upon the trochanteric until it has worn for itself a shallow socket three inches and a half long; the approximated surfaces being smooth and polished like ivory.

The trochanter major is usually turned backwards, the shaft of the femur being rotated in this direction, the same as is usually observed in other fractures of the neck of the femur. I have seen one exception to this general rule in a specimen belonging to Dr. Mütter (No. 29); the trochanter in this instance is turned forwards, so that the neck is shorter in front than behind.

The upper fragments of the trochanter major, whenever the lines of fracture are transverse, are generally inclined inwards toward the neck, as if displaced in this direction by the force of the blow, or perhaps by the resistance offered by certain muscles and ligamentous bands which find an insertion upon its summit.

The neck is found, in most cases, standing inwards at nearly a right angle with the shaft, the head being much more depressed than the outer extremity of the neck, in consequence of which the lower margin of its broken extremity is driven much deeper into the trochanteric fragment than is the upper margin.

Malgaigne believes that impaction with consequent fracture of the trochanters, is never absent in true extra-capsular fractures, unless it be in that very unusual variety in which the trochanter forms a part of the inner fragment (fractures through the trochanter major and base of the neck). Robert Smith entertains the same opinion, although Malgaigne does not seem to have so understood him. I cannot agree, however, with either of these gentlemen that the rule is so invariable, since I am confident that no such splitting has occurred in either of the two specimens to which I have referred as belonging respectively to Drs. Mütter and Neill. It is true these are both old fractures, and to some extent the signs of fracture may have become obliterated, but in Mütter's specimen an abundant callus indicates plainly enough where the shaft separated from the neck, while the trochanter major is smooth as in its normal condition, nor does its summit incline either way from its usual position. Neill's specimen, though less satisfactory, does not fail to convince me that neither impaction nor splitting of the trochanters ever occurred.

It is certain, however, that impaction and comminution of the outer fragment are very constant, and that, whether the fracture is produced by a fall upon the feet or upon the trochanter major. But the impaction does not necessarily continue; sometimes, indeed, it does, and the position of the limb, whatever it may be at the moment, remains unalterably fixed; either very little or considerably shortened, according to the degree of impaction; rotated outwards or inwards, or in neither direction, perhaps, according to the direction of the force and of the fracture. In other cases, owing to the extreme comminution, and to the wide separation of the trochanteric fragments, or to the contraction of the muscles inserted into the top of the femur, or to the weight of the body in attempts to walk, or to injudicious handling on the part of the surgeon, such as forcible rotation, by which the neck is made to act as a lever, and to actually pry the fragments apart, or to violent extension, by which the impaction is overcome—owing to some one or several of these causes it often happens that the fragments separate, and the leg becomes immediately more shortened, movable, and more inclined to rotate outwards.

Symptoms.—The symptoms which indicate a fracture of the neck of the femur without the capsule, are pain, mobility, crepitus, shortening and eversion of the limb. The trochanter major is not as prominent as upon the opposite side, and it rotates upon a shorter axis. There are also several other signs to which I shall refer when considering the differential diagnosis.

The pain and tenderness, accompanied sometimes with swelling and discoloration, are situated chiefly in front of the neck of the bone.

Mobility exists in a majority of cases, even when the fragments are impacted; that is, the limb can be moved pretty easily in any direction by the surgeon, but not without producing pain or provoking muscular spasms, yet the patient himself is unable to move the limb by his own volition, or he can only move it slightly.

Crepitus is present whenever there exists a moderate but not complete impaction. It is also present generally when, the trochanteric fragment having been extensively comminuted and loosened, the impaction becomes excessive; and it is only absent when the impaction is such that the fragments are completely and firmly locked into each other.

A shortening is inevitable, at least in all cases accompanied with either temporary or permanent impaction, and we have seen that one of these conditions seldom fails. According to Sir Astley Cooper the shortening varies from half an inch to three-quarters of an inch, but Robert Smith has established the following distinction. When the fracture is extra-capsular and impacted, that is, when it remains impacted, the shortening is only moderate, varying from one quarter of an inch to one inch and a half; in fourteen cases measured by him the average was a fraction over three-quarters of an inch; but when it does not remain impacted it ranges from one inch to two inches and a half; indeed, Mr. Smith mentions one example in which the shortening reached four inches, and forty-two cases gave an average shortening of something more than one inch and a quarter.

Eversion of the toes is very constant; but in a few instances upon record the toes have been found turned in, or even directed forwards. In the specimen referred to as being found in Dr. Mütter's collection, with an inward or forward rotation of the trochanter major, the same relative position of the whole limb must have existed.

Fig. 120.

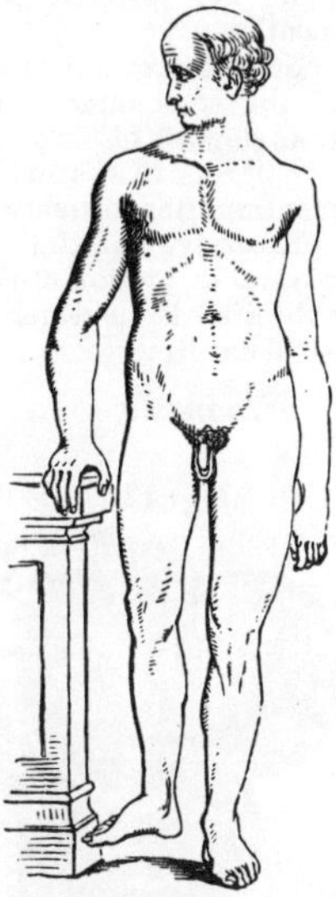

Fracture of the neck of the femur. (Fergusson.)

The trochanter major usually seems depressed or driven in, and, when the two main fragments are completely separated, if the limb is rotated, the trochanter will be found to turn almost upon its own axis, or upon a very short radius.

In enumerating the signs of extra-capsular fracture, it will be seen that I have, with only slight variations, repeated the signs of a fracture within the capsule. It will become necessary, therefore, to indicate, as far as possible, a differential diagnosis. And without pretending that all of the differential signs which I shall enumerate are thoroughly established, or that in every case, even after a careful grouping of all the symptoms, a satisfactory diagnosis can be made out, I shall state briefly my own conclusions, or, rather, what seem to me to be the probable facts.

SIGNS OF A FRACTURE WITHIN THE CAPSULE.	SIGNS OF A FRACTURE WITHOUT THE CAPSULE.
Produced by slight violence.	Produced by greater violence.
A fall upon the foot or knee, or a trip upon the carpet, &c.	A fall upon the trochanter major.
Generally over fifty years of age.	Often under fifty years of age.
More frequent in females.	Relative frequency in males or females not established.
Pain, tenderness and swelling less, and deeper.	Pain, swelling, and tenderness greater and more superficial. It is especially painful to press upon and around the trochanter.
(The two following measurements to be made from the anterior superior spinous process of the ilium to the inner condyle of the femur.)	
Shortening at first less than in extra-capsular fractures, often not any.	Shortening at first greater, almost always some.
Shortening after a few days or weeks greater than in extra-capsular fractures; sometimes this takes place suddenly, as when the limb is moved, or the patient steps upon it.	Shortening after a few days or weeks less than in intra-capsular fractures. That is, the amount of shortening changes but little, if at all; if the impaction continues, not at all; if it does not continue it may shorten more.
Measuring from the top of the trochanter to the inner condyle or to the malleolus internus the femur is not shortened.	Measuring from the top of the trochanter to the inner condyle or to the malleolus internus the femur may be found a little shortened.
More mobility of limb, at joint.	Less mobility.
Trochanter major moves upon a longer radius.	Trochanter major moves upon a shorter radius.

25

SIGNS OF A FRACTURE WITHIN THE CAPSULE.—(*Continued.*)	SIGNS OF A FRACTURE WITHOUT THE CAPSULE.—(*Continued.*)
If the patient recovers the use of the limb, not restored under three or four months.	If the patient recovers the use of the limb, restored in six or eight weeks.
No enlargement or apparent expansion of the trochanter major, after recovery, from deposit of bony callus.	Enlargement or irregular expansion of trochanter, which may be felt sometimes distinctly through the skin and muscles.
Progressive wasting of the limb for many months after recovery.	The limb preserving its natural strength and size.
Excessive halting, accompanied with a peculiar motion of the pelvis, such as is exhibited in persons who walk with an artificial limb.	Slight halt, motions of hip natural.

Prognosis.—In attempting to establish the differential diagnosis we have necessarily been led to consider most of the essential points of prognosis. Very little, therefore, remains to be said upon this subject.

Fig. 121.

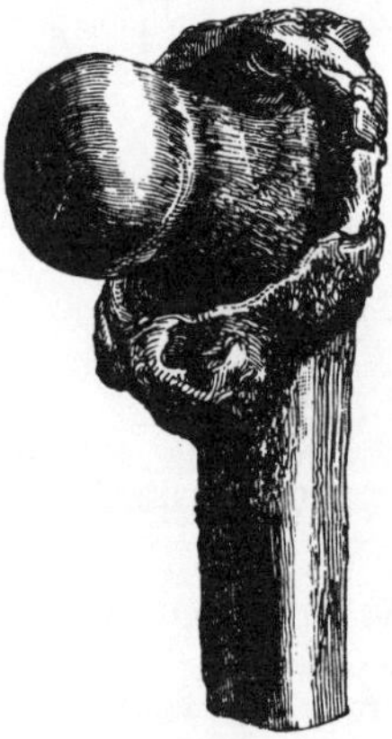

Fracture of neck without the capsule. (Erichsen.)

Union generally occurs as rapidly in this fracture as in fractures of the shaft, and, perhaps, even sometimes more promptly, owing to the existence of impaction.

But whether it occurs promptly or slowly, or, indeed, if it does not occur at all, a remarkable deposit of ossific matter almost invariably takes place along the inter-trochanteric lines, where the bone has separated from the shaft, and also, not unfrequently, along the lines of the other fractures of the trochanter.

This deposit is no less remarkable for its abundance than for its irregularity, long spines of bone often rising up toward the pelvis and forming a kind of knobby or spiculated crown, within which the acetabular fragment reposes.

Fig. 122.

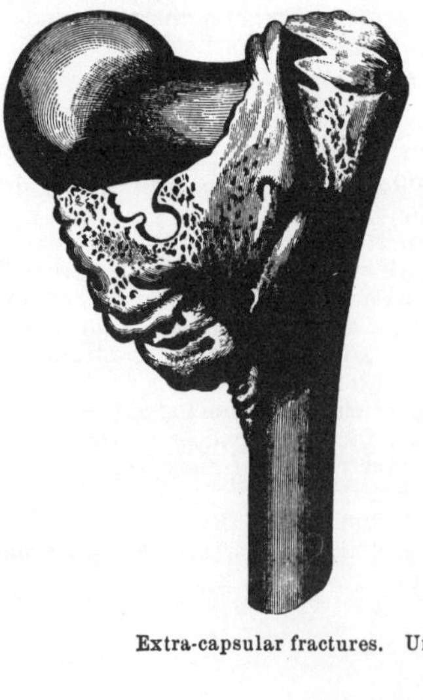

Fig. 123.

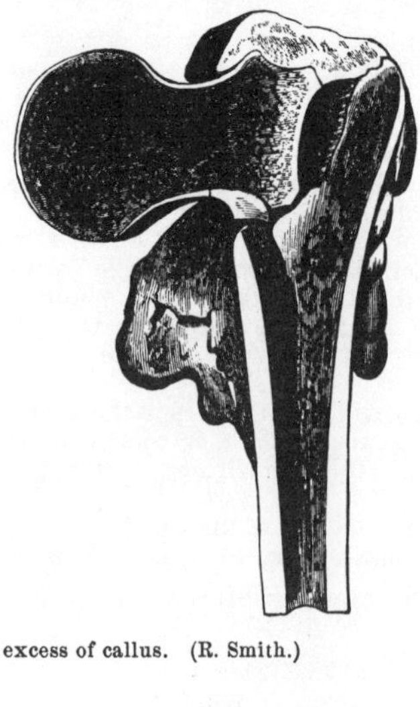

Extra-capsular fractures. Union with excess of callus. (R. Smith.)

Fig. 124.

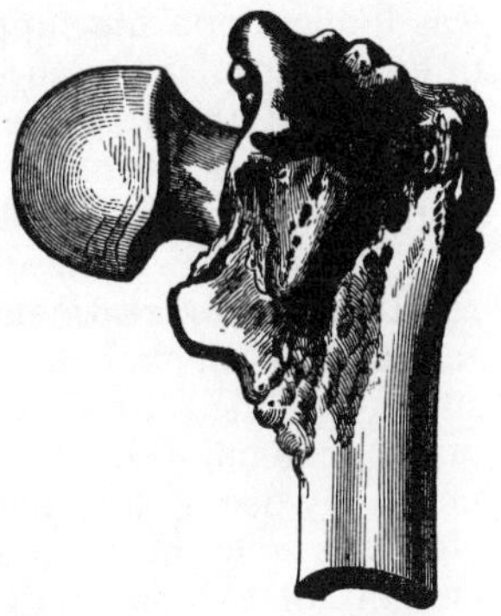

In a few instances these osteophites have reached even to the bones of the pelvis, and formed powerful abutments which seemed to prevent any farther displacement of the limb in this direction, and, by some writers, they have been supposed thus to fulfil a positive design. A sufficient explanation of their existence, however, we think can be found in the fact that they proceed entirely from the trochanteric fragment, whose extensive comminution and great vascularity would naturally lead to such results. The same, but in a less degree, has already been noticed as occurring in impacted fractures at the anatomical neck of the humerus, where certainly such bony abutments could not serve any useful purpose.

Treatment.—The same principles of treatment are applicable here as in fractures of the neck within the capsule; by which I mean to say that, as in all of those examples of fracture within the capsule where the relation of the fragments is such as to warrant a hope that a bony union may be consummated, namely, where the fragments are not displaced or are impacted, the straight splint, with only moderate extension, constitutes the most rational mode of treatment; so also in this fracture, whenever the fragments are impacted and remain impacted, a straight splint, employed only as a retentive apparatus, is the most suitable. It is only by employing this plan of treatment, which no one has yet shown to be inapplicable to either of these two varieties of accidents—I do not speak of the opinions which men may have entertained, but of the practical testimony—it is only, I say, by employing this uniform plan of treatment in both cases that those serious misfortunes to the patient can be avoided which would necessarily continue to occur if Sir Astley Cooper's advice was followed, namely, to allow the patient in the one case to dispense with splints wholly, and to get upon his crutches as soon as the condition of his limb and of his body will permit, when it is certain that in the other case some retentive apparatus is generally necessary. This conclusion is based upon the admitted difficulty of diagnosis. If, as is well understood, the diagnosis between these two varieties of fracture can seldom be made out satisfactorily during the life of the patient, then how shall we know in any given case which of the two plans to adopt. If we act upon the supposition that it is within the capsule, adopting Sir Astley Cooper's method, and it proves to have been a fracture without the capsule, we have, I fear, done irreparable injury to our patient. It is precisely here that this distinguished surgeon committed his great error, not in denying that certain specimens were fractures of the neck of the femur within the capsule united by bone, nor in constantly urging upon his contemporaries the improbability of such an event, but in that while he admitted its possibility, he chose to recommend a plan of treatment which was unlikely to insure such a union, and which, in the uncertainty if not impossibility of diagnosis, was liable, upon his supposed authority, to be adopted in many cases of extra-capsular fractures.

Again, if the fracture be extra-capsular and not impacted, or the impaction has been, for any cause, overcome; or, if the fracture be intra-capsular and not impacted, or if the capsule is lacerated and the fragments are in consequence displaced; then again no injury need result from the treatment, if we adopt the straight splint with moderate extension, such as may be obtained from the use of Hagedorn's splint modified by Gibson. That it is not impacted we may know often, or generally, by the amount of displacement, although we may not easily decide whether the fracture is within or without the capsule. Now the amount of shortening will determine, properly enough, the amount of extension to be employed. In either case we shall not employ, because the patient will not permit, as much extension as in fractures of the shaft; and while in the one case we shall only gain a shorter and firmer ligamentous union, in the other we shall insure a better and more speedy bony union.

Fig. 125.

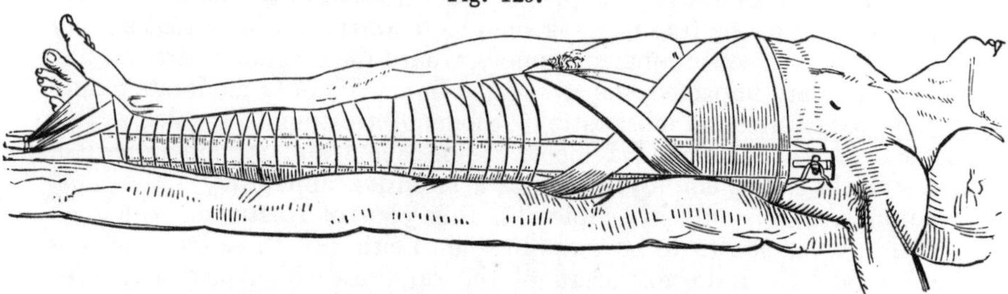

Miller's splint for extıa-capsular fractures. (From Miller.)

If any surgeon, acting upon the suggestions here made, shall confine a feeble or an aged person in the horizontal posture, and in a straight splint until the powers of nature have become exhausted, and death ensues, as our readers have already been admonished may happen, we are not to be held responsible for his want of judgment or of skill. We have advised this plan of treatment only for so long a period as the condition of the patient renders it entirely safe. No doubt, then, in a large number of cases it will have to be abandoned very early, and in not an inconsiderable proportion all constraint will be plainly inadmissible *from the beginning;* and it is for such examples that the treatment recommended by Sir Astley Cooper for all intra-capsular fractures, ought to be reserved.

(c.) *Fractures of the Neck partly within and partly without the Capsule.*

It is scarcely necessary to say that the line of fracture through the neck of the femur may be such, that it shall be in part within and in part without the capsule; and such fractures will be even more difficult to diagnosticate than either of those forms of which we have just spoken. The symptoms will be mainly, however, those which characterize fractures within the capsule, while the treatment ought to be such as we would adopt in those fractures which are wholly without the capsule. The chances for bony union are increased in proportion as the line of separation extends outside of the capsule, and we ought to be diligent in our efforts, if we have made ourselves certain that the fracture is partly extra-capsular, to secure a good bony union; a result which experience has shown may be reasonably anticipated.

The necessity for some extension, and of a firm retentive apparatus in this form of fracture, furnishes another argument in favor of the employment of the same means in fractures wholly within the capsule. We shall thus avoid the mischief which might arise from mistaking a fracture of the character of which we are now speaking, for a fracture wholly within the capsule.

§ 2. Fracture through the Trochanter Major and Base of the Neck of the Femur.

This fracture, which Sir Astley Cooper calls a "fracture of the femur through the trochanter major,"[1] passes obliquely upwards and outwards from the lower portion of the neck, but instead of traversing the neck completely, it penetrates the base of the trochanter major; the line of fracture being such as to separate the femur into two fragments, one of which is composed of the head, neck and trochanter major, and the other of the shaft with the remaining portions of the femur.

The following two examples are all in relation to which we possess any positive information, or in which the diagnosis has been confirmed by an autopsy. The first is thus related by Sir Astley Cooper.

"The first case of this kind I ever saw, was in St. Thomas's Hospital, about the year 1786. It was supposed to be a fracture of the neck of the thigh-bone within the capsule, and the limb was extended over a pillow rolled under the knee, with splints on each side of the limb, by Mr. Cline's direction. An ossific union succeeded, with scarcely any deformity, excepting that the foot was somewhat everted, and the man walked extremely well. When he was to be discharged from the hospital, a fever attacked him, of which he died; and upon dissection, the fracture was found through the trochanter major, and the bone was united with very little deformity, so that his limb would have been equally useful as before."[2]

The second example is reported by Mr. Stanley.

"A woman, in her sixtieth year, fell in the street and injured her right hip. On examination, the limb was found slightly everted, and shortened to the extent of three-quarters of an inch, but movable in every direction. The extremity of the shaft of the femur was in its natural situation; but behind the femur, and at a little distance from it, a bony prominence was discovered, resting upon the ilium, toward the great sciatic notch, strongly resembling the head of the femur. Various opinions were entertained as to the nature of the injury, some

[1] Sir Astley Cooper, op. cit., p. 183. [2] Op. cit., p. 184.

believing it to be dislocation, and others a fracture. After a confinement of several months to her bed, the woman was sufficiently recovered to walk with the assistance of a crutch, and in this state she continued till her death, which took place about three years after the accident, during the whole of which period I had watched the progress of the case. Having obtained permission to examine the seat of the injury, I ascertained that there had been a fracture extending obliquely through the trochanter major, and through the basis of the neck into the shaft of the femur, and that the prominence which had been mistaken for the head of the bone was occasioned by the posterior and larger portion of the trochanter drawn backwards toward the ischiatic notch."[1]

Sir Astley relates three other examples in which he believes the fractures to have been of the character above described; and he details the peculiar plans of treatment which, in each case, he saw fit to recommend. I can see no reason, however, why the treatment need differ from that which has already been recommended for fractures of the neck, since the indications are nearly identical in all of these cases; namely, moderate extension, and steady support of the limb in its natural position.

§ 3. Fracture of the Epiphysis of the Trochanter Major.

So far as I know, the only well-authenticated example of this accident is the one reported by Mr. Key to Sir Astley Cooper.[2] The subject of this case was a girl, aged about sixteen years, who fell, March 15, 1822, upon the side-walk, and struck her trochanter violently against the curb-stone. She arose, and, without much pain or difficulty, walked home. On the 20th she was received into Guy's Hospital, and the limb was examined by Mr. Key. The right leg, which was the one injured, was considerably everted, and appeared to be about half an inch longer than the sound limb. It could be moved in all directions, but abduction gave her considerable pain. She had perfect command over all the muscles, except the rotators inwards. No crepitus could be detected. Four days after admission she died, having succumbed to the irritative fever which followed the injury.

The autopsy disclosed a fracture through the base of the trochanter major, but without laceration of the tendinous expansions which cover the outside of this process, so that no displacement of the epiphysis had occurred, nor could it be moved, except to a small extent upwards and downwards. A considerable collection of pus was found also below and in front of the trochanter.

The absence of displacement in the fragment, with its peculiar and limited motion, sufficiently explained why the fracture could not be detected during life.

In the eighth volume of the *Transactions of the Medical and Physical Society of Calcutta* (1835), J. Clarke, Esq., reports a case of comminuted

[1] Stanley, Med.-Chir. Trans., vol. xiii.

[2] Sir Astley Cooper on Dislocations and Fractures, etc., Amer. ed., 1851, p. 192.

fracture of the trochanter major, which has been mentioned by Malgaigne as an example of simple fracture of the trochanter; but, after reading the case carefully, I cannot avoid the conclusion that it was an example of fracture of the neck without the capsule, accompanied with impaction and extensive comminution. "Extravasation," says Mr. Clarke, "was discovered within the capsular ligament and around the trochanter major; and, on clearing away the muscles, the trochanter was found crushed and shattered, several pieces entirely detached, and fissures extending deeply into the shaft of the bone."[1]

I shall venture to express the same opinion in relation to the case reported by Bransby Cooper.[2] The diagnosis was not confirmed by an autopsy, and the testimony drawn from Mr. Cooper's account of the case is far from being, to my mind, conclusive. It may, indeed, have been a simple fracture of the epiphysis; but there is nothing in the narrative to render it improbable that there existed also an impacted extra-capsular fracture of the neck.

I have also myself reported one example of this fracture as having come under my own observation,[3] but of which I wish now to speak somewhat less confidently. The patient, James Redwick, a travelling showman, æt. 23, fell, in August, 1848, from a high wagon, striking upon his left hip. When he got upon his feet, he found himself unable to walk, and was carried to his room. Dr. Wilcox, of this city, was called to see him, and applied a long straight splint. Fourteen days after the accident I saw the patient with Dr. Wilcox. The thigh was not appreciably shortened, nor was there either eversion or inversion; but the epiphysis of the trochanter major was carried upwards toward the crest of the ilium half an inch, and slightly sent in. No crepitus could be detected. The splint was continued five weeks; and about a month after, I found the fragment in the same place, but he was able to walk with only a slight halt.

I think this also may have been an extra-capsular impacted fracture.

With the small amount of positive information which we possess in relation to this fracture, we might venture a few conjectures as to what would constitute its symptoms, or as to the probable results and the

Fig. 126.

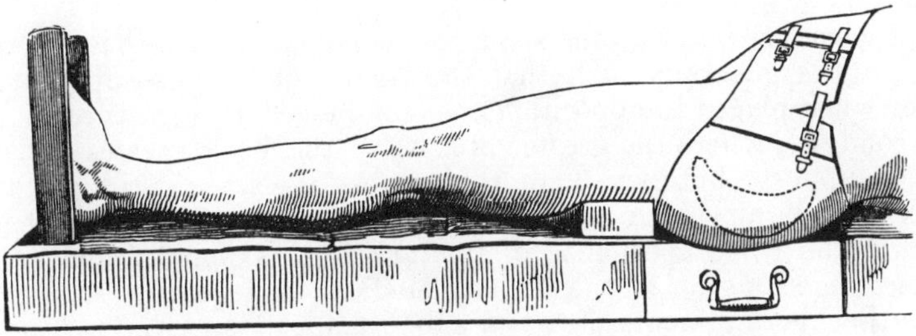

Sir Astley Cooper's mode of treating fractures of the trochanter major. (From A. Cooper)

[1] Clarke, Amer. Journ. Med. Sci., Nov. 1836, vol. ix. p. 181.
[2] B. Cooper, A. Cooper on Dislocations, &c., op. cit., p. 192.
[3] Hamilton, Trans. Amer. Med. Assoc., op. cit., vol. x. p. 254.

most suitable treatment; but we prefer to occupy ourselves with a simple statement of the facts, so far as they are known, leaving all mere speculative inferences to those who choose to make them.

§ 4. Fractures of the Shaft of the Femur.

Etiology.—Unless the fracture has taken place just above the condyles, or immediately below the trochanter minor, in a very large proportion of cases it has been produced by a direct blow, such as the passage of a loaded vehicle across the thigh, or the fall of a piece of timber directly upon it. An analysis of twenty-one cases, taken indiscriminately, presents three fractures immediately above the condyles, and these were all produced by falls upon the feet; but of the remaining eighteen, all of which occurred higher in the limb, only two were the result of falls upon the feet or of indirect blows, and one of these was a fracture just below the trochanter minor.

Pathology.—It has already been remarked that this bone is most frequently broken in its middle third: thus, of eighty-nine fractures of the shaft, eighteen occurred in the upper third, twenty-one in the lower third, and fifty in the middle third. I have made the same observation in an examination of specimens belonging to Dr. Mütter. In his cabinet, of twenty four fractures of the shaft, three belonged to the upper third, two to the lower, and nineteen to the middle third.

In the adult, these fractures are, with only an exceedingly rare exception, oblique; and the obliquity is generally greater than in the case of other bones. This fact, which it is very difficult to determine, in most cases, upon the living subject, I have established by a considerable number of observations made upon cabinet specimens. A transverse fracture is found only twice in Dr. Mussey's collection, containing thirty examples of fracture of the shaft; and in Dr. Mütter's collection, specimen B 71 is an adult femur, broken nearly transversely through its middle third; and it is united with a shortening of about one inch. Indeed, it is more common to find a transverse fracture in the middle third than at any other point of the bone; but in the upper third the obliquity is extreme and almost constant.

At whatever point of the shaft the bone is broken, the degree of obliquity is generally such that the fragments cannot support each other when placed in apposition; unless indeed the fracture is near the condyles, where the greater breadth of the bone creates an additional support; but even here, the cabinet specimens still present a striking obliquity with more or less overlapping. I believe that in each of the three specimens of fracture at this point found in the collection belonging to the Albany Medical College, the obliquity is such that the fragments were not supported, and an overlapping has taken place. In specimen 719 the fracture extends into the joint; and although it is united by bone, a shortening of about one inch has occurred.

In the case of children, and especially of infants, the rule is reversed;

the bone is either broken transversely or nearly transversely, or it is serrated or denticulated, so that complete lateral displacement is much less frequent.

The same remark is probably true of some fractures occurring in extreme old age; but as the shaft of the femur is not often broken in very old persons, owing to the readiness with which the neck yields to violence, I have not had any opportunity to verify this opinion.

The direction of the obliquity varies exceedingly, especially in the middle and upper thirds; in the middle third, however, it is generally downwards and inwards; but in the lower third, its direction is, with only rare exceptions, downwards and forwards, and the superior fragment is found lying in front of the inferior.

In one instance I have found both femurs broken at the same point, and in the same manner. Mr. L. Brittin, aged about fifty-five years, while employed upon a building, fell from a fourth story window upon the stone pavement below, striking upon his feet. In addition to several other fractures, I found both femurs broken obliquely downwards and forwards, just above the condyles. Very little inflammation ensued, and although it was found impossible to employ extension, union occurred readily, and with only a moderate overlapping. In the left limb, however, the upper fragment pressed down sufficiently to interfere somewhat with the patella, and the patient is unable now, after the lapse of several months, to straighten the knee completely. The motions of the right knee are unimpaired.

Fig. 127.

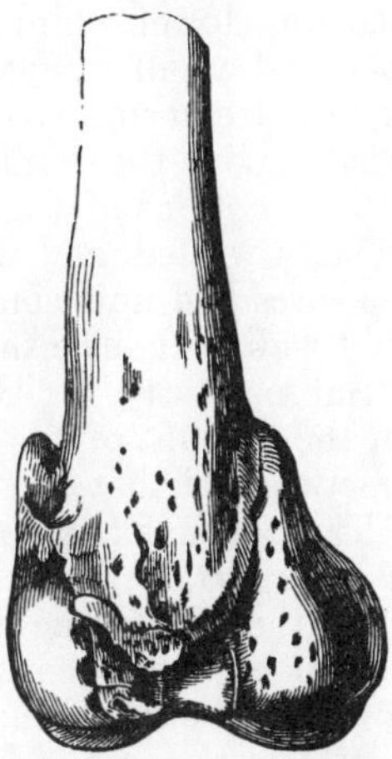

Fracture at base of condyles.

I have only once met with a fracture at this point, in which the line of separation was downwards and backwards. As the case presents several points of interest, it will be proper to narrate the facts somewhat at length.

George Taylor Aikin, of Lockport, N. Y., æt. 7. May 18, 1854, in jumping down a bank of about three feet in height, he broke the right thigh obliquely, just above the knee-joint. Direction of the fracture obliquely downwards and backwards.

Dr. G., an accomplished surgeon, residing in Lockport, was called. The limb was not then much swollen. He applied side splints, rollers, &c., carefully, and then laid the limb over a double inclined plane. The knee was elevated about six or eight inches. Before applying the splints, suitable extension had been made, and after completing the dressings, the two limbs seemed to be of the same length.

On the second or third day, Dr. G. noticed that the toes looked unnaturally white, and were cold.

Counsel was now called at the request of Dr. G., when it was determined to abandon all dressings and direct their efforts solely to saving the limb.

The result was that slowly a considerable portion of his foot died and sloughed away, leaving only the tarsal bones. The fracture united, but with considerable overlapping and deformity.

Feb. 26, 1856, the boy was brought to me by his father. On examining the fracture I noticed that the anterior line of the femur seemed nearly straight, and this appearance was owing in some degree to the muscles, which covered and concealed the bone, and in some degree, also, to the manner in which the fragments rested upon each other: the pointed superior end of the lower fragment resting snugly upon the front of the upper fragment, so that no abrupt angle existed in front. On the back of the limb, however, the lower end of the upper fragment, quite sharp, projected freely downwards and backwards into the popliteal space, so that its extreme point was only about half an inch above the line of the articulation. The limb had shortened one inch, and this enabled us to determine accurately that the lower point or the commencement of the fracture was one inch and a half above the articulation, while the point where the line of fracture terminated in front, was probably quite three inches and a half above the joint.

The motions of the knee-joint were pretty free. The leg was extremely wasted, and the anterior half of the foot having sloughed off, the sores had now completely healed over. He was able to walk tolerably well without either crutch or cane.

Subsequently, Dr. G. found it necessary to sue the father of the child for the amount of his services, when Mr. Aikin put in a plea of malpractice, and that consequently the services were without value.

The case was tried in the March term of the Niagara circuit of 1856, at Lockport, N. Y., the Hon. Benj. F. Greene presiding.

On the part of the defence it was claimed that the death of the foot was in consequence of the bandages being too tight. They failed, however, to show that they were extraordinarily or unduly tight. While on the part of Dr. G., the prosecutor, it was shown that the death of the toes was preceded by a total loss of color, and that it was not accompanied with either venous or arterial congestion. The medical gentlemen examined as witnesses, declared that this circumstance furnished the most positive evidence which could be desired, that the death of the toes was not due to the tightness of the bandages, but that its cause must be looked for in an arrest of the arterial or nervous currents supplying the limb, or in both. They believed, also, that the projection of the superior fragment into the popliteal space was sufficient to cause this arrest. They also believed that overlapping and consequent projection could not have been prevented in this case, and that, therefore, the treatment was not responsible for this unfortunate result: indeed, they regarded the treatment as correct, and the result as a triumph of skill, in that any portion of the limb was saved; the leg and foot now remaining being far more useful than any artificial leg and foot could be.

The Hon. Judge, in a speech remarkable for its clearness and liberality, sought to impress upon the jury the value of the medical testimony. The jury returned a verdict for Dr. G., allowing the amount of his claim for services, with the costs of suit.

Specimen 121, in Dr. March's collection at Albany, presents a similar disposition of the fragments. The fracture is oblique, from above downwards and backwards, and the upper portion lies behind the lower. It is firmly united by bone, but with an overlapping of from two and a half to three inches. The young gentleman who showed me the specimen remarked that it had been found impossible, owing to an ulcer upon the heel, and to other causes, to employ in the treatment any degree of extension.

These two are the only examples which have come under my observation in which a fracture at this point has taken this direction.

Sir Astley Cooper does not seem to have recognized this form of fracture and displacement. Amesbury has, however, recorded one case, which came under his own observation, where, although the bloodvessels and nerves escaped, the bone projected through the skin in the ham, and finally exfoliated.[1] And he thinks the point of bone may sometimes so penetrate the artery and injure the nerves as to render amputation necessary, in order to save the life of the patient.

M. Coural also has related a case in which an epiphysary disjunction, occurring in a child twelve years old, was attended with a displacement of the upper fragment backwards, and amputation became necessary.[2]

I know of no other cases of this rare accident which have been reported. Lonsdale refers to it as "the rarest direction for a fracture to take;" and thinks that in case of its occurrence, the vessels in the popliteal space will stand a chance of being wounded; but he mentions no example. The popliteal artery hugs the bone so closely at this point, that a displacement of the upper fragment in a direction downwards and backwards must always greatly endanger its integrity. Indeed, it is here that the artery and vein are in the closest contact with each other, and with the bone; an anatomical fact, which has been used by Richerand and others to explain the greater frequency of aneurisms in the ham.

The direction of the displacement, however, in fractures of the shaft of the femur, does not always depend upon the direction of the line of fracture. In fractures of the upper third, whatever may be the direction of the line of fracture, the lower end of the upper fragment inclines forwards and outwards, and the upper end of the lower fragment inwards; unless, indeed, this inclination is controlled by actual entanglement of the broken ends with each other.

In the middle third the fragments also generally take the same relative position, whatever may be the direction of the fracture; but when the fracture takes place at or near the condyles, where the diameter of the bone is much greater, the direction of the obliquity determines pretty uniformly the direction of the displacement.

Symptoms.—The symptoms which characterize a fracture of the shaft of the femur are those which are common to all fractures, namely, mobility, crepitus, displacement of the fragments, pain, and

[1] Remarks on Fractures, &c., by Joseph Amesbury, vol. i. p. 293. London, 1831.
[2] Archiv Gén. de Méd., tom. ix. p. 267.

swelling, to which are added generally a shortening of the limb, with eversion of the foot and leg.

Owing to the great amount of muscle covering the thigh, and sometimes to the swelling which immediately follows the injury, it is often very difficult to determine at what precise point the fracture has occurred, and still more difficult to say whether the fracture is oblique or transverse; indeed, this latter question is sometimes decided approximatively by a reference to the age of the patient rather than by the examination of the limb.

The immediate shortening varies from half an inch to an inch and a half, or even more, and it will average about one inch in the case of healthy adults.

Prognosis.—Whatever may have been the general opinion of experienced surgeons as to the question of shortening in other fractures, very few certainly have ever claimed that in fractures of the femur a complete restoration of the bone to its original length was generally to be expected. There seems, however, to have existed only certain vague and indefinite notions as to the proportion and amount of this shortening, and which have had for their basis nothing better than a few imperfectly analyzed observations.

Says Scultetus (quoting first from Hippocrates): "'For the bones of the thigh, though you do draw them out by force of extension, cannot be held so by any hands; but when the first intension slacks, they will run together again; for here the thick and strong flesh are above binding, and binding cannot keep them down.'—*Hippocrates de fract.* Which Celsus seems to confirm, *Lib.* 8, *cap.* 10, where he writes as follows of the cure of legs and thighs: 'For we must not be ignorant that if the thigh be broken, that it will be made shorter, because it never returns to its former state.' And Avicenna, *Lib.* 4, *Fen.* 5, saith 'that it is a rare thing for the thigh once broken, to be perfectly cured again.'

"These words admonish us," continues Scultetus, "that we should never promise a perfect cure of the thigh; but rather, using all diligence, we should foretell that it is doubtful that the patient will be always lame; but when this shall happen from the nature of the fracture, or which most frequently falls out, from the impatience of the sick person, it may be imputed to our mistake; and instead of a reward, bring us a disgrace."[1]

Says Chelius: "Fracture of the thigh-bone is always a severe accident, as the broken ends are retained in proper contact with great difficulty. The cure takes place most commonly with deformity and shortening of the limb, especially in oblique fractures, and those which occur in the upper and lower third of the thigh-bone. Compound fractures are so much more difficult to treat."[2]

Maclise, while commenting somewhat indefinitely upon certain plans of treatment, takes occasion to say: "Out of every six fractures of either clavicle or thigh-bone, I believe that as the result of our treatment by the present forms of mechanical contrivances, there would not be

[1] The Chirurgeon's Store-house, by Johannes Scultetus, a Famous Physician, and Chirurgeon of Ulme in Suevia. London, 1674.

[2] System of Surgery, by J. M. Chelius, translated, &c., by South. First Amer. ed., vol. i. p. 627, 1847. See also p. 625, paragraph 679.

found three cases of coaptation of the broken ends of the bone so complete as to do credit to the surgeon."[1]

Says John Bell: "The machine is not yet invented by which a fractured thigh-bone can be perfectly secured." And Benjamin Bell declares that "an effectual method of securing oblique fractures in the bones of the extremities, and especially of the thigh-bone, is perhaps one of the greatest desiderata in modern surgery." "In all ages," he adds, "the difficulty of this has been confessedly great; and frequent lameness produced by shortened limbs arising from this cause, evidently shows that we are still deficient in this branch of practice."[2]

Colles observes, that "although three or four methods of treatment are practised, the pieces at the conclusion are often found overlapped."[3] One reason for which, in his opinion, is a too blind adherence to the principles recommended by Pott.

Velpeau says, that "after fractures of the femur, there is no limping unless the shortening exceeds three-quarters of an inch; and the same is true if the shortening occurs in the tibia." The reason is, that the pelvis inclines toward the shorter limb, and thus compensates for the deficiency in length. In speaking of the various contrivances for dressing the fractured femur, he remarks that "most of them fail to obviate the shortening, and produce eschars, anchylosis, or troublesome arrests of the circulation. This is the price that is usually paid for the employment of these complicated machines, and a shortening of a quarter to three-quarters of an inch is not avoided after all. The simplest apparatus that will maintain the adjustment of the fractured femur, so that union may take place with shortening of only half an inch, is the best."[4]

Nélaton holds the following language:—

"A fracture of the body of the femur, with an adult, is always a grave accident, inasmuch as it demands so long a confinement to the bed, and especially on account of the shortening of the limb, which it is almost impossible wholly to prevent; accordingly, Boyer recommends to the surgeon, from the first day, to announce to the parents of the patient the possibility of this accident. With infants, on the contrary, it is almost always easy to avoid the shortening."[5]

While Malgaigne declares his opinion on this subject thus, at length:—

"When we do not succeed in drawing back the displaced fragments, end to end, so that they may oppose themselves to the action of the muscles, it is impossible to preserve to the member its normal length, whatever may be the appareil or method employed. Surgeons are not sufficiently agreed upon this question.

[1] Surgical Anatomy, by Joseph Maclise, Surgeon. First Amer. ed. Part I. p. 36, 1851.

[2] System of Surgery, by Benjamin Bell, vol. vii. p. 21. Edinburgh, 1801.

[3] Lectures on the Theory and Practice of Surgery, by Abraham Colles (Dublin), p. 321. Philadelphia ed., 1845.

[4] Peninsular Journ. of Med., vol. iii. p. 384; also Memphis Med. Journ., vol. iv. p. 254, 1856.

[5] Elémens de Pathologie Chirurgicale, par A. Nélaton, tom. prem., p. 752. Paris, 1844.

"Hippocrates gives us to understand, that we can always correct the shortening; Celsus, falling into the opposite error, declared, that a broken thigh always remains shorter than the other. At a period quite recent, Desault pretended to cure all fractures without shortening, and his journal contains several examples. In imitation of Desault, various practitioners have modified, corrected, and improved the apparatus for permanent extension, and they claim to have themselves obtained as complete success. I ought then to declare here in the most positive manner, that I have never obtained like results, either in the use of my own apparatus, or with that of others, nor indeed where in pursuance of my invitation, several inventors have applied their apparatus in my wards. I have examined, more than once, persons declared cured without shortening, and yet, upon measurement, the shortening was always manifest. The misfortune of all those who believe that they have obtained those miraculous cures, is that they have not even thought of instituting a comparative measurement of the two limbs; I will say even more, that they are most generally ignorant of the conditions of a good and faithful measurement. Sometimes, also, they have been deceived in another way; in falling upon fractures which were not displaced, especially with young persons, and they have believed that they have cured with their apparatus a shortening which had never existed. In short, when the fragments are not displaced, or even when they are brought again into a contact maintained by their reciprocal denticulations, it is easy to cure the fracture of the femur without shortening; aside of those two conditions, the thing is simply impossible.

"Several distinguished surgeons of our day have acknowledged this impossibility, and have renounced, in consequence, permanent extension. They allege, moreover, that an overriding of even three centimetres is of little importance, and occasions no limping. I cannot agree with this opinion. I have seen persons walk very well with a shortening of one centimetre; beyond this limit, either they limp, or they have lifted the heel of the shoe, or, in short, the limping is only concealed by a lateral deviation of the spine.[1] We thus are made to comprehend how a fracture with overlapping is always serious, and how cautious we ought to be in our prognosis."[2]

That the foregoing remarks are intended by the author to be equally applicable to other fractures of the shaft of the femur than to those of the middle third, is made evident by what he has said before, when speaking of fractures of the upper third.

"The prognosis is sufficiently favorable when the fragments are denticulated (engrenées): when they ride, on the contrary, we must look for a shortening as almost inevitable."—*Ibid.*, p. 718.

In our own country several of the most distinguished surgeons have testified to the constant difficulty, if not impossibility, of curing frac-

[1] Dr. Buck, of New York, thinks that with a shortening of one inch, or even one inch and a half, the patient may have "a useful limb, with little or no halting in his gait." N. Y. Journ. of Med., vol. xvi. p. 294.

[2] Traité des Fractures et des Luxations, par J. M. Malgaigne, tom. prem. pp. 723, 724. Paris, 1847.

tures of this bone without a shortening. In a suit instituted against a surgeon in New York city, for alleged malpractice in the treatment of an oblique, comminuted, and otherwise complicated fracture of the femur near its condyles, Dr. Mott is reported to have testified that "more or less shortening of the limb is uniformly the result after fractured thigh, even in the most favorable circumstances."[1]

In a very interesting communication made to the author by Jonathan Knight, of New Haven, late President of the American Medical Association, occurs the following passage:—

"I have seen but few fractures of the femur in the adult, unless of the most simple kind, in which there was not some remaining deformity; often slight, so as not to impair the usefulness of the limb, and in others considerable and apparently unavoidable." Dr. Knight adds, however: "In the greater proportion of the fractures in children, the recovery has been so nearly perfect that no marked deformity or lameness has followed."

Says Dr. Gibson: "Had the surgeon no other difficulties to encounter than such as present themselves after simple transverse fracture of the shaft of the thigh-bone, he would have little reason to complain of the defectiveness of art, or of the power of nature in promoting a cure. So different, however, from this is the result of an oblique fracture of the body of the bone, or of a transverse fracture of its neck, that it is hardly possible in any case to calculate with certainty upon reunion without more or less shortening and deformity of the limb."[2]

Dr. Detmold, in his remarks made before the New York Academy of Medicine, at its meeting in March, 1855, declared his belief that a shortening of the femur always occurs after fracture, and that "but one inch of shortening in an average of twenty cases is a good result."[3]

Dr. J. Mason Warren, of Boston, writes to me as follows: "As you are making observations on fractures, I would state that, after a long and very careful observation, I have never yet seen, either in Boston or elsewhere, an oblique fracture of the thigh, in a patient over seventeen years of age, in which there was not some shortening. I have had cases shown to me in which it was averred that the limb was not shortened, but on measuring myself I have found the fact otherwise. In children, I believe that union without shortening may be accomplished."

In a paper published by Dr. Lente in the number of the *New York Journal of Medicine* for September, 1851, he states that he believes the average shortening after treatment in the New York Hospital to be three-quarters of an inch; but subsequently Dr. Buck, one of the hospital surgeons, has furnished Dr. Lente with more exact statistics. Says Dr. Buck:—

"After carefully scrutinizing over one hundred cases of fracture of the femur, taken from the register of the N. Y. Hospital, and elimi-

[1] Boston Med. and Surg. Journ., vol. xxxiv. p. 450. See also opinions of Drs. Reese, Post, Parker, Cheeseman, Wood, &c., in relation to the prognosis in this particular case.

[2] Institutes and Practice of Surgery. by Wm. Gibson, 8th ed., vol. i. p. 297. Philadelphia, 1841.

[3] New York Journ. of Med., second series, vol. xvi. p. 261.

nating such as involved the cervix, or condyles, or belonged to the class of compound fractures, there remained an aggregate of seventy-four cases, of both sexes, and of all ages from 3 to 63, in which the shaft of the femur alone was fractured. In all these cases, the difference in the length of the fractured limb resulting from the treatment was ascertained by careful measurement with a graduated tape, and the following deductions were drawn from the analysis:—

Of the 74 cases of all ages, 19 resulted without any shortening, a proportion of about one-fourth. The average shortening of the remaining 55 cases was a fraction less than $\frac{3}{4}$ of an inch.

Seventeen cases in the above aggregate were under 12 years of age, of which six resulted without any shortening, a proportion of about one-third. The average shortening in the remaining 11 cases, was a fraction less than one-half an inch.

Of the 57 cases over 12 years of age, 13 resulted without any shortening, a proportion of about one-fourth; and the average shortening in the remaining 44 cases was a fraction over $\frac{3}{4}$ of an inch.[1]

It is not to be denied, however, that a few surgeons in all parts of the world have claimed, and still continue to claim, in their own practice, or from the adoption of their own peculiar plans of treatment, much better success. Indeed, some of them do not hesitate to affirm that, as a general rule, any degree of shortening is quite unnecessary.

Mr. Amesbury declares, that when the fracture is in the "middle or lower third," under a "judiciously managed" application of his own splint, "consolidation of the bone takes place without the occurrence of shortening of the limb, or any other deformity deserving of particular notice."[2]

Mr. South, in a note commenting upon an opposite sentiment expressed by Chelius, and already quoted, remarks: "In simple fractures of the thigh-bone, except with great obliquity, I have rarely found difficulty in retaining broken ends in place, and in effecting the union without deformity, and with very little, and sometimes without any shortening. For the contrary results the medical attendant is mostly to be blamed, as they are usually consequent upon his carelessness or ignorance."[3]

Mr. Hunt, of the Queen's Hospital, at Birmingham, who treats all fractures with the *apparatus inmobile* of Suetin, has published the results of his observations; and of the simple fractures of the femur only one presented, after the cure, any degree of shortening; and he adds, that all other fractures which he has treated by this method were followed by "equally good results."[4] In relation to which statements, Mr. Gamgee exclaims: "This is conservative surgery. What other mode of treatment would have given such results? And those cases are not exceptional. Mr. Hunt tells us he has selected them from

[1] Buffalo Med. Journ., vol. xv. p. 22, June, 1859.

[2] Practical Remarks on Fractures, by Joseph Amesbury, vol. i. p. 384. London ed., 1831.

[3] Op. cit., vol. i. p. 627.

[4] Researches on Pathological Anatomy and Clinical Surgery, by Joseph Sampson Gamgee. London ed., pp. 159, 160.

amongst many others equally successful. They accord with the experience recorded in my little treatise on this subject; and the works of Suetin, Burggræve, Crocq, Velpeau, and Salvagnoli Marchetti, record numerous cases no less remarkable and demonstratively conclusive."[1]

Desault, also, according to the passage from Malgaigne, which I have already quoted, "pretended to cure all fractures without shortening." I do not find, however, any other authority for this statement, as here made; neither in his *Treatise on Fractures and Luxations*, edited by Bichat, nor elsewhere. Bichat even says positively, that "Desault himself did not always prevent the shortening of the limb."[2] He declares, however, that "Desault has cured, at the Hôtel Dieu, a vast number of fractures of the os femoris, without the least remaining deformity."[3]

Dr. Dorsey, of Philadelphia, who employed the apparatus of Desault, as modified by Physick and Hutchinson (Fig. 128), was equally successful.[4]

Fig. 128.

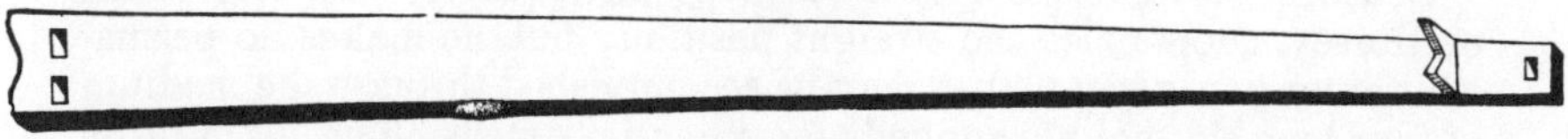

PHYSICK'S SPLINT.—The splint is intended to reach to the axilla, but the counter-extension is made by a perineal band. Physick employed also a second, long, inside splint.

Dr. Scott, of Montreal, Prof. of Clinical Surgery in the McGill College, and Physician to the Montreal General Hospital, has reported 19 cases of fractures of the long bones, taken promiscuously and without selection, from his hospital service, of which 3 belonged to the clavicle, 7 to the femur, 8 to the tibia and fibula, and 1 to the condyles of the humerus. All of which recovered without any degree of shortening or deformity; except the case of fracture of the condyles of the humerus, which resulted in death.[5]

It is never a pleasant duty to call in question the accuracy of another's statements, as to what he has himself alone seen and experienced. The circumstances which would justify such an expression of scepticism, where the witnesses, as in this case, are presumed to be intelligent and honest men, must be extraordinary. Such, however, I conceive to be the circumstances in this instance. It is certainly very extraordinary that a few gentlemen of acknowledged skill, but whose means and appliances are concealed from no one, are able to do what nearly the whole world besides, with the same means, acknowledges itself unable to accomplish. Such is the fact nevertheless; and our lack of faith in their testimony is only a necessary result of our experience, and of the experience of the vast majority of practical surgeons, as opposed to theirs.

[1] Op. cit., p. 167.
[2] A Treatise on Fractures and Luxations, etc., by P. J. Desault, edited by Xav. Bichat. Amer. ed., p. 251. 1805.
[3] Op. cit., p. 223.
[4] Elements of Surgery, by John Syng Dorsey, vol. i. p. 163. Philadelphia, 1813.
[5] "Medical Chronicle" of Montreal, vol. i. No. 7, 1853.

I might properly enough dismiss this subject with no further argument than may be found in the overwhelming testimony of practical surgeons, that broken femurs do in their experience rarely unite without more or less shortening; but I cannot avoid calling attention to the evidence of the falsity of the opposite opinion, which is furnished by the testimony of the very persons who themselves claim to have obtained such fortunate results.

It is not, as might have been supposed, one particular form of dressing, which, in itself peculiar, and more perfect than all others, has furnished these results. On the contrary, the plans of treatment have been constantly unlike, and sometimes quite opposite. Thus: Desault used a straight splint, with extension and counter-extension, and he refused to adopt the flexed position recommended by Pott, because his experience, and the experience of other French surgeons, had taught him its inutility.[1] Adopting the straight position, he made perfect limbs; with the flexed position, he found it impossible to do so.

Dorsey used the splint of Desault, as modified by Physick and Hutchinson.

South, whose success seems to have been equal to that of Desault or Dorsey, adopts also the straight position; but he makes no permanent extension, except what may be accomplished through the medium of four long side splints applied after "gentle" extension has been made by the assistants.

Mr. Amesbury, on the other hand, made perfect limbs only with his own double inclined plane; and speaking in general of the various plans hitherto contrived, not excepting that invented by Desault, or the method practised by South, which had already been recommended by several surgeons, he declares that "they are seldom able to prevent the riding of the bone, and preserve the natural figure of the limb. Indeed, so commonly does retraction of the limb occur under the use of the different contrivances usually employed, that I have heard a celebrated lecturer (now retired) in this town, publicly assert, that he never saw a fractured thigh-bone that had united, without riding of the fractured ends!"[2] And in his "*General Inferences*," he uses the following emphatic language: "The contrivances which are commonly used in the treatment of these fractures do not sufficiently resist the operation of the forces above mentioned, but suffer their influence to be exerted upon the bone, in all cases more or less injuriously, and at the same time often assist in *producing* displacement of the fractured ends; so that deformity, differing in kind and degree in different cases, is almost the constant result of fractures of the femur treated by these means."[3]

While Mr. Gamgee, a writer of much talent and industry, thus broadly contradicts the statements of Desault, South, Dorsey, and Amesbury, and administers a severe rebuke even upon the illustrious Liston: "Pott's plan, the long splint, M'Intyre, and their modifications, as a rule entail sensible deformity, which in many cases is very

[1] Works of Desault. Op. cit., p. 225.

[2] Amesbury on Fractures, &c., vol. i. p. 310.

[3] Op. cit., vol. i. p. 384.

considerable. It is a significant fact, that, though the example established in University College Hospital by the late Mr. Liston, of treating fractures of the thigh by the long splint (Fig. 129), and of the leg by the modified M'Intyre, which are admitted equal, if not superior, to other splints, was rigidly followed in that institution, the patients admitted with broken thighs or legs were frequently discharged with manifest deformity."[1]

Fig. 129.

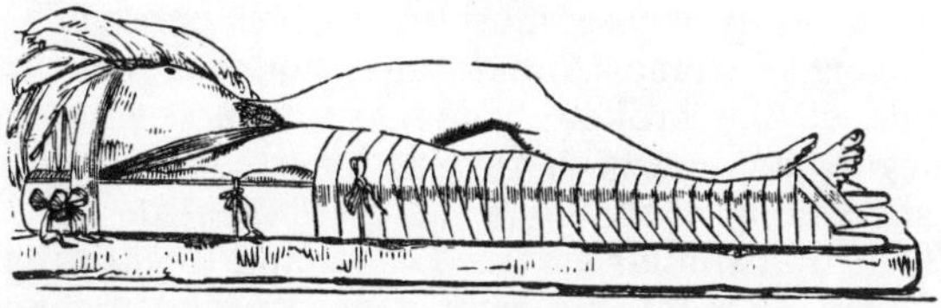

Liston's method, recommended by Samuel Cooper, Fergusson, Pirrie, and others.

With how much force his own remarks as to the experience of the University College Hospital will apply to the starched bandages used by himself, the reader will be able to determine when referred to the opinion of Velpeau, already quoted, who claims no result better than an average shortening of half an inch. It is true, however, that M. Velpeau prefers and advocates the starched bandage, but it is not true that he claims to be able to prevent a shortening of the bone.

"What other modes of treatment would have given such results?" This question, propounded, no doubt honestly, by Mr. Gamgee, has here its fair and satisfactory answer. Almost any of the various modes named; for if we must receive his testimony, we are equally bound to receive the testimony of Desault, South, Dorsey, Amesbury, and Scott. If we give credit to Mr. Gamgee, so far as to doubt the statements of these latter as to the degree of success claimed by them, by the same rule we must doubt his own statements also, as to the degree of success claimed by himself. This I say with all sincerity and kindness, fully believing that these gentlemen are mistaken, and not that they intentionally misrepresent the facts.

By a reference to my "Report on Deformities after Fractures," it will be seen that the average shortening in fractures of the upper third of the femur, in the cases examined by me, was about four-fifths of an inch; in the lower third it was a fraction over three-quarters, and in the middle third, a fraction less than three-quarters of an inch; and the average of the whole number was almost exactly three-quarters of an inch (three-quarters and $\frac{1}{47}$). These analyses were made upon simple fractures, and were exclusive of those in which no shortening at all occurred. An analysis which included also those which had not shortened, reduced the average shortening to half an inch and about one-tenth.

An examination of cabinet specimens does not present a result so

[1] Advantages of the Starched Apparatus, by Joseph Sampson Gamgee. London, 1853, pp. 54, 55.

favorable even as this. Of nineteen fractures of the shaft of the femur contained in Dr. Mütter's cabinet, not one seems to have been shortened less than one inch. Specimen B 63, a fracture of the middle third, is united with a shortening of two inches and a quarter; and specimen B 130, imperfectly united after a fracture through the middle third, is overlapped three and a half or four inches.

In conclusion, I wish to say briefly, that in view of all the testimony which is now before me, I am convinced—

First. That in the case of an oblique fracture of the shaft of the femur occurring in an adult, whose muscles are not paralyzed, but which offer the ordinary resistance to extension and counter-extension, and where the ends of the broken bone have once been completely displaced, no means have yet been devised by which an overlapping and consequent shortening of the bone can be prevented.

Second. That in a similar fracture occurring in children, or in persons under fifteen or eighteen years of age, the bone may sometimes be made to unite with so little shortening that it cannot be detected by measurement; but whether in such cases there is in fact no shortening, since with children especially it is exceedingly difficult to measure very accurately, I cannot say.

Third. That in transverse fractures, or oblique and denticulated, occurring in adults, and in which the broken fragments have become completely displaced, it will generally be found equally impossible to prevent shortening; because it will be found generally impossible to bring the broken ends again into such apposition as that they will rest upon and support each other.

Fourth. That in all fractures, whether occurring in adults or in children, where the fragments have never been completely or at all displaced, constituting only a very small proportion of the whole number of these fractures, a union without shortening may always be expected.

Fifth. That when, in consequence of displacement, an overlapping occurs, the average shortening in simple fractures, where the best appliances and the utmost skill have been employed, is about three-quarters of an inch.

If we consider the muscles alone as the cause of the displacement in the direction of the long axis of the shaft, the shortening of the limb, other things being equal, must be proportioned to the number and power of the muscles which draw upwards the lower fragment. This will vary in different portions of the limb, but nowhere will this cause cease to operate, nor will its variations essentially change the prognosis.

I have not intended to say that other causes do not operate occasionally in the production of shortening, but only that muscular contraction is the cause by which this result is chiefly determined, and that its power will be ordinarily the measure of the shortening.

Treatment.—All the early surgeons, so far as we know, adopted the straight position in the treatment of fractures of this bone; either with simple lateral splints, or with long splints, with or without extension, or with only rollers and compresses, or with extension alone.

Such was the unanimous opinion and practice of surgeons until about the middle of the last century, at which time Percival Pott wrote his remarkable treatise on fractures, a work distinguished for the originality and boldness of its sentiments, and which was destined soon to revolutionize the old notions as to the treatment of fractures, and to establish in their stead, at least for a time, what has been called, not inappropriately, the "physiological doctrine;" the peculiarity of which doctrine consisted in its assumption that the resistance of those muscles which tend to produce shortening can generally be sufficiently overcome by posture, without the aid of extension, and that for this purpose, for example, in the case of a broken femur, it was only necessary to flex the leg upon the thigh, and the thigh upon the body, laying the limb afterwards quietly on its outside upon the bed.

Very few surgeons, even of his own day, ever gave in their full ad-

Fig. 130.

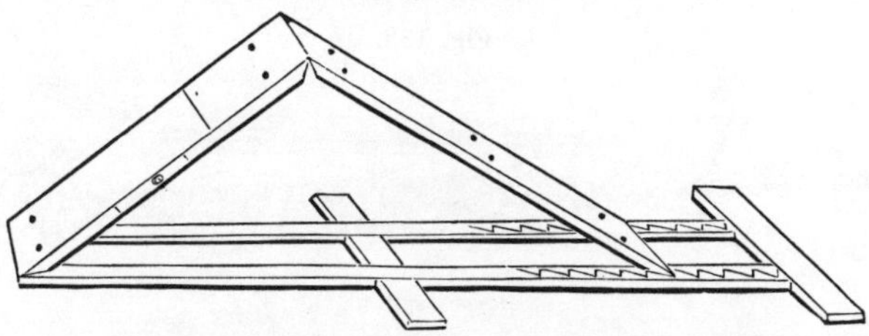

Double inclined plane employed in Middlesex Hospital, London.

hesion to the exclusive physiological system as taught and practised by Pott himself, but multitudes, especially among the English, adopted in general his views, only choosing to place the patients upon their

Fig. 131.

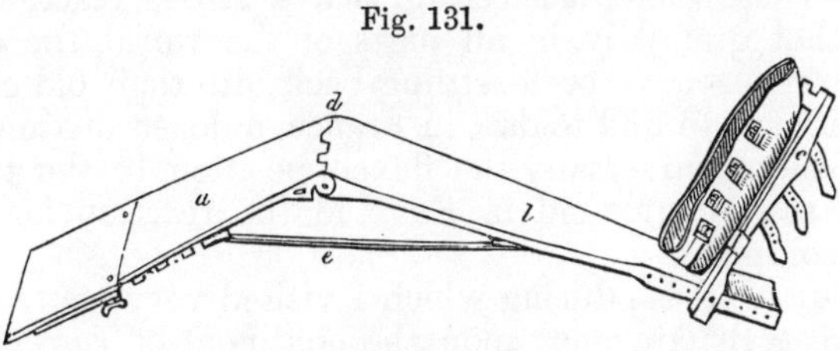

Amesbury's splint.

Fig. 132.

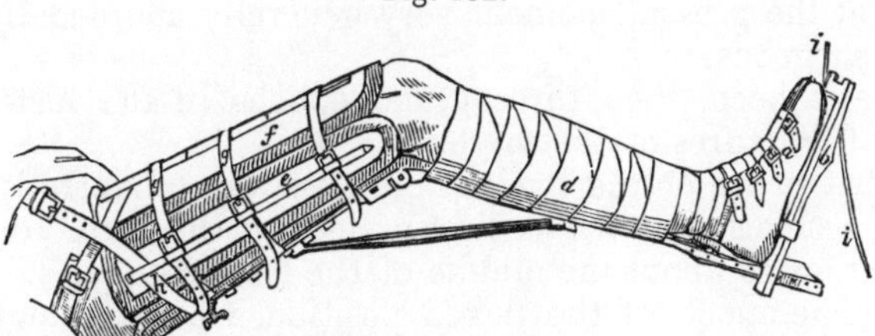

Amesbury's splint applied.

backs rather than upon their sides, and laying the limbs flexed over a double inclined plane. (Fig. 130.) To the support of this system of Pott's, thus modified, Sir Astley Cooper, C. Bell, John Bell, Earle, White, Sharp, and Amesbury (Figs. 131, 132), lent the influence of their great names, and its triumph, so far as the judgment of British surgeons was concerned, soon became complete.

In France, and upon the continent generally, the reception of this system was more slow and reluctant; but Dupuytren now for once taking ground with his great rival, Sir Astley, adopted almost without qualification these novel views. The decision of Dupuytren determined the opinions of a large portion of the continental surgeons; and had it not been for the early and decisive opposition of Desault and Boyer (Fig. 133), the great surgeon of St. Bartholomew might have continued for a long time to have enjoyed a triumph upon the continent, and perhaps throughout the world, equal to that which had already been decreed to him in Great Britain.

Fig. 133.

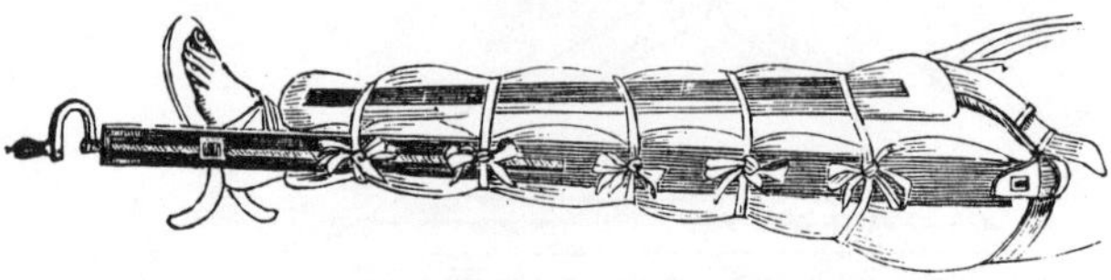

Boyer's splint.

On this side of the Atlantic, the practice of Pott, at least in so far as it applied to the treatment of fractures of the thigh, never gained a distinguished advocate; and but few ever adopted the practice as modified by White, Amesbury, Bell, A. Cooper, &c.

But whatever may have been the early success of these doctrines, either here or elsewhere, it is certain that a strong reaction has taken place, and that gradually, in all parts of the world, the opinions of practical surgeons have been settling back into their old channel. It would be difficult to find to-day, in France, a dozen distinguished surgeons who adopt universally the flexed position in the treatment of fractures of the femur; and in England the reaction is, if possible, even more complete.

In my tour of 1844, during which I visited very many of the hospitals of Great Britain and upon the continent of Europe, I do not remember to have seen the flexed position once employed in the treatment of a broken thigh; and I shall presently show that the straight position is at the present moment very generally adopted by the best American surgeons.

There have been, then, three grand epochs in the history of the treatment of fractures of the thigh.

First. That in which the straight position was universally adopted, and which reaches from the earliest periods to the period of the writings of Pott, or to about the middle of the last century.

Second. The epoch of the flexed position, which, inaugurated by Pott, had already begun to decline at the beginning of the present century, and which may be said to have been completed within less than one hundred years from the date of its first announcement.

Third. The epoch of the restoration, or that in which surgeons, by the vote of an overwhelming majority, have declared again in favor of the straight position. This is the epoch of our own day.

Although American surgeons have generally adopted the straight splint in the treatment of fractures of the thigh, yet the form and construction of the splint have been greatly varied. The simple long splint of Desault and the more complicated apparatus of Boyer (Fig. 133), have each their advocates; but it is seldom that we meet with these, or with any of the other forms of apparatus originally employed in foreign countries, without noticing that they have been subjected to considerable modifications; indeed, most of the straight splints as well as double-inclined planes in use at present among American surgeons, may farily be regarded as original inventions.

Nathan Smith, of New Haven;[1] Nathan R. Smith, of Baltimore[2] (Fig. 134); Nott, of Mobile[3] (Fig. 136); McNaughton, of Albany,[4] and Valentine Mott, of New York, are the only American surgeons of

Fig. 134.

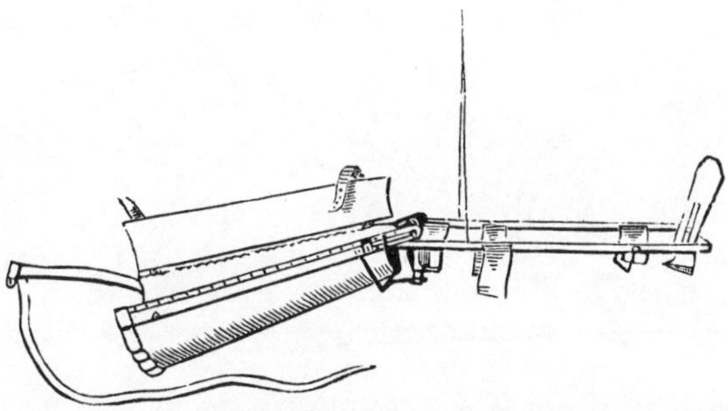

Nathan R. Smith's suspending apparatus, or double inclined plane.

distinguished reputation, and with whose practice I am familiar, who recommend exclusively the double-inclined plane; and perhaps we have a right to infer from the following paragraphs, copied from a letter addressed to the author a year or two since, that the opinions of Dr. Mott have undergone some modification in view of the improvements recently made in the construction of straight splints, and in the means of extension and counter-extension.

"Many years since I introduced into the New York Hospital Boyer's long splint, and continued to use it there, and in private practice, for a long time. I found, however, in many cases, that I had more or less trouble at the foot and groin from the points of extension and counter-extension. I then gradually laid it aside, and for some years have again taken up the double inclined plane.

"From the abundance which I have seen, I am free to say that, if I

[1] Amer. Med. Rev. Published at Philadelphia, 1825, vol. ii. p. 355. Also Medical and Surgical Memoirs of Nathan Smith. Published at Baltimore, pp. 129–141.

[2] Med. and Surg. Memoirs, pp. 143–162. See also Geddings, Baltimore Med. and Surg. Journ., vol. i. 1833; and Sargent's Minor Surgery, p. 171.

[3] Amer. Journ. Med. Sciences, vol. xxiii. p. 21.

[4] Trans. Amer. Med. Assoc., vol. x. p. 317. Rep. on Defor. after Frac.

had my own femur broken, I would be treated upon the double inclined plane.

Fig. 135.

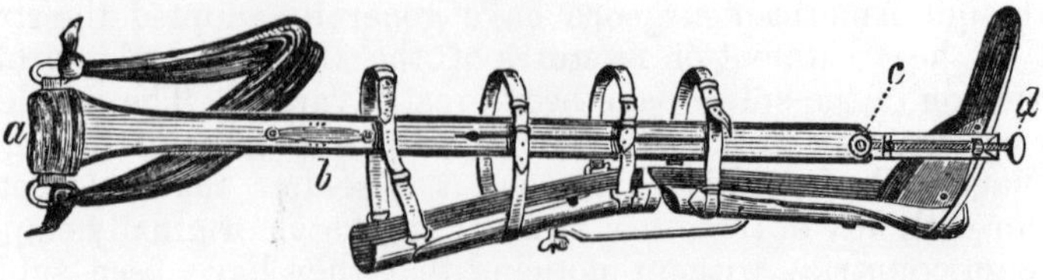

B. Welch's Thigh Apparatus.

a. Upper extremity, broad and well cushioned so as to rest easily over against the side of the body. *b* Brace for fixing a joint; to be used only in packing. *c.* Screw for adjusting a sliding joint, for the purpose of lengthening or shortening the splint. *d.* The thumb-screw for making extension.

The hollow splints suspended below can be moved upon each other by a joint opposite the ham, and their position secured by a movable bar. They may also be lengthened or shortened. There is a joint corresponding to the heel, and another opposite the sole of the foot.

This apparatus may be used as a double inclined plane, or as a straight splint. Lateral splints accompany the apparatus, all of which are made of gutta percha veneered with mahogany.

Fig. 136.

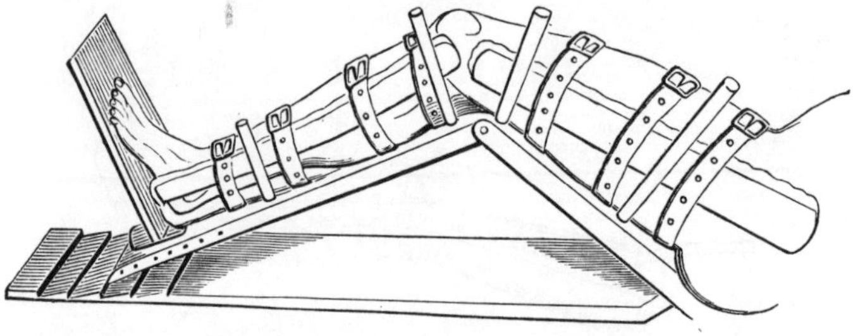

Josiah C. Nott's Double Inclined Plane.

In this apparatus the limb is secured to the splint by vertical pins and leather straps; the upper surface of the thigh splint is carved out a little, to fit the thigh; the two portions are articulated by a joint like that of a carpenter's rule, and this joint may be steadied by a horizontal bar underneath. For the rest, the drawing sufficiently explains itself.

"The Drs. Burges, Brothers, Court St., Brooklyn, Long Island, have made an improvement upon the extended principle (Figs. 137, 138). Their apparatus is now complete, and is in use at the Bellevue Hospital, where I advised, some time since, that it should be tried. It has succeeded admirably in two cases."

While, on the other hand, among the advocates of the straight splint are found the names of Physick,[1] Dorsey,[2] Gibson,[3] Horner,[4] J. Hartshorne,[5] H. H. Smith,[6] Neill,[7] R. Coates,[8] H. Hartshorne,[9] Norris,[10] Gross.[11]

[1] Elements of Surgery, by John Syng Dorsey. Philadelphia, 1813, p. 175.
[2] Ibid.
[3] Institutes and Practice of Surgery, by Wm. Gibson, 6th edit., vol. i. Phila.
[4] Treatise on the Practice of Surgery, by Henry H. Smith. Phila., 1856.
[5] Ibid. [6] Ibid.
[7] Philadelphia Med. Examiner. October, 1855.
[8] Amer. Journ. Med. Sciences, vol. xx. p. 18.
[9] Trans. Amer. Med. Assoc., vol. v. Rep. on Deg. after Frac.
[10] Ibid. [11] Ibid.

Fig. 137.

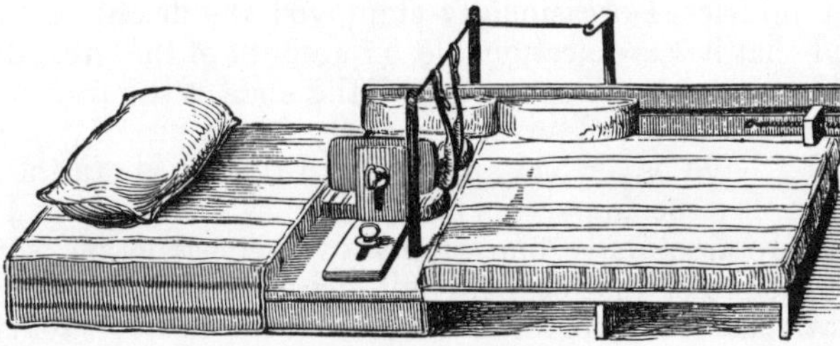

BURGE'S APPARATUS.

Fig. 138.

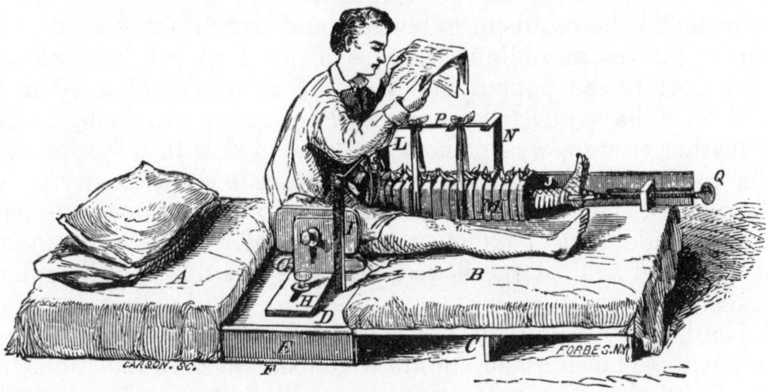

BURGE'S APPARATUS APPLIED.

"*A.* Thick mattress. *B.* Thin mattress. *C.* Wooden platform upon which the thin mattress is laid. This platform is made in two pieces and hinged together so as to fold upon itself for convenience of transportation, and when in use is merely hooked upon the central platform *D.*

"*D.* Central or cushioned platform supported at either end by wooden strips marked *E*, which rests upon *F.* A second platform of same extent as *D.* This constitutes a shelf for the bed pan, which may be introduced below from either side.

"*G.* Hair cushion, upon which the hips of the patient rest. This cushion, as well as the platform *D*, to which it is buttoned, has a semicircular opening at its lower margin for convenience of defecation.

"*H.* A rectangular wooden slide, exactly corresponding to its fellow upon the opposite side of the pelvis. These slides are so arranged upon the platform *D* as to be separated or approximated at will, and, by a thumb-screw which passes through a fissure in the horizontal portion of each, they may be fixed at the desired point so as exactly to embrace the pelvis of any patient. There is also a fissure in the perpendicular portion of each rectangular slide, and a screw passing through the same. One of these is to secure the upper end of the long splint *J*, and the other for the attachment of a short splint *I*, upon the side of the pelvis corresponding to the uninjured limb. Both of these splints are well padded upon one surface and may be elevated or depressed at will, in order to bring them to the level of the limbs, and fixed at the proper attitude by the screws already mentioned. They are also mutually transferable, thus adapting the apparatus to fractures of either thigh.

"*SS.* Counter-extending pads. These are attached by leather straps to the upper surface of the platform *D*, about twelve inches apart. Passing under the cushion *G*, and becoming well-rounded pads, they traverse the tuberosities of the ischia, pass between the thighs and thence perpendicularly to the horizontal iron rod or *crossbar L.* The crossbar *L* is supported at each end by a perpendicular bar extending upwards from the platform *D.* Attached by one extremity to the crossbar *L*, is a rod *P*, running parallel with and situated directly above the thigh. The other end of this rod *P*, is supported by an arched iron bar *N*, extending upwards from the outer side of the long splint *J.* The rod *P* is designed to afford special support to the injured limb whenever such support is deemed advisable. Two or three strips of cotton cloth, of suitable width, may be passed around the limb, either internally or externally to the splints of coäptation, and tied over the supporting rod *P.* Splints of coäptation are to be applied according to the exigencies of the case.

"*M.* An inside splint covered by the bandages. *Q.* The screw by which extension is effected in the ordinary way, having at one extremity a swivel and hook tied to a strip of wood in the loop of adhesive plaster below the foot."

Says Dr. Gross: "Many years ago, before I had much experience in this class of injuries, I occasionally employed the flexed position, but I soon found that it was objectionable, on account of the great difficulty in maintaining so accurate apposition of the ends of the fragments. Of late years I have confined myself entirely to the use of the straight position, and I have never had any cause to regret it. In the adult, I sometimes employ the apparatus of Desault, as modified by Physick, but much more frequently one of my own construction, somewhat upon the principle of that of Dr. Neill, described in the *Philadelphia Medical Examiner* for 1855. I have used it for nearly twenty years, and it has generally answered the purpose most admirably in my hands. It consists simply of a box for the thigh and leg, with a foot-piece, and two crutches, one for the axilla and the other for the perineum, to make the requisite extension and counter-extension. With such an apparatus, an oblique fracture of the thigh can be treated with great comfort to the patient, and with the assurance of a good limb. In children, I have effected some excellent cures simply by means of a sole leather trough, well padded and provided with a foot-piece.

"The great objection to the flexed position is the difficulty of keeping the ends of the broken bones in apposition; the upper one having a constant tendency to pass away from the inferior. Other objections might be urged against the flexed position, but this is quite sufficient to induce me to reject it."[1]

Dr. Neill, of Philadelphia, has contrived a very ingenious mode of making both extension and counter-extension at the same moment, by means of a twisted rope which is fastened by its two ends respectively, to the perineal band above and the extending bands below (Fig. 139).

Fig. 139.

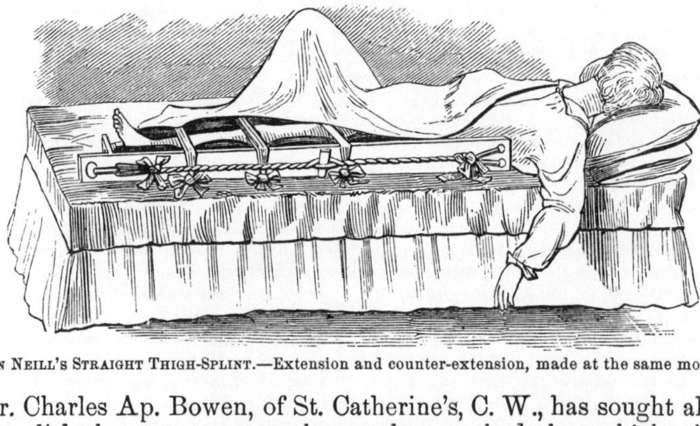

John Neill's Straight Thigh-Splint.—Extension and counter-extension, made at the same moment.

Dr. Charles Ap. Bowen, of St. Catherine's, C. W., has sought also to accomplish the same purpose by another method; but which will be best understood by a reference to the accompanying drawing (Fig. 140). The projection of the foot-piece on both sides of the splint is intended to give additional security to the splint, and to render the instrument applicable to either the right or left limb.

[1] Trans. Am. Med. Assoc., vol. x.; also System of Surg., by S. D. Gross, 1859, p. 221.

Fig. 140.

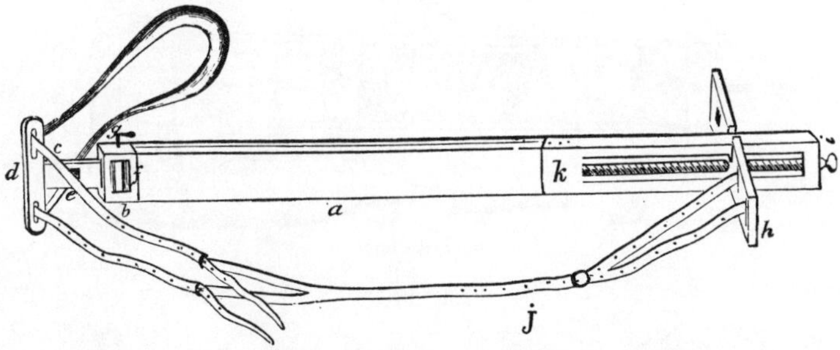

CHARLES AP. BOWEN'S THIGH-SPLINT.

a. Splint composed of two thin pieces of board screwed together. *b.* Brass band. *c.* Sliding bar, for increasing the length of the splint. *d.* Crutch-head, with slots for counter-extending bands. *e.* Transverse grooves in sliding bar. *f.* Eccentric roller, which, being turned by its handle *g*, is made to fasten itself in the transverse grooves and secure the sliding bar. *h.* Foot-piece with slots for extending bands on one side, and for counter-extending bands on the other. *i.* Screw. *j.* Martingale counter-extension straps. *k.* Pin which holds the screw in place. By taking out the pin *k*, the screw and the foot-piece can be removed, and then the whole apparatus may be packed in a very small space.

J. F. Flagg's thigh apparatus, as used in the Massachusetts General Hospital, by Warren, Bigelow and others (Figs. 141 to 149 inclusive).

Fig. 141.

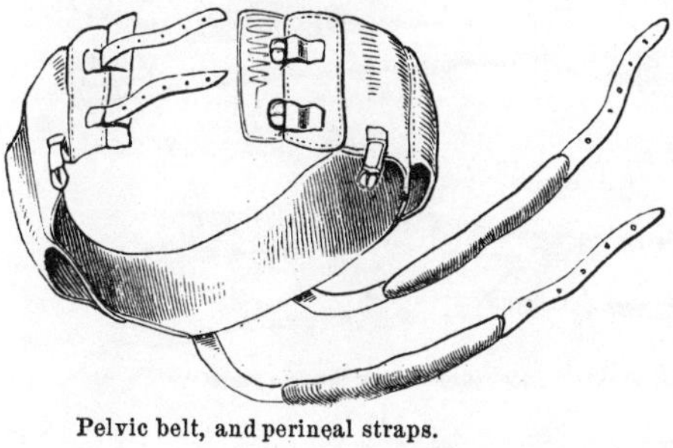

Pelvic belt, and perineal straps.

Fig. 142.

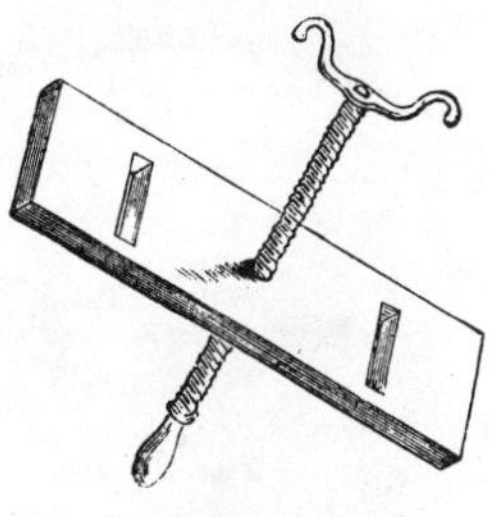

Foot-piece and screw.

Fig. 143.

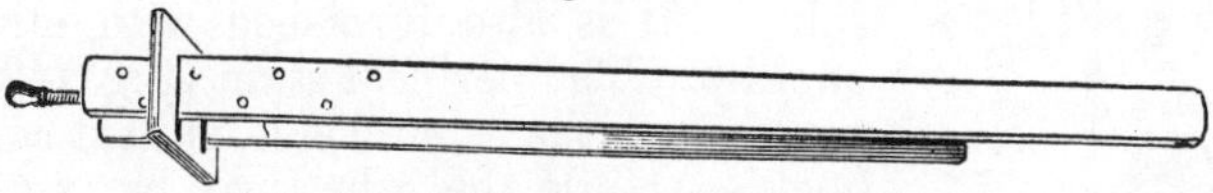

Lateral view of the apparatus, without the belt.

Fig. 144.

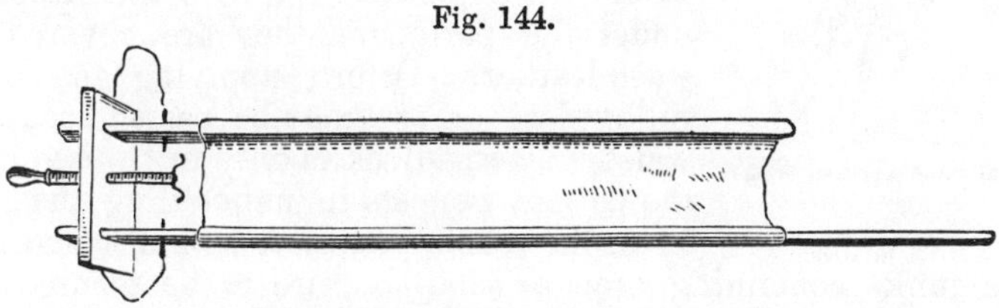

Front view, with folded sheet laid across.

Fig. 145.

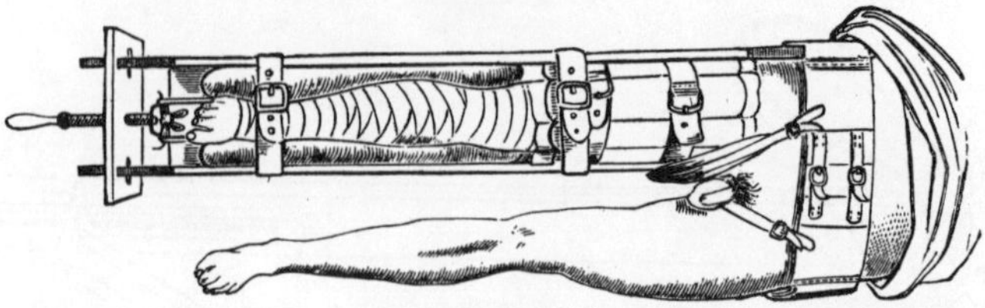

Apparatus applied.

Fig. 146.

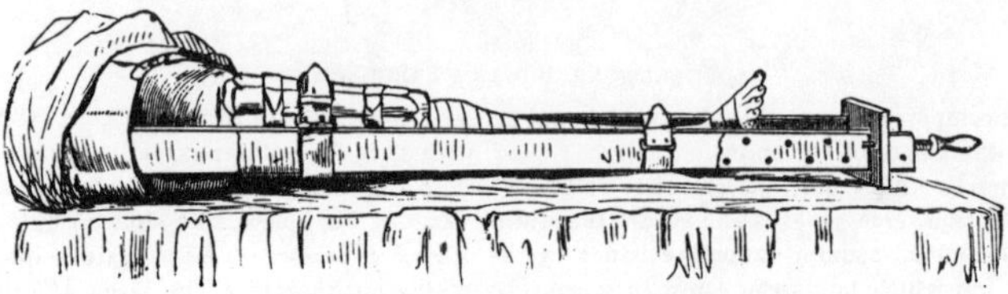

Side view of appa●atus applied.

Fig. 147.

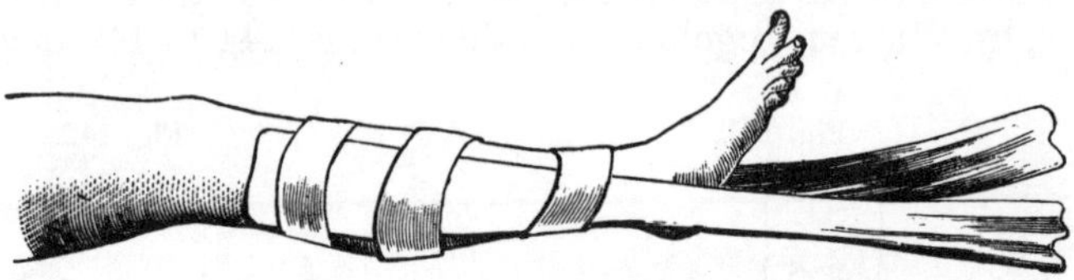

Fig. 148.

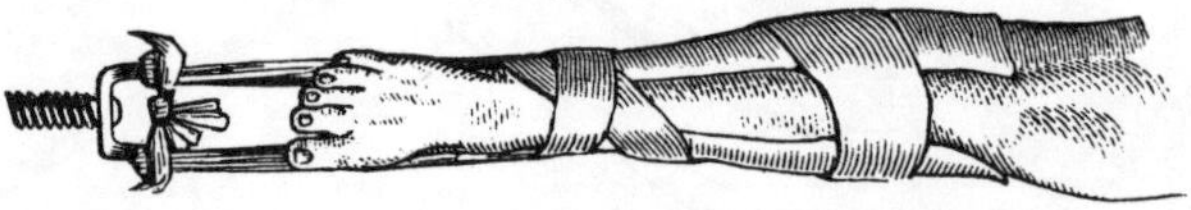

Figs. 147, 148. Mode of making extension with adhesive plaster.

Fig. 149.

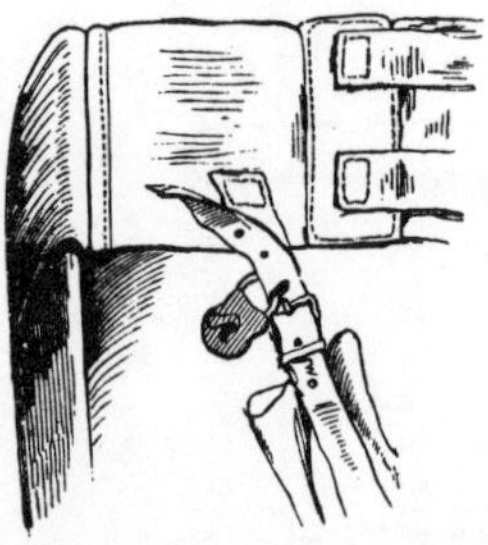

Perineal band secured with a padlock.

"The belt is made of strong webbing, having pockets on each side, to receive the long splint. It is also furnished with straps and buckles. The perineal strap (Fig. 149), corresponding to the injured side, is kept constantly buckled, while the other may be occasionally loosened, or left off, as its purpose is only to steady the apparatus. Where the straps pass under the perineum, they are covered with wash-leather. Before applying the belt, a pillow-case or two may be passed around the waist. The padlock is only to be used in case the patient persists in unbuckling the straps. The splints being applied, with also short side splints, junks, containing bran or sand, &c., are to be secured more firmly to the limb by bands of webbing and buckles."

The two Warrens, father and son, of Boston, Kimball, of Lowell, Sanborn, of Lowell, Mass., Mussey, of Cincinnati, Ohio, J. B. Flint, of Louisville, Ky., Armsby, of Albany,[1] also recommend some form of the straight splint. Says Dr. Mussey:—

"For all fractures of the thigh-bone, I employ the extended position of the limb. There are but few cases in which extending force is not necessary to prevent the degree of deformity or shortening which would occur without it. Of thirty specimens of fracture of the shaft, in my collection, only two are transverse. In fractures of the neck, especially with old subjects, I sometimes avoid the application of any kind of apparatus for permanent extension; but in all cases, whether of the neck or shaft, where such extension is attempted, I have found the straight position of the limb to be the most reliable."

And Dr. Kimball, who employs generally, Sanborn's splint (Fig. 150), uses the following emphatic language:—

"If I should be asked under what circumstances I would use the double inclined plane in case of fracture of the femur, I would unhesitatingly answer, never! I have long since abjured the double inclined plane in every form of fracture of this bone, finding the straight splint fully adequate to all purposes for which any apparatus of this kind is required. In support of this statement, I could furnish a great number of cases showing that the locality of the fracture, the importance of which is so much dwelt upon in the books, constituted, in no case, a valid objection to it use."

Fig. 150.

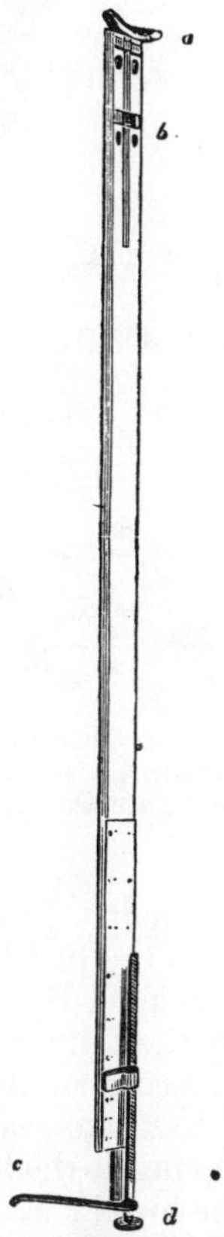

SANBORN'S SPLINT. *a.* The movable crutch. *b.* The screw which fixes the crutch. *c.* The crossbar, to which the ends of the strap are fastened. *d.* The moving screw.

Extension in Sanborn's apparatus is effected by means of adhesive straps, and counter-extension by a perineal band; but the patient may at any moment relieve the pressure in the perineum by esting his axilla upon the head of the crutch.

Daniell, of Savannah, Georgia, recommends the straight position, the limb being laid in a kind of long box, and the extension being made with a weight and pulley.[2] Dugas, of Augusta, Georgia, employs the pulley and weight also, but uses the long side splint instead of the box.[3]

Says Dr. Dugas: "Suitable compresses having been placed upon the thigh, apply over them four wooden splints a little shorter than the femur (one in front, one in the rear, and one on either side),

[1] Trans. Am. Med. Assoc., vol. x. Report on Deformities after Fractures.
[2] Amer. Journ. Med. Sciences, vol. iv. p. 330, 1829.
[3] Southern Med. and Surg. Journ. Feb. 1854.

Fig. 151.

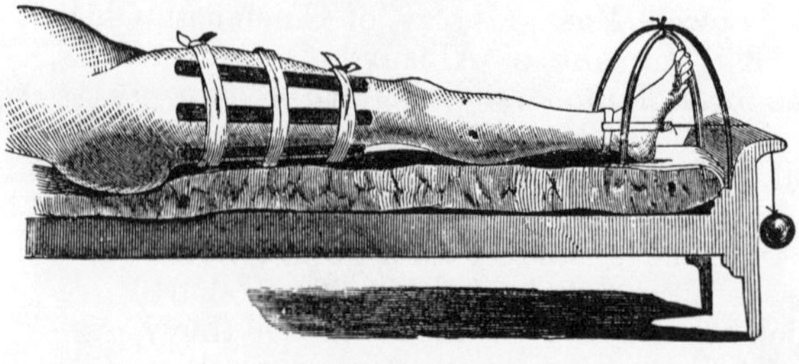

L. A. Dugas' method. The long splint omitted because it would mask the drawing.

and secure these with many-tailed bandages or with single ties. A two or three pound weight should then be fixed to the foot and hung over the foot-board of the bed, as indicated in the annexed figures (Figs. 151, 152), so as to keep up extension, while the resistance of the patient's body will effect counter-extension. A splint four inches wide, and extending from the side of the thorax to a little below the foot, will now serve to keep the limb straight and to maintain the foot in a proper position. This splint should be secured by separate ties passed around the abdomen, pelvis, thigh, leg, and foot. Finally, an arch of crossed hoops should protect the toes from the bedclothes."

Fig. 152.

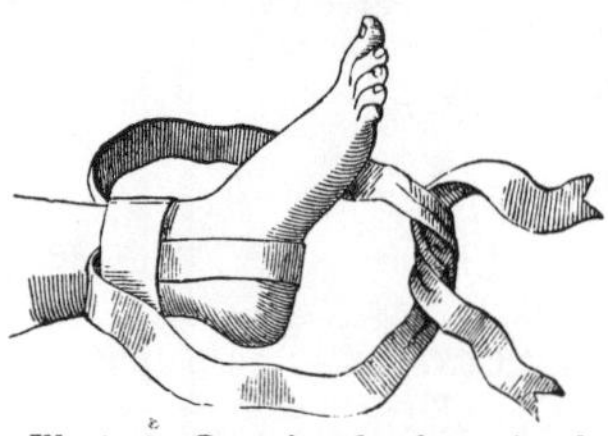

Illustrates Dugas' mode of securing the weight without fatigue to the ankle-joint.

Joshua B. Flint, of Louisville, Ky., has sometimes, as will be seen by the following quotation from a letter addressed to the author, employed a similar apparatus with excellent results.

"Of late years I have generally employed Liston's single long splint; having it thickly padded, and then applying a roller from the foot to the hip, in such a manner as to secure the limb firmly to the splint. This is about the only case in which I now wrap a fractured limb with a roller." * * * * * * *

"I have repeatedly used, and with much satisfaction, extension by means of the pulley, having the co-operation only of short lateral splints at the place of the fracture. With a mattress slightly inclined toward the head, and moderate, but persistent traction made on the injured limb by a weight made fast to the foot by means of a cord passing over a pulley—the pulley being secured to the foot-board—I have conducted some tolerably oblique fractures to a satisfactory termination, and with much more comfort to the patients than attends any other equally effectual method of extension."

Wm. E. Horner, of Philadelphia, employed a long outside splint (Fig. 153, *a*), extending into the axilla, and padded, so as to avoid the necessity of junks; with fenestræ, for extending and counter-extending bands; and also a foot-piece; and a short inside splint (*b*), made to extend from the perineum to the bottom of the foot. Across the ex-

Fig. 153.

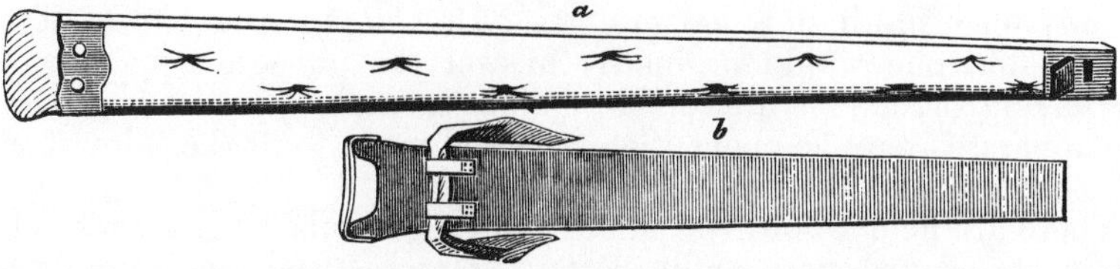

W. E. Horner's thigh-splint.

cavated upper end of this splint, a strip of leather is stretched to receive the pressure of the perineum, while the perineal band is made to pass through two firm leather loops on the outside of the splint.

Dr. Joseph E. Hartshorne, of Philadelphia, rejected the perineal band altogether, and sought to make the counter-extension by means of the internal long splint alone; and for this purpose, he cushioned the head of the inside splint, as will be seen in the accompanying drawing (Fig. 154). The head of the outside splint may also be cushioned,

Fig. 154.

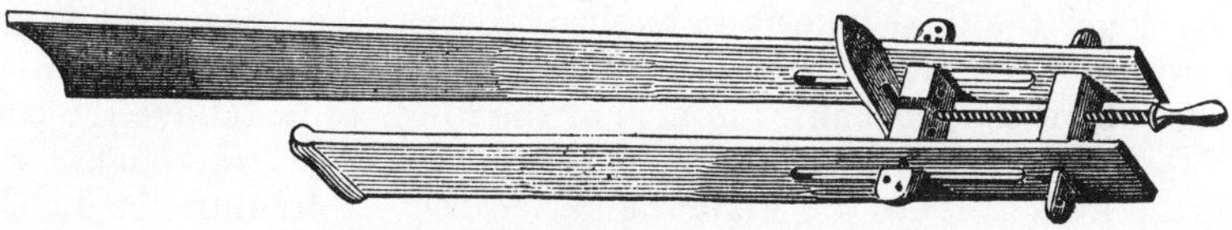

Joseph Hartshorne's thigh-splint.

but not for the purpose of employing it as a means of counter-extension. The outside splint is so adjusted to the foot-piece, that it may be removed, in case of a compound fracture, without disturbing either the extension or counter-extension.[2]

The accompanying drawings (Fig. 155, 1, 2, 3, 4), representing a very simple and easily-constructed apparatus devised by Dr. Alonzo Chapin, of Massachusetts, has many points of real excellence.[3] It will serve at least to instruct the reader how he may furnish himself extemporaneously with a complete apparatus when he is not otherwise pre-

Fig. 155.

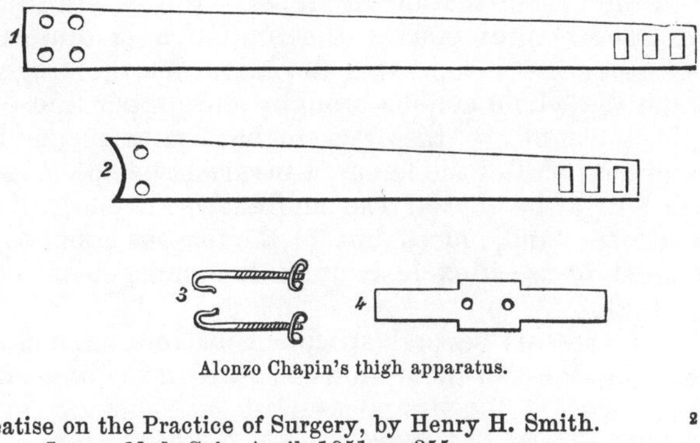

Alonzo Chapin's thigh apparatus.

[1] Treatise on the Practice of Surgery, by Henry H. Smith. [2] Ibid.
[3] Amer. Journ. Med. Sci., April, 1851, p. 355.

pared. The iron screw and swivel for making extension can be made by any blacksmith in a few minutes. Dr. Chapin uses two of these screws, but one would ordinarily answer the purpose equally well. By having the tenons in the side splints instead of in the foot-piece, the apparatus may be opened laterally and made to fit the sides of the limb more or less closely.

There are many, however, of our most distinguished surgeons, who retain the flexed position in certain fractures, such as an oblique downward and forward fracture, occurring just below the trochanter minor, and a similar fracture just above the condyles, or in certain cases of fractures in children, or in very old people, but who, nevertheless, give a decided preference to the straight splint in those oblique fractures of the shaft which constitute by far the greatest proportion of all these accidents. Among these, I will mention the names of Post, of New York,[1] De Lamater, of Cleveland, Ohio,[1] Pope, of St. Louis, Mo.,[1] Knight, of New Haven,[1] and Eve, of Nashville, Tenn.[1]

Dr. Pope has given us his views upon this subject very much at length:—

"In the treatment of fractures of the femur, I employ neither the straight nor the flexed position exclusively, but the one or the other, according to the site of fracture. If the fracture involves either the upper (below the trochanter minor) or the lower third (above the condyles) of the femur, I make use of the double inclined plane of Sir Charles Bell. If, on the other hand, the seat of fracture be in the middle third of the thigh, I greatly prefer the straight, long splint of Mr. Liston.

"My reasons are briefly the following: In fractures below the trochanter minor, the upper fragment is tilted forwards and upwards, by the unrestrained action of the psoas muscle, so that no extension in the straight direction will avail to draw down the upper in a line with the lower portion of the lever.

"The same thing results in fractures of the lower third, but in opposite directions. Here the heel becomes the fixed point, and the gastrocnemii draw the lower fragment backwards and downwards, whilst the upper fragment projects in front. Rectilinear extension can no more correct the malposition of the lower fragment in this case, than it can in the former that of the upper. But in both (upper and lower third fractures), by placing the limb over a double inclined plane, these otherwise insuperable deviations of the fragments are prevented, and the whole bone is brought into proper line.

"When, on the contrary, the fracture implicates the middle third or even the middle half of the femur, I invariably employ the straight splint, which I regard as by far the simplest, most effectual, and best means of treatment; and, indeed, but for the reasons assigned, I should only be too glad to use it exclusively in the management of all fractures of the thigh.

"My cabinet presents several specimens of broken femurs, which illustrate the soundness of these views: in which the abnormal direc-

[1] Trans. Amer. Med. Assoc., vol. x.; Rep. on Def., etc.

tion of the fragments alluded to as occurring in fractures of the upper and lower thirds, is very marked; the deformities having resulted from treatment in the straight position. So far as function and symmetry are concerned, the lower deformity is altogether the most serious. The unseemly projection above the knee, the unnatural exposure in front of the articular surfaces of the condyles, which are not set bluffly on those of the tibia, together with the altered site of the patella, and the diminished power of the quadriceps muscle, both weaken and deform the joint.

"With regard to the management of fractures below the trochanter minor, or at other points of the femur, by means of the double inclined plane, I am well aware of the difficulty of properly confining the pelvis, but this objection I am far from considering as insuperable. So, too, the outward tendency of the upper fragment, caused by the gluteus, may be humored by carrying the limb off at an oblique angle to the axis of the body.

"It is, perhaps, needless to add, that in fractures of the condyles, of the inter-trochanteric portion, as well as of the neck of the femur (when osseous union is attempted), whether within or without the capsule, I likewise give preference to the straight position."

The practice of Dr. Pancoast, of Philadelphia, is peculiar, and will be best described by himself.

"I treat all thighs, fractured in their middle part, by the long splint, and in the straight position. In fractures occurring at either end of the bone, I resort at first to the angular splint and the flexed position, and thus place the muscles more at rest; in which position, also, there is less tendency to angular displacement and shortening. After the lapse of a few days, when the disturbed muscles have lost their tendency to spasm, and the hardened cellular tissue about the fracture has formed a sort of bond between the ends of the broken bone, I gently bring the limb down to the straight position, and apply the long splint."[1]

The practice of treating fractures of the thigh, as well as all other fractures of the long bones, with the roller alone, and without either lateral splints or extending apparatus, first suggested by Radley, has found in this country but one distinguished advocate, Dr. Dudley, of Lexington, Ky.[2] Nor, with all my respect for that venerable and truly great surgeon, can I persuade myself that the practice is able to accomplish, in a majority of cases, the indications proposed, nor indeed that it is, at least in the hands of inexperienced surgeons, wholly safe. Dr. D., of Aberdeen, Miss., has reported to me one example in which, after the application of this bandage, by a pupil of Dr. Dudley's, to a negro slave, who had a fracture of the femur, death of the limb ensued, and amputation became necessary. The negro was sixteen years old, and healthy; the fracture was caused by the fall of a tree or of a branch, and was simple. The bandage was applied from the toes upwards to the groin, and was not opened for several days, at which time the

[1] Trans. Am. Med. Assoc., vol. x. Rep. on Def., etc.

[2] Amer. Journ. of the Med. Sci., vol. xix. p. 270; Transylvania Journal, April, 1836; Boston Med. and Surg. Journ., vol. xxxiv. p. 35.

whole limb was found to be in a state of dry gangrene, with the exception of the upper two-thirds of the thigh, which was swollen enormously, and partially gangrenous as high up as the groin.

Dr. D. says: "Having heard the history of the case carefully stated, observing the leg and the lower part of the thigh to be in a state of dry gangrene, and seeing the marks of the bandage visibly impressed on the surface, my opinion was made up at the time that the gangrene had resulted from pressure of the bandage. The femoral artery at the groin was in a sound and natural state, and, if I mistake not, after the limb was removed, it was traced to the point of obliteration where the gangrene commenced, and where the impression of the bandage was observed; thus far, I think, it was of natural size and calibre. Hence the conclusion is inevitable, that the death of the limb resulted from the pressure of the bandage, and not of one of the fragments. It was a curious specimen of dry mortification, and I regret that I did not use the means of preserving it. I was then engaged in a very laborious practice, thirty miles from home, on horseback, and consequently could not conveniently spare the time to attend to it as an object of surgical curiosity. Dr. H. and myself cut into the leg in various places in order to examine the muscles, arteries, nerves, etc., but found the integuments so hard that it was really difficult to penetrate them with a knife; the resistance to the knife was more like that of dry hickory wood than anything else."[1]

In relation to other plans of treatment, I shall content myself by declaring my belief that the starched bandage of Suetin, Velpeau, Gamgee, and others, cannot be regarded as a safe or effectual apparatus; and that extension alone, without either side splints or long splints, which I have seen practised by Jobert, of Paris, and other French surgeons occasionally, is inefficient. My remarks hereafter will therefore be confined to a more full declaration of the principles involved in, and the proper mode of using, the long splint.

Without limiting ourselves to the consideration of any one of the special forms of apparatus, we may say that the following ought to be regarded as essential elements in the construction of the long straight splint (Fig. 162): Length sufficient to extend at least several inches above the ala of the pelvis, and the same distance below the foot; such thickness as that it shall be firm and unyielding; width sufficient to make it serve as one of the lateral splints, since over all the more properly called lateral splints it possesses this advantage, that it can never become displaced downwards or upwards; its width ought seldom to be less than three and half inches, nor should its width diminish as it descends toward the foot, as, in consequence of this construction, the roller, which is intended to secure the limb to the splint, has a constant tendency to slide in the same direction.

A foot-piece, or transverse block to which the foot may be attached for the purpose of making extension as nearly as possible in the axis of the limb. If this foot-piece is movable, it will serve only the single purpose above mentioned, and no rule need govern its width. But in

[1] For a more complete account of this interesting case, see Buffalo Med. Journ., vol. xiv. p. 193, Sept. 1858.

this case there must be another block attached to the bottom of the long splint, at a right angle with the shaft, and of the same width as the splint; the object of which will be to support and steady the side splint, and to prevent its rolling inwards or outwards. Where this is neglected, frequent disturbance of the broken fragments, and a deformity from inclination of the foot outwards or inwards, are apt to ensue. If the foot-piece is not movable, then it may be of the same width as the side splint, and serve both to steady the side splint and as a means of extension. The length of the foot-piece ought not to be such as to interfere with a long inner splint, in case its use should be deemed advisable. With two fenestræ placed at the upper part of the splint, for the reception of the counter-extending band, the long outside splint is now complete.

These are, so to speak, its simple elements, and compose the splint in its rudest form, without which no splint can be perfect, yet upon which many real improvements may be based. Thus, it must be regarded as an improvement to have the splint so constructed as that it may be readily lengthened or made shorter, to accommodate itself to the size of the patient; or that the foot-piece should be furnished with a screw, for the purpose of making the extension more uniformly; or that the same mode of operating should apply also to the counter-extension.

The adhesive plaster bands are beyond all comparison the best means of making a permanent extension which are at present known to surgeons. Hitherto, one of the most serious difficulties in the way of extension, and the objection which has been most effectively urged against its adoption, has been the excoriations, ulcerations, and even sloughing, which so often occurred from the use of the various extending bands about the ankle. This, together with the injuries occasionally inflicted by the perineal band, has been regarded by other surgeons than Dr. Mott, whose opinion we have already quoted, as a sufficient reason for preferring the flexed position. But no one who has employed the adhesive plaster extending bands will doubt that, so far as injuries to the foot and ankle are concerned, this objection is now entirely disposed of. It is adopted in many, perhaps most of the American hospitals, and in no case where it has been employed have I known the slightest excoriations to have been produced. I regard this simple invention, therefore, as one of the most important improvements in the treatment of fractures of the thigh, and it is not surprising that several claimants have appeared for the original suggestion. By Dr. Brinton it has been claimed for Dr. Ellerslie Wallace, of Philadelphia;[1] and by Dr. Sargent for Dr. Gross, of the same city;[2] while by American surgeons generally the invention has been conceded to Dr. Josiah Crosby, of New Hampshire, to whom certainly is due the credit of having brought it into notice, if not, indeed, of the first suggestion.[3]

[1] Note to first American edition of Erichsen's Surgery, p. 225.

[2] Note to 3d American edition of Miller's Practice of Surgery, p. 653. See also N. Y. Med. Gaz., vol. iv. p. 87.

[3] See case reported in N. H. Journ. of Med., for 1851; also, N. Y. Journ. of Med., vol. vi. 2d series, p. 137. See also, Trans. Amer. Med. Assoc., vol. iii. p. 382.

The mode of using adhesive plaster for extension is briefly as follows:—

A single band, long enough to extend from a point just below the knee to twelve or sixteen inches beyond the foot, and about three inches wide, is to be applied along each side of the leg. Instead of one band on each side, two may be employed; which shall traverse each other somewhat obliquely, so that one band shall fall a little in front of the malleolus and one a little behind. Having wrapped the whole circumference of the ankle, including the malleoli and heel, in a heavy pledget of cotton, laid underneath the adhesive bands, a roller is now to be applied from the toes upwards as far as the knee, and secured with a little flour paste or starch. Before fastening the bands to the foot-block, each band should be twisted into a rope below the foot; and to prevent any degree of lateral pressure upon the sides of the ankle and foot, already tolerably protected by the cotton, a piece of thin board, longer than the width of the ankle, and notched at each extremity, should be placed between the bands below the bottom of the foot.

The attempt to use the adhesive plaster also as a perineal band, for the purpose of making counter-extension, does not seem to have been equally successful, unless I except the experience of that very excellent surgeon, Dr. David Gilbert, of Philadelphia, and of one or two other gentlemen mentioned by him, whose practice I will presently describe more particularly. For my own part I never could succeed to any purpose with these bands in the perineum, or at least no better than with the ordinary perineal bands; and I very much fear that, notwithstanding the ingenious contrivances of my friend Dr. Gilbert, we have still to incur the risk of ulcerations, &c., from this portion of our dressings; fortunately, however, the perineal band never completely ligates the limb, and it has rarely, therefore, been found so mischievous as the ordinary extending bands at the ankle.[1] In the fracture apparatus lately invented by the Burges, the peculiar mode of action of the perineal band, avoiding, as it does, pressure upon the front of the groin, diminishes still further this danger; and in the construction of my own splint, I have long had regard to the importance of this principle by attaching the anterior portion of the perineal band to an upright crutch-head, which is made to rise more or less from the top of the splint, according to the size or obesity of the patient. In Burges' and Lente's apparatus this principle is, however, most fully recognized, and the indication is most completely accomplished.

I will take this occasion to mention that with large fat people, I have sometimes found it necessary to dispense with the perineal band altogether, and in such cases I have succeeded very well in making counter-extension by lifting the foot of the bed one or two feet, and trusting alone to the weight of the body.

Dr. Gilbert, as I have already stated, believes also that the adhesive plaster may be employed as successfully in making counter-extension as in extension. He published his first case of treatment

[1] For cases of sloughing, &c., from perineal band, see N. Y. Journ. of Med., vol. xvi., 2d ser., p. 261, March, 1856; also same journal, Jan. 1840, p. 239.

by this method in the *American Journal of Medical Science* for 1851, and since then he has used it in every case of fracture, not only of the thigh, but of the leg, as he affirms, with the happiest results. Drs. Kerr, Kenderdine, and Hunt, of Pennsylvania, who have also adopted Dr. Gilbert's method, speak of it in terms of commendation. In the first of the accompanying wood-cuts (Fig. 156) nothing is intended to be shown but the long splint and the adhesive straps employed in extension and counter-extension. It will be seen also that Dr. Gilbert employs the ordinary tourniquet of Petit for the purpose of making the extension. The "pelvic band" is a broad strip of adhesive plaster, and serves to bind down the perineal bands more closely to the skin. If necessary, additional strips of adhesive plaster may be applied, and in order to increase their strength they may be doubled.[1]

In compound fractures Dr. Gilbert recommends a modification of the common fracture box (Fig. 158). In this apparatus the foot-board is omitted, and a block for the reception of the frame of the tourniquet is substituted. Each side of the box consists of three separate segments. Of these the upper and lower are permanently screwed to the bottom-

Fig. 156.

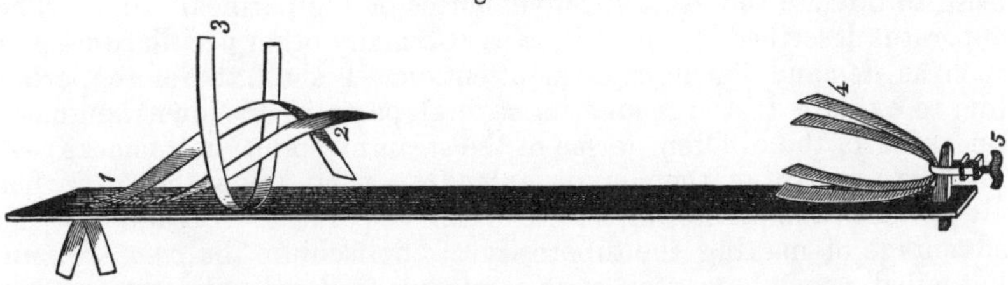

D. GILBERT'S MODE OF MAKING COUNTER-EXTENSION, AND EXTENSION.

1. Anterior and posterior counter-extending adhesive bands, two and a half inches wide, crossing each other before they pass through the mortise holes. 2. The same, crossing at the upper part of thigh and perineum. 3. Horizontal pelvic band, which may be three inches wide. 4. Extending bands, receiving strap of tourniquet in the hollow of the foot. 5. Tourniquet.

Fig. 157.

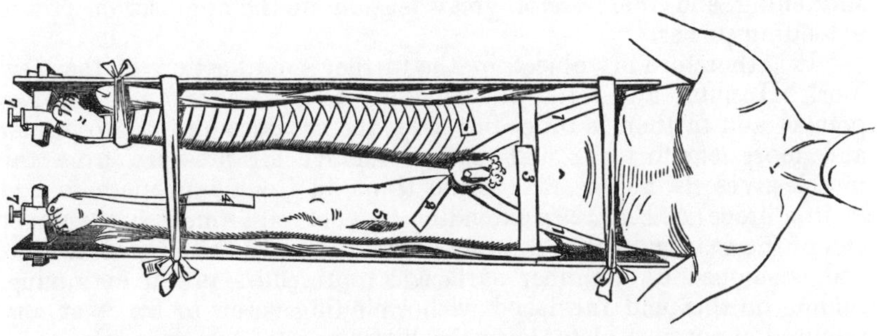

GILBERT'S APPARATUS APPLIED IN A CASE OF FRACTURE OF BOTH THIGHS.

1, 1. Anterior adhesive counter-extending strips. 2. Distal extremity of posterior adhesive strip of left side. 3. Adhesive strip surrounding pelvis, binding the anterior and posterior strips to pelvis. 4. Inner extremity of the extending adhesive strip, forming stirrup under the foot to receive the strap of the tourniquet. 5. Cicatrix of left thigh. 7, 7. Petit's tourniquet, by which the power was applied.

[1] Gilbert, Amer. Journ. Med. Sci., April, 1859, pp. 410–424.

board, and the central one is attached by hinges. By this arrangement there is full access to the wound, which may be dressed from day to day without disturbing the extension and counter-extension, maintained by the permanently attached upper and lower segments.

Fig. 158.

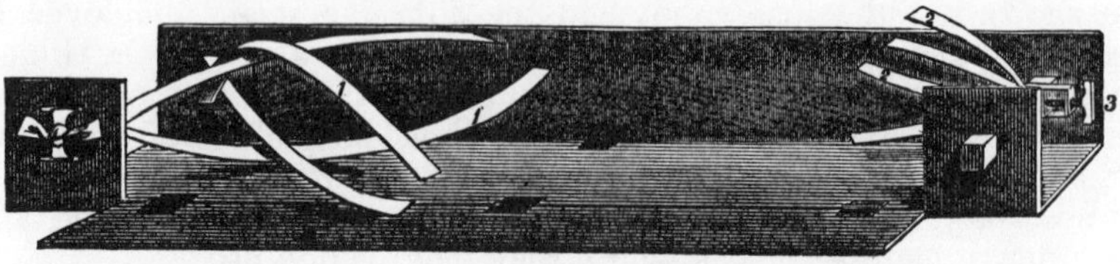

Gilbert's Box for Compound Fractures of the Thigh.

1. The four counter-extending adhesive strips, as if encircling the knee and upper part of leg. 2. The two extending adhesive strips crossing at the bottom of the foot, ready to be applied to the foot. 3. Tourniquet.

Lente, of Cold Spring, N. Y., has also occupied himself with the invention of an apparatus by which he hopes, in some measure at least, to obviate the usual inconveniences of the perineal band. The apparatus described by him possesses also many other peculiarities, and such as demand for it especial attention. I shall, therefore, permit him to explain to the reader its several parts in his own language. Speaking of the different forms of the straight splint, he remarks:—

"The pressure of the counter-extending band upon the groin has always been the stumbling block of this apparatus. Desault saw the advantage of making the tuberosity of the ischium the *point d'appui*, but failed, as we have seen, in his attempt to do so; and various surgeons have since contrived as many different plans for effectually carrying out his idea, but without complete success. No one, however, has approached this nearer than the Burges. However, the fact seems to be that neither the groin nor the tuberosity is fitted to bear alone the pressure of the counter-extension in cases of considerable shortening, and therefore of great tension in the application of the extending power.

"It is therefore my object, in the further modification of the New York Hospital apparatus, to distribute the pressure on these two points; and further, in order to render the pressure on the groin safer and more comfortable, and also to remove all pressure from the muscles, vessels, nerves, &c., of the thigh in front, I propose to add an iron brace (A, Fig. 159), extending, in a curved form, from the upper end of the external splint directly across the body to the median line, and cushioned on its inner surface as represented in the engraving. Sliding on this, and furnished with a binding screw to fix it at any required point, is a plate, P, to the lower part of which is attached a buckle for securing the anterior extremity of the perineal band. By this arrangement, I am enabled to make the direction of the counter-extending force of this portion of the band correspond to the axis of the limb, instead of oblique; and, furthermore, it allows me to dispense with all that portion of the outer splint between the crest of the ilium and the axilla; thus reducing it to the original length of Desault, obviating the constriction of the chest by the body-band, and producing a less irksome confinement of the upper part of the body. In lieu of the body-band, there is a pelvic strap extending from the end of the iron brace, to the movable plate of which it is secured by buckles, around the back to the top of the splint, thus binding the apparatus firmly to the pelvis, if found necessary. It should be mentioned that the brace is so attached to the splint, through the ingenuity of Mr. Tiemann, surgical instrument maker, of New York, as to allow of its being shifted to either side according as the fracture is on the right or left, or of being removed for packing. He has also made the long splint in two portions sliding on each other so as to shorten or lengthen it according to the size of the patient, and to facilitate its package and transportation. Desault attached the posterior as well as the anterior extremity of the perineal band to the long splint; but it will be found that, by so doing, he does not grasp with it, as he intended, the tuberosity; on the contrary, when extension is applied, it slips under it or above it, and is thus almost totally ineffectual in relieving the groin. To be effective, it should be attached to the splint at a point considerably lower down; and it is necessary that the medium of attachment should be movable, in order that, when the upper end of the splint is placed opposite the crista ilii, it may be shifted, if necessary, a trifle upwards or downwards, that the band may exactly grasp the tuberosity. I therefore provide a button (B, Fig. 159),

Fig. 159.

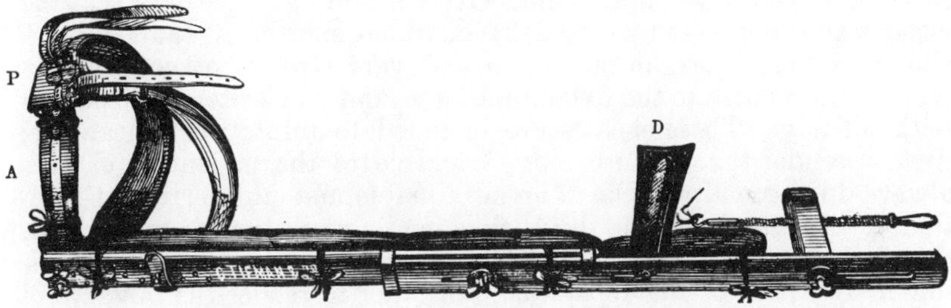

secured by a thumb-screw, and several holes at different contiguous points in the splint, to which it may be shifted with facility. The posterior end of the perineal band is either passed under the outer splint and buttoned, as shown at B, Fig. 159, or carried between the cushion and splint, over the top of the latter to the button, as indicated at E, Fig. 160. The latter arrangement is applicable especially to fat and muscular subjects, particularly females, who have an abundance of fat and other tissues covering the tuberosity, which might allow the band to slip by the bone, unless attached in this manner. I propose, also, to attach both the extending and counter-extending bands to the apparatus through the medium of elastics. Upon suggesting this to Mr. Tiemann, I found that some one had anticipated me with regard to the extending band; and Mr. T. has arranged a strong spiral spring in the ferule of the screw, which supplies the

Fig. 160.

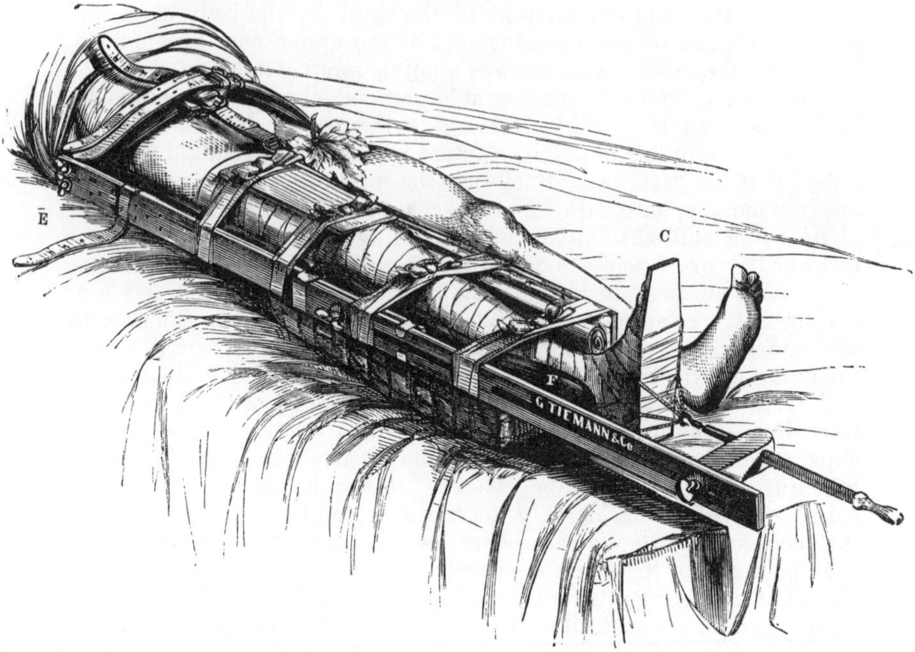

place of the elastic at that point. It is absolutely necessary that the elastics attached to the perineal band, which may be of India rubber, should be very short, an inch or so, and very strong; otherwise, they will give too much to the extending force, and had better be dispensed with entirely. These elastics are intended to fulfil two indications; first, to render the pressure more tolerable to the patient, as elastics always do; secondly, to keep up an equable and uninterrupted traction on the muscles of the thigh, thus tending still further to diminish the shortening, and to counteract the effect of any stretching or yielding in any part of the apparatus. In order to render the pressure of the perineal band still less unpleasant, and less likely to cause excoriation of the groin, it might be of service to apply several coatings of a mixture of collodion 25 parts, castor oil 1 part, which has been found to form, in other parts of the body, and might form here a smooth and enduring cuticle.

"My remaining modification of the splint is a foot-piece (D, Fig. 159), attached by a slide and thumb-screw to the mortise in the external splint, and capable of removal at pleasure. This is intended to obviate two inconveniences of the old arrangement; first, to prevent a tendency to eversion of the foot, which almost always exists, sometimes to a great extent; and, secondly, by projecting a little beyond the toes, to take off the pressure of the bedclothes, which tends still further to evert the foot, and is, besides, exceedingly uncomfortable to the patient. In Fig. 160 this arrangement is dispensed with, and its place supplied by a foot-piece (C), which also obviates the necessity for the block for preserving the parallelism of the adhesive bands, since these bands pass from the leg, on either side, around this piece, binding firmly to the sole of the foot. The cords connecting it with the screw are so arranged as to draw uniformly on this, so as not to tilt it against the 'ball' of the foot. By resting below the heel on the mattress, it serves to support the weight of the clothes, and also prevents eversion of the foot. This contrivance is an imitation of Boyer's, and may, by some surgeons, be preferred; although it is, in my opinion, not so efficient as the foot-piece (D, Fig. 159). (F) is a wedge-shaped cushion, very useful in maintaining the whole apparatus in a level position, and taking off the pressure from the heel and tendo Achillis. An inside splint, extending from the perineum to the inner malleolus, and a guttered splint for the upper and lower surfaces of the thigh respectively, with suitable cushions for the splints, complete this apparatus."

Following the suggestion made by Dr. Neill,[1] who uses for this purpose a Spanish windlass, I have had the foot-block of my own splint (Fig. 161) so constructed as that counter-extension may be made at the same moment with the extension. The principle is the same as that employed in the ancient "glossocomon," described by most of the early surgical writers. The advantages of this method are that the counter-extension, as well as the extension, can be made slowly, steadily, and firmly; the patient cannot, if disposed to interfere with the dressings, loosen or disturb them; the limb is acted upon equally in each direction, and the rollers which secure the limb to the splint do not become drawn obliquely and disarranged by the daily attempts to increase or continue the extension. The only danger is, that, in the hands of inexperienced surgeons, too much force will be applied, and perineal ulcerations ensue.

In constructing the perineal band, I now usually adopt the suggestion made to me some time since by Dr. Boardman, of this city. A sheet of foolscap, or the half of a newspaper is folded into a ribbon of about one inch and a half in width; this is intended to give firmness to the perineal band, and to prevent its corrugation. The surface which is to be laid against the skin is then covered with cotton wadding, and the whole enveloped in a long, narrow strip of cotton cloth, and neatly stitched. The strip of cotton cloth must be much longer than the padded portion of the band, in order to tie through the fenestræ. Before securing the band in place, a strip of patent lint should be laid in the perineum with its soft side against the skin. This may be occasionally renewed.

With children I often employ only the simple splint figured in Fig. 162, yet if the little patient is restless and disposed to throw himself about the bed, I prefer the double splint shown in Fig. 163, to which is attached a screw of peculiar construction, called the "endless screw," (Figs. 164, 165, 166, 167), the pattern for which was sent to me by some gentleman in Boston, whose name, I regret to say, I cannot now recall.

It will be found necessary, generally, to confine both limbs to the

[1] Philadelphia Med. Exam., vol. xi. p. 579.

Fig. 161.

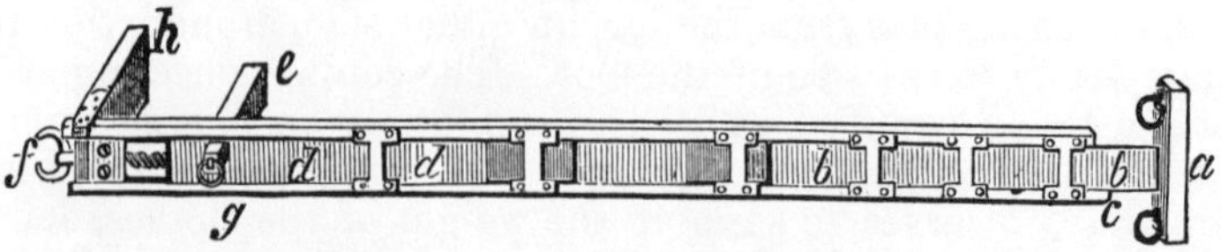

The Author's Single Straight Thigh-Splint, for Children or Adults.—*a.* Crutch-head, with two rings for the passage of the perineal band. *b*, *b*. Upper sliding portion of the splint. *c.* Ratchet to secure the upper portion of the splint when drawn out. *d*, *d*. Lower sliding portion of the splint, to which is attached the foot-block. *e.* Foot-block, which, with the lower sliding portion of the splint, *d*, is moved upwards or downwards by the screw, *f.* *g.* Brass ring fastened to the outer end of the foot-block. The perineal band having passed through the rings in the crutch-head, is made fast to this ring; so that when the foot-block descends, extension and counter-extension are made at the same moment. *h.* Cross-piece, to steady the long splint.

Fig. 162.

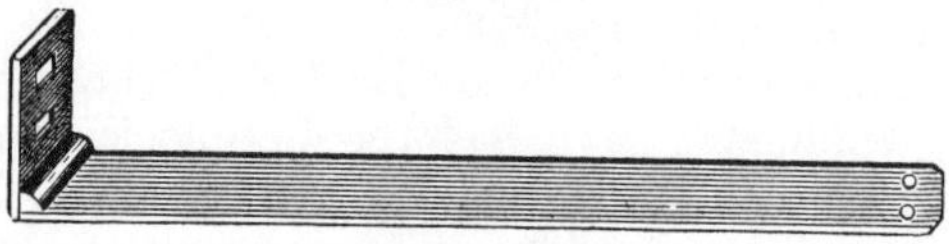

The Author's Single Straight Thigh-Splint, for Children, or the straight splint in its simplest and elementary form.

Fig. 163.

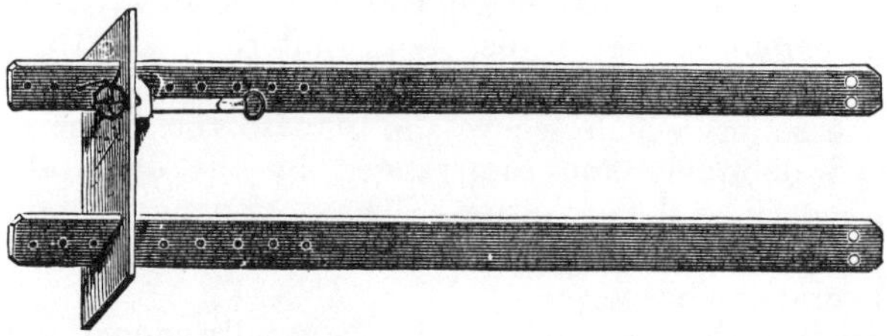

The Author's Double Straight Thigh-Splint, for Children or Adults.—Both of the long splints are laid outside of the two thighs.

Fig. 164.

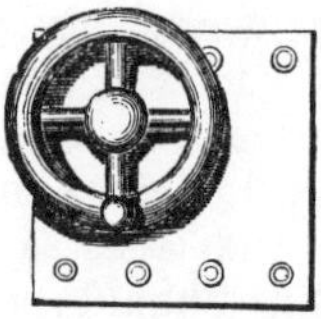

Fig. 165.

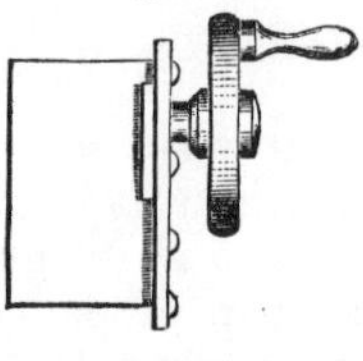

Fig. 166.

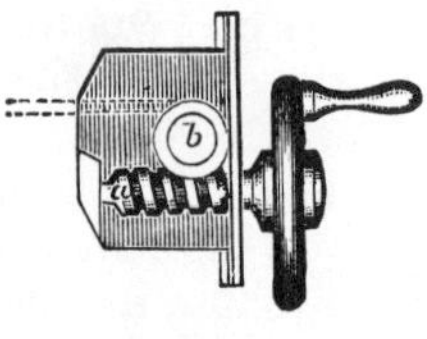

Fig. 167.

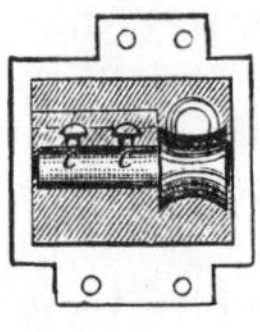

SCALE ONE-FOURTH OF FULL SIZE.

Endless Screw, used by the Author for making Extension in the Double Straight Splint.—Fig. 164. Front view. Fig. 165. Side view. Fig. 166. End view; *a* is a screw working in a toothed wheel, *b.* Fig. 167. Front removed, showing the plane part of toothed wheel for extension strap. *c*, *c*. Two small screws to fasten extension strap.

long side splints with rollers, over junks, the rollers being carefully applied from the foot to the groin. In this way alone can children be prevented from constantly disturbing the dressings. When thus secured, these patients become completely manageable, and can be readily moved at any time from the bed to a lounge or even into the open air.

In all cases one should prefer to use side splints, carefully fitted;

the whole, both side and long splints, being applied to the limb over neatly-made cotton pads or junks, of which there ought to be laid upon every part of the leg and thigh as many as may be necessary to prevent unequal pressure.

I am especially careful to place a thick but soft pad underneath the knee, since if this is not done the forced extension into which the hamstrings are thrown soon becomes irksome and even painful. A thick compress ought also to be placed under the back of the leg, just above the heel, to prevent the weight of the limb from producing ulceration.

To this general plan of treatment now recommended for fractures of the femur the writer makes no exceptions, unless it be in the case of a fracture of the neck of the femur occurring in very old persons, or in fractures just above the condyles, where the direction of the fracture is obliquely downwards and forwards; in the former of which often no rule can be adopted, except that the patient should be placed in that position which may be found most comfortable; and in the latter of which the flexed position seems indeed the most rational, yet, according to the evidences furnished by Malgaigne, its advantages over the straight position are far from being established. In fractures occurring just below the trochanter minor, my own experience agrees with that of the distinguished author just quoted, that the straight position is still the best; an experience which seems to me also to admit of a satisfactory explanation. It is not directly upwards, but rather outwards and upwards (Fig. 168), that the lower end of the proximal fragment is thrown by the action of the psoas magnus and iliacus internus, so that in order to meet the supposed indication it will be necessary to carry the lower part of the limb outwards also, a position which would certainly be found very inconvenient, if not actually impracticable, in the majority of cases.

Fig. 168.

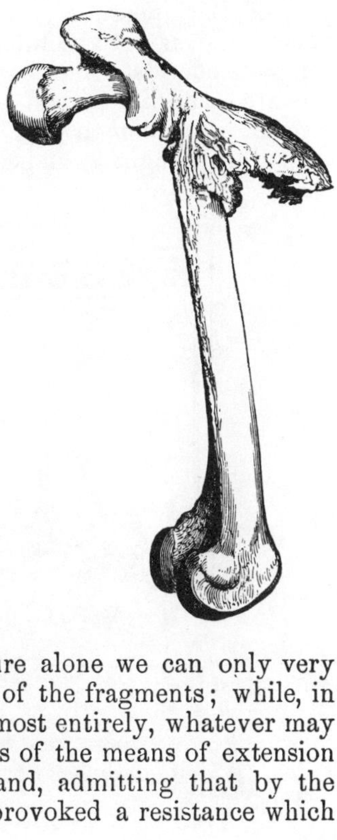

Nor can the tendency of the upper fragment to rise, and consequently to separate from the lower, be effectually met by posture alone, unless the thigh is completely flexed upon the body; a position, again, which will be found inconvenient, if not impossible.

It is apparent, therefore, that by posture alone we can only very imperfectly accomplish an approximation of the fragments; while, in adopting the flexed position, we have almost entirely, whatever may be said to the contrary, deprived ourselves of the means of extension and counter-extension. On the other hand, admitting that by the straight position we have momentarily provoked a resistance which flexion of the limb might have prevented, we shall be able, slowly but effectually, to overcome this resistance by steady and continued extension. In the one case we have made a present gain, but a final loss; and in the other a present loss results in our final gain. So it is that experience has shown in more than one case which has come under our observation, that although for a few moments, or perhaps for several hours, after the straight position has been assumed in these fractures, the upper fragment will rise spasmodically, after a time, longer or shorter, and especially after the application of the side splints and bandages, this tendency will cease altogether.

My convictions upon this subject are clear, but since they do not correspond with the convictions of a pretty large proportion of practical surgeons, I am compelled to regard the question of posture in this particular fracture as still open. I will take the liberty to suggest, however, that it is by the results of carefully recorded experience alone that it can ever be determined, and not by any reference to physiological or anatomical arguments, which I suspect have had hitherto much more influence with surgeons in respect to this question than personal observation.

In hospitals, and in private practice whenever the circumstances of the patient will warrant the expense, a bed constructed with especial view to fractures of the thigh ought to be regarded as an essential part of the apparatus; always contributing to the comfort of the patient, if it is not absolutely necessary to the attainment of the most complete success. Indeed, where some form of fracture-bed cannot be procured, and the patient is compelled to lie upon a common cot bed instead, or a common post bedstead, or upon the floor, I cannot think the surgeon ought to be held in any degree responsible for the result.

Fig. 169.

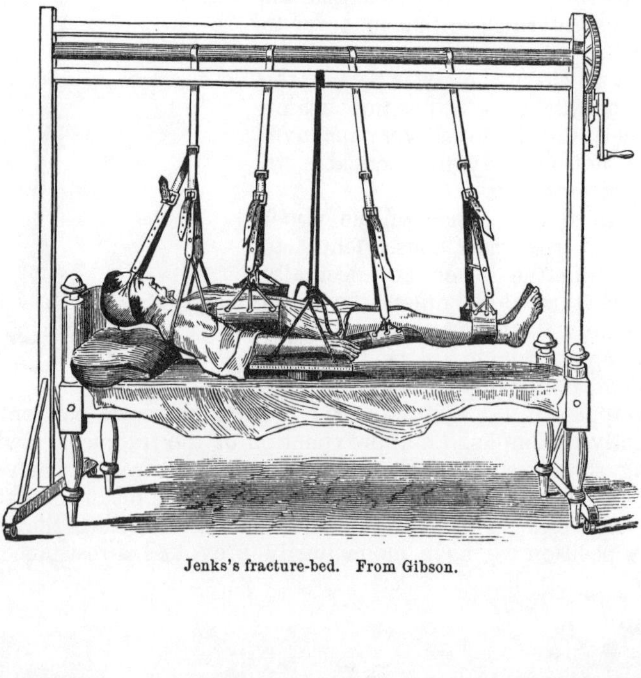

Jenks's fracture-bed. From Gibson.

The fracture-beds in use among American surgeons are exceedingly various, among which I will mention, as being especially ingenious, the beds invented by Jenks, Daniels, the Burges, Addinell Hewson, of Philadelphia,[1] J. Rhea Barton, and B. H. Coates, of the same city.[2]

Of these several contrivances, Jenks's bed (Fig. 169) has been for the longest period in use among American surgeons, and its excellencies most thoroughly tested. It is composed of "two upright posts about six feet high, supported each by a pedestal; of two horizontal bars at the top, somewhat longer than a common bedstead; of a windlass of the same length placed six inches below the upper bar; of a cog-wheel and handle; of linen belts, from six to twelve inches wide; of straps secured at one end to the windlass, and at the other having hooks attached to corresponding eyes in the linen belts; of a head-piece made of netting; of a piece of sheet-iron twelve inches long, and hollowed out to fit and surround the thigh; of a bed-pan, box and cushion to support it, and of some other minor parts.

"The patient lying on his mattress, and his limb surrounded by the apparatus of Desault, Hagedorn, or any other that may be preferred, the surgeon, or any common attendant, will only find it requisite to pass the linen belts beneath his body [attaching them to the hooks on the ends of the straps, and adjusting the whole at the proper distance and length, so as to balance the body exactly], and raise it from the mattress by turning the handle of the windlass. While the patient is thus suspended, the bed can be made up, and the feces and urine evacuated. To lower the patient again, and replace him on the mattress, the windlass must be reversed. The linen belts may then be removed, and the body brought in contact with the sheet."[3]

But in my own experience no bed has proved so complete and universally applicable as the fracture-bed invented more recently by Daniels (Figs. 170, 171, 172); and which may be used either as a double inclined plane, or as a single horizontal plane suitable for the support of the patient when his limb is dressed with the straight splint.

Sometimes I have had constructed a simple frame, covered with a stout canvas sacking, having a hole at a point corresponding with the position of the nates, and this I have laid directly upon a common four-post bedstead. A mattress and one or two quilts must be placed upon the boards of the bedstead underneath the sacking, and a sheet or two above the sacking, upon which last the patient is to be laid. In arranging the linen underneath the patient the most convenient plan is, instead of using only one sheet, which will require that a hole shall be made in it corresponding to the hole in the sacking, to employ two sheets, and, doubling them separately, to bring the folded margin of each from above and from below to the centre of the opening. When the patient has occasion to use the bed-pan it is only necessary that two or four persons should lift this frame, and place under each corner a block about one foot in height, or it may be raised by a pulley and ropes suspended from the ceiling.

[1] Hewson, Amer. Journ. Med. Sci., July, 1858, p. 101.
[2] Eclectic Repertory, 5th and 9th vols.
[3] Gibson's Surgery, vol. i. p. 320.

Fig. 170.

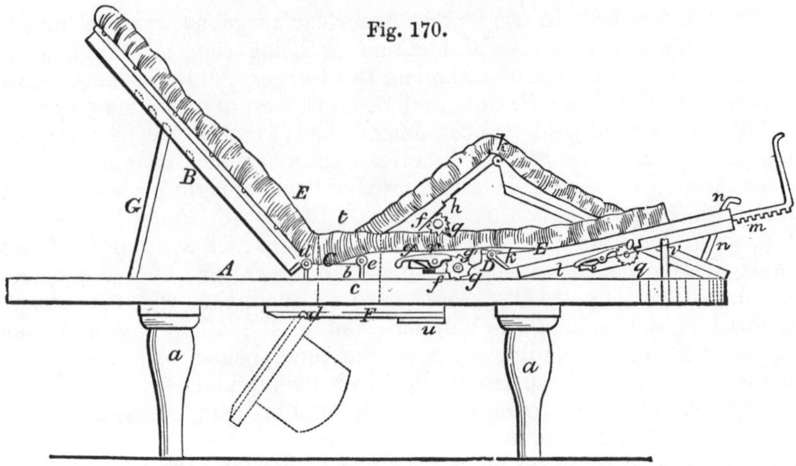

Fig. 171.

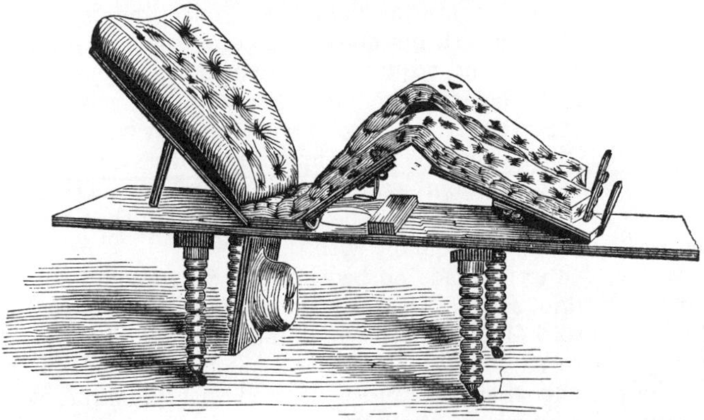

Fig. 172.

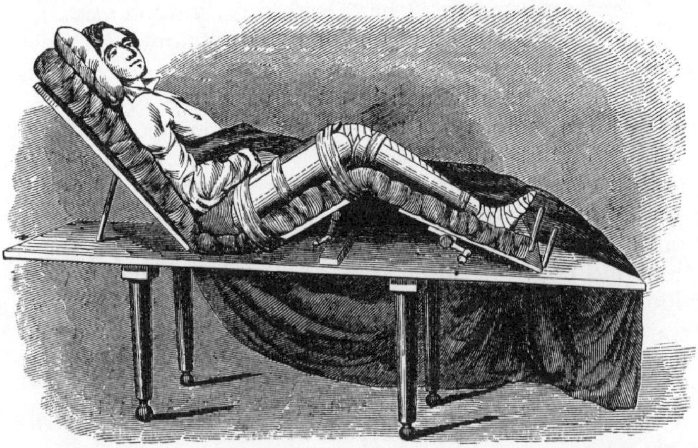

E. DANIEL'S FRACTURE-BED.

"*A* represents a platform of a suitable length and width, and supported by four legs, *a*. To the upper surface of the platform *A* there is attached a cross-piece, *b*, at a short distance from the centre, and directly through the centre of the platform there is made a circular hole or aperture, *c* (in dotted lines), said hole or aperture having a semicircular cut or recess in the cross-piece *b*. To the straight edge of the cross-piece *b* there is attached, by hinges, *d*, a board, *B*, termed the body plane, the width of which may correspond with that of the platform *A*, and when depressed its outer edge may be even with the edge of the platform. The sides of the body plane may be elevated, or raised so as to be slightly concave on its outer surface. To the opposite side or edge of the cross-piece *b*, and at each side of the semicircular cut or recess formed by the hole or aperture *c*, there are attached by hinges, *e*, cast-iron plates, *C C*, which are provided with grooves or ways at their sides, in or between which plates, *D D*, work. The plates *C C*, *D D* (one on each side) are thigh planes, and their edges are provided with ease or projections, *f*, in which a shaft, *g*, works, one on each plate *C*. On each shaft *g* there is placed a pinion, which gears into a rack attached to the under surface of the plates *D D*. At one end of the shafts *g* there are attached ratchets, *g'*, in which pawls, *j*, catch, said pawls being attached to the sides of the plates *C C*. To the outer edges of the plates *D D* there are attached by hinges, *k*, boards, *E E;* these boards are leg planes, and are slightly raised at their inner ends, where they are connected to the plates *D*, in order to form depressions to correspond to the shape of the legs. To the under surface of each leg plane there is attached a metal guide, *l*, in which a rack, *m*, works; the outer ends of the racks have bars, *n*, projecting from them at right angles. To each leg plane there is attached a shaft, *o*, having a pinion, *p*, and ratchet, *q*, thereon, and pawls, *r*, which catch into the ratchets *q*, the pawls being attached to the outer sides of the leg planes. The pinions gear into the racks *m*. The body plane, and also the thigh and leg planes, are covered by a suitable mattress, *E*, with a hole made through it to correspond with the hole or aperture *c* in the platform *A*, and the mattress is slit or cut to cover properly the thigh and leg planes without interfering with their movements. To the under side of the platform *A* there is attached by hinges a flap, *F*, having a stuffed pad or cushion, *t*, upon it, which, when the flap *F* is secured upwards against the platform *A*, fits in the hole or aperture *c* in the platform and mattress. The flap is secured against the platform by a button, *u*."

We may also floor over a common bedstead, having previously, in case it is an adult whom we have to treat, removed the foot-board, so that we may extend the floor two or three feet beyond the usual length of the bedstead. In the centre of this floor we may make an opening, so arranged as to be closed by a board slid underneath, or by a door fastened with a couple of leathern hinges, and closed by a spring catch.

A very comfortable bed, especially for children, can sometimes be made from a cot. But it will be necessary, always, to nail a piece of board firmly across the top and bottom of the bedstead when the sacking is at its utmost tension, in order to prevent the side rails from falling together. The top board must be nailed on vertically like an ordinary head-board, so as to prevent the pillows from falling off, but the bottom piece should be at least one foot wide, and laid horizontally to support and steady the apparatus as it extends beyond the foot.

Having had occasion, lately, to assist Dr. Treat, of this city, in the management of a fracture of the thigh, in the case of a little girl not quite three years old, I was struck with the simplicity and completeness of an arrangement which he had made to prevent the bed and the dressings from becoming soiled with the urine. It was only to leave directly underneath the nates a complete opening through to the floor for the escape of the urine, and to protect the margins of the sacking and sheets, which came nearly together at the opening, with pieces of oiled cloth folded upon themselves. It was found that not only the bed was in this way kept dry, but the dressings also; it being now observed that the dressings had become wet heretofore by soaking up the moisture from the bed rather than by the direct fall of the urine upon them.

Having prepared the bed for the reception of the patient, we may proceed as follows in the case of a simple fracture.

Lay the perineal band in its place, and four pieces of bandage transversely where the broken thigh is to repose; over the four transverse bands lay a firm splint, long enough to reach from the tuberosity of the ischium to the lower margin of the ham, and nearly as wide as the diameter of the thigh. This may be made of a board covered with cotton cloth, and carefully stuffed, so as to fit all the inequalities of the several portions of the limb. It can be fitted with sufficient accuracy by comparing and trying it upon the sound limb. Of all the side splints this is the most important, and the greatest care ought to be exercised in its construction.

The patient, having been previously stripped and washed with warm water and soap, is laid upon the bed with his thigh reposing upon the back splint; the head and trunk being at first moderately raised to prevent any strain upon the muscles of the front of the thigh. An assistant seizes the knee firmly with both hands and makes moderate traction so as to steady the limb, and at the same time prevent the fragments from penetrating the flesh; while the surgeon lays his long strips of adhesive plaster upon each side of the leg in the manner which has already been described, protecting the ankles with small pads made of cotton batting. Elevating the foot a little more, he proceeds to apply a roller from the toes up to the ham. Everything is now ready for the long splint, which, in case only one is used, is laid outside the broken limb, and the perineal band adjusted and tied temporarily in a bow knot: one long junk is pressed between the splint and the limb, reaching from the hip to the heel, and immediately the surgeon fastens the extending bands to the foot-piece or to the extending screw, and tightens it moderately so that the assistant may release his hold upon the knee.

The whole limb is now steadied and at rest, and the patient seldom fails to declare himself relieved; after which, the surgeon may proceed more at leisure to complete his dressings.

A padded splint should next be laid upon the inside of the thigh, extending from the groin to immediately below the knee, but it must not be allowed to press much upon the knee, as it would be likely to become painful, and perhaps, vesicate the skin over the projecting bones. Another splint in front, extending from the groin to within one inch of the knee, completes the inclosure of the limb; and the whole are to be retained in place by tying the four transverse bands, previously laid under the limb, around the three short lateral splints, and the long outside splint. In some cases I prefer to secure the short lateral splints to the limb independently of the long splint, and then it is necessary to lay a fourth short splint upon the outside of the limb, between it and the long splint, otherwise the transverse bands will cut into the flesh.

The perineal band ought now to be made permanently fast, and the extension carried to the point of utmost tolerance on the part of the patient, while the surgeon proceeds to apply a roller from the instep to the groin, enveloping at the same time the splint and the limb in its successive turns; but as he progresses upwards, he should lay between the limb and the splint and underneath the limb as many soft, cotton pads as may be needed to fill up all the inequalities; these pads it will be found necessary to extend from the malleolus externus to near the middle of the leg, and to lay them under the tendo-Achillis and knee, outside of the knee, above the trochanter major, &c.

Before the surgeon leaves he should ascertain whether the extension is too violent, or whether it is quite painful, and in either case it must be a little slackened.

If the patient is a child, or an intractable adult, the double splint ought to be preferred, and the unbroken limb be secured to the opposite long splint in the same manner as the broken, only that no perineal band or extending straps are needed for the sound limb.

The rules which have now been laid down in relation to the order and manner of dressing, are the results of my own personal experience as to what method is generally the most convenient and useful; but circumstances must occasionally require that they should be somewhat varied or modified; and when other forms of apparatus are employed than those for which I have already indicated my preference, the rules of procedure must be determined by the peculiarities of the apparatus. In short, much must always be left to the discretion of the surgeon, only that he never can be at liberty to dress a broken thigh in a hasty or slovenly manner.

During the first two or three weeks the limb ought to be seen daily, and at each visit a careful examination of every portion of the apparel should be made, so far as this can be done without opening or removing the dressings; and whenever anything is disarranged, or has become too tight or too loose, so far as may be necessary to correct these faults, the bandages should be removed and readjusted. Generally they can be tightened by over-stitching or by additional bandages. If the patient complains of pain at any point where a splint presses, his complaints should receive prompt attention, and the cause should be ascertained and removed if possible. Especially ought the surgeon to look to the condition of the perineum; and generally no harm comes of slackening or removing the band whenever this part is to be inspected, since the weight of the body alone is sufficient, during the few minutes it is removed, to prevent any shortening of the limb.

During the first week the extension should be increased, according to the ability of the patient to endure it, each day; and after that, steadily maintained until union has taken place.

In the case of an adult, we ought never to encourage a hope that he can be released from his splints in less than eight weeks, although we may find it safe to remove them as early as the end of the sixth week; but the patient seldom wears the splints too long, while they are often removed too soon. Remember that the fragments are in nine cases out of ten uniting side by side and not end to end; the muscles which act upon them are powerful, and the weight of the limb is great, so that the time within which the limb can be safely trusted alone is never short.

The extension may, however, be relaxed as soon, generally, as the twenty-eighth day, and the leg may be lifted daily after this, and the knee and ankle very gently flexed and rubbed, but never so early as this period can the short side splints be abandoned safely. Still more important do I regard the continuance of the long side splint—no longer now as a means of extension, but only of retention—lest the weight of the limb should turn the foot gradually out, or occasion some other deformity.

It is true that in some cases, where patients are remarkably careful and everything has gone along well, I have, at the end of four weeks, applied a paste bandage from the toes to the groin, and permitted them to get up upon crutches; but I would not dare to recommend this practice to the inexperienced surgeon or to the incautious patient. It has often done well, but sometimes it has proved disastrous. It is an extra hazard which the surgeon should be reluctant to incur.

When at length the patient is permitted to leave his bed, a pair of crutches becomes indispensable, and during the following two months but little weight should be borne upon the limb; and in rising from the bed care must be taken lest the limb should be so situated as that its weight would make it bend.

§ 5. Fractures of the Condyles.

(a.) *Fractures of the External Condyle.*

Dr. Alph. B. Crosby, of New Hampshire, has published an account of a case of simple fracture of the external condyle, in a young man twenty-one years of age, and which happened from a sudden twist of the limb, while he was undressing himself to bathe. He was "standing on a shelving bank, with the right leg flexed over the left in order to remove his pantaloons: he lost his balance, partially twisted the leg, and fell to the ground." Six months after, the fragment was removed by Dr. Crosby, through an incision below the condyle. The recovery of the young man has been complete.

Fig. 173.

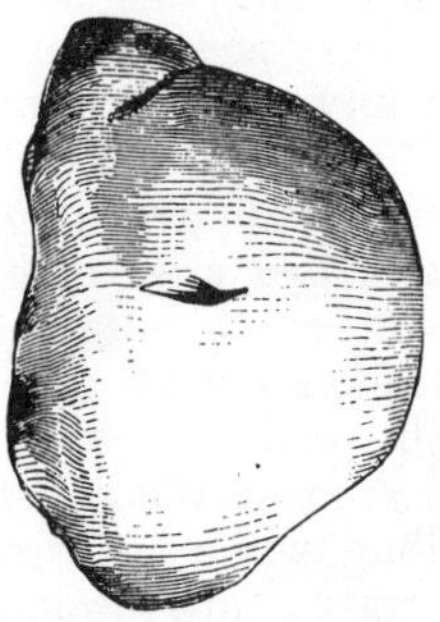

Dr. Crosby's specimen of fracture of the external condyle.

The accompanying drawing represents the specimen as seen from its lower or cartilaginous surface, and of its actual size.

Dr. T. S. Kirkbride has also reported an example of simple fracture of this condyle, which was produced by the kick of a horse, the blow having been received upon the inside of the knee. When this patient entered the Pennsylvania Hospital, Dec., 1834, the knee was much swollen and crepitus was plainly felt, but the fragment was not much displaced; the muscles upon the outer side, however, were so strongly contracted as to abduct the leg and produce considerable angular deformity. The limb could be easily made straight, but it returned to its former position of abduction, as

[1] Crosby, New Hampshire Journ. of Med., 1857.

soon as it was released. When fully extended, slight bending of the joint did not give severe pain, but when in any degree flexed all motion was very painful.

The limb was placed in a long straight fracture box, and cold applications were made: great swelling followed. It was kept extended in this manner, or in the long splint of Desault, twenty-eight days; at which time union seemed to have taken place, but the motions at the joint were very limited and productive of great pain. From this period the limb was laid in a splint so constructed as that the angle at the knee could be changed daily. At the end of about six weeks he began to walk on crutches, and he could then flex the leg to a right angle.[1]

Fig. 174.

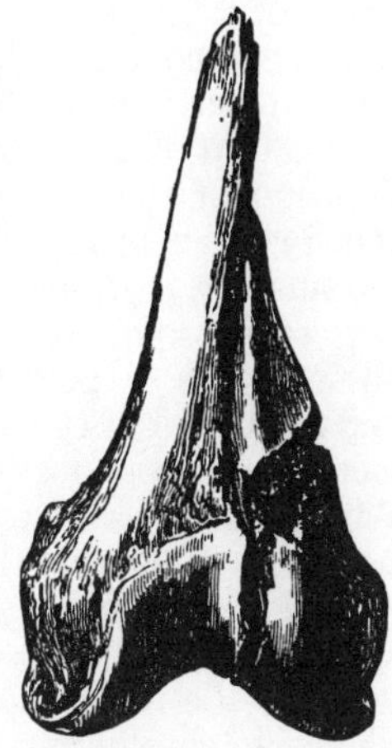

Sir Astley Cooper's case of fracture of the external condyle.

Sir Astley has related a case of compound fracture of the same condyle, produced by falling from a curb-stone upon the knee. The man died on the 24th day. On examination after death the external condyle was found to be broken off, and also a considerable fragment was detached from the shaft higher up.[2]

(b.) *Fractures of the Internal Condyle.*

Dr. Thomas Wells, of Columbia, S. C., has reported an example of fracture of the internal condyle, accompanied with a dislocation of the head of the tibia outwards and backwards. The man was about forty years old, and intemperate. Dr. Wells was not called until two days after the injury was received, when he found the limb greatly swollen and gangrenous. The man's account of himself was that while walking in the back yard he fell, and thus dislocated his knee, and that he was then brought into the house, being unable to stand upon his feet. It does not appear that any attempt was made to reduce the limb, probably because his general condition indicated that speedy death was inevitable. On the fourth day he died. The autopsy disclosed, in addition to the dislocation of the tibia, that a thick scale of bone was broken from the inner part of the inner condyle, but it remained attached to the ligaments.[3]

Treatment of Fractures of either Condyle.—The few cases of these accidents which have been reported have been, with one or two exceptions, treated in the straight position. In Kirkbride's case any degree of flexion was painful, although there was little or no displacement of the fragment; and we think we can see, in the relative position of the articular surfaces of the tibia and femur, a sufficient reason why the straight or nearly straight position must generally be preferred. Whichever

[1] Kirkbride, Amer. Journ. Med. Sci., May, 1835, vol. xvi. p. 32.
[2] Sir Astley Cooper, On Disloc., &c., op. cit., p. 239.
[3] Wells, Amer. Journ. Med. Sci., May, 1832, vol. x. p. 25.

condyle is broken, the remaining condyle will be sufficient to prevent a dislocation and consequent shortening of the limb, unless, indeed, the dislocation has already occurred as an immediate consequence of the injury. It is very certain that it would not take place from the action of the muscles when the limb was straight. In the flexed position, I can conceive that it might take place, but yet not easily. It is not a dislocation of the limb, then, that we seek chiefly to avoid, but a deflection of the leg to the right or to the left, according as one or the other of the condyles has been broken. It will be readily seen that, in order to resist this tendency, nothing but the straight position will answer, and that for this purpose it will be necessary to lay a long splint upon one or both sides of the limb, and to secure the whole length of both thigh and leg to this splint. The long fracture-box used by Kirkbride, if well cushioned on all sides, seems to me at once to answer most completely this important indication, rendering it even unnecessary to employ a bandage, since the opposite sides of the box will compel the limb to adopt the proper position.

I need scarcely say that neither extension nor counter-extension will be demanded.

As to the remainder of the treatment, it must consist essentially in the active employment of such means as are calculated to prevent and allay inflammation; especially ought the surgeon not to omit to avail himself of so valuable an antiphlogistic agent as cool water lotions.

As soon as the union is consummated the joint surfaces should be submitted to passive motion in order to prevent anchylosis; and it would be better to commence this so early as to hazard somewhat a displacement of the fragment than to wait too long. It may not, in some cases, be improper as early as the fourteenth day, and in nearly all cases it should be practised as early as the twenty-eighth.

(c.) *Fractures between the Condyles and across the Base.*

Etiology.—A fracture of this character may be produced by a blow received upon the side of the limb or upon the lower extremity of the femur; sometimes the blow has been received directly upon the patella when the knee was bent, and Bichat mentions a case in which it was produced by a fall upon the feet.

Symptoms.—This fracture is easily distinguished from the preceding by the much greater mobility of the fragments and by the palpable shortening of the limb, since an overlapping of the broken ends is here almost inevitable. Each fragment may be felt to move separately, and the motion will be accompanied with crepitus.

Prognosis.—The danger of violent inflammation in the joint is imminent, and anchylosis of the knee is to be anticipated as the most favorable result, since the joint surfaces are likely to be rendered immovable by fibrinous deposits in their immediate vicinity, and also by the adhesion of the muscles to one another and to the bone higher up, where the fracture of the shaft has occurred. More fortunate results than these may, indeed, be hoped for, inasmuch as they have occasionally been noticed, but they cannot fairly be expected.

In a majority of cases, such accidents have demanded, either immediately or at a later period, amputation. If recovery takes place, a shortening of the thigh is inevitable.

Treatment.—Malgaigne saw a patient who had been treated by Guerbois with the aid of extension and counter-extension, who was confined to his bed five months, and who had at the end of eight years very little motion in the joint, and he seems disposed to charge in some measure these unfortunate consequences to the position in which the limb was placed, namely, the straight position. But in my opinion, it is much more reasonable to suppose, that if the treatment was at all responsible for the results, the error consisted in too long and unnecessary confinement, and in too much extension. I suspect that the mere matter of position had nothing to do with the anchylosis. Malgaigne does not, however, himself recommend anything more than a very slight amount of flexion at the knee; and to this practice I am prepared to give my assent; since it will give to the limb the best position in case anchylosis does occur, and it is not inconsistent with the employment of the moderate amount of extension which alone is justifiable after this accident. If the young surgeon should differ with me in opinion as to the necessity or propriety of using great force to retain the fragments in place and prevent overlapping, I beg him to consider that this accident never happens except from the application of an extraordinary force, and that consequently intense inflammation and swelling are almost certain to ensue; and that in some cases, the very fact that immediately after the accident, or for some hours succeeding, no swelling occurs, or muscular contraction, and that replacement of the fragments is easily accomplished, is evidence only of the great severity of the injury, and that the whole system is lying under the shock: to which, if the patient does not succumb, sooner or later reaction will ensue, and the fragments will be gradually drawn up with a resistless power. The surgeon ought to remember also that to make extension in this case, he is obliged to pull upon those very ligaments and tendons about the joint which, having been torn or bruised, must soon become exquisitely sensitive.

The long straight box, already recommended when speaking of fracture of one condyle, is equally applicable here; only that it needs a foot-board, or some sort of foot-piece to which an extending apparatus may be secured, and that a pillow should be placed under the knee to give the limb the proper flexion.

Case.—A man was admitted into St. Thomas's Hospital, London, Sept. 17, 1816, with a fracture between the condyles, accompanied also with a fracture through the shaft higher up, occasioned by being caught in the wheels of a carriage while in motion. There was a small wound opposite the point of fracture, and the external condyle was displaced outwards.

The limb was laid in a fracture box, and in a position of semiflexion.

On the 18th of Nov., the external condyle, having protruded through the skin, and being dead, was removed with the forceps, bringing with it a portion of the articular surface.

On the 6th of Dec. he was discharged from the hospital, and in February following he was walking without any support, and with the free use of the joint.[1]

Case.—While I am writing, a gentleman living about eighty miles from town has been thrown from his carriage, breaking the left femur just above the condyles into many fragments, so that when I saw him, on the following day, the attending physician showed me about four or five inches of the entire thickness of the shaft which he had removed. The external condyle was completely separated from the internal, and was quite movable.

In this case the attempt to save the limb resulted in the loss of the patient's life on the sixth or seventh day.

CHAPTER XXIX.

FRACTURES OF THE PATELLA.

Causes.—Of fourteen fractures of the patella which have come under my observation, thirteen were the result of direct blows, or of falls upon the knee. In the remaining example the fracture was due solely to muscular action: A sailor, aged about thirty years, had caught the heel of his boot in a knot-hole in the floor, which threw him backwards, and in the effort to sustain himself the patella was broken transversely. Dr. Kirkbride has reported a case in which both patellæ were broken in a similar manner but at different periods. The patient was a girl, æt. 29, who was admitted into the Pennsylvania Hospital, Oct. 16, 1833. "In falling backwards, and making an effort to save herself," the right patella had been fractured. She was dismissed cured on the second of Dec., and on the 20th of April following she was readmitted, with a fracture of the left patella, produced in the same manner as before; but in her effort to save the right limb, the left received all the strain and the patella gave way.[2] Dr. Kirkbride records another instance of fracture from muscular exertion in a man æt. 32, who attempted to jump into a cart, by raising his body, with his hands resting upon the bottom of the vehicle;[2] and Dr. Hayward, of Boston, saw a case in the Mass. Gen. Hospital, in a man æt. 67, which occurred in consequence of a false step in descending a flight of stairs.[3]

Pathology.—All the fractures produced by muscular action have been found to be transverse, and the same is true generally of fractures

[1] A. Cooper on Disloc., &c., op. cit., p. 239.
[2] Kirkbride, Amer. Journ. Med. Sci., Aug. 1835, vol. xvi. p. 330.
[3] Hayward, Am. Journ. Med. Sci., vol. xxx., from New Eng. Quart. Journ , July, 1842.

produced by direct blows; occasionally, however, we meet with longitudinal fractures, or with fractures more or less oblique and comminuted. Eleven of the fractures seen by me were simple and transverse; one was simple and oblique, and one was comminuted. The

Fig. 175.

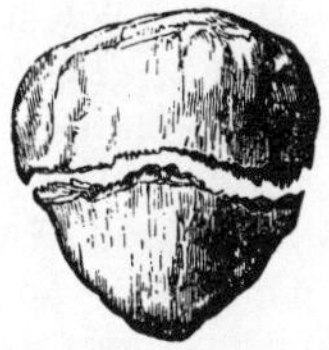

Fig. 176.

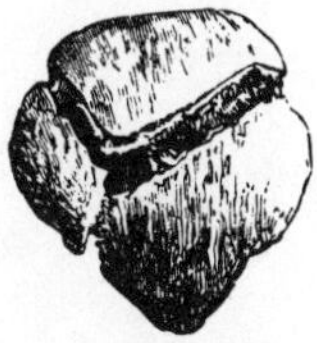

oblique fracture was in the person of a child five years old, who fell on his left knee, Jan. 31, 1848, breaking off a small fragment from the upper and inner margin of the patella. It did not separate from the main fragment except when the knee was flexed, and it was then thrown directly forwards, presenting to the finger a sharp point. Dr. Flint, who was with myself in attendance, kept the leg extended and had the knee constantly moistened with cool lotions. Six months after, I could not discover any traces of the accident. There is a specimen, illustrating a similar fracture, but not united, in the collection at St. Thomas's Hospital, London.[1] Dupuytren, A. Cooper and others have also mentioned cases of longitudinal fracture.

I have seen a double transverse fracture, or a fracture of both patellæ in a man æt. 22, who fell from a third story window, striking, he says, upon his knees. He was taken to the Hospital of the Sisters of Charity, in this city, and, after a few weeks, made an excellent recovery.

Fig. 177.

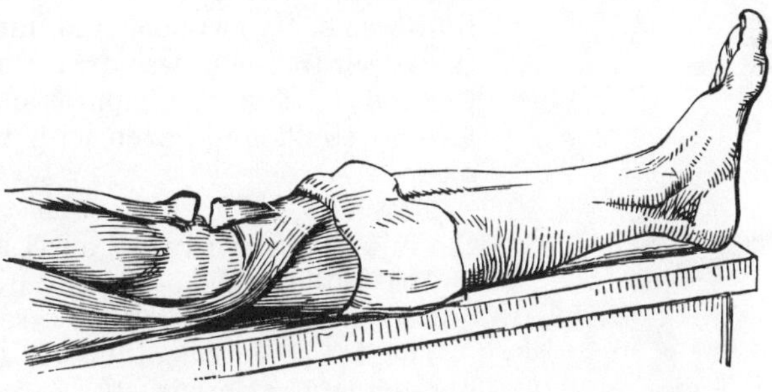

Symptoms.—The symptoms which characterize a transverse fracture of the patella are sufficiently diagnostic. The fragments are separated from each other, the superior fragment being drawn upwards more or less, according to the power and activity of the muscles, or the degree to which the ligamentous covering of the patella has been torn. In

[1] A. Cooper, On disloc., &c., op. cit., p. 232.

some cases, also, the violent flexion of the knee, Fig. 178, has completed the separation which otherwise might have been only partial. By passing the finger along the anterior surface of the limb with a moderate degree of firmness, the depression between the fragments will be made manifest.

Fig. 178.

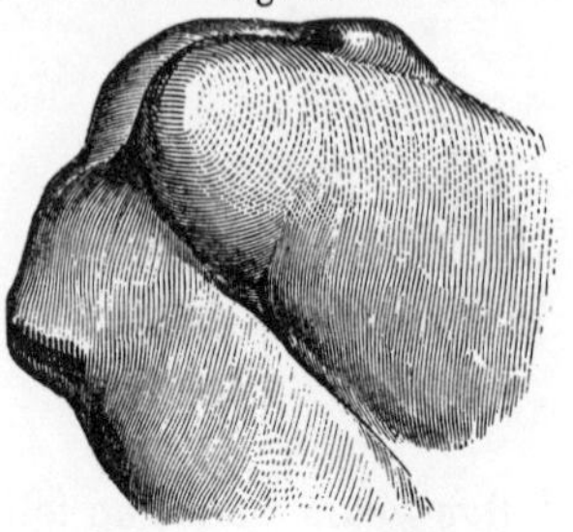

Fragments separated by flexion of the knee.

No crepitus can be expected unless the fragments remain in contact, a condition which is very unusual. The patient is unable to stand, and especially is the power of extending the leg upon the thigh completely lost. Usually a good deal of swelling immediately succeeds the accident, and after a time the skin becomes more or less discolored from effusions of blood. If the fracture is longitudinal or oblique, a slight lateral separation is usually present, but not always very easily detected.

Prognosis.—One of my patients, who had a comminuted fracture, with other serious injuries, died, but not as a consequence of the fracture. In the following case the fragments appear never to have united, although the patient recovered.

John Sharkie, æt. 24, a soldier in the British service, while serving in the East Indies, was struck on the right knee while he was in a sitting posture, with his leg bent under him.

He was immediately placed under the charge of the surgeon of the 89th regiment of infantry. During the first eleven days no splints or bandages were applied, on account of the severe inflammation and swelling. A compress was then placed over both fragments, and they were bound together by rollers, &c. The whole limb was suspended on an inclined plane, the foot being made fast to a foot-board. This treatment was continued four months. When the bandages were removed the limb was badly swollen; and immediately the upper fragment was drawn up toward the body. Eighteen months elapsed before he could walk, even with the aid of a cane.

Fig. 179.

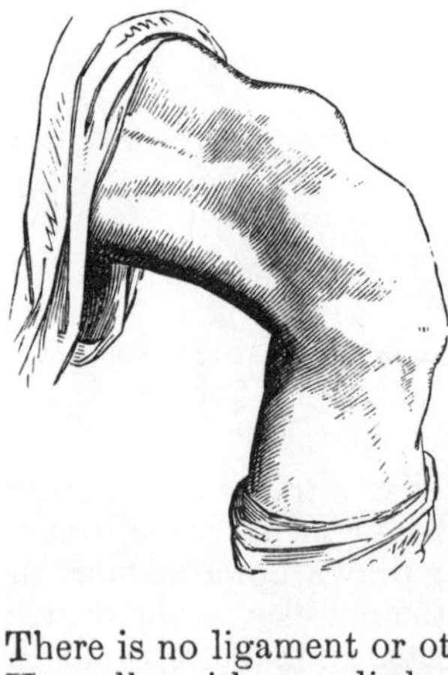

March 27, 1855, twenty-nine years after the injury was received, he was an inmate of the Buffalo Hospital, and I was permitted to examine his knee carefully.

The lower fragment is not displaced, but when the leg is straight upon the thigh the upper fragment lies two and a half inches from the lower, and when it is flexed upon the thigh the upper fragment is removed five inches from the lower. There is no ligament or other bond of union, so far as I can discover. He walks with very little or no halt, but he cannot walk fast.

In every other instance which has come under my notice union has taken place at periods varying from twenty-four to fifty-eight days, the average being thirty-eight days. Eleven cases have united by a ligament varying in length from one-quarter to one-half an inch. These measurements, made upon the living subject, may not be mathematically accurate, but they cannot be far from the truth.

In one instance, the case of a man æt. 40, the fracture having been treated by another surgeon, the ligamentous union, at first complete, seems to have subsequently given way in part. He called upon me for advice nine weeks after the fracture had occurred. The patella was surrounded with bony callus, so that it was considerably wider than the other. The fragments seemed to be united by a short ligament, except on the inner side, where there was a separation or rupture of the ligament to the extent of one-quarter of an inch. The patient explained this by saying that the splint was removed at the end of four weeks, and that after a week more he began to walk, but that he almost immediately felt it tear or give way on the inner side.

Dr. Kirkbride has reported a case of ligamentous union of the patella, in which the ligament was two and a half inches long, and was attached only to the inner margins of the fracture. "He was able to walk as rapidly as ever, and without perceptible limping."[1] A similar case is reported by Dr. Watson, of New York, in which the fragments became separated three and a half inches.[2] In both instances the fragments were supposed to have united by a short ligament, which had become lengthened by premature use of the limb; in the case reported by Kirkbride, the ligament seemed to have partly torn, as in the case reported by myself. Dr. Coale presented to the Boston Society for Medical Improvement, at its April meeting in 1856, a specimen of a fractured patella taken from a man sixty-five years old, the fracture having occurred ten years before. The fragments were at first so closely united that no division between them could be discovered, but subsequently they became separated at their outer edges one inch, and at their inner edges one-eighth of an inch.[3]

Twice, I believe, I have seen a bony union of the patella. The first instance is that to which I have already referred as an oblique or longitudinal fracture across one corner of the patella; and in the other example the action of the muscles upon the upper fragment was prevented by the occurrence of a fracture of the shaft of the femur at the same time, which permitted the thigh to shorten upon itself. The man was about twenty-five years old, and in a fall from a scaffold had broken his left femur, and also the patella. The patella was broken transversely, near its middle, and also longitudinally, near its inner margin. The fragments were all distinctly made out. Drs. Lewis and Dayton, of this city, were in attendance, and on the fifth day I was called in consultation. We dressed the limb with a long straight splint, employing moderate extension and counter-extension. The patella was covered with strips of adhesive plaster. On the fifty-eighth day I found the fragments of the patella united.

1 Kirkbride, Amer. Journ. of Med. Sciences, vol. xvi. p. 32.
2 Watson, N. Y. Journ. of Med. and Surgery, vol. iii., first series, p. 366.
3 Coale, Boston Med. and Surg. Journal, vol. liv. p. 402.

June 3, 1854, five months after the accident, I examined the limb carefully. The femur was shortened half an inch, and, although the two main fragments of the patella were separated half an inch, the bond of union seemed to be bone. It was hard, and allowed of no motion in the upper fragment separate from the lower. The lateral fragment was also apparently united by bone and in place. He had but little motion in the knee-joint, yet he walked very well, and was able to pursue his trade, as a carpenter, without much inconvenience.

Sir Astley Cooper succeeded in obtaining a bony union in some longitudinal fractures, but in a majority of cases it failed, owing to the want of apposition in the fragments. It might seem that it would be easy to accomplish apposition in all longitudinal fractures, but experience has shown that it is not always, the fragments being kept asunder partly by the action of the oblique fibres of the vasti and partly by the pressure of the condyles of the femur, especially when the leg is slightly flexed.

Whether the fracture is transverse or longitudinal, a bony union may occasionally be obtained when the fragments are retained in absolute contact for a sufficient length of time; but the failure to procure a bony union is not a matter of consequence, since a short ligament is equally useful.

Post, of New York, has reported three cases of compound fracture of the patella extending into the knee-joint, brought to a successful termination.[1]

In a case mentioned by Dr. Eve, of Augusta, occasioned by the kick of a horse, and in which amputation became necessary on the tenth day, "the knee-joint was found filled with dark grumous blood; a portion of the cartilage of the internal condyle of the os femoris was chipped off, and the patella broken into a number of fragments."[2]

Dr. Lewitt, of Michigan, has related a case of fracture in a lad æt. 16, produced by striking his knee against a piece of timber, which resulted in suppuration of the knee-joint, but from which he finally recovered with the perfect use of the limb. The fracture of the patella was oblique, traversing only its upper and outer margin, and it was never much displaced.[3]

Treatment.—Dr. Sanborn, of Lowell, Mass., has contrived a method of treating transverse fractures of the patella, Figs. 180, 181, and also cases of rupture of the ligamentum patellæ, which I shall take the liberty of describing in his own language.

"While repairing one of the public buildings of this city, two men, masons by trade, were precipitated, by the breaking of a staging, a distance of twenty-five feet on to a plank floor. One of the men received a fracture of the base of the skull, and died in consequence; the other escaped with a rupture of the ligamentum patellæ. The man was conveyed home, and a neighboring physician applied the usual dressing of a 'figure-of-eight' bandage, with a splint behind the

[1] Post, New York Journ. of Med., vol. ii., first series, p. 367.

[2] Eve, Southern Med. and Surg. Journ., 1848; also Bost. Med. Journ., vol. xxxvii. p. 427.

[3] Lewitt, Medical Independent, Sept. 1856.

joint. In the course of the following night, the pain in the knee became intolerable from the swelling and consequent tightness of the bandage, and all dressings were removed. The following day the case was transferred to my care by the attending physician. I found the knee a good deal swollen and inflamed, and there was evidence of extensive extravasation of blood into the joint and surrounding tissue. The patella was drawn up the thigh for a distance of four inches; and, although it could be brought down nearly to its proper situation by the hand, a bandage sufficiently tight to keep it there could not be borne. The object to be accomplished, then, was to bring a sufficient force to bear on the patella, without making pressure on the joint or impeding the circulation of the limb. And it was accomplished in this manner: A strip of ordinary adhesive plaster, four feet long and two and a half inches wide, was applied to the limb from the upper portion of the thigh to the middle of the leg, leaving at the knee a free loop. A roller bandage was then applied above and below the knee, for the purpose of securing the plaster and controlling the circulation and muscular contraction. A small stick, six or eight inches in length, then being put through the loop over the knee, the plaster was twisted until the patella was brought nearly down to its proper situation. Before applying the *twist*, a hard compress was placed above the edge of the patella in such a manner as to bring the force to bear directly upon that bone. * * * * Leeches and fomentations were applied to the joint, and, as the inflammation subsided, the plaster was tightened, until (at about the sixth day) the bone was brought fully down to its normal situation. It was there held, without the slightest uneasiness to the patient, until union took place. In

Fig. 180.

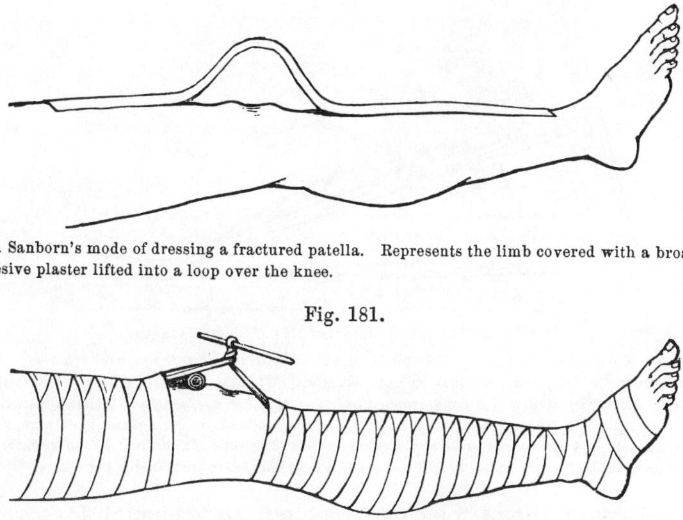

E. K. Sanborn's mode of dressing a fractured patella. Represents the limb covered with a broad band of adhesive plaster lifted into a loop over the knee.

Fig. 181.

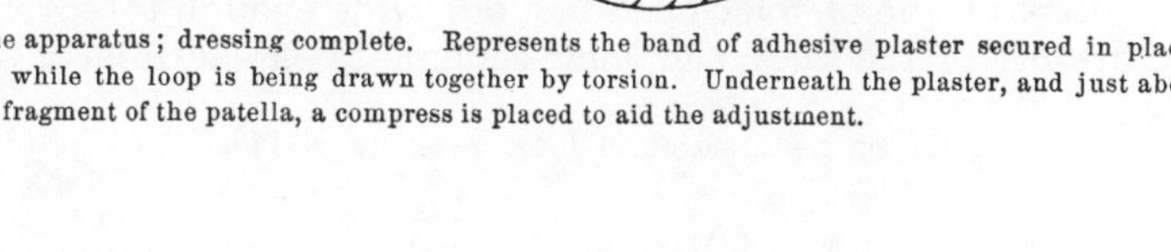

Same apparatus; dressing complete. Represents the band of adhesive plaster secured in place by a roller, while the loop is being drawn together by torsion. Underneath the plaster, and just above the upper fragment of the patella, a compress is placed to aid the adjustment.

three weeks the man was able to walk alone, with the plaster still applied, and the recovery was ultimately perfect. There is now no perceptible halt in the gait.

"Within the last two years several cases of transverse fracture of the patella have been treated by this method, both by myself and others in this vicinity, and with perfect success."[1]

The dressing which I have usually employed in the treatment of this fracture, consists of a single inclined plane, of sufficient length to support the thigh and leg, and about six inches wider than the limb at the knee. This plane rises from a horizontal floor of the same length and breadth, and is supported at its distal end by an upright piece of board, which serves both to lift the plane and to support and steady the foot. The distal end of the inclined plane may be elevated from six to eighteen inches, according to the length of the limb and other circumstances. Upon either side, about four inches below the knee, is cut a deep notch. The foot-piece stands at right angles with the inclined plane, and not at right angles with the horizontal floor; it may be perforated with holes for the passage of tapes or bandages to secure the foot.

Having covered the apparatus with a thick and soft cushion carefully adapted to all the irregularities of the thigh and leg, especial care being taken to fill completely the space under the knee, the whole limb is now laid upon it, and the foot secured gently to the foot-board, between which and the foot another cushion is placed.

The body of the patient should also be flexed upon the thigh, so as the more effectually to relax the quadriceps femoris muscle.

Fig. 182.

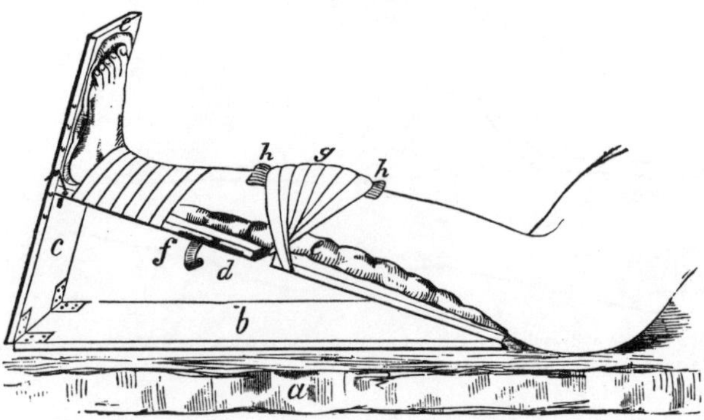

THE AUTHOR'S MODE OF DRESSING A FRACTURED PATELLA.

a. Bed. *b.* Floor of apparatus. *c.* Foot-piece, furnished with fenestræ through which straps may be passed to secure the foot, and with pins on each margin. *d.* Single inclined plane fastened to the foot-piece at any height, by means of a hook dropped over the pins. *e, e.* Cushion: thicker under the knee than at either end. *f.* Roller to secure leg and thigh to the inclined plane; not completely applied. *g.* Adhesive plasters laid over a compress and crossed under the splint. Those from above pass through a notch in the splint below the knee. *h, h.* Ends of the compresses, seen from under the adhesive plasters.

A compress made of folded cotton cloth, wide enough to cover the whole breadth of the knee, and long enough to extend from a point

[1] Boston Med. and Surg. Journ., vol. liv. p. 174.

four inches above the patella to the tuberosity of the tibia, and one-quarter of an inch thick, is now placed on the front of, and above the knee. While an assistant presses down the upper fragment of the patella, the surgeon proceeds to secure it in place with bands of adhesive plaster. Each band should be two or two and a half inches wide, and sufficiently long to inclose the limb and splint obliquely. The centre of the first band is laid upon the compress partly above and partly upon the upper fragment, and its extremities are brought down so as to pass through the two notches on the side of the splint and close upon each other underneath. The second band, imbricating the first, descends a little lower upon the patella and is secured below in the same manner. The third, and so on successively until the whole extent of the compress and knee is covered, is carried more nearly at right angles around the leg and splint; the last bands passing obliquely from below the ligamentum patellæ upwards and backwards. The dressing is now completed by passing a cotton roller around the whole length of the limb and splint, commencing at the toes and ending at the groin. This is to be applied lightly, as its object is only to support and steady the limb upon the splint.

The great advantage which this mode of dressing possesses is, that it does not ligate the leg or thigh completely, since, on either side, between the broad margins of the splint and the points where the straps and bandages touch the limb, there is a space, more or less considerable, against which no pressure is made, and through which the circulation may go on without impediment; so that, however firmly the bands are drawn across the knee, no swelling occurs in the foot. As to its efficiency, the best testimony which can be presented is the simple fact that of six cases treated by this method, four have united by a ligament of only one-quarter of an inch in length, and two by a ligament of half an inch.

The following example of a fracture of both patellæ will illustrate the general advantages of this dressing:—

John Dundas, æt. 22, fell, October 22, 1852, in the night while asleep, from a window in the third story of a dwelling-house, striking with his knees upon the stone side-walk.

On the tenth day I took charge of him at the Buffalo Hospital of the Sisters of Charity. I found both limbs in Gibson's modification of Hagedorn's splint for fractured thighs, with a figure-of-8 bandage loosely applied. The fragments were very much displaced. I immediately proceeded to inclose each leg, from the toes upwards as far as the knee, with a paste bandage, and then, having properly cushioned the limbs and laid them over two separate inclined planes, I secured the fragments in place with adhesive plaster; subsequently the limbs and planes were made fast together by successive turns of a roller.

The knees were examined frequently, and the dressings occasionally renewed.

November 28, 1852, thirty-seven days after the fractures had occurred, the splints and bandages were finally removed. Both patellæ had united by ligamentous tissue, the length of which was about one-quarter of an inch.

In a few weeks more he left the hospital, walking with only a slight impairment of the motions of the joints.

The plan adopted by M. Gama, of Val de Grace,[1] is similar to that which I have now described, but the splint upon which the limb reposes is not so wide, while width is an essential point in the attainment of the objects which I propose. Dr. Neill, of Philadelphia, uses also the adhesive plaster straps, but they are not placed outside of the splint.[2] Such, also, I understand to be Mr. Alcock's method of using the adhesive plaster.[3]

The dressing and apparatus employed by Wood, of King's College Hospital, is very similar to my own, but, as will be seen by the accompanying drawing (Fig. 183), the splint is only five or six inches wide. Dr. Wood has substituted hooks for the notches.[4]

Fig. 183.

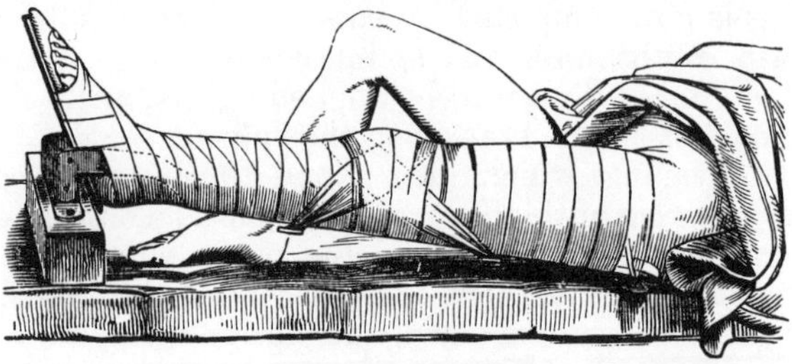

Wood's apparatus.

Dr. Dorsey, of Philadelphia, employed a very simple apparatus, Fig. 184, which will serve to illustrate the general plan adopted by many surgeons, both at home and abroad. It is liable, however, to the objec-

Fig. 184.

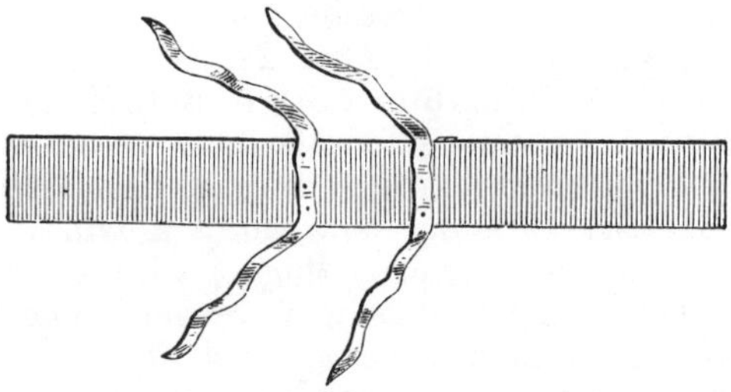

John Syng Dorsey's patella splint.

tion already stated—namely, that it interrupts too much the circulation of the limb. His apparatus consists of a piece of wood half an inch thick and two or three inches wide, and long enough to extend from the

[1] Malgaigne, Traité des Fractures, etc., op. cit., p. 764.

[2] Philadelphia Med. Examiner, vol. x. p. 1.

[3] Practical Observations on Fractures of the Patella and of the Olecranon, by Thomas Alcock, p. 296.

[4] Fergusson's Surgery, p. 307.

buttock to the heel; near the middle of this splint, and six inches apart, two bands of strong doubled muslin, a yard long, are nailed. The splint is then cushioned, and the limb being laid upon it, a roller being first applied from the ankle to the groin, encompassing the knee in the form of the figure-of-8; after which the two muslin bands are secured across the knee in such a manner as that the lower one shall draw down the upper fragment, and the upper one elevate the lower fragment.

A single instance will explain the danger of ligation to which I have alluded, and which, although it may be greater in case a starch or dextrine bandage is used, exists in some degree, whatever material for bandaging is employed, if it is applied to the whole circumference of the limb, and constant attention is not paid to the progress of the swelling.

"A vine-dresser, æt. 40, of a good constitution, fell and received a simple transverse fracture of the patella on the 15th of January. The medical officer called upon to attend him applied first a bandage for the purpose of drawing together the fragments, and afterwards a starched bandage extending from the toes to the upper part of the thigh; the limb was then put upon an inclined plane. The patient was visited a few times, but, as he scarcely suffered, the apparatus was in no way disturbed. On the first of March (sixteenth day) the attendant returned to remove the bandage, when the odor arising from the limb led him to believe that gangrene had taken place, and Dr. Defer was sent for. Dr. Defer found the limb in the following state: The toes which were not covered by the bandage were completely insensible and mummified. The bandage being removed, the gangrene was perceived to extend within seven inches of the knee, and was arrested in its progress. The foot was cold, and was totally insensible; the epidermis was raised up, and was beginning to be separated from the skin. The articulation of the ankle was exposed, and the ligaments destroyed. The bones of the leg were also exposed in their lower third, and the tendons were in a sloughy state. Amputation was performed, and the patient recovered."[1]

Very little better than the starch bandage, and exposing the patient in a still greater degree to the dangers of ligation and strangulation, are either of the methods recommended by Sir Astley Cooper, Figs. 185, 186.

Fig. 185.

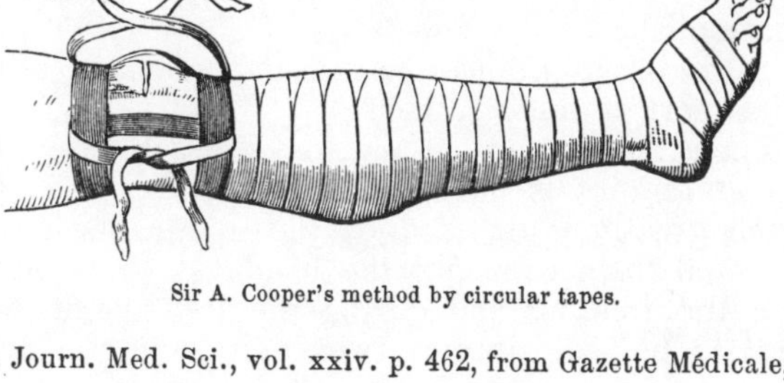

Sir A. Cooper's method by circular tapes.

[1] Amer. Journ. Med. Sci., vol. xxiv. p. 462, from Gazette Médicale, No. 28.

Fig. 186.

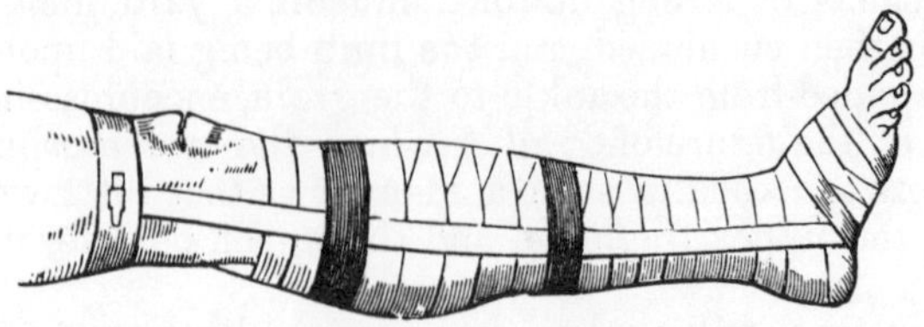

Sir A. Cooper's method by a leather counter-strap.

Mr. Lonsdale's instrument, Fig. 187, is ingenious, but too complicated and expensive. It is also liable to the serious objection that it forbids almost entirely the use of bandages, which, while they are capable of doing great mischief when they bind the limb too closely, are capable also of proving eminently serviceable when they press upon certain portions of the limb, and not with too much force.

Fig. 187.

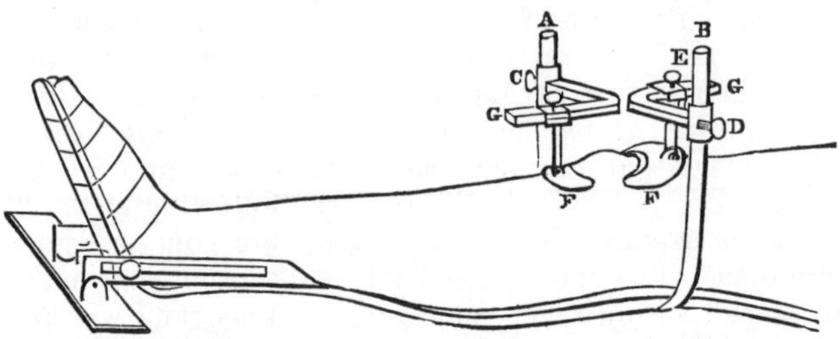

Lonsdale's Apparatus for Fractured Patella.—A B. Two vertical iron bars, each supporting a horizontal one; these horizontal arms slide upon the vertical bars, but can be secured at any point by the screws C D. To the horizontal beams are attached other vertical rods, which are movable, and yet fixable by screws, as at E. Finally, to each of these last upright pieces is fixed an iron plate, F F, by means of a hinge point, which keeps the patella in place. The foot-piece is movable up and down upon the main body of the apparatus, and can be made fast at any point, so as to adapt the splint to limbs of different length.

In case the fracture is oblique or longitudinal, it will be only necessary to lay the limb in a straight position, so as to prevent that lateral displacement of the fragments which has been shown to occur when the limb is flexed. It will not be necessary to employ a splint, unless the patient is unmanageable and demands restraint, nor to elevate the foot. After the swelling has subsided, a slight amount of lateral pressure, accomplished by a few turns of a roller, with or without compresses, as the circumstances may seem to demand, will complete the mechanical part of the treatment.

I have not mentioned the rapid and sometimes intense inflammation to which the knee-joint is liable after a fracture of the patella; and which is often greatly aggravated by the injudicious application of bandages. In no instance ought the bandages to be applied very tightly at the first dressing, and during the first five or six days the patient ought to be seen once or twice daily, and the most prompt attention given to any complaints of pain or soreness about the knee. From the beginning, cloths moistened in cool water should be constantly laid over the dressings; but in case adhesive plaster is used, we must be careful not to soak the straps sufficiently to loosen them.

If the swelling and inflammation increase rapidly, it would be far better to remove the straps or bandages altogether for a few days, than to take the risks consequent upon their continuance.

The anchylosis which usually follows the recovery of the patient, and which is often almost complete, is to be overcome by long continued passive motion; but great care must be taken not to rupture the ligament, as we have already seen happen in some cases.

Dr. Alfred C. Post, of the New York Hospital, has excised the knee-joint in a case of anchylosis of long standing; the limb being so much flexed in consequence of a comminuted fracture of the patella, as to be not merely useless, but an intolerable incumbrance. The patient was a laboring man of about forty years of age. This operation was made in preference to amputation, at the request of the man himself.[1]

CHAPTER XXX.

FRACTURES OF THE TIBIA.

Etiology.—Fractures of the tibia alone are, in a large majority of cases, produced by direct blows, such as the kick of a horse, or a blow from a stick of wood; in one instance I have seen it broken by a kick from a Dutchman's boot. It is occasionally broken by a fall upon the foot, the force of the impulse being expended before the fibula gives way, but almost always the fibula breaks at the same moment, or immediately after the fracture has taken place in the tibia.

Dr. Proudfoot, of New York, has reported an example of fracture of the tibia *in utero*, produced in the sixth month of pregnancy, by violent pressure upon the abdomen.[2]

Pathology, Division, &c.—In an analysis of twenty fractures of the tibia, five were found to have occurred in the upper third, seventeen in the middle third, and three in the lower third; of which latter, one was a fracture of the malleolus.

Four of the twenty are known to have been transverse or only slightly oblique. It is probable, also, that several of the remainder were transverse. In this respect, therefore, fractures of the tibia alone

[1] Post, New York Med. Gazette, vol. i. p. 309, Nov. 1850.

[2] Proudfoot, Bost. Med. and Surg. Journ., vol. xxxv. p. 268, 1846; from New York Journ. Med.

will be found to differ materially from fractures of the tibia and fibula; but it is only in accordance with the general observation that indirect blows produce almost constantly oblique fractures, and direct blows, somewhat more frequently, transverse.

Dr. James L. Van Ingen, of Schenectady, has reported a case of oblique fracture of the upper end of the tibia extending into the joint, accompanied with a slight displacement of the fibula at its upper end, and also a fracture of the external condyle of the femur. This was in the person of a man who had fallen from a load of hay upon the frozen ground.[1] Many other examples of fractures of the tibia extending into the knee-joint are recorded by surgeons, most of which were compound, or otherwise seriously complicated so as to render amputation necessary, and the consideration of which scarcely belongs properly to a treatise upon fractures.

Prognosis.—No shortening can occur in this fracture unless one or both ends of the fibula are displaced, a complication which I have noticed in two instances; but in neither case did the shortening exceed one-quarter of an inch.

Occasionally the upper fragment has been slightly displaced forwards. With these exceptions, and one other of delayed union which I shall presently mention, this bone in my experience has been found to unite promptly and without any appreciable deformity. Other surgeons have noticed occasionally that the upper end of the lower fragment has become displaced toward the fibula. Dr. Donne, of Louisville, has reported an example of delayed union in a simple, transverse fracture of the upper end of the tibia. The man was intemperate. Ten weeks after the accident no union had occurred, and Dr. Donne introduced a seton, and in about six weeks the fragments were firm.[2]

If the fracture extends into either the knee or ankle-joint, the danger of anchylosis is imminent, yet experience has shown that it may sometimes be avoided. In the case of Dr. Van Ingen's patient already mentioned, the motions of the knee-joint were almost completely restored, although the accident was serious and complicated.

When the malleolus is broken off, it generally becomes slightly displaced downwards, and in this position a complete bony or ligamentous union takes place.

Treatment.—The tendency to displacement, in a fracture of the tibia, is so slight, if it exists at all, that simple dressings, light splints of felt or binder's board, with rest in the horizontal posture upon a pillow, fulfil nearly all of the indications which are usually present. The following cases will illustrate the usual course of these accidents.

Mrs. W., of Buffalo, æt. 58, fell, Oct. 19, 1848, striking on her right knee, breaking the tibia transversely just below the tuberosity.

The fall was the result of a misstep on level ground, and was attended with only slight bruising of the soft parts. She says, that on attempting to rise she discovered what had happened, the bone pro-

[1] Van Ingen, Report of an action brought to recover for surgical services, 1855.

[2] Donne, Amer. Journ. Med., vol. xxviii. p. 524; from Western Journ. Med. and Surg., Aug. 1841.

jecting very distinctly, and she pushed and pulled it into place with her own hands.

Dr. Barnes, who was the family physician, requested me to see it on the same day. Mrs. W. was large, with a leucophlegmatic temperament. The limb was already swollen and œdematous. The fragments were in place, but motion and crepitus were distinct.

I dressed the limb by laying it upon a pillow outside of which were placed two broad deal splints, tying the whole snugly together with several strips of bandage. At a later period the leg and thigh were laid over a double inclined plane.

At the end of six weeks all dressings were removed, and the fragments were found to have united firmly, and so perfectly as that the point of fracture could not be traced.

Peter Hamil, of Buffalo, æt. 29, was admitted into the hospital Aug. 31, 1849, with an injury to his left leg, which had occurred two days before. A young surgeon had examined the limb, and thought the femur was broken just above the joint. He had applied a roller from the toes to the thigh; and to the thigh were applied lateral splints. These dressings were on the limb at the time of his admission, and were not removed until the next day. I could not then discover any fracture or displacement, and the dressings were discontinued, the limb being merely laid upon pillows. After about eight days, however, when the swelling of the foot, consequent upon the bandaging, had subsided, I reapplied side splints, believing it possible that I might have overlooked a transverse fracture of the lower end of the femur. On the 26th of Sept., I discontinued them altogether.

Oct. 4, when examining the limb, I detected a slipping sensation, like that produced in a false joint, through the upper end of the tibia, and I now easily understood what had been mistaken for a fracture of the femur. It was a transverse fracture through the upper end of the tibia, and without displacement.

No splints were afterwards applied, and on the 25th of Nov., three months after admission, he was dismissed, the motion between the fragments having ceased, but the knee still remaining quite stiff.

The presence of inflammation, with other complications, may, however, occasionally render the treatment more difficult and the results less satisfactory.

John Mahan, æt. 39. Admitted to the Buffalo Hospital, Feb. 16, 1853, with a compound fracture of the right tibia, near the middle of the leg. The bone was broken by the kick of a Dutchman. I found the limb much swollen and very painful, and I laid it carefully over a double inclined plane, and directed cold water irrigations; I also directed morphine in full doses. The inflammation for several days threatened the complete loss of his limb. On the tenth day, the distal end of the upper fragment was projecting in front of the lower, and I depressed the angle of the splint and made moderate pressure upon the upper fragment. On the twentieth day, the fragments were bent backwards, and I placed a compress behind. On the thirty-seventh day, we took the limb from the inclined plane and trusted alone to side splints. On the forty-fifth day, we removed all dressings. The fragments had not united. The limb was then laid upon a pillow, and six days later a firm gutta-percha splint was applied for the purpose of steadying the bone, but the splint was removed daily in order that the leg might be bathed and rubbed. He was allowed to sit up. On the fifty-ninth day, motion could still be perceived between the fragments, and he was directed to use crutches. On the ninety-third day, the union was found to be firm, the upper fragment remaining slightly displaced forwards.

In case the fracture extends into the knee-joint, it is best to lay the limb upon pillows or in a nicely-cushioned box, and nearly straight. No extension or counter-extension is necessary here any more than in other fractures of the tibia alone, nor are lateral splints or rollers necessary or proper at first, as a general rule; but especial attention ought constantly be given to the prevention of inflammation, and of subsequent anchylosis. The omission to employ splints in a case of this kind was charged against a surgeon in Vermont as evidence of malpractice. I am happy to say, however, that, in this particular case, he was sustained by the testimony of the medical men and by the verdict of the jury; but the attempt which the reporter has made to defend this as a universal practice in fractures of the legs, or of the tibia alone, is unfortunate, and evinces a lack of practical experience.[1]

Whatever position is adopted, and whatever means of support or retention are employed, if bandages and splints are applied tightly or injudiciously, great suffering and irreparable mischief to the knee-joint may be the consequence.

A man, æt. 23, entered the Pennsylvania Hospital July 18, 1839, with an oblique fracture through the head of the tibia. A physician had applied a bandage and splint to the leg, and sent him twenty miles to the city, and on examination after his arrival, the whole limb as high as the groin was much swollen, red, and excessively painful. The knee-joint was distended and very tender. All dressings were immediately removed and the limb laid in a long fracture-box, slightly elevated at the foot; cool lotions were applied, and the patient was freely bled, both from the arm and by the application of leeches. The limb was kept in this position about six weeks, and, at the end of two or three weeks more he was dismissed cured. Dr. Norris, who was the hospital surgeon in attendance, has, in his report of the case, very properly taken this occasion to warn surgeons of the danger of excessive bandaging and splinting in this kind of fracture, as well as in all other fractures of the lower extremities.[2]

Fractures of the malleolus demand only that the limb should be laid upon its outer, or fibular side, with the foot so supported as that it shall incline inwards toward the tibia. In this simple disposition of the limb we have done all that can be done by any mechanical contrivance toward approaching the lower fragment to the shaft from which it has been broken.

[1] Boston Med. Journ., vol. liv. p. 1, March, 1856.

[2] Norris, Amer. Journ. of Med. Sci., vol. xxiii. p. 291.

CHAPTER XXXI.

FRACTURES OF THE FIBULA.

Causes.—In a record of thirty-two cases, I have been able to ascertain the cause satisfactorily in eighteen, of which number three were the results of falls directly upon the bottom of the foot, four of a slip of the foot in walking on level ground, or on ground only slightly irregular, and twelve of direct blows.

Pathology.—In all of the fractures which have been produced by falls upon the bottom of the foot, and in all, except one, produced by a slip of the foot, the accident was accompanied with a dislocation of the ankle; the foot being turned outwards. In the one exceptional case mentioned, the dislocation may also have occurred, but the fact is not known.

Both Malgaigne and Dupuytren have noticed a dislocation in the opposite direction, or a turning of the foot inwards, more often than a turning outwards. I cannot think their observations were carefully made.

Moreover, in at least seven of the twelve fractures produced by direct blows the tibia has been thrown more or less inwards, and consequently the foot has turned out.

In twenty-four examples the fracture of the fibula has taken place within from two to five inches of the lower end of the bone. Twice I have found the external malleolus broken off, and seven times the internal malleolus.

Fig. 188.

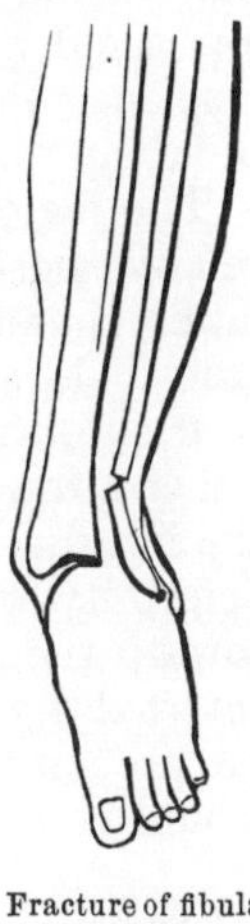

Fracture of fibula near lower end.

Four of the fractures occurring in consequence of direct blows were compound, and one was also comminuted.

Prognosis.—In a majority of cases, where the fibula has been broken from two to five inches above the lower end, the fragments have united inclined toward or resting against the tibia; occasionally I have seen them displaced backwards. Once the fibula refused to unite altogether.

The malleoli have generally united nearly or quite in place, but in two instances the external malleolus has been found displaced very much downwards.

Of the compound fractures, two required amputation, one was treated by resection of the lower end of the tibia, and one died without any operation. Douglas has reported a case of compound dislocation with fracture of the fibula, which being reduced, he was able to save the limb, but not without much difficulty, and the ankle remained stiff.[1] Other surgeons have met with similar success, but I shall refer to this subject again under the head of compound dislocations.

Of those which recovered, twenty-eight in number, ten have been found to have more or less unnatural prominence of the internal malleolus, and in two of these the malleolus, or lower end of the tibia, projects very much. In nearly all of these examples the foot appears somewhat inclined outwards.

Generally the ankle-joint has remained stiff for some time after the bandages have been removed; and probably in all cases in which the accident was accompanied with a dislocation of the tibia. But this stiffness has usually disappeared after a few weeks or months. Twice I have noticed considerable stiffness after about six months; three times after one year; in one case after two years, and in one case after twenty years the ankle would occasionally swell and become quite stiff. In one case it remained almost immovable after twenty years; and in a still more remarkable instance, I examined the limb thirty years after the accident, when the man was sixty-three years old, and although there existed no swelling or deformity, yet this leg was not as muscular as the other, and he declared that up to this time the ankle remained quite tender to the touch, and that occasionally it became painful.

When I come to speak of dislocations of the ankle, I shall adopt the usual nomenclature, and shall name all those dislocations in which the tibia projects inwards from the foot, "inward dislocations of the tibia," yet I have some doubts as to the propriety of this appellation. This accident seems to me to have been in general rather a lateral *rotation* of the foot, or of the astragalus, upon the lower articulating surfaces of the tibia and fibula. Of all the ginglymoid joints, the ankle approaches most nearly in form to a ball and socket joint, in consequence especially of the marked prolongations of the malleolus internus and externus. In other ginglymoid articulations lateral displacements are not unfrequent, but lateral rotation can scarcely by any accident occur. Here, however, the reverse holds true; lateral displacement is difficult, while lateral rotation is comparatively easy of accomplishment.

The majority of cases which occur involving a disturbance of the relative position of the ankle-joint surfaces, are, I am satisfied, of this latter character, viz., lateral rotations within the capsule, rather than true dislocations; and although the restoration of the joint surfaces to position is, in general, easily accomplished; yet, in consequence of either a fracture of the fibula, or malleolus internus, or of a rupture of the internal lateral ligaments, it will almost always happen that some deformity will remain. The fragments of the fibula will fall inwards toward the tibia, and the foot, unsupported by either its fibula or its internal ligaments, will incline perceptibly outwards. Nor can this be prevented, usually, by any mechanical contrivance. Indeed, it would be easy to demonstrate, as I have often done to my pupils, that

[1] Boston Med. and Surg. Journ., vol. xxxiv. p. 336, from Southern Journ. of Med.

even Dupuytren's splint, usually employed in this accident, must fail of success in a great majority of cases; since the subsequent deformity is due, less to the fracture of the fibula and its consequent displacement, than to the loss of the internal ligaments, which loss nature can seldom fully repair. The whole apparatus of the joint has suffered greatly, and its form and functions, therefore, are not likely to be completely restored, whether the fibula has participated in the injury or not. As further evidence of the correctness of this view, I will state that in three of the examples in which I have found the fractured fibula united and resting against the tibia, the motions of the ankle-joint have been completely recovered.

If, however, it were true that a fracture and displacement of the fibula is the sole or essential cause of the subsequent deformity, it would still be found often impracticable to avoid the maiming, since it would still remain impossible to lift the broken ends from the tibia, against which, or in the direction toward which, they are so prone to fall. Inversion of the foot does not accomplish it, nor have I ever been able to make anything but the most trivial impression upon the upper end of the lower fragment by pressure upon the lower extremity of the fibula.

I think too much confidence has been placed in the efficiency of "Dupuytren's splint." I believe, indeed, that this splint ought generally to be preferred as a means of support and retention after this accident, and I have myself usually employed it; but I doubt whether it is able to accomplish more than a moiety of all that its illustrious inventor proposed.

Treatment.—I have already expressed my preference for Dupuytren's mode of dressing as a general practice, and especially would I give it the preference whenever the accident has been accompanied with an outward luxation of the foot, and a consequent rupture of the internal lateral ligaments, or a fracture of the internal malleolus.

This mode of dressing is essentially as follows:—

A pad, or long junk, made of a piece of cotton cloth, stuffed with cotton batting, is constructed of sufficient length to extend from the condyles of the femur to a point just above the malleolus internus. This pad must be about five or six inches in width, and thicker by one or two inches at its lower than its upper end. This is to be laid upon the inside of the leg, with its base or thickest portion resting against the tibia just above the internal malleolus. Over this pad is

Fig. 189.

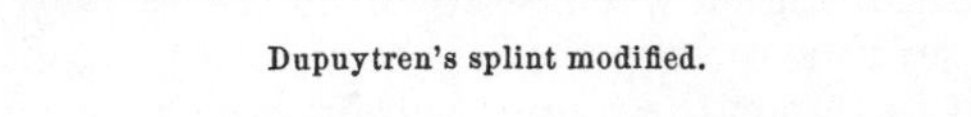

Dupuytren's splint modified.

to be placed a long firm splint, extending also from above the knee to three inches beyond the bottom of the foot. With a few turns of a oller the upper end of the splint will now be made fast to the knee, and with a second roller the lower end must be secured to the foot. The application of this last bandage requires, however, some care in its adjustment. Its purpose is simply to rotate the foot inwards, while at the same time the tibia is pressed outwards; and to this end it must be applied in the form of a figure-of-8 over both splint and foot, embracing alternately the heel and the instep. In order to be effectual, it must be drawn pretty firmly, and no portion of the bandage must pass higher than the malleolus externus. In some surgical books I have seen this apparatus represented with a roller embracing the whole length of the leg; and in others it is represented as encircling the limb two or three inches above the malleolus (Fig. 190), but it is evident that these modes of dressing must defeat the great object which Dupuytren had in view, namely, the throwing out of the upper end of the lower fragment.

Fig. 190.

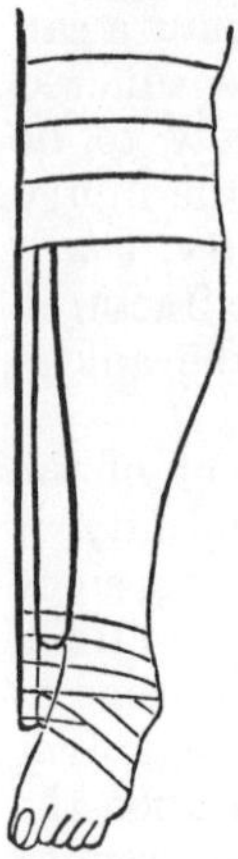

Dupuytren's splint incorrectly applied.

When the limb is thus dressed, the knee may be flexed and the leg laid upon its outside, supported by a pillow, or upon its inside, as in the accompanying engraving. (Fig. 191.)

If it is only a fracture of the external malleolus, or if the fracture has occurred in the middle or upper third of the bone, this treatment is no longer appropriate, and it will generally be found sufficient to place the limb at rest for a few days upon a suitable cushion or upon a pillow.

Fig. 191.

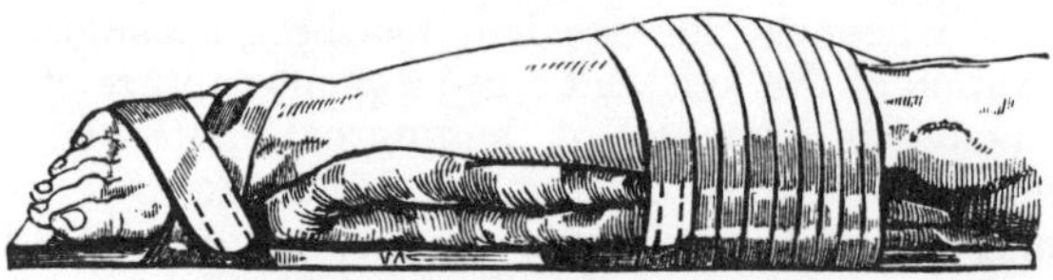

Dupuytren's splint as originally applied by himself.

It is scarcely necessary to say that, since after this accident anchylosis is so frequent, early and unremitting attention should be given to the establishment of passive motion in the joint. Indeed, I cannot but think that a desire to accomplish the indications recognized and urged by Dupuytren has led to the neglect of the indication which ought to have been regarded as of equal, if not of the greatest, importance, namely, the prevention of contractions and adhesions around and between the joint surfaces.

As a general rule, the dressings ought to be wholly laid aside by the end of the third or fourth week; and although it may be well for a somewhat longer time to keep the foot turned in by having it properly supported as it lies upon the pillow, yet after this date I regard the use of splints and bandages as only pernicious.

CHAPTER XXXII.

FRACTURES OF THE TIBIA AND FIBULA.

Causes.—Probably four-fifths of these fractures are the results of direct blows, or of crushing accidents, such as the kick of a horse, the passage of a loaded vehicle across the limb, the fall of heavy stones or timbers, &c.

In an analysis of eighty-three cases, I find the bones broken in the upper third from a direct cause four times, and from an indirect cause once. In the middle third thirty-three have been referred to a direct cause, and one to an indirect; and in the lower third thirty-three to a direct cause, and twelve to an indirect. An observation which does not sustain the remark of Malgaigne, based upon his analysis of sixty-seven cases, that fractures of the upper third are produced by direct causes alone, those of the middle third much more frequently by indirect causes, and that those of the lower third are especially due to indirect causes. Direct causes produce a large majority of the fractures of the lower third, but the proportion is smaller than in the middle third.

Of the indirect causes, falls upon the feet from a considerable height—as from a scaffolding, or from the top of a building—are by far the most common. Four times I have found the bones broken by muscular action alone, as in the following example:—

Mrs. W., of Buffalo, aged about twenty-five years, and weighing at this time nearly two hundred pounds, was descending her door-steps with an infant in her arms, when, the steps being covered with ice, she slipped and fell, breaking her right leg just above the ankle. Mrs. W. says she felt and heard the bones snap before she touched the steps. Of this she is certain.

We found the tibia broken obliquely, the fragments being quite movable, but not much, if at all, displaced. The limb was dressed with a carefully moulded and well-padded gutta-percha splint, and then laid in a pillow upon the bed. Mrs. W. experienced unusual pain from the fracture for several days, for the relief of which we were compelled at times to permit her to inhale chloroform. She was of a nervous temperament, and had frequently resorted to chloroform before to relieve neuralgic pains. The limb became very much swollen, and remained so for a week or two. No extension was ever employed.

Within the usual time the bones united in perfect apposition, and in about four months she was able to walk without any halt.

Pathology, Symptoms, &c.—We have seen that fractures of both bones through some part of the lower third are most frequent. Thus, of one hundred and forty-two fractures, eleven belonged to the upper third, forty to the middle, and eighty-five to the lower. In six cases the two bones were broken in different divisions. It is probable that in this analysis some errors have occurred, and that in a larger proportion than here stated, the two bones have given way at opposite extremities, since it is often difficult, and sometimes quite impossible to determine precisely where the fibula is broken; but the analysis is sufficiently correct to illustrate the much greater frequency of fractures of the lower third, and also the fact that the two bones generally break nearly on the same level; usually the point of fracture in the tibia is between two and three inches above the joint, where the bone is the weakest.

In an examination of twenty museum specimens I have found both bones broken at the same point, or within two or three inches of the same point, sixteen times, and at extreme points, four times; and in these last examples, the tibia has always been broken in the lower third, while the fibula has been broken in the upper third.

In thirteen of the fractures mentioned as belonging to the lower third, only the malleolus of the tibia was broken, while the fibula was broken two or three inches above its lower end. Some of these were, perhaps, examples of dislocation of the ankle.

I have seldom seen a transverse fracture of the tibia except in its lower or upper extremity, in the expanded portions of the bone, and even in those examples which we are accustomed to call transverse, because they are sufficiently so to prevent any sliding or overlapping of the fragments, there has existed, generally, a marked inclination of the line of fracture in one direction or another.

The examples of fracture produced by muscular action have, without an exception, occurred in adults. Three of them were in the lower third of the leg, and one in the middle third. I think they were, all of them, nearly transverse, since they never became much, if at all displaced.

Most of the fractures of the tibia produced by falls upon the feet are very oblique, and the direction of the fracture is generally downwards, forwards, and inwards; but I have found almost every conceivable variation from this general rule.

The fracture in the fibula is even more constantly oblique than the fracture in the tibia; but this is a point of very little practical consequence, and one which we can seldom determine positively, unless one of the fractured ends protrudes through the flesh.

Compound and comminuted fractures are more frequent here than in any other of the bones of the body. My tables, which have rejected all fractures demanding immediate amputation, most of which are compound, do not for this reason give a just idea of their proportion to simple fractures; yet even in these tables of one hundred and forty-four fractures, fifty-four were compound, and also, generally, more or less comminuted. Of eighty cases reported by W. W. Morland, of Boston, from the Massachusetts General Hospital, and in which the character of the accident is recorded, thirty-nine were compound.[1]

The symptoms indicating a fracture of both bones of the leg are the same which are usually present in other fractures, namely, mobility, crepitus, shortening of the limb, distortion, swelling, &c. Generally

Fig. 192.

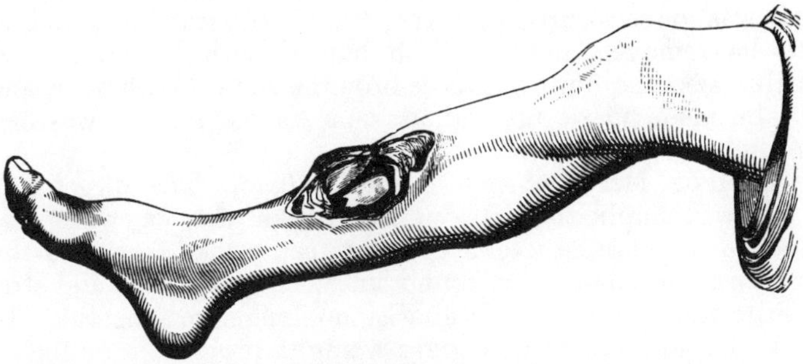

Compound and comminuted fracture of the leg.

the lower end of the upper fragment projects in front, and can be seen or felt; but in some instances the swelling follows so rapidly that it is impossible to feel distinctly the point of fracture, and its existence can only be determined by the crepitus, mobility, and shortening of the limb, or, perhaps, by the marked deformity or deviation from the natural axis.

The shortening, where it exists at all, varies at the first from a line or two to a half or three-quarters of an inch. Generally, it is about half an inch.

Prognosis.—The average period of perfect union in twenty-nine cases, including those in which union was delayed by extraordinary causes beyond the usual time, was forty days. The general average under ordinary circumstances may be stated at about thirty days.

Union has been delayed in six cases, four of which were simple fractures, and two were compound. The longest period was seventeen weeks.

F. C. T., of Erie Co., N. Y., æt. 35, broke his right leg in jumping from a buggy in June, 1852. Fractures oblique in both bones; near the lower end of the upper third; simple.

The limb was dressed with lateral splints, made of white wood, and with compresses and bandages, and then laid upon a pillow.

Eight weeks after the fracture had occurred, the gentlemen in attendance wished me to see the limb with them. I found Mr. T. still in bed, and the fragments not at all united.

Mr. T. had enjoyed average health heretofore, but he was never very robust. When I was called to see him he looked pale; his skin was cold and moist, pulse 120, and appetite poor. The broken leg

[1] Transac. of Mass. Med. Soc. for 1840; Fractures, by A. L. Pierson.

and foot were greatly swollen. The swelling was œdematous. Considerable excoriations existed on the back of the leg. The fragments were quite movable, and were overlapped three-quarters of an inch.

We agreed that the patient ought, as soon as possible, to be got out of bed, so as to enable him to recover his strength, which had sadly declined. To this end, a gutta-percha splint was made to fit accurately the whole length of the leg; and, having attached a large number of tapes, it was to be secured upon the limb. Several times each day it was to be removed, and the limb bathed with brandy and water. Gradually, also, the limb was to be brought down to the floor, and the patient be made to sit up, and, as soon as possible, he was to walk with crutches, or to ride.

Nov. 4, 1852, Mr. T. visited me at Buffalo. The directions had been followed implicitly. About two weeks after my visit, he rode out, and in about nine weeks, or seventeen weeks from the time of the fracture, the bones were found united. His health and strength were quite restored, and the limb was no longer œdematous. It was found to be straight, or with only a slight projection of the upper fragment in front of the lower, and shortened three-quarters of an inch.

A gentleman, æt. 33, from Bergen, N. Y., was struck by a billet of wood on the 3d of August, 1856, breaking his left leg nearly transversely, three and a half inches above the joint. The fracture was simple. A surgeon was called immediately, who applied bandages and side splints, and then laid the limb over a double inclined plane. At the end of six weeks the dressings were removed, but the bones had not united. Seven months after the accident, this gentleman consulted me at Buffalo. I found him in good health, but no union had yet taken place. This is the only example, except where amputation or death interposed, in which the union has been so long delayed as to entitle it to be considered as a case of non-union. My own observation would, therefore, incline me to think that, while non-union is a rare event in fractures of the leg, delayed union is more frequent than in most other fractures.

It has once occurred to me to see a complete non-union of the fibula after a period of several years, while the tibia had united well. This circumstance occasioned no inconvenience to the patient, and was not known to him until I had made the discovery.

A little more than one-half of those cases in which an accurate note of the result has been made, have been found to be more or less shortened by overlapping, namely, sixty-one cases out of one hundred and ten. The greatest amount of shortening in any one case has been one inch and a half; and the average shortening of the sixty-one cases has been half an inch and a fraction over. This analysis includes both simple and compound fractures; but a pretty large proportion of the simple fractures have also been found shortened, as in the following extreme illustration.

John Granger, of Hungerford, England, æt. 43, was tripped by a stone while walking, breaking his right leg through its lower third. Fracture simple and oblique. It was treated by Richard Barker, surgeon, of Hungerford, England. He employed only side splints.

Two years after, I found the leg shortened one inch, the upper fragment riding upon the front and inner side of the lower.

Generally, when a shortening has occurred, I have found the upper fragment in front of the lower, and oftener a little upon the inner than upon the outer side.

The deviation from the natural axis of the limb has been noticed by me in a good many instances. Seven times the lower part of the limb has fallen backwards, and five times it has, in a degree much less marked, inclined inwards. Once I have seen it inclined outwards, and twice forwards.

Ulcers upon the back of the heel, seen by me five times, as a result of undue pressure upon this part, have, however, been presented but once in a case of simple fracture.

It is not very unusual to find, also, over the exact point of fracture, and after the lapse of several months, or even years, an ulcer, or sinus, which is due sometimes to the presence of a small fragment of bone which has remained in the wound from the time of the accident, or to a thin scale which has subsequently exfoliated. In other cases it is due to the prominence of the salient angle when the lower part of the limb inclines considerably backwards, and in still other cases, no doubt, to the general dyscrasy of the system, and to the same causes which produce chronic ulcers in the lower extremities where only the skin has been originally injured. I have reported elsewhere examples of this complication existing after five months, two, and three years,[1] and in the remarkable case which I shall now briefly relate, an ulcer existed at the end of twenty-three years.

Thurstone Carpenter, when four years old, received an injury, breaking both bones of one of his legs near its middle. The fracture was compound. It was dressed and treated by an excellent surgeon, then residing in this city, but long since dead.

Twenty-three years after the accident, Mr. Carpenter called upon me on account of a paralysis of his lower extremities, which had recently occurred. He stated that from the time of the fracture until within about one year, an open ulcer had existed over the seat of fracture, and that soon after it had closed over completely he began to lose the use of his limbs. During the time it was open, small scales of bone have frequently been thrown off. The limb is half an inch shorter than the other, but straight.

Two years since, I amputated the leg of a gentleman residing in Quincy, Chatauqua Co., N. Y., which had been broken a little above the ankle in 1844. The accident was produced by the wheel of a carriage, and the skin was considerably lacerated. The wounds, however, healed kindly, and the broken bones united in the usual time without any apparent deformity, but the limb continued swollen and

[1] Trans. Amer. Med. Assoc. Report on Deformities after Fractures.

painful, until finally suppuration took place. After twelve years of great suffering, I amputated the leg near its middle, from which time he made a speedy recovery. I found the lower end of the tibia inflamed, softened, and expanded, and containing in its interior about three ounces of pus, but no sequestrum.

Anchylosis of the knee or ankle-joint may follow as a result of the accident or of improper treatment; and at one or both of these joints I have found more or less anchylosis at the end of nine months, one year, six years, twenty-five, thirty, and forty years. Generally, however, it disappears in a few weeks, and seldom remains, to any considerable extent, in the knee-joint after the dressings have been removed two or three weeks; but an Irishman called upon me in 1853 whose leg had been broken about three inches below the knee-joint six years before. It was a simple fracture. A surgeon in Ireland had treated the case. I found the limb shortened one inch and a half, the fragments being overlapped and displaced backwards at the point of fracture. The knee was also partly anchylosed. I could not learn what the treatment had been.

In other cases, where no permanent anchylosis has followed, the ankle-joint has been occasionally painful, and subject to swellings, after the lapse of many years.

After all that has been said as to the occasionally serious nature of the consequences of these accidents, as shown in the shortening of the limbs, in their deviations from their natural axes, in the stiff ankles, ulcers and abscesses, it must still be admitted that in another point of view these results are not extraordinary, and may hereafter continue to be fairly anticipated in a certain proportion of cases, even under the best management; since it must be understood that more fractures of the leg are attended with serious complications than of any other limb; and that while many produce death rapidly from the severity of the shock, and very many are condemned at once to amputation, a large number of those which are saved have been in that condition which has rendered the application of bandages or splints impossible for many days. Indeed, not a few of these crooked limbs may still be presented as real triumphs of the art of surgery, inasmuch as by consummate skill alone have they been saved.

Treatment.—Without being able, in a case which presents so many forms and complications, to establish any rule of universal application, I nevertheless do not hesitate, after considerable experience, in declaring a plan of treatment which in my opinion ought to be adopted with only occasional exceptions, that is, I mean to say, in simple fractures. The plan to which we choose to give so general a preference is well known as that recommended and practised by Pott, the distinguished surgeon of St. Bartholomew's Hospital; and with only slight modifications, it will be found applicable to probably nine-tenths of all the simple fractures of the leg, and to some of the compound fractures.

The apparatus will consist of two splints with pads and bandages.

First we are to construct a splint (Fig. 193), made of a thin piece of board, long enough to extend from a little above the knee, to a point two inches beyond the sole of the foot, about seven inches in width, and reaching forwards at the lower end, so as to support the foot. This splint is to be covered heavily with cotton batting in order that it may fit all the inequalities of the outer side of the leg and foot, taking, however, especial care that there should be a depression at a point corresponding to the external malleolus, so deep as that even when the limb is bound down to the splint the malleolus shall not touch. The splint with its padding must then be covered with cotton cloth neatly sewed on.

The remaining splint may be made of binder's board, felt, or gutta percha; but in either case it need not extend higher than the bend of the knee or lower than the upper margin of the malleolus internus,

Fig. 193.

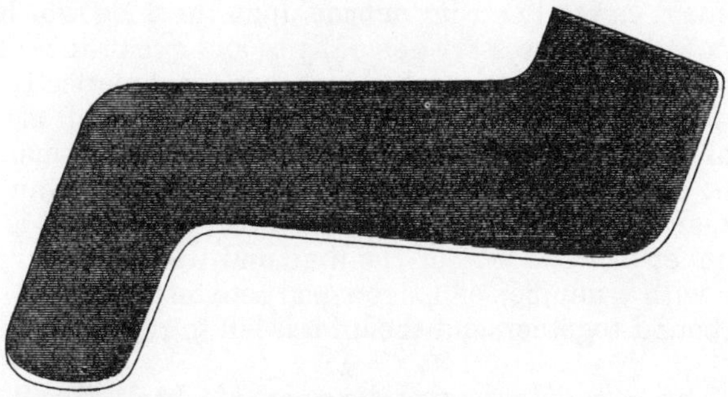

Long splint for treatment of a fracture of the leg in Pott's position.

unless the fracture should be near one of these extremities; and in case it does extend lower, the same precautions must be taken to protect the malleolus internus from pressure. Whichever also of the materials is employed, the splint never ought to be applied directly to the skin, but a thin pad made of a few layers of cotton sheeting covered with cotton cloth must be laid underneath.

It is seldom that I have found it necessary or useful to apply any bandages directly to the skin; but in certain cases of compound fractures where dressings have been applied which needed support and protection, a bandage has been of service. The roller, unless the patient is a child, whose limb can be easily lifted and managed, is always objectionable; but the many-tailed bandage, made of narrow strips of cloth, laid upon each other as we have already described in our general remarks upon bandages, &c., is much to be preferred.

Having made these preparations, we proceed to flex the leg to a right angle with the thigh, and, by the hands, make extension and counter-extension as much as the patient will bear, or as much as may be necessary to restore the fragments to place. If the fracture is compound, and the point of bone protrudes through the skin, it is often difficult to replace it. That is, we are unable to overcome the action of the muscles sufficiently to make the limb of its natural length, and for this reason, mainly, we are unable to get the point of bone beneath the skin. If we cannot then "set" the bone, or bring the ends into apposition, and this will be the fact pretty often, we still have no apology generally for leaving the bone outside of the skin. First an attempt must be made to accomplish this reduction by pulling aside the skin with the fingers, or with a blunt hook. This simple procedure has often succeeded with me in a moment, when others have been trying in vain to accomplish the same end by pulling upon the limb. If this fails, then the skin should be cut sufficiently to allow the bone to retire, or if the point is sharp, and especially if it is stripped of its periosteum, it may be sawn off. Resecting thus the end of an oblique fragment does not generally affect in any degree the length of the limb, or interfere with a prompt and perfect cure, but on the contrary it often is advantageous in every point of view.

Having restored the fragments to their places as well as we may, the limb is laid carefully on its outside upon the long wooden splint. We shall now find it necessary generally to add two or three thin pads, in order to supply vacancies which we have not perfectly provided for in the preparation of the splint. Generally we shall also see the necessity of placing a pretty thick pad under the outer margin of the foot or toes, so as to bring the great toe in line with the inner edge of the patella, and spine of the tibia. The other side splint is now laid along the inner or tibial side of the limb and with successive turns of a roller, or with a number of narrow and separate strips of cloth, the whole are bound together, and the limb is left to repose upon its outer side.

The patient may, if necessary, lie upon his back, but it is better that he should be turned a little toward the side of the broken limb. The danger of twisting the fragments upon each other is lessened by lying upon the same side with the broken limb, but I have frequently permitted patients to lie upon their backs and found no such result. If the long under splint extends a little way upon the thigh and is well fastened to the thigh, the twist cannot very well occur.

By adopting this general plan of treatment we avoid all chances of gangrene or swelling of the foot from excessive ligation, and it is to these accidents, especially, that the remarks of Dr. Norris, already quoted, are applicable. The large size, and irregular form, of the bones of the leg, the small amount of muscular tissue covering them, especially near the articulations, the severity of the injuries to which they are liable, with their remoteness from the centre of circulation—these circumstances, altogether, render them exceedingly exposed to injury from the too great or unequal pressure of splints or of bandages; and it has often occurred to myself, as it has to Dr. Norris, to find the skin vesicated, or even ulcerated and sloughing, when the patients are first admitted to the hospital; a condition which, in nine cases out of ten, is due to the mal-adjustment of the splints, or to the tightness of the bandages.

If bandages are used under the splints, and next to the skin, they must be applied very moderately tight, and loosened or cut as the swelling augments; and from the first day of the treatment to the last, the surgeon must be careful to loosen or tighten the dressings when the swelling increases or subsides, just as the prudent boatman trims his sails to the rising and falling breeze.

The following case, which has been communicated to me by Dr. Fuller, of Wyoming, N. Y., with permission to make such use of it as I choose, is sufficiently pertinent for the instruction of others, and deserves a public record.

A man, æt. 71, fell from a tree, striking upon his foot, Aug. 27, 1855, producing a backward dislocation of both the tibia and fibula upon the os calcis, and also a fracture of both bones of the leg a few inches above the ankle.

An empiric took charge of this unfortunate man, and immediately applied lateral splints and a firm roller from the toes to the knee. Notwithstanding the remonstrances and prayers of the patient to have the bandage loosened, it was kept on until the ninth day, when the doctor cut the bandage upon the top of the foot, and it was found vesicated. Ignorant, however, as to the cause of this vesication, and of the danger which it threatened, he omitted to loosen the remainder of the bandages, and the limb was left in this condition until the twenty-third day, when Dr. Fuller being called and having removed all the dressings, found the integuments covering the whole foot dead and dried down to the bones. The dislocations had not been reduced. Soon after this the limb became œdematous, and on the twenty-seventh of October the leg was amputated by Dr. Barrett, of Le Roy; from which time the patient recovered rapidly.

But it is to the advantages of the posture recommended by Pott that I wish especially to direct attention. The position hitherto generally preferred by surgeons has been that in which the limb rests upon its back, either in a box or upon a double inclined plane; but all of the five examples of ulcers upon the heel which I have seen have been after treatment in this position. Indeed, it is almost impossible for this accident to happen in any other way, and it has therefore never occurred to me to see it in cases treated by Pott's method. It is true that, with great care, such a result might generally be prevented while the leg is resting upon its calf, yet experience shows that it is by no means easy to avoid it always. And if, in our anxiety to obviate this evil, we place pads underneath the tendo Achillis, above the heel, we incur the risk of pressing the fragments forwards, and of compelling them to unite with the whole lower part of the leg inclined backwards. I have mentioned already that this has happened in cases that have subsequently come under my observation no less than seven times, while an attempt to correct this fault by placing the support under the heel has either produced ulcers of the heel, or driven the lower part of the limb in the opposite direction.

The same thing—that is, a deviation backwards or forwards—might happen in any posture, but I am sure it is much less liable to in Pott's position than in any other.

Then, again, a twist or rotation of the lower fragment is more liable to take place when the toes point upwards, and the limb rests upon the calf and heel, than when the limb reposes upon its side. In the one case it is resting upon a narrow surface, with the whole weight of the foot disposing it to either eversion or inversion, while in the other it lies upon a broad surface, with the foot entirely at rest, and demanding no extraordinary support.

In short, Pott's position is less irksome to the patient, and vastly less troublesome to the surgeon. Ugly and crooked limbs are sometimes inevitable, and they are often the consequences of unskilful management or of inattention on the part of the surgeon; but, other things being equal, the best legs have, in my experience, come out of Pott's position, and the worst out of the double inclined plane and the box.

As to the tendency of the upper fragment to rise at the point of fracture, it depends, no doubt, upon the usual direction of the fracture, and the action of the muscles both in front and behind; so far as the former circumstance is the cause—that is, the direction of the line of fracture—no position is sufficient to remedy it, and in relation to the action of the muscles, the indications are as easily and naturally fulfilled with the limb upon its side as upon its back. Generally the leg needs to be flexed upon the thigh; but if the fracture is high up, and its direction is obliquely downwards and forwards, it must be made nearly or quite straight, so as to overcome the action of the anterior muscles of the thigh, acting, through the ligamentum patellæ, upon the upper fragment. The simple rule which I recommend and adopt is, to flex or extend the limb more or less until it is ascertained in what position the apposition of the fragments is most complete.

In such few cases as demand or warrant a resort to extension and counter-extension, a double inclined plane furnishes the most convenient mode for its accomplishment; but it is only occasionally that, in fractures of the leg, permanent extension and counter-extension can be employed, an assertion which, however much it may excite surprise, experience will prove true. If the fracture is near the middle of the leg, quite remote from the points upon which the appliances for extension, &c., are to be made fast, and the inflammation is moderate, something may be done in this way; but when the point of fracture approaches the ankle-joint, as it actually does in a great majority of cases, a gaiter, made of any material whatever, if it has sufficient firmness to overcome completely the action of the muscles, will inevitably cause congestion and swelling, accompanied sooner or later with great pain and with ulcerations, and simply because the extension is made directly upon parts already tender and inflamed from the accident itself; and when we add to this complete and violent ligation of the limb near the seat of fracture, a similar ligation of the limb just below the knee, for the purpose of making counter-extension, as is done in what is known among American surgeons as "Hutchinson's splint"[1] (Fig. 194), we are prepared to understand how the worst consequences may ensue. I have once seen, when this abominable apparatus had been used, a complete ring of ulceration below the knee, and another as complete around the foot and ankle. The limb was twice girdled,

[1] Elements of Surgery, by John Syng Dorsey, vol. i. p. 181. Philadelphia, 1813.

and yet the surgeon thought he was performing a duty for the omission of which he would scarcely have been regarded as excusable.

Fig. 194.

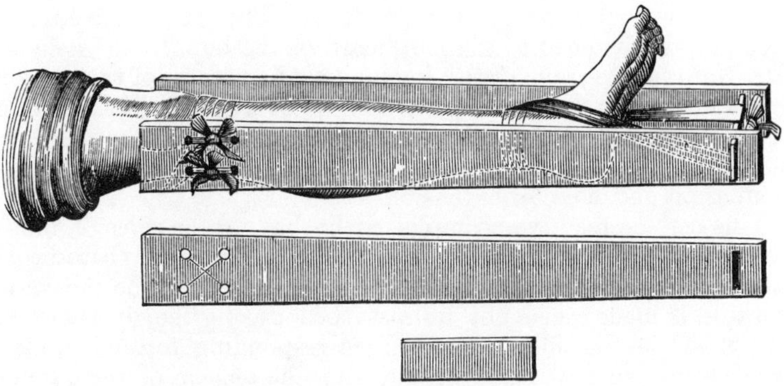

James Hutchinson's splint for extension, etc., in fractures of the leg. (From Gibson.)

Jarvis's adjuster, a still more mischievous, inasmuch as it is a more powerful, instrument, operating in a similar manner, has been productive of like consequences; but Jarvis's adjuster is liable to the additional objection that by its great weight it drags off the limb, turning the toes outwards, an objection which no care or diligence can generally overcome.

I could wish that neither of these appliances would ever again be impressed into the service of broken legs.

Neill, of Philadelphia, Crandall, of New York, and Daniels, of Broome Co., N. Y., have each sought to overcome some of the difficulties in the way of making extension in fractures of the legs, by substituting adhesive plaster for the usual extending or counter-extending bands.

Says Dr. Neill: "For simple fractures of both bones of the leg, attended with shortening and deformity not easily overcome, the limb should be placed in a long fracture-box (Fig. 195), with sides extending as high as the middle of the thigh, and a pillow should be used for compresses.

Fig. 195.

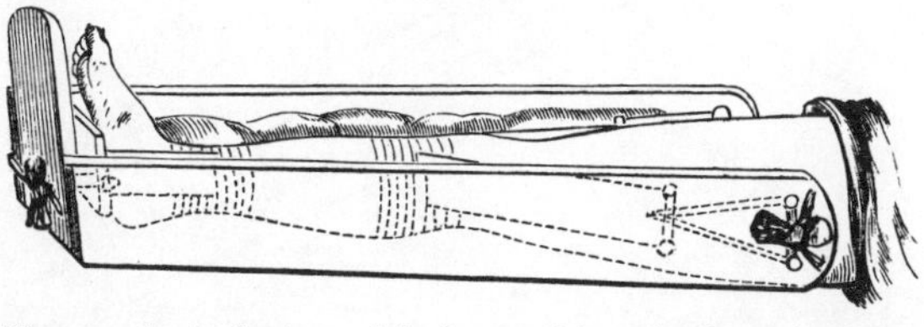

John Neill's apparatus for fractures of the leg, requiring extension and counter-extension.

"The counter-extension is made by strips of adhesive plaster, one inch and a half in breadth, secured on each side of the leg below the knee, and above the seat of fracture, by narrower strips of plaster applied circularly. The end of the counter-extending strips may then be secured to holes in the upper end of the sides of the fracture-box, by which the *line of the counter-extension is rendered nearly parallel with the limb.*

"The extension is also to be made by adhesive strips, in a mode which is now well known and understood. The ends of the extending bands may be fastened to the foot-board of the box."[1]

Dr. Neill further remarks: "In compound fractures of the leg, shortening and deformity are often difficult to overcome, as is well known to experienced surgeons. In such cases we may wish to dress the wounded soft parts, and, at the same time, maintain a certain amount of extension and counter-extension.

"This can be readily accomplished by having the sides of the fracture-box (Fig. 196) sawed in two parts at the knee, so that the sides of the box above the knee, from the upper ends of which the counter-extension is made, need not be disturbed during the dressing, while that portion of the side of the box, corresponding to the leg, may be opened at pleasure, without diminishing the tension of the extending or counter-extending bands."

Fig. 196.

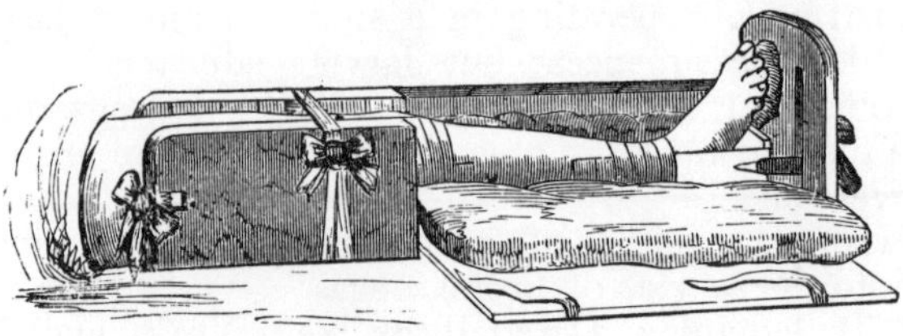

John Neill's apparatus for compound fractures of the leg.

The following wood-cuts (Figs. 197, 198, 199) are intended to illustrate the apparatus invented by R. O. Crandall, for the purpose of making permanent extension. The extension is represented as being made by a gaiter, but Dr. Crandall leaves it to the choice of the surgeon whether he shall employ the gaiter or adhesive straps.[2]

Fig. 197.

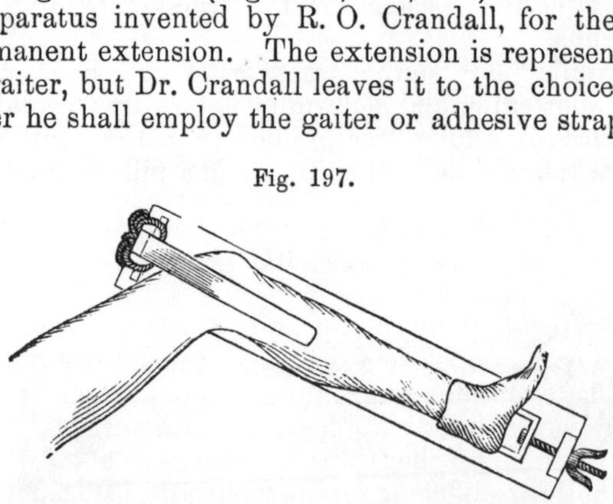

Section of Crandall's apparatus, applied to the limb; showing adhesive plaster counter-extending band, gaiter for extension, &c.

[1] Philadelphia Med. Exam., vol. xi. p. 580, 1855.

[2] Crandall, Phil. Med. Journ., vol. iv. p. 193, Jan. 1856; also Transac. of Med. Assoc. of Southern and Central New York, 1855, pp. 81, 82.

Fig. 198.

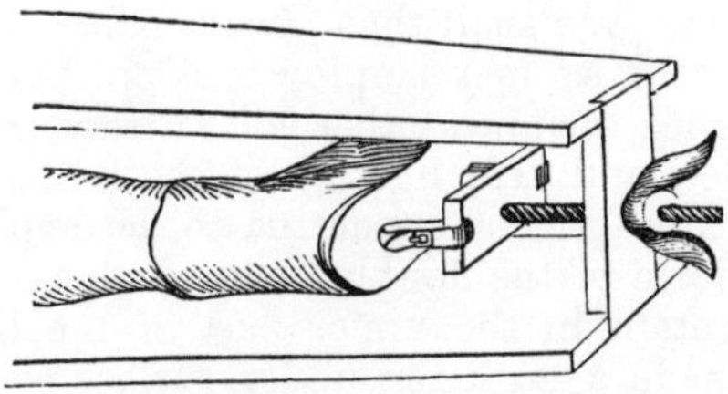

Posterior view of the lower portion of Crandall's apparatus.

Fig. 199.

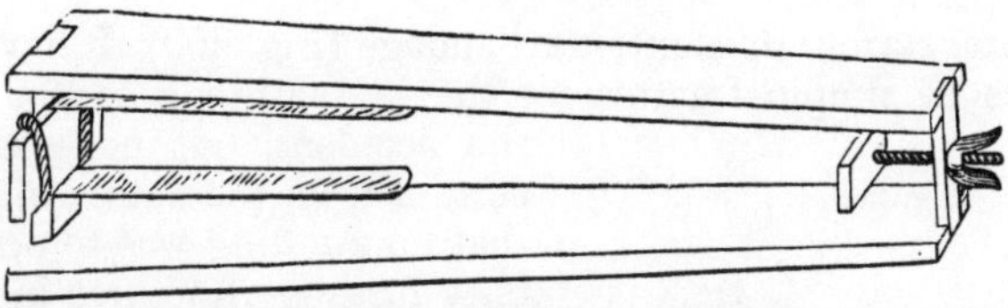

Crandall's apparatus complete. The counter-extending straps are passed over a block of wood supported above the knee, to prevent their pressure upon the sides of the knee.

Without intending to deny to these contrivances much ingenuity and considerable practical value, I am far from conceding that they will be found capable of overcoming altogether the action of the muscles where the ends of the fragments do not support each other. Their mode of action is such that they can scarcely do more than to steady the limb, and if they operate upon the fragments at all in the direction of their axes, it must be only in the most inconsiderable degree. The adhesive plasters are substituted for the circular knee bands and the gaiters with a view to avoid the ligation; but in order to do this they must not encircle the limb, but only be laid parallel to its long axis. The leg of an adult or that portion to which the adhesive plasters can be applied, supposing the fracture to be exactly at the centre, may be sixteen inches, that is, eight inches for extension and eight for counter-extension; but when we employ the same means for extension in fractures of the thigh, we find it necessary to apply the straps over the whole of these sixteen inches, the entire length of the leg, or they will not hold. It will be apparent also that we cannot use even the eight inches which we have, for the purposes of argument, allowed these gentlemen in fractures of the leg. There must be at least a space of eight inches between the ends of the two opposing straps in order that they may operate at all upon the fragments; indeed I do not believe that even then their influence would reach beyond the skin to which they were directly applied; but if a space of eight inches is left, only four remain for the straps at either end; and this is an amount of surface wholly insufficient for our purpose. What then shall we do when the fracture is near one of the extremities of the bone? These gentlemen seem to have forgotten, moreover, that the whole leg is tender and that the skin easily vesicates. In short, they have not seen the many points of difference between the application of these means in fractures of the thigh and leg, and which, while they allow us to accomplish all that we could desire with the one, are of little or no use in the other. We shall then always come to the same conclusion; whatever means we may employ to make permanent extension in fractures of the leg, we must either fail entirely or incur the hazards incident to complete and firm ligation of the limb; and if the preference is given to any form of apparatus to accomplish these ends, it must be to some form of the double inclined plane, by which we may at least avoid ligation in the upper part of the limb, the counter-extension being made against the under surface of the thigh while it is resting upon the thigh piece; or to one of the long straight thigh splints which will enable us to make the counter-extension from the thigh and perineum.

The paste, starch, or dextrine bandage (Fig. 200), I have used in a few cases of simple fracture of the leg within a day or two after the accident, but not unless I felt certain from the nature of the injury that no swelling was to occur. It is only in those fractures in which the bones do not become displaced, or only very slightly, that I would recommend its employment at a period so early.

Fig. 200.

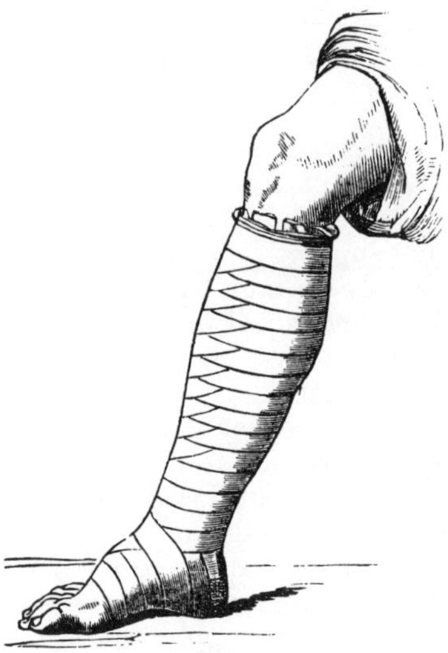

"Immovable" apparatus: applied to the leg. (From Fergusson.)

But as soon as the fragments have united, in almost any form of fracture of the leg, it will not be improper to put on the paste bandage and allow the patient to go about carefully upon crutches; or if, indeed, the fragments have not united, but the swelling has completely subsided and the wounds healed, it cannot be regarded as unsafe to adopt this practice. The young surgeon cannot, however, be too much impressed with the danger of this mode of treatment, as a universal or general plan, employed without discrimination. Its most devoted advocates, Suetin, Velpeau, Gamgee, and others, will not deny the necessity of caution in its use; and the numerous accounts of crooked limbs, ulcerations, and even of gangrene which have been attributed fairly, I think, to one or another of the forms of the immovable dressing, ought to be sufficient to place us fully upon our guard.[1]

The majority of such cases as in my judgment may be safely intrusted to a paste bandage, will also do well enough in almost any form of dressing; and not a few of the examples of simple fracture of the leg without much if any displacement, which have come under

[1] Accidents resulting from the use of the immovable apparatus. Amer. Journ. Med. Sci., vol. xxv. p. 460, Feb. 1840; from Gazette des Hôpitaux.

my notice, I have treated by simply inclosing the leg neatly in a pillow, tied against the limb with tapes, only that I have taken care that the pillow shall be so fastened around the foot and leg as to keep the limb steady. At other times I have laid outside of the pillow thus arranged, two broad side splints, and bound these against the limb, with the pillow interposed; or I have in the summer used splints made of rolls of straw inclosed in pieces of cloth—"straw junks." In all these cases I have laid the leg upon its back, and I cannot say but that the limbs have done well.

If a double inclined plane is used, I prefer either a plain apparatus, such as we have already described as in use for fractures of the thigh, constructed of boards, joined together by hinges opposite the knee, and with an upright foot-board, upon which a carefully arranged and thick cushion has been placed, or the more elegant double inclined plane of Liston (Fig. 201) or of Welch (Fig. 202).

Fig. 201.

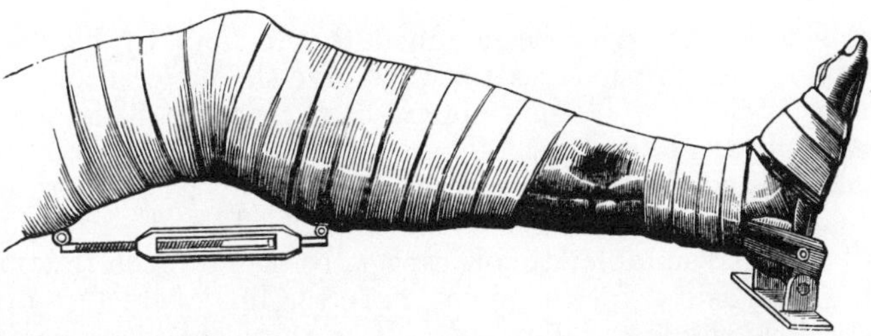

Liston's double inclined plane; applied to the leg in a case of compound fracture. (From Miller.)

If Welch's splint is preferred, a piece of narrow board should be placed transversely under the heel of the apparatus, and made fast, as may be seen in Liston's splint, so as to prevent its tendency to fall over to one side or the other.

Fig. 202.

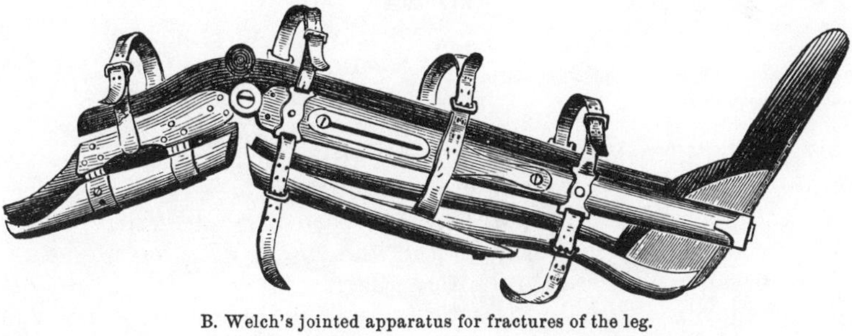

B. Welch's jointed apparatus for fractures of the leg.

The apparatus may be flexed or extended, and fixed in the position required, by the hinges. This is done by means of pinion-like teeth at the circumference of the hinges, which are held in contact by screws forming the pivots of the joints. It is fitted to limbs differing in length by sliding joints at the sides of the limb, and in the splint which supports the under side of the limb. The depth is increased or diminished by turning a screw at the bottom of the foot-piece.

Welch's side splints, also (Fig. 203), made of veneered gutta percha, may be used in connection with his double inclined plane, and are especially useful in fractures occurring near the ankle-joint.

Fig. 203.

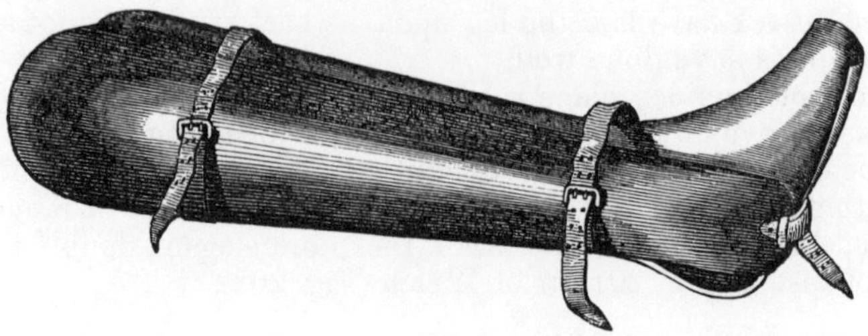

B. Welch's flexible side splints.

These side splints may be confined to the limb by bandages or straps, and indeed to bandages I always give the preference.

In using Welch's or Liston's apparatus, it must not be inferred that the knee is always to be bent. These splints are designed to be used occasionally as single planes or as straight splints; and there will be found many cases of fractures of the legs in which the straight position will be most suitable: this is especially true of such fractures as, occurring just below the knee-joint, have the line of fracture directed obliquely downwards and forwards. But there are many compound fractures which demand the same extended position; and in nearly all cases where this form of apparatus is used as a double inclined plane, the lower end of the splint should be elevated so that the heel shall not be much below the level of the knee.

Bauer's wire splints, used also for side splints (Fig. 204), when they are formed to fit the limb accurately, possess some advantages which

Fig. 204.

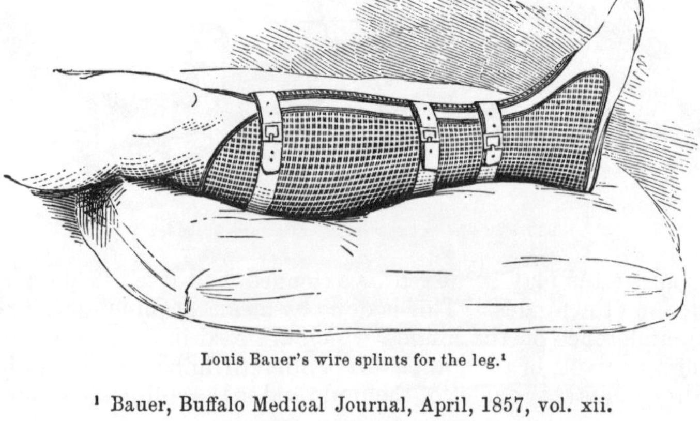

Louis Bauer's wire splints for the leg.[1]

[1] Bauer, Buffalo Medical Journal, April, 1857, vol. xii.

must recommend them to the attention of surgeons; but neither these splints nor any others, however accurately fitted, ought to be applied directly to the naked skin. They require always the interposition of a well-padded lining.

Boxes are rarely useful except in certain compound fractures. They are heavy and awkward machines, which prevent the patient from moving readily in bed; or which being fixed, if he does move, allow the upper fragment only to descend, or to move upon the lower as a fixed point. If used at all, they ought generally to be suspended (Fig. 205), or made to move on a suspended railway (Fig. 206). But, however they are arranged, the limb is a great part of the time concealed from sight, and the surgeon is prevented from making use of such means to rectify deviations in the line of the bone, as he would probably have otherwise employed.

Fig. 205.

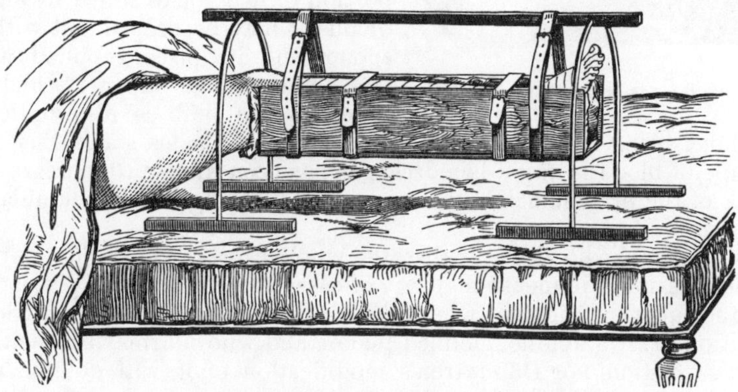

Swing box or "cradle." (From Skey.)

The swing invented by James Salter, of London (Fig. 206), is constructed so as to allow not only a lateral motion, but also a more com-

Fig. 206.

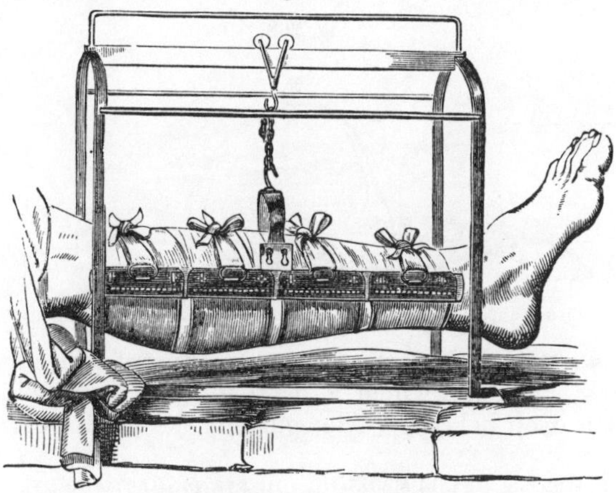

Salter's cradle. (From Fergusson.)

plete motion in the direction of the axis of the limb, by which the danger of pushing the fragments upon each other is obviated. This is accomplished by the rolling of two pulley-wheels upon a horizontal bar. The case in which the leg rests may be made of metal or of wood, and the frame of iron for the sake of lightness and strength.

These boxes are sometimes filled with bran, the bran being closely packed upon all sides so as to support the limb uniformly and gently. This method of treating compound fractures of the leg was first suggested by J. Rhea Barton, of Philadelphia,[1] and has been much used in the Pennsylvania Hospital. It possesses the advantage of affording a perfect protection against flies in the summer season, and of absorbing the matter as it escapes. Whenever any portion of it becomes soiled by blood or pus it may be dipped out with a spoon, and its place supplied with fresh bran. The support which it gives to the limb is also uniform without being at any time excessive, and Dr. Coates states that the escape of blood in rapid hemorrhages has been known to increase the bulk of the bran sufficiently to arrest the bleeding by its accumulated pressure.

Fig. 207.

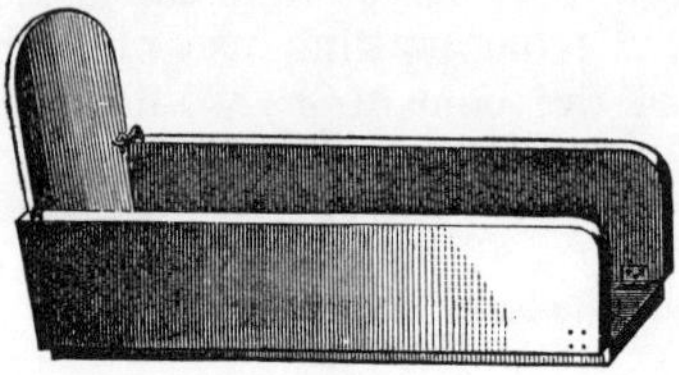

Fracture box, with movable sides.

Malgaigne, who declares that the whole world knows how impossible it is, in an immense majority of cases, to overcome the projection of the superior fragment when the limb is placed in the extended position (over a double inclined plane), and who affirms that neither Pott's position, nor Dupuytren's modification of it, will do much, if any better, nor, indeed, that Laugier's plan of cutting the tendo Achillis possesses in this respect any real advantage, concludes at last to resort to a new and really ingenious method, the value of which, also, he claims to have already fully demonstrated. His apparatus (Fig. 208) consists simply of a steel band of sufficient size to encircle three-fourths of the limb, at the two extremities of which are two horizontal mortises through which a band is passed, and which may be buckled upon itself behind. The centre of the metallic arch, in front,

Fig. 208.

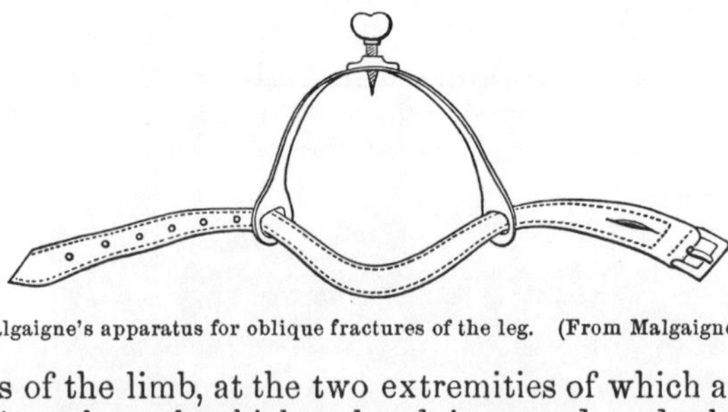

Malgaigne's apparatus for oblique fractures of the leg. (From Malgaigne.)

[1] Barton, Amer. Journ. of Med. Sci., vol. xvi. p. 31, and vol. xix. p. 515.

is penetrated with a firm, metallic screw, terminating in a very sharp point, and which is moved by a flat thumb-piece.

The limb being laid over a double inclined plane, and the pads being carefully adjusted, as we have already directed when speaking of other forms of apparatus, and the limb properly extended, the apparatus of Malgaigne is placed over the limb, with the sharp point of the screw resting upon the upper fragment, a few lines above the point of fracture; and at the same moment that this point is pressed firmly down to the bone, the fragments being held together by an assistant, the strap is buckled as tightly as possible under the splint. A few turns of the screw will now make its point penetrate more deeply into the bone, and insure the most complete apposition of the broken extremities. "This is accomplished," says Malgaigne, "with very little pain to the patient;" and, as will be seen (Fig. 209), the steel arch effectually prevents any ligation of the limb.

Fig. 209.

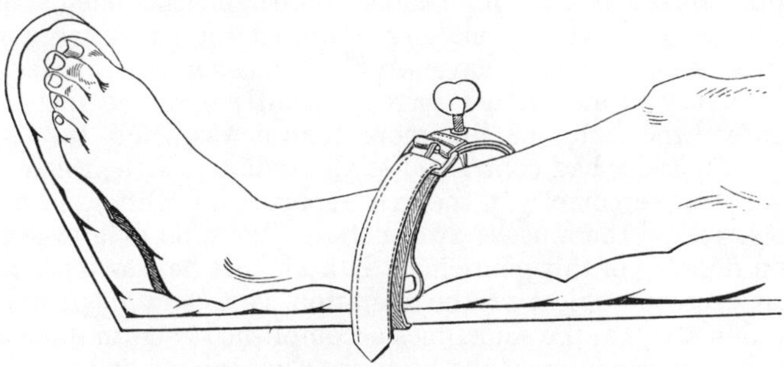

Malgaigne's apparatus applied. (From Malgaigne.)

Although I have had for some time this instrument in my possession, I confess that I have been reluctant to make use of it in any case which has presented itself to me. My friend, Dr. March, of Albany, has, however, employed it in his practice, and he expresses himself as much pleased with its operation.

The authority of either of these distinguished gentlemen is, in my judgment, a sufficient guarantee of its excellence, and I think I shall only wait for another favorable opportunity to give it a fair trial.

In some cases of extreme deformity of the legs consequent upon badly united fractures, resection of the bones has been practised with more or less success.

The first case of which I have seen any mention made where the bones were actually resected, is reported by Charles Parry, of Indianapolis, Ind. A young man, æt. 15, having broken his leg near its middle, the fragments united, from some cause, nearly at right angles with each other. Some years afterwards, on the 15th day of January, 1838, Dr. Parry operated, by removing a wedge-shaped portion from both the tibia and fibula. The recovery was tedious, but satisfactory.[1]

[1] Parry, Amer. Journ. Med. Sci., Aug. 1839, p. 334.

Mr. Key, of London, made an operation of this kind upon a gentleman who had suffered a fracture of the right tibia from a musket ball. The limb was nearly useless, since he could only bring his toes to the ground. Mr. Key operated in Oct. 1838, and when the report of the case was made five months subsequently, the patient was doing well.[1]

In Sept., 1840, Dr. Mütter, of Philadelphia, made a similar operation upon a patient whose leg was shortened three inches and a half and very much deformed, by which operation, when the recovery was complete, the shortening was considerably reduced.[2]

Cases may occur which will justify a resort to these extreme measures, or in which they may be preferred to amputation; but an examination of the several examples reported will show that these operations are not unattended with danger to the life of the patient; indeed, in this respect, amputation has greatly the advantage. If, moreover, the surgeon expects by this method to lengthen a limb, where it is merely overlapped and shortened, he is I am certain destined to disappointment, at least in all cases where sufficient time has elapsed for the bones to have become firmly united. I have never myself refractured a bone, but I have several times met with cases of old fractures newly broken, and I have constantly observed that I could never extend the limb one line more than it was before the last fracture. The muscles had contracted to that point, and their contraction would not be overcome. In the case reported by Mütter, he believed that he stretched the muscles two inches. With all deference for the skill and honesty of this gentleman, I think that he was mistaken.

If, however, the object of the operation is to straighten the limb, then no doubt it may be sometimes accomplished; and in some degree also by the straightening of the limb, the shortening may be overcome; but in our opinion, such procedures ought to be reserved for extraordinary circumstances.

An instructive case of refracture is reported by Dr. Horner, of Philadelphia, in the *Medical Examiner*. The limb had been broken eight weeks and was quite crooked, but was not very firmly united, and Dr. Horner having refractured it, was able at once to restore it to a nearly straight line.[3]

[1] Key, Amer. Journ. Med. Sci., Aug. 1839, p. 339, from Guy's Hospital Reports, April, 1839.

[2] Mütter, Amer. Journ. Med. Sci., April, 1842, p. 359. Three similar cases may also be found in the Oct. No. for 1841, and the April No. for 1842 of the same journal, in which the operations were made by Portal, of Palermo. Malgaigne mentions two other examples.

[3] Horner, New York Journ. Med., May, 1851, p. 432.

CHAPTER XXXIII.

FRACTURES OF THE TARSAL BONES.

Causes.—The astragalus is generally broken by a fall from a height, the patient having struck upon the bottom of the foot. Monahan in an analysis of ten cases, found it had been broken by a fall upon the foot nine times,[1] and only once by a crushing accident.

The calcaneum is also occasionally broken by violent lateral pressure but much more often by a fall upon the foot, or rather upon the heel. In some instances both heel bones have been broken at the same moment; but Malgaigne has collected eight cases of fracture of this bone by muscular action, as in jumping upon the toes; the posterior portion of the bone being thus violently acted upon by the tendo Achillis. South, in his notes to Chelius, has mentioned two other cases, one of which was seen by Lawrence, and has been reported in the second volume of the *Lancet.* This person had received the injury by jumping off a stage coach. The fragment was found to be drawn upwards slightly, but not so far as to prevent crepitus when the muscles on the back of the leg were relaxed. The other example mentioned by South, is a cabinet specimen contained in the museum of St. Bartholomew's Hospital. The fracture had taken place just below the attachment of the tendo Achillis, but the upper fragment was not displaced.[2] Mr. Cooper mentions two other cases, both produced by violent efforts on the part of the patients to sustain themselves when falling. In one of these the fragment was immediately drawn up three inches.[3]

The other bones of the tarsus are generally broken by crushing accidents, such as the fall of heavy weights upon them, by the passage of loaded vehicles, &c.

Pathology.—The astragalus often, indeed generally, escapes without injury in those crushing accidents which break many or most of the other bones of the foot, and, as we have seen, it is seldom broken except when the patient has fallen upon the bottom of his foot; but at the same moment, the foot being turned forcibly out or in, a dislocation of the tibia takes place, and the fibula is broken. In nine of the cases collected by Monahan, one or the other of these forms of dislocation had occurred, in eight of which the dislocation was compound. The direction of the fracture is found to vary greatly; thus, it has been found broken in its length, antero-posteriorly, in its breadth or transversely, and in one instance it has been divided nearly hori-

[1] Fracture of the astragalus, with an analysis of the recorded cases of this injury. An inaugural thesis, presented to the Faculty of the Buffalo Med. Col., March, 1858, by Bernard Monahan, M. D.

[2] South, Notes to Chelius's Surgery, vol. i. p. 639, Amer. ed.

[3] B. Cooper's ed. of Sir Astley, Amer. ed., p. 311.

zontally, so as to separate the upper face completely from the lower. Sometimes it suffers a species of impaction, the fragments being actually driven into each other; at other times, as in one case related by Amesbury, the bone may be split without the occurrence of any displacement.

The calcaneum also may be broken in any direction, and it is equally with the astragalus liable to impaction, by which its vertical diameter is sensibly diminished, while its transverse diameter is increased. If the fracture is a consequence of muscular action, the line of fracture is always posterior to the astragalus, and in some cases only that portion is broken off to which the tendo Achillis has its attachment. It may be broken also vertically, directly underneath the astragalus, in which case the lateral and interosseous ligaments will prevent anything more than a slight displacement of the posterior fragment. When the fracture takes place posterior to the lateral ligaments, the detached fragment is liable to be drawn very far from the body of the bone, even to the extent of four or five inches, and possibly further when the leg is extended upon the thigh and the foot flexed upon the leg. Constance relates a case in which the tuberosity, having been broken off by a direct blow, was drawn up five inches.[1]

Fractures of the calcaneum produced by contraction of the sural muscles are generally simple, but those which result from a crushing of the bone are more often compound. The same remark is applicable also to the other bones of the tarsus, the fractures of which, being only produced by direct blows, are generally complicated with external wounds.

Symptoms.—All fractures of the bones of the tarsus demand especial care in their diagnosis, since only a few of the usual signs of fracture are in a majority of the cases presented. The explanation of this fact will be found in the number, size, and strength of the bones of the tarsus, and in their close and firm union by ligaments, by which they give to each other a mutual support, so that the fracture of a single bone does not necessarily or usually result in displacement or deformity, and even crepitus is with difficulty detected; and when we consider, moreover, that the fracture is generally produced by great violence, directly applied, in consequence of which the foot in most cases becomes rapidly and enormously swollen, we shall understand the true nature of the difficulties which are usually presented in the way of an accurate diagnosis.

Of all the usual signs of fracture, crepitus alone is pretty generally present, but even this often fails to tell us which bone is broken, and still more often does it fail to inform us as to the direction and extent of the bony lesions.

If the whole or a portion of the tuberosity of the calcaneum is separated by the action of the muscles, and the fragment is drawn upwards, it may be discovered in its new position, and the heel will be flattened or shortened, but no crepitus can be felt unless the fragments are again brought into contact.

[1] Constance, Amer. Journ. Med. Sci., vol. v. p. 222, Nov. 1829, from the Midland Med. and Surg. Reporter.

Treatment.—Not any of the fractures of the tarsal bones in themselves demand the use of splints, and it is only when complicated with a dislocation of the ankle and fracture of the fibula that it is proper to employ apparatus of this sort; certainly the exceptions to this rule must be very rare; so that our practice in these cases will be confined chiefly to the prevention and reduction of inflammation. The limb must be placed in the most easy position, and cool water lotions assiduously applied. This will be the sum of the treatment demanded during the first few days after the receipt of the injury in probably all cases of simple fracture, and in many cases of compound fracture.

If single bones, or fragments of single bones, are displaced to any considerable extent, and there is an external wound communicating with the fracture, I have no doubt it would be best in all cases to remove at once by dissection the projecting bone, even although it were possible, or perhaps easy, to force it back again to its place. The same rule I would apply to examples of fracture uncomplicated with any external wound, if the fragments were very much displaced, and could not by the application of moderate force be replaced, since the bone left to project would prevent the patient from ever wearing a boot with comfort, and would entail as much weakness upon the limb as would be likely to follow from its complete separation. But such cases as I have last supposed are exceedingly rare; indeed, I have never met with a simple fracture of a tarsal bone accompanied with displacement.

Norris has, however, reported a case of fracture of the astragalus accompanied with displacement of about one-half of the bone, but without any lesion of the soft parts. This was in the person of a man æt. 30, who was admitted into the Pennsylvania Hospital on the 26th of Sept. 1831. "An hour previous to admission, while descending a ladder, he slipped and fell in such a manner as to throw the entire weight of his body upon the outer part of his left foot. Upon examination, the foot was found to be turned inwards and nearly immovable. A slight depression existed immediately below the lower end of the tibia, and there was a considerable hard and rounded projection on the outer part of the foot, a little below and in front of the extremity of the fibula. The skin covering this projection was reddened, but not excoriated. There was no fracture of either bones of the leg."

These appearances led Drs. Norris and Barton, under whose care the patient was placed, to regard the accident as a simple luxation of the astragalus forwards and outwards; and a short time after admission efforts were made to reduce it. "This was done after relaxing in as great a degree as possible, the muscles of the leg, by fixing the knee and having assistants to keep up extension, by seizing the heel and front part of the foot; at the same time the bone being pushed inwards and toward the joint by the surgeon. These efforts were continued for a considerable time, but had no effect in changing the position of the bone.

"Six hours afterwards, Drs. Huston and Harris saw the patient in consultation, when efforts were again made at reduction, which not proving more effectual than in the first trial, the excision of the bone was determined on.

"The patient being properly placed, an incision was made through the integuments, parallel with the course of the tendons, commencing a short distance above the projection on the foot, and extending down far enough to expose fairly the astragalus and its torn ligaments. The bone was then seized with forceps and easily removed after the division of a few ligamentous fibres, that continued to connect it to the adjoining parts.

"Very little hemorrhage occurred, two small vessels only requiring the ligature.

"After removal, it was discovered that about one-half of the surface which plays in the lower end of the tibia had been fractured, and remained firmly attached to the extremity of that bone, and as it was judged that the efforts to remove this would be likely to produce more injury to the joint than would arise from allowing it to remain, no attempt was made to extract it.

"The joint being carefully sponged out, the sides of the incision were brought accurately together by means of sutures and adhesive straps, after which simple dressings and a roller were applied, and the foot, restored to its natural situation, placed in a fracture box."

Subsequently that portion of the astragalus which was permitted to remain, having become carious and loosened, was removed also.

The case continued to do badly; all the bones of the tarsus and even the lower ends of the tibia and fibula becoming eventually carious; and on the 27th of March, 1853, more than a year and a half after the receipt of the injury, the leg was amputated; but no healthy action ensued, and the patient soon died.[1]

The result of this case can scarcely be regarded as having settled anything in reference to the value of the procedure which I have recommended. For reasons which seemed satisfactory to the surgeons who made the operation, only one-half of the broken bone was removed; whether the result would have been different if the whole had been at once taken away, we cannot now determine. I have related it, however, as the only example of a simple fracture with displacement which I have been able to find upon record; and in this case, several surgeons of merited distinction concurred in the opinion that the protruding fragment ought to be removed.

A fracture of the posterior portion of the calcaneum, especially when it has been produced by muscular action, constitutes an exception to fractures of the tarsal bones generally, and demands usually that apparatus of some kind should be employed in its treatment.

In order to replace the posterior fragment when displaced, or to maintain it in apposition until a bony union is accomplished, it will be necessary to shorten the gastrocnemii by flexing the leg upon the thigh and extending the foot upon the leg. But to retain the limb in this position it will be expedient always to employ apparatus. A

[1] Norris, Amer. Journ. Med. Sci., vol. xx. p. 379.

very simple contrivance, however, will generally answer all the indications. A bandage, padded strap, or a stuffed collar, may be fastened about the thigh just above the knee, and made fast to the heel of a slipper by a tape (Fig. 210). The apparatus is the same which has been recommended for a rupture of the tendo Achillis.

Fig. 210.

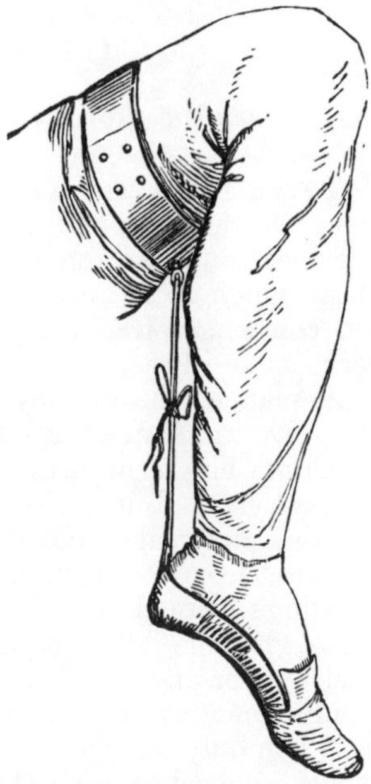

Apparatus for fracture of the tuberosity of the calcaneum.

In addition to this, the limb ought to be covered from the foot upwards as far as the knee with a snug roller, underneath which, on each side of and above the detached fragment, ought to be placed suitable compresses, the object of the roller being to diminish muscular contraction, and the compresses being intended to retain the detached piece in contact with the main body of the bone.

Some surgeons have not found it necessary to flex the leg upon the thigh, and they have contented themselves with extending the foot upon the leg, and confining it in this position by a splint of wood or gutta percha laid along the front of the leg, ankle, and foot. In still other cases, the fragment has shown so little disposition to become displaced as to render no precautions of any kind necessary, except to impose upon the patient complete quiet, with the limb resting upon its outside and flexed, as in Pott's fracture of the fibula. As soon as the inflammation has sufficiently subsided, passive motion must be given to the ankle in order to prevent, as far as possible, the anchylosis which is an almost constant result of these accidents. Indeed, the patient is fortunate who recovers a tolerable use of his foot after the lapse of many months, nor can he be assured that the inflammation will leave these bones and their dense fibrous envelops for a long period, and that it may not result in caries of more or less of the tarsal bones, demanding finally amputation of the whole foot.

We have not intended to speak in this place of those severer accidents, accompanied with comminution and extensive laceration, which forbid the hope of saving the foot, and for which immediate amputation is the only proper resource, but which constitute, in fact, the great majority of all the fractures of the tarsal bones.

CHAPTER XXXIV.

FRACTURES OF THE METATARSAL BONES.

THESE bones can scarcely be broken except by direct blows, and the great majority of their fractures are the results of severe crushing accidents, such as render amputation sooner or later necessary. Of those which do not demand amputation, by far the largest proportion are compound fractures; of which class the following example will serve as an illustration.

A man in the employ of one of the railroads which connect with this city was run over by a loaded car on the 14th of June, 1856, crushing his right arm so as to render its immediate amputation necessary. I found also a compound comminuted fracture of the fourth metatarsal bone of the right foot. Considerable hemorrhage occurred from the wound, but this ceased spontaneously. Cool water dressings were diligently applied, without splints or bandages, and, although some inflammation and suppuration ensued, the parts finally healed over and the fragments united, with only a slight backward displacement at the seat of fracture.

When only one bone is broken, the displacement is usually very trivial; but when several are broken, it may be considerable. Malgaigne relates an example of this latter accident in which, the three middle bones being broken by the wheel of a carriage, and the integuments being badly torn and bruised, it was found impossible to retain the fragments in place. The patient recovered, and was able to place the foot well to the ground, but the proximal fragments continued to project upwards upon the top of the foot to such a degree as to require a special shoe.

In a majority of cases, the direction of the displacement is backwards or upwards, especially when the middle metatarsal bones are the subjects of the fracture.

I have in my cabinet a second metatarsal bone broken obliquely near its middle, with only a very slight displacement of the lower fragment backwards; and also a cast of a bone which has united with an enormous backward projection.

In one instance I have seen the metacarpal bone of the little toe cut in two with an axe, and the fragments united in about thirty days, but with the lower fragment slightly displaced outwards.

Delamotte relates a case also in which the first four metatarsal bones were cut off, and complete union was accomplished on the fortieth day: at the end of two months the patient walked without lameness.

If the fragments are not displaced, nothing is required except that the foot shall be kept at rest, and the inflammation controlled by suitable means.

In case, however, a displacement exists, it ought to be remedied if possible, since if only very slight it may become the source of a serious annoyance. If the fragments project upwards they interfere with the wearing of a boot, and if they sink toward the sole, the skin beneath is liable to remain constantly tender, and the patient may thus be seriously maimed for life.

In case the displacement is not due to the action of the muscles, but only to the nature and direction of the force producing the fracture or to entanglement of the broken ends, and it is likely to cause any of the inconveniences which I have mentioned if permitted to remain, it will be advisable at once to employ considerable force in the way of pressure, or to elevate the fragments through an opening previously made upon the dorsum of the foot, calling to our aid even the saw or bone cutters, if necessary. After which the fragments may be retained in place by carefully applied pasteboard splints and compresses.

CHAPTER XXXV.

FRACTURES OF THE PHALANGES OF THE TOES.

If fractures of the other bones of the foot are generally of such a character as to require immediate amputation, these fractures demand this extreme resort still more often. Our experience, therefore, in the treatment of fractures of the phalanges of the toes is extremely limited.

Lonsdale observes that it is not uncommon to find great irritation arise after fracture of the great toe; an inflammation extending along the absorbents on the inside of the leg to the groin, causing abscesses to form in different parts of the limb, and producing sometimes great constitutional disturbance. An illustrative case has come under my own observation at the Buffalo Hospital of the Sisters of Charity. The patient, Morgan McMann, æt. 18, was admitted Dec. 23, 1853, having several days before received an injury upon the great toe which contused the flesh severely and broke the first phalanx. He was then suffering from severe pain in the foot and leg, and the absorbents were inflamed quite to the groin. Poultices being applied to the foot and cool lotions to the limb, the inflammation soon subsided, but not until a portion of the toe had sloughed away. Eventually also it became necessary to remove some portion of the phalanx, which had died; after which the wounds healed kindly.

When any of the smaller toes are broken, it will be found easier to support the fragments by a broad and long splint which shall cover the whole sole of the foot and all the toes at the same time, than to attempt to apply a splint to the broken toe alone. If, however, we prefer this latter mode, a thin piece of gutta percha will be found altogether the most convenient material for the purpose.

If the great toe is broken, its great breadth may prevent any displacement, and a well-moulded gutta-percha splint will generally secure a perfect and rapid union.

PART II.

DISLOCATIONS.

DISLOCATIONS.

CHAPTER I.

GENERAL CONSIDERATIONS.

§ 1. General Division and Nomenclature.

A dislocation is the displacement of one bone from another at its place of natural articulation.

Dislocations may be divided into accidental or traumatic, spontaneous or pathologic, and congenital.

Our remarks upon the etiology, pathology, symptomatology, prognosis, and treatment of these injuries must be considered as applicable only to accidental or traumatic dislocations, unless the fact is in any case otherwise stated.

"Accidental" dislocations are those in which the bones have suffered displacement in consequence of the application of a sudden force; and surgeons have divided these accidents into Complete and Partial, Simple, Compound, and Complicated, Recent and Ancient, Primitive and Consecutive.

A "complete" dislocation is one in which no portions of the articular surfaces remain in contact.

A "partial" dislocation is one in which the articular surfaces are not completely removed from each other.

A "simple" dislocation is that form of the accident in which the bone has only slid from its articulation, and is accompanied with the least or only an average amount of injury to the soft parts or to the bones adjacent to the joint.

A "compound" dislocation implies that the articulating surface of the bone has been thrust through the flesh and skin, or that in some other way a wound has been made which communicates with the joint.

"Complicated" dislocation is a term employed by some writers to designate a condition wholly differing from a compound dislocation, or, in some cases, a condition of extra complication. Thus, a simple dislocation may be complicated with a fracture, or with the laceration of an important bloodvessel, &c.; and a compound dislocation may be complicated in the same way, and with the addition, perhaps, of extensive laceration and destruction of integument, muscles, nerves, &c.

A "recent" luxation has taken place within a period of a few days, or, at most, of a few weeks; and an "ancient" luxation has existed during a longer period; the exact point of time at which a dislocation shall be called recent or ancient not being fully determined by surgeons, and the application of these terms is therefore always somewhat arbitrary.

By "primitive" luxation we mean that the bone remains nearly or precisely in the position into which it was at first thrown; while by "secondary" or "consecutive" luxation we understand that it has subsequently, in consequence of the action of the muscles, or from unsuccessful efforts at reduction, or from some other cause, changed its position sufficiently to entitle it to a new designation. Thus a primitive dislocation upon the ischiatic notch may become a secondary dislocation upon the dorsum ilii, or the reverse.

§ 2. General Predisposing Causes.

Age.—According to Malgaigne, whose conclusions are based upon an analysis of six hundred and forty-three cases, dislocations are very rare in infancy, only one having occurred under five years; but the frequency increases gradually up to the fifteenth year, from this period more rapidly up to the sixty-fifth year, and from this time onward again dislocations become more rare. He has mentioned none after the ninetieth year; and the period of greatest frequency is between the thirtieth and sixty-fifth year. To this middle period belong four hundred and seven of the whole number.

The inference from this analysis may be thus briefly stated: age, as a predisposing cause, is most active in middle life, less active in advanced life, and least active of all in early life.

It is proper, however, to observe that while such statistics may be relied upon as indicating the relative frequency of these accidents at different periods of life, they cannot be regarded as determining absolutely the value of age alone as a predisposing cause, since the direct or exciting causes may be more active at one period than another, and in some measure these latter causes may be, and doubtless are, responsible for such results.

Constitution and Condition of the Muscles and Ligaments.—It may be stated as a general fact that persons of feeble constitutions, and whose muscular systems are much weakened, suffer dislocation from slighter causes than those who are in health, and whose muscular systems are firm and vigorous; and that a relaxation of the ligaments which surround a joint, however this may have been occasioned, predisposes to dislocation. Thus, a paralyzed and atrophied limb is predisposed to luxation; a joint in which the capsule has become stretched by effusions, or by violent extension, or weakened by laceration from a previous dislocation, or by ulceration, or if in any other way the articulation is deprived of these natural protections, we need scarcely say that it is thereby rendered more liable to luxation.

Ball and socket joints, other things being equal, are more liable to displacement than ginglymoid; but then much more depends upon the relative exposure of the joint than upon its anatomical structure, so that the elbow is much more frequently dislocated than the hip, the shoulder-joint, however, being, from its position and extent of motion, peculiarly exposed, and being also a ball and socket joint, is, of all others, most liable to dislocation.

§ 3. Direct or Exciting Causes.

These may be classed under two general heads, namely, external violence and muscular action.

External violence operates either directly or indirectly. When a person falls upon the knee and dislocates the head of the femur, the force is said to have acted indirectly, and this is by far the most frequent mode of dislocation; but when the blow is received upon the upper end of the humerus, and its head is sent into the axilla, it is said to have been dislocated by direct violence.

Muscular action produces a dislocation slowly, as in some cases of chronic rheumatism, and then it is called a spontaneous or pathologic dislocation; or suddenly, as in the violent spasmodic contractions which accompany convulsions; or sometimes by the mere voluntary effort of the muscles; and these latter are true accidental luxations.

It is very probable that external force can seldom be regarded as the sole cause of a dislocation, but that, in a large majority of cases, muscular action consenting with the shock, performs an important rôle in the history of the accident. The limb being driven obliquely across its socket by the external violence, is seized by the stretched and excited muscles with such vigor as to contribute not a little to the unfortunate result. Thus it will be found that the same force which is adequate to the production of a dislocation in the living and healthy subject is wholly insufficient to accomplish the same in the dead; and a man who is fully intoxicated seldom suffers a dislocation.

§ 4. General Symptoms.

As fractures are characterized by preternatural mobility and crepitus, to which may be generally added the circumstance that, when reduced, the fragments will not remain in place without external support, so, on the other hand, dislocations are characterized by preternatural rigidity, an absence of crepitus, and by the fact that, when reduced, the bone does not generally require support to maintain it in position.

These three are the usual, and they may be termed the common, signs of distinction between fractures and dislocations, but no one of them can be alone depended upon as positively diagnostic. Generally, when a bone has been dislocated, we shall find the limb in a certain position, which is uniform for all dislocations of the same character, and almost immovably fixed; but when the ligaments and muscles about the joint have been extensively torn, or the whole body is still suffering under the shock, or in any other circumstances where the power of the muscles is weakened, this rigidity may give place to extreme mobility.

True crepitus does not exist without a fracture, but it is not always present in fractures, and there is often a sensation produced in the rubbing and chafing of dislocated bones which very much resembles certain kinds of crepitus, and by the inexperienced has been often mistaken for it. I allude to the subdued rasping sound or sensation which is found generally on the second or third day, and sometimes earlier, and which is the result of fibrinous effusions, or, perhaps, in some instances, of the mere rubbing of firmly compressed ligamentous and cartilaginous surfaces upon each other. The crepitus of a recent fracture can be scarcely confounded with this obscure sensation, unless it is in some cases of incomplete fracture, or of a fracture situated remote from the surface, as in the case of the hip; but a fracture which is a few days old, whose surface has become softened by inflammation and more or less covered with lymph, and, when the rigidity is great, may sometimes deceive the most experienced surgeon, so exactly will it be found to imitate the sensations produced by the chafing of an inflamed joint, or of closely approximated fibrous surfaces.

I have said that a true crepitus does not exist without a fracture; but then a very minute fracture, such as the detachment of a scale of bone by the tearing away of a tendon or of a ligament, may produce crepitus; or even the separation of a piece of cartilage may sufficiently expose the bone to determine the presence of this phenomenon. These are, however, no longer examples of simple dislocation.

Nor are the two reverse propositions, in relation to the retention of the bones in place, invariable in their application. A broken bone, well reduced, does not always manifest a tendency to displacement, nor does a dislocated limb, when restored to its socket, in all cases maintain its position without support.

The other general signs of dislocation are pain, swelling, and discoloration. The pain is generally more intense in dislocations than in fractures, the expanded end of the bone resting often upon one or more large nerves, which usually, with the arteries, approach very near the joints, this pressure being also greatly increased by the extreme tension of the muscles. Not unfrequently numbness and temporary paralysis of the whole limb are the consequences. In other cases the pain is due solely to the pressure upon the muscles or to the tension of the muscles, or, perhaps, to the tension of the untorn ligaments and capsule.

Generally, the limb is shortened, but in a few cases it is found slightly lengthened, while the natural axis of the bone with its socket is always changed. If examined early, and before the supervention of swelling, the joint end of the displaced bone may be felt in its unnatural position, and a corresponding depression may be discovered in the situation of the articulation, especially if the bones are superficial.

§ 5. Pathology.

The dissection of recent dislocations produced by external violence, shows the capsular ligament more or less torn, and also a rupture of some of the lateral and other short ligaments, with a complete rupture in most cases of some of the tendons which immediately surround the joint, or of those which are attached to the capsule: the muscles, nerves, arteries, &c., through which the bone in its passage has passed, or upon which it is found resting, being also contused, stretched, or torn asunder.

This description, however, does not apply to dislocations produced by muscular action alone, in a majority of which cases the capsule is only stretched, and not torn, and no lesions of other structures are necessarily present.

If the fracture remains unreduced, the margins of the old socket, in the case of enarthrodial articulations, become gradually depressed while the concavity of the socket is filling in with a fibrous or bony tissue, until at length the whole of this portion of the joint apparatus is nearly or entirely removed. This process is generally very slow, and may not be consummated until after the lapse of many years.

At the same time, but with much greater rapidity, the head of the bone in its new position, and the soft or hard parts upon which it rests, are undergoing certain changes to adapt them to their new relations, and calculated in some measure to restore the limb to its normal functions. If the head of the bone rests upon muscle, the cellular and fibrous tissues which enter into the composition of the muscle become condensed and thickened, forming a shallow or elongated cup, whose margins are attached to the neck or shaft of the bone, and whose walls are lubricated with synovia. If it rests upon bone, by a process of interstitial absorption a true socket is formed, sometimes deep and sometimes shallow, whose edges, receiving additional ossific depositions, become lifted so as to form a rim. At the same time the head of the bone is undergoing corresponding changes, to adapt itself to the newly-formed socket; it is flattened or otherwise changed in form, and in the progress of this change its natural secreting and cartilaginous surfaces are gradually removed, a porcellanous deposit taking its place. The same kind of hard, polished, ivory-like deposit is found also in those portions of the new socket which have been especially exposed to pressure and friction. Instead of the eburnation, an imperfect fibro-serous surface or synovial capsule may be formed.

I have in my cabinet an example of ancient luxation of the hip-joint in which the head of the femur, having rested upon the dorsum ilii, has formed a nearly flat but smooth surface—a kind of elevated plateau; in other cases I have seen the margins of the new socket so elevated as to rest against the neck of the femur, and completely lock it in.

Consenting with these changes, and in consequence partly of the disuse of the limb, the muscles, and even the bones sometimes, suffer a gradual atrophy. In some measure these alterations may be due also to the pressure of the dislocated bone upon arterial and nervous trunks, by which their functions become partially or completely annihilated, and their structure even may be wholly obliterated. In consequence also of the inflammation which immediately results, we ought not to omit to notice that the large trunk of an artery sometimes becomes firmly adherent to the capsule or periosteum of a displaced bone, and its reduction is attended with imminent danger of laceration and of a fatal hemorrhage. Numerous instances of this grave accident, especially in attempts to reduce old dislocations of the shoulder-joint, are upon record.

§ 6. General Prognosis.

We shall study the prognosis of these accidents to better advantage when we come to speak of the individual bones and their various forms of dislocation; but it is proper to state in this place, generally, that very few joints, having been once completely displaced from their sockets by external violence, are ever so completely restored as not to leave some traces of the accident for many years, if not for the whole of the subsequent life of the patient, either in the partial limitation of their motions, or in the diminished size and power of the muscles of the limbs, or in the presence of an occasional arthritic pain: the degree and permanence of these sequences depending upon the joint which is the subject of the displacement, the extent of the original injury, the length of time it has remained unreduced, the means employed in its reduction, the health and condition of the patient, with so many other contingent circumstances as to preclude the idea of a complete specification.

If the bone is not reduced, a permanent maiming is inevitable; but it is surprising how much time and the intelligent processes of nature can eventually accomplish toward a restoration of the natural functions, especially when aided by a good constitution and judicious treatment. If the symmetry of form and grace of motion are never replaced, the value of the limb, for all the practical purposes of life, is not unfrequently completely re-established.

§ 7. General Treatment.

The first indication of treatment is to reduce the bone. Whatever delays may be proper or justifiable in certain cases of fracture, such delays are never to be argued in cases of dislocation. The sooner the reduction is accomplished, the better. For this purpose we resort at once to such manipulations or mechanical contrivances as the nature of the case demands; and if these fail, or if at the first they are deemed insufficient, we invoke the aid of constitutional means, or such as are calculated to diminish the power and antagonism of the muscles.

Many dislocations may be reduced promptly by manipulation alone; which mode is always to be preferred when it will prove sufficient, for the reasons that it is generally the least painful to the patient, and the least apt to inflict additional injury upon the muscles and ligaments.

A person wholly unacquainted with anatomy or surgery, may occasionally succeed in reducing a dislocated limb; indeed, it frequently happens that the patient himself, by mere accident in getting up or in lying down, accomplishes the reduction; and even in a very large majority of cases force and perseverance will finally succeed by whomever they may be employed; but the observing student of surgery will soon discover the difference between accident and brute force on the one hand, and intelligent manipulation on the other. The charlatan bone-setter does not often allow himself to fail, unless the courage of his patient gives out, or he ignorantly supposes the reduction to be effected when it is not; but his success, achieved through great and unnecessary suffering, is often obtained, also, at the expense of the limb. While the surgeon whose knowledge of anatomy enables him to understand in what direction the muscles are offering resistance, and through what ligaments the head of the bone must be guided, lifts the limb gently in his hands, and the bone seeks its socket promptly and without disturbance, as if it needed only the opportunity that it might demonstrate its willingness to return.

We must understand not only what muscles and ligaments antagonize the reduction, if we would be most successful, but also what muscles, by being provoked to contraction, will themselves aid in the reduction. In short, to become expert bone-setters in the department of dislocations, one must possess a complete knowledge of the physiognomy or the external aspect of joints, acquired only by repeated and careful examinations, he must be familiar with the anatomy and functions of the muscles, he must understand thoroughly the ligaments, he must have experience, tact, and fertility of resource.

Without these qualifications he will do better never to undertake to treat dislocations, since he is constantly liable to mistake fractures for dislocations, and dislocations for fractures; he will submit a sprained wrist to violent extensions under the conviction that the joint is displaced; he will mistake natural projections for deformities, and fail to recognize the real deformity when it actually exists; he will leave bones unreduced, fully believing that they are reduced; and he will all in all, within a few years, accomplish vastly more evil than he can ever do good. Let a man practice any other branch of surgery if he will, without experience or scientific knowledge, but he must not attempt to reduce dislocated bones. The most learned and the most skilful we shall find falling into error, embarrassed by the uncertainty of the diagnosis, or successfully resisted by the power of the opposing agents; what then can be expected of those who are both ignorant and inexperienced, but failures and disasters?

As a means of disarming the muscles, or of placing them off their guard, we often practise successfully the diversion of the mind of the patient. At the very moment that the limb is moved or extension is made, a question is addressed to him, or he may be suddenly surprised by some unexpected intelligence.

Fig. 211.

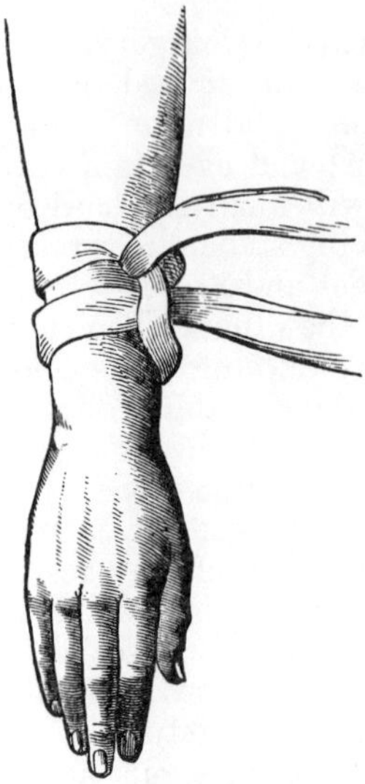

Clove hitch. (From Erichsen.)

Extension and counter-extension, made with our own hands or with the hands of assistants, constitute the second resort where manipulation alone has failed. The surgeon, seizing upon the limb firmly with his hands, makes the extension, while the assistants make the counter-extension; or, instead of grasping the limb directly, the operator may use for this purpose circular and longitudinal bandages, or the bandage or handkerchief tied in the form of the clove hitch (Fig. 211). Extension is thus applied in connection with manipulation, aided, perhaps, by direct pressure upon the head of the displaced bone. Failing in this, we employ some one of the various mechanical contrivances which, while they are capable of exerting much more power, possess also the important advantage of operating gradually and steadily, by which mode the resistance of the muscles is always more speedily and more completely overcome.

For this purpose surgeons employ generally in the case of the large limbs, the compound pulleys (Fig. 212), or the simple rope windlass, which is thus described by Dr. Gilbert, of Philadelphia: "Place the patient, and adjust the extending and counter-extending bands as for

Fig. 212.

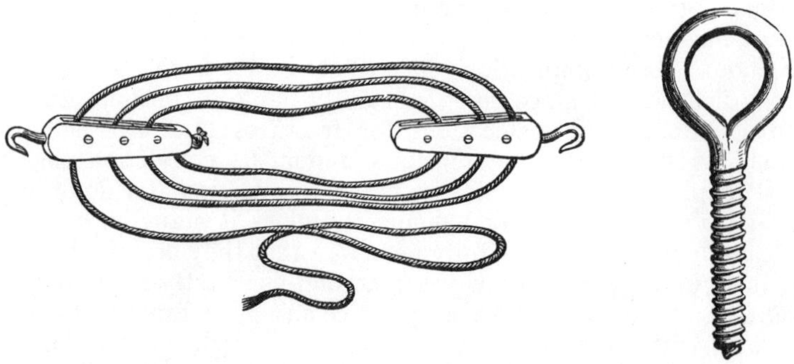

Compound pulleys and ring to which one end of the pulley rope is fastened.

the pulleys; then procure an ordinary bed-cord or a wash-line, tie the ends together and again double it upon itself, pass it through the extending tapes or towels, doubling the whole once more, and fasten the distal end, consisting of four loops of rope, to a window-sill, door-sill, or staple, so that the cords are drawn moderately tight; finally, pass a stick through the centre of the double rope, then by revolving the stick as an axis or double lever, the power is produced precisely as it should be in such cases, viz., slowly, steadily, and continuously."

Jarvis's adjuster, although very complex and expensive, possesses some advantages over the pulleys, which may, perhaps, entitle it to the preference in some cases.

Among the constitutional means, ether and chloroform occupy the first rank; indeed they are, at the present day, almost the only means of this class to which surgeons resort, and their value in this point of view can scarcely be over-estimated. Only when some unusual circumstance or condition of the patient forbade the use of an anæsthetic, would the surgeon return to the ancient practice of bleeding *ad deliquium*, of prostrating the system with antimony, or to the use of those vastly less efficient agents, opium and the warm bath.

CHAPTER II.

DISLOCATIONS OF THE LOWER JAW.

THERE are two principal forms of this dislocation, namely, the double or bilateral dislocation, and the single or unilateral; in both of which the direction of the displacement is forwards. To these there has been added one example of an outward displacement accompanied with a fracture.[1]

§ 1. DOUBLE OR BILATERAL DISLOCATION.

This form of dislocation of the lower jaw is much the most frequent, being met with in about two out of every three cases. It appears also to occur oftener in women than in men, and usually between the twentieth and thirtieth year of life. In infancy and extreme old age it is exceedingly rare; yet Sir Astley Cooper mentions a case in which "two boys" being at play, one had an apple thrust into his mouth, producing a double dislocation; and Nélaton saw the same accident in an old man of seventy-two years, who was toothless.

This comparative immunity in youth and old age has been ascribed to certain peculiarities in the form of the jaw at these periods of life. Nélaton attributes its more frequent occurrence in middle life to the great length and strong anterior inclination of the coronoid process.

In a majority of cases the direct or immediate cause has seemed to be muscular action alone. Malgaigne found this cause to prevail in

[1] Robert, Journal de Chir., 1844.

twenty-five out of forty cases; and of the twenty-five cases fifteen were occasioned by gaping, five by convulsions, four by vomiting, and one by rage. Dr. Physick, of Philadelphia, found both condyles dislocated in a woman in consequence of the violent gesticulation of her jaw while scolding her husband. But in a more remarkable case still, this surgeon found the jaw dislocated after recovery from a profuse salivation, and of the cause of which, or the time of its occurrence, the patient, a young girl, could give no account. Dr. Physick made several ineffectual attempts at reduction, and only succeeded at last after he had made her completely intoxicated with ardent spirits.[1]

Dr. E. Andrews, of Michigan, found both condyles dislocated by a lobelia emetic. The patient had often taken these emetics before, and had frequently experienced a sensation "of catching" at the joint, but the jaw had always until this time resumed its position spontaneously.[2]

Among the causes from outward violence, the introduction of some foreign body into the mouth, and the extraction of teeth, occupy the most important place. In fifteen cases, seven were from the former and six from the latter cause.

My late pupil, A. W. Gilbert, has related a case which came under his own observation, produced by a similar cause. During his apprenticeship with Dr. Parsons, a dentist, he was requested to insert a set of teeth for a young man residing in Cattaraugus Co., N. Y., and while opening his mouth to take an impression of his gums, he dislocated "both condyles forwards, under the zygomatic arches;" but so perfectly were the muscles relaxed, that he immediately reduced them, without the least difficulty, by placing his thumbs as far back as possible upon the molar teeth, depressing the back part of the jaw, and at the same moment elevating the chin.[3]

The late Prof. James Webster, of Rochester, N. Y., dislocated the jaw of a lady while attempting to pry out a root of one of the molars.

Pathology.—In order that we may better understand the pathology of this accident, it will be proper to say a few words in relation to the anatomy of the temporo-maxillary articulation and the other parts concerned in the dislocation now under consideration.

The articulation is formed by the condyloid process of the inferior maxilla and the glenoid fossa of the temporal bone, in front of which fossa, and at the root of the zygomatic arch, is a slight elevation, called the articular eminence. Between the joint surfaces, both of which are covered with a cartilage of incrustation, is placed an interarticular cartilage, which divides the joint into two cavities, one corresponding to the condyle of the inferior maxilla, and the other to the glenoid fossa, each of which is furnished with a distinct synovial membrane.

Properly there is but one ligament—namely, the external lateral—which passes from the outer surface of the articular eminence to the corresponding surface of the neck of the condyle. What is called the internal lateral ligament arises from the apex of the spinous process of the sphenoid bone, and is inserted into the margin of the dental fora-

[1] Physick, Dorsey's Elements of Surgery, vol. i. p. 202. Philadelphia, 1813.
[2] Andrews, Peninsular Journ. Med., vol. iii. p. 101. 1855.
[3] Gilbert, Thesis, on Dislocation of the Inf. Max. University of Buffalo, 1858.

men, and has therefore no immediate connection with the articulation, although it tends to strengthen the joint. The same is true of the stylo-maxillary ligaments.

The lower jaw is drawn upwards, or closed upon the upper jaw, by the action of the temporal, masseter, and internal pterygoid muscles; it is drawn downwards by the action of the digastricus, mylo-hyoideus, and genio-hyoglossus muscles; forwards by a few fibres of the masseter and by the external pterygoid muscles; and laterally by the alternate action of the external and internal pterygoid muscles.

When the mouth is open to its utmost extent, the maxillary condyle rises upon the articular eminence until it rests upon its very summit. Indeed, it is probable that in most persons it advances rather in front of the centre of the eminence; so that in order to become actually dislocated it only needs that the capsule shall be somewhat relaxed, or that it shall actually give way in front, when the condyles slide forwards and occupy a position directly in front instead of behind this eminence.

It is easy to comprehend how the combined action of the two external pterygoid muscles, with a portion of the fibres of the masseter, may alone produce the dislocation when the mouth is wide open, and especially when, in consequence of a slight blow upon the chin, the anterior portion of the capsule becomes lacerated; for it must be noticed that the ascending ramus, with its prolonged condyloid process, constitutes a lever of the first kind, in which the temporal muscle, attached to the coronoid process, the masseter, and even the mastoid process, constitute the fulcrum, the anterior portion of the capsule, the weight, and the force acting against the front of the chin, the power.

Fig. 213.

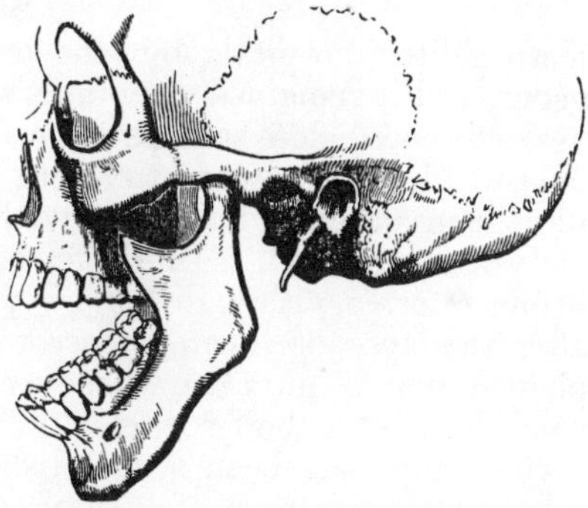

Double dislocation of the inferior maxilla.

In this position of the condyle, drawn upwards and forwards by the action of the pterygoid and temporal muscles, the chin descends toward the neck, and the coronoid process rests against the back of the superior maxilla, or against the malar bone at the point of its junction with the upper maxillary. The temporal, masseter, and internal pterygoid muscles are very much upon the stretch, if not more or less lacerated.

Symptoms.—The mouth is widely open and the jaw nearly immovable. It has been noticed generally that the chin may be slightly depressed, but that, owing probably to the pressure of the coronoid process against the body of the upper maxilla, or against the malar bone, it is generally impossible to elevate the jaw in any degree whatever.

The jaw is also slightly advanced; a depression, covering a considerable space, exists between the auditory canal and the posterior margin of the condyle. A slight fulness is observed in the temporal fossa and also upon the side of the cheek in the region of the masseter muscle.

Ordinarily the patient suffers considerable pain, but not always, from the pressure of the condyles upon the branches of the temporal nerves. There is a constant flowing of the saliva from the mouth; the patient is unable to articulate, and even deglutition is performed with great difficulty.

Fig. 214.

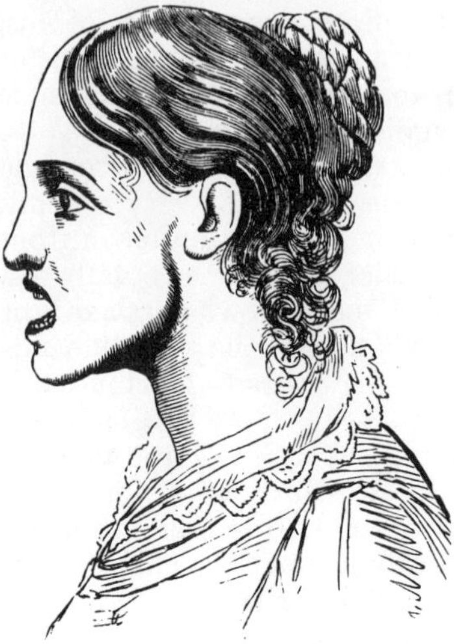

Double dislocation of the inferior maxilla.

Prognosis.—When the dislocation remains unreduced, the lower jaw gradually approximates the upper, and its anterior projection sensibly diminishes, the saliva ceases to dribble from the mouth, deglutition and speech are restored, mastication is performed with considerable ease, and in short, the patient comes at length to experience no great inconvenience from the displacement.

Robert Smith relates the case of a woman whose lower jaw was dislocated during an epileptic convulsion. She was at the time in one of the metropolitan hospitals, but the accident was not noticed by the surgeons, and it remained ever afterwards unreduced. At the end of a year she could close the lips perfectly, but was able to open the mouth only to a limited extent; the teeth of the lower jaw remained advanced, but the involuntary flow of saliva had ceased, and the faculty of speech had been regained.[1] In Professor Webster's case, to which I have before referred, although the jaw was immediately and easily reduced, after the lapse of several years when I saw the lady, she still complained that it hurt her whenever she eat, and that she often felt the condyles slip in their sockets.

Reduction has been accomplished by Physick in the case already related after the lapse of several weeks; Sir Astley reduced a double dislocation after one month and five days, which had been overlooked by the surgeon in attendance;[2] and Donovan succeeded after ninety-eight days.[3]

Treatment.—Reduction may generally be accomplished with ease in cases of recent luxation, in the following manner: The patient being seated upon the floor with his head between the knees of the operator, a couple of pieces of cork, gutta percha, or pine wood are placed as far back between the molars as possible, when the surgeon seizing upon the chin draws it steadily upwards, taking care not to draw it

[1] Robert Smith, on Fractures and Dislocations. Dublin, 1854, p. 288.

[2] Sir Astley Cooper, on Disloc. and Frac.; Amer. ed., p. 316.

[3] Donovan, Amer. Journ. Med. Sci., Oct. 1842, p. 470; from Dublin Med. Press, May 25, 1842.

forwards at the same time, since by this movement he would resist the action of the muscles which naturally tend to restore it to place whenever the condyloid processes are lifted sufficiently from the zygomatic fossæ. Many surgeons prefer to sit or stand in front of the patient, and depress the condyles by means of the thumbs placed inside of the mouth and upon the tops of the molars. If the thumbs are used in this way, it would be well to protect them with a piece of leather, or to slip them off from the teeth suddenly when the condyles are gliding into their places, as the muscles sometimes close the mouth with sufficient violence to bruise severely anything which might at this moment be interposed between the teeth.

The method practiced by Ravaton, of simply lifting the chin gradually and forcibly toward the upper jaw, was essentially the same, but far less efficient; for although he placed nothing between the molars to serve as a fulcrum, the backmost teeth themselves must in some degree perform this service whenever the lower jaw being dislocated and drawn upwards, the chin is forcibly approximated toward the upper.

In other cases it has been found necessary first to disengage the coronoid process, by depressing the chin gently, and then pressing backwards in the direction of the articulation; a method which would certainly deserve a trial in case of the failure of that first described. This was the method practiced by Hippocrates.

A more effectual expedient, however, consists in reducing one side at a time; taking good care always that the side first reduced is not reluxated while the attempt is being made to reduce the other, a thing which happened in one of the cases treated by Sir Astley Cooper, and has happened many times in the practice of other surgeons.

Finally, if all other expedients fail, we ought not to hesitate to resort to anæsthetics, nor indeed could any objection exist to their employment at any period of the treatment, were it not that in a large majority of cases the reduction is effected so easily and promptly as to render their employment wholly unnecessary.

After the reduction is accomplished, it will be a matter of wise precaution to sustain the jaw by a double-headed bandage passed under the chin, and secured upon the top of the head, so as to prevent the mouth from being accidentally opened too far, especially during sleep, since experience has shown that a tendency to a reproduction of the dislocation remains for some time. It will be prudent to continue these measures of protection for at least one week; after which the danger of anchylosis should be borne in mind, and the extent of passive motion should be gradually and cautiously increased. In illustration of this tendency to reluxation, Malgaigne refers to the case mentioned by Putégnat of a woman whose jaw for many years became luxated at least once a month; but she was always able to reduce it herself.

§ 2. Single, or Unilateral Dislocations.

The causes of this accident are in general the same as those which produce double dislocations, and it occurs most often in middle life. Tartra has seen one exceptional example in a child only fifteen months old, and Levison saw a case in an old man who had lost all his teeth.[1]

Symptoms.—The mouth is open, but not so widely as in double dislocation; the jaw is nearly immovable; the teeth are advanced; the condyloid process can be felt in front of the articular eminence, leaving a depression in its natural situation, and the coronoid process is more prominent than in the bilateral dislocation.

It will be remembered that we have already pointed out an important diagnostic mark between a fracture of the neck of the vertical ramus and a dislocation of one condyle. In the latter the chin inclines to the opposite side, while in the former it falls toward the side upon which the accident has occurred. According to Hey, this lateral deviation of the chin is not always present in dislocations; and Robert Smith mentions one case in which the surgeon was misled by this circumstance so far as to attempt a reduction upon the left side when the dislocation was upon the right.

Treatment.—The same rules of treatment which we have established for dislocations of both condyles will be applicable to the single dislocations, with only such modifications as will be naturally suggested to the surgeon.

In the case mentioned by Levison, the dislocation was constantly recurring upon the left side; and it was especially liable to happen when just awaking from sleep. "He would then pull his jaw, press it backwards, when, after about half an hour's work, bang it seemed to go, and all was right again." This old gentleman was finally relieved of these annoyances by a band fastened under the chin. In such a case, an apparatus constructed after the same plan as my lower jaw fracture apparatus might perhaps serve a useful purpose.

§ 3. Conditions of the Jaw simulating Luxations.

There is a condition of the temporo-maxillary articulation called by Sir Astley Cooper "subluxation of the jaw," in which it is assumed that the condyles slip before the anterior margins of the inter-articular cartilages, and thus for the time render the jaw immovable. No positive evidence, however, has ever been presented, either by Sir Astley or others, that any such derangement of the joint apparatus does actually take place, the opinion being based, not upon dissections, but only upon the symptoms which are known to accompany the accident. It is quite probable that this explanation of the phenomenon in question is the true one, yet it is not impossible that it has no

[1] Levison, Boston Med. and Surg. Journ., vol. xxxiv., 1846, p. 388, from London Lancet.

relation whatever to the inter-articular cartilages, but that it indicates a true subluxation of the inferior maxilla upon the zygomatic eminences.

It occurs mostly in young people, and in those of a feeble or scrofulous diathesis. Relaxation of the capsule, ligaments, and muscles about the joint may, therefore, be regarded as the principal predisposing causes. The exciting causes are generally yawning or biting upon some very hard substance.

The symptoms are a sudden arrest of the motions of the jaw, with the mouth about half open, the arrest of motion being accompanied or preceded generally with a sensation of slipping in one of the articulations. The chin is slightly inclined to the opposite side. The condyle may be felt somewhat advanced in its socket, and while it remains in this position the patient experiences some pain.

Frequently the condyle resumes its place spontaneously, or after a slight lateral motion of the jaw; but at other times it requires some little manual force to replace it.

I have myself, during several years of my early life, while pursuing my studies at college, experienced this accident many times. It was peculiarly prone to occur in the morning, and it became necessary that I should eat with some care at my first meal. Sometimes the locking of the jaw was upon the right and sometimes upon the left side; it was always painful. Generally the condyle was made to fall into place by a voluntary lateral motion of the jaw, but occasionally I was obliged to press gently against the chin with my hand. I never adopted any measures to remove the predisposition, but as I became older the annoyance gradually ceased.

Benevoli, in a dissertation published at Florence, Italy, in the year 1747, describes another condition very analogous to this which we have now described, but which evidently depended upon a contraction of the muscles. A priest having opened his mouth very widely in gaping, found himself unable to close it. A surgeon who was called diagnosticated a dislocation of the jaw, and attempted to reduce it, but failing, Benevoli was called, who, observing "that the jaw was not absolutely immovable, that the articulations were not separated, and that the chin did not incline outwards or toward the sternum," concluded that it was only a contraction of the depressing muscles. He therefore prescribed fomentations and oily unctions. The same night the temporal muscles had acquired the size of a couple of eggs, from contraction, but the next day the patient could shut his mouth, and by the following day the tumefaction of the temporal muscles had also disappeared, and the restoration of the functions of the mouth was complete.

Malgaigne, to whom I am indebted for the above case, relates two others, one in the person of the surgeon Mothe, and the other in a young man who was suffering from paralysis and spasmodic contractions of the muscles. Mothe observes that it had occurred to him very often, and that it still continued to happen sometimes, that when he gaped pretty widely, the genio-hyoid and mylo-hyoid muscles contracted with so much force as to render it impossible for him to close his mouth; these muscles being thus in a state of cramp, their bellies became hard under the chin, and so painful that he was obliged immediately to press upwards against the under surface of the chin in order to oppose their action. This condition would last from one to three minutes, and was relieved, generally, by frictions made with the hand over the contracted muscles. Sometimes he actually believed that the lower jaw was dislocated, although the result always convinced him that it was not.

CHAPTER III.

DISLOCATIONS OF THE SPINE.

DELPECH and Abernethy denied the possibility of a dislocation of the spine, either in the cervical, dorsal, or lumbar region, without the concurrence of a fracture.

Says Sir Astley Cooper: "I have never witnessed a separation of one vertebra from another through the inter-vertebral substance, without fracture of the articular processes; or, if those processes remain unbroken, without a fracture through the bodies of the vertebræ." He would not, however, be understood to deny the possibility of a dislocation of the cervical vertebræ, their articular processes being placed more obliquely than those of the other vertebræ.

The accident is, no doubt, exceedingly rare, at least without the complication of a fracture, and it is not improbable that the actual number is smaller than the reported examples would indicate. Those who make autopsies do not always perform their duties with that exact fidelity which might be necessary to determine so nice a point as a fracture of an oblique process, and it is quite likely that the circumstance may have been overlooked in some cases; but a considerable number of well authenticated examples of simple dislocations of cervical vertebræ have accumulated within the last fifty years. The reported examples of simple dislocations of the other vertebræ are not so numerous, nor as well attested.

The causes are in general the same with those which produce fractures of the vertebræ, such as falls upon the head, feet, or back, and violent flexions of the spine backwards or to the one side or the other.

Several examples are recorded of "spontaneous" dislocations, the result of some morbid changes in the bones or in the ligaments of the spinal column; which accidents seem to belong more properly to general treatises upon surgery.

The symptoms, also, partake of the same general character with fractures; the accident being accompanied with more or less complete paralysis of those portions of the body which receive their nervous supply from below the point at which the dislocation has occurred; the spinal column presenting at the seat of displacement an angular projection or some form of irregularity; and the distortion being attended with pain, especially when an attempt is made to move the body.

In very many cases the symptoms are so nearly like those presented in a case of fracture, that the diagnosis is rendered exceedingly difficult. The presence or absence of crepitus may aid in the diagnosis, and yet it is well understood that this symptom is often absent in simple fractures, and that it may be present in all those examples of dislocation which are accompanied with a fracture of an oblique process, or of any other portion of the vertebræ, which class of examples constitutes a large majority of the whole number.

There is usually present, however, in the dislocation, whether partial or complete, a peculiar fixedness or rigidity of the spine, which serves to distinguish this accident from a fracture of the spine as plainly as the preternatural rigidity of the limb in dislocations of the long bones serves to distinguish these accidents from fractures of the same bones. The head, or upper portion of the spinal column is bent forwards, or backwards, or more commonly to one side, and in this position it remains immovably fixed until the reduction is accomplished. Sometimes, also, the surgeon may feel distinctly the lateral deviation of the spinous process, and, in the neck, the transverse processes become an important guide in the diagnosis.

After these few general remarks, I shall proceed to speak of dislocations of the spine in the same order in which I have treated of fractures of the spine.

§ 1. Dislocations of the Lumbar Vertebræ.

Sir Astley Cooper plainly intimates that he does not believe a dislocation can occur in either the dorsal or lumbar region without the concurrence of a fracture, and Boyer affirms positively that it is "entirely impossible."

Without wishing ourselves to insist upon the actual impossibility of these accidents, we are prepared to affirm that no well-authenticated case has yet been reported; at least of a complete dislocation, unaccompanied with a fracture of the articulating apophyses. We can even conceive it possible that a lumbar vertebra may be dislocated forwards or backwards, and that a dorsal vertebra may be dislocated laterally, without a fracture; yet we hardly think either of these events probable. What we urge, however, is that no evidence appears to be furnished that such a dislocation has actually occurred.

Cloquet mentions the case of a "tiler" who fell from the roof of a house backwards, and dislocated one of the lumbar vertebræ. This patient lived many years after the accident, and at the autopsy it was found that the second lumbar vertebra had been luxated to the right by a movement of rotation about the left articular process, the two oblique processes of the left side preserving their connection, while those of the right were separated quite half an inch. The right vertebral plate was broken, and the canal of the vertebra was thus thrown open and widened.[1]

Dupuytren says that a man was crushed by the falling of a bank of earth upon his loins, when in the act of bending forwards. On the third day he was brought to Hôtel Dieu, when it was observed that his lower extremities were completely paralyzed, and that there existed in the upper part of the lumbar region, a hard tumor, by pressure upon which a crepitus was manifest. A second tumor could be distinctly felt in front through the abdominal parietes, and the length of the spine was evidently diminished. This man died on the sixth day from a gradual asphyxia. When the body was examined it was found that the last dorsal and first lumbar vertebræ had been pushed forwards more than one inch, lacerating the spinal marrow, breaking the transverse and oblique processes of the last dorsal and first two lumbar vertebræ, and tearing off a small fragment of the body of one of the vertebræ where the intervertebral substance adhered to it.[2]

These are all the cases of dislocation of the lumbar vertebræ of which I am able to find any record. Both were accompanied with fractures. In neither case was any attempt made to reduce the dislocations. In the second, it is scarcely probable that any means could have been employed which would have succeeded in restoring the bones to their places; nor is it probable that if the bones had been restored to place, the patient would have survived the accident a day longer, probably not so long. The cord was greatly lacerated, and the diaphragm torn up and displaced, rendering a recovery almost impossible.

In the first example, where the dislocation was less complete, and the complications less grave, could reduction have offered any reasonable chance for relief? By extension, combined with a movement of rotation in a direction opposite to that in which the displacement had taken place, it is possible that a reduction might have been accomplished. The attempt certainly would have been justifiable; but since the man lived "many years" without the reduction, it is doubtful whether the result of a reduction would have been more fortunate.

§ 2. Dislocations of the Dorsal Vertebræ.

Malgaigne enumerates twelve examples of dislocations of the dorsal vertebræ. I have found reported by American surgeons, at dates too recent to have been included in his analysis, two other examples; but of this number only three are claimed to have been simple dislocations, unaccompanied with fracture. One of the fourteen was a dislocation of the fifth dorsal vertebra upon the sixth, one of the eighth, two of the ninth, five of the eleventh, and five of the twelfth. The relative frequency of their occurrence in the different vertebræ corresponding

[1] Cloquet, Malgaigne, from Journ. des Difformités de Maisonabe, tom. i. p. 453.

[2] Dupuytren, Injuries and Dis. of Bones, Syd. ed., p. 340.

with the observation of Weber, as to the points of the spinal marrow which allow of the greatest freedom of motion, and are consequently most liable to dislocations. The direction of the displacement in ten cases, was observed to be six times forwards, twice backwards, and twice to the one side.

Two of those which were unaccompanied with fracture, occurring respectively in the tenth and sixth dorsal vertebræ, were examples of a dislocation forwards, and the third, belonging to the ninth vertebra, was a dislocation backwards. A lateral luxation without fracture has not been recorded. It is worthy of remark, also, that these three examples, being all which our science up to this moment possesses, have happened in the experience of the same surgeon.[1]

A moment's consideration of the anatomy of these processes will render it apparent that even a partial luxation forwards without a fracture of the oblique apophyses is impossible, and that in the direction backwards, the luxation can only occur to the extent of about one-quarter of an inch, constituting only a spècies of articular diastasis, without breaking off the articulating apophyses of the lower corresponding vertebra. The first two examples, therefore, notwithstanding they have been received without question by Malgaigne, I shall unhesitatingly reject. The third, which alone carries evidence of its having been correctly reported, and which was only a partial dislocation, is related as follows: "A mason having fallen from a height in such a manner as that the lower part of his back struck upon the angle of the upper step of a ladder, died on the following day. After death it was observed that the spinous processes of the dorsal vertebræ were prominent down to the tenth; and that the tenth process with all of the processes below were depressed. It was also noticed that this depression, very marked when the trunk was thrown backwards, gradually diminished and finally disappeared altogether when the body was bent forwards. On removing the soft parts it was found that the ligaments were extensively torn asunder and detached, so as to permit the articulating apophyses of the tenth vertebra to be carried into contact with the back of the ninth. The spinal marrow had undergone no visible alteration.[2]

Malgaigne thinks he has once observed the same thing on a living subject, and that by simply bending the body forwards he accomplished the reduction and effected a perfect cure, except that a slight curvature remained at the point of injury.

Among the cases reported as having been complicated with fracture, the following example, reported by Dr. Graves, of New Hampshire, to Dr. Parker, of New York, possesses unusual interest.

On the second day of Jan. 1852, a man, æt. 25, was struck on the back while in a stooping posture by a falling mass of timber, causing a dislocation of the last dorsal upon the first lumbar vertebra. His lower extremities were completely paralyzed, and priapism continued for several hours. The surgeon determined to make an attempt at reduction, and for this purpose he placed the patient upon his face, and

[1] Melchiori, Gaz. Medica, stati sardi, 1850. [2] Melchiori, loc. cit.

secured a folded sheet under his armpits and another around his hips, directing four strong men to make extension and counter-extension by these sheets. Chloroform was administered, and when the patient was completely under its influence, the extending and counter-extending forces were applied, and in a few minutes the vertebræ glided into place with a distinct bony crepitus. The restoration of the line of the vertebral column was found to be nearly but not quite perfect.

On the sixteenth day he began to have slight sensations in his feet, and at the end of six or eight weeks he was able to control the evacuations from the bladder and rectum. Several months later he had recovered so completely as to walk with only the aid of a cane.[1]

I know of only one similar case. Rudiger has published an account of a dislocation obliquely backwards and to the right side, which occurred at the same point in the spinal column. The subject was a musketeer, who had been struck upon his back by a falling wall which he was endeavoring to pull down. Rudiger laid him upon his belly, and by the assistance of others he was able, but not without causing pain, to reduce the bones. Immediately, however, when the extension was discontinued, the action of the muscles caused the displacement to recur. The surgeon then directed four men to make extension, while another man retained the bones in place by pressing upon them with his hands. After several hours this method of pressure was replaced by a board underlaid with compresses and sustaining a weight of more than fifty livres. On the following day it was found sufficient to bind compresses over the projecting bone, and in this condition the patient remained fifteen days; during all of which time he lay upon his belly with his shoulders more elevated than his pelvis. On the twentieth day he could lie upon his back, and in about six weeks he was so completely restored as to be able to pursue his trade as before![2] This is certainly a very extraordinary case, whether considered in reference to the means employed to restore the bones to place, or to its results: and if the statements are to be received at all, it must be with some hesitation and allowance.

On the other hand, we are able to present at least one example in which, although no reduction has been accomplished, the patient has survived the accident many years; yet it must be admitted that his recovery is far from having been as complete as in the two cases just mentioned.

Joseph Stocks, æt. 11, in the spring of 1826, was crushed under the body of an ox-cart in such a manner as to produce a dislocation of the last dorsal from the first lumbar vertebra, causing immediately almost complete paralysis of all the parts below. This young man was seen by Dr. Swan, of Springfield, Mass., in the summer of 1834, at which time he was occupied as a portrait painter. His lower extremities remained paralyzed and of the same size as at the time of the receipt of the injury. He was unable to sit erect owing to the mobility of the spine at the seat of dislocation, and he had therefore lain con-

[1] Graves, N. Y. Journ. Med., March, 1852, p. 190.
[2] Rudiger, Journ. de Chir. de Desault, tom. iii. p. 59.

stantly upon his side. The upper portion of his body was well developed, and his intellectual faculties were of a high order.[1]

It is not, however, with a life of perpetual deformity that the two examples of reduction already described are to be contrasted. A result so fortunate as this, where the bones remain unreduced, is unique; in all the other cases reported the patients died miserably after periods ranging from a few days to one year or a little more.

Charles Bell has related the case of an infant who was run over by a diligence, and who died thirteen months after the accident. On examination after death the last dorsal vertebra was found to be completely luxated backwards and to the left, upon the first lumbar vertebra.[2]

With these facts before us, I think we cannot hesitate when the nature of the accident is fully made out, and especially when the dislocation has occurred in the lower dorsal vertebræ, to attempt the reduction by forcible extension, united with judicious lateral motion, or with a certain amount of direct pressure upon the projecting spines.

§ 3. Dislocations of the Six Lower Cervical Vertebræ.

It is much more common to meet with simple luxations of the vertebræ of the neck uncomplicated with fractures, than of either of the other vertebral divisions. This is doubtless owing to the greater extent of motion which their articulating surfaces enjoy.

They may be dislocated forwards or backwards. The forward luxation may be complete or incomplete; with both sides equally advanced ("bilateral" of Malgaigne), or one of the articulating apophyses may be dislocated forwards, leaving the opposite apophysis in its place ("unilateral" of Malgaigne).

Schranth[3] has collected twenty-four examples of luxation of the cervical vertebræ, of which four are recorded as dislocations forwards, two back, and six to the one side or the other. Three of this number were dislocations of the atlas; two were dislocations of the second vertebra; five of the fourth; two of the fifth; two of the sixth, and one of the seventh. In the other cases the seat was not stated.

Malgaigne has brought together forty-five examples; of which twenty-one were complete forward luxations, nine incomplete forward luxations, nine unilateral and forwards, and four were backward luxations. Three were dislocations of the second vertebra upon the third, four were dislocations of the third vertebra, ten of the fourth, eleven of the fifth, fifteen of the sixth, and two of the seventh.

The bilateral forward luxations are generally caused by a fall upon the top and back of the head, or upon the top of the head while the neck is very much flexed forwards. The unilateral is caused generally by a direct blow upon the back of the neck, the blow being

[1] Swan, Bost. Med. and Surg. Journ., vol. xxii. p. 102, March, 1840.
[2] Charles Bell, on Injuries of the Spine. 1824.
[3] Schranth, Amer. Journ. Med. Sci., May, 1848, from Archiv. for Phys. Heilkunde.

probably directed somewhat to one side or the other. The number of backward luxations which have been reported are too few to enable us to indicate very accurately the general causes, but it seems probable that they are most often occasioned by a fall upon the fore and top part of the head, received while the neck is bent forcibly back.

In dislocations of the cervical vertebræ forwards, the head is usually depressed toward the sternum; in dislocations backwards the head is thrown back, and in unilateral dislocations the head is turned over one of the shoulders. Neither of these malpositions of the head is uniformly present in these several dislocations, and indeed not unfrequently, especially in case the system is greatly shocked by the accident, the head and neck assume a preternatural mobility, and may be turned easily in any direction.

The spinous process, unless the patient is very fleshy or considerable swelling has supervened, can easily be felt, and its deviations to the right or to the left, forwards or backwards, furnish us with the most valuable and important sign of the dislocation. Even the transverse processes may be felt sometimes, especially in the upper part of the neck, with sufficient distinctness to render them useful in the diagnosis.

To these circumstances we may add paralysis of the body below the seat of injury, with pain and swelling at the point of dislocation. In some cases also the patient has himself distinctly felt a cracking or sudden giving way in the neck at the moment of the accident.

Prognosis.—The complete bilateral luxations, whether backwards or forwards, have in most cases terminated fatally within a short time, generally within forty-eight hours. Unilateral luxations are less speedy in their results, but when the dislocation remains unreduced, death generally takes place in a month or two. Lente, of New York, relates a case of incomplete dislocation of the fifth cervical vertebra backwards, unaccompanied with fracture, which accident the patient survived five days.[1] A patient of Roux's lived eight days; but in the case of a second patient mentioned by Lente, with a complete luxation, without fracture, of the fifth vertebra, the patient survived the injury only two hours.[2]

On the other hand, occasional examples are presented of partial or complete recovery with the luxation unreduced.

Horner, of Philadelphia, presented to the class of medical students of the University of Pennsylvania in 1842, a lad æt. 10, who had fallen a distance of twenty feet, alighting upon his head. He was found senseless and motionless, with his head bent under his body. He gradually recovered from the shock, but his neck was stiff, distorted, and motionless, his face being inclined downwards to the right side. Two days after, his "common and accurate perceptions returned, but he was affected for some time with tingling and numbness in his left arm." When presented to the class the transverse processes, from the fifth upwards, were about half an inch in front of those below, showing that the left oblique process of the fourth was dislocated forwards

[1] Lente, New York Journ. Med., May, 1850, p. 284. [2] Lente, ibid., p. 397.

upon the fifth. The rotary motions of the neck could now be executed to some extent, but much more freely to the right than to the left. Professor Horner refused to make any attempt to reduce the dislocation.[1]

Dr. Purple, of New York, has reported a case of what was called a dislocation of the fifth and sixth cervical vertebræ, producing complete paralysis of the lower part of the body, in which the patient survived the accident many years; but his lower extremities were so useless and cumbersome as to induce him, in the year 1851, six years after the injury had been received, to submit to the amputation of both at the hip-joint. In 1852, having become very intemperate, he died, but no autopsy was obtained, so that the exact character of the injury was never ascertained.[2] Sanson, of Paris, has reported also a case which came under his observation at Hôtel-Dieu, of dislocation of the "third cervical vertebra backwards," from which, although unreduced, the patient partially recovered. The character of this accident was not much better determined; for, although he felt a severe and sharp pain at the moment of the injury, which was greatly aggravated by motion, and his head was bent forwards and to the left, "the chin being fixed on the upper part of the sternum," there was no paralysis of either the motor or sentient nerves. After the lapse of about four months he left the hospital, still unable to lift his chin more than four inches from the sternum; after which he resumed his usual occupations, suffering no further inconvenience than what was occasioned by the unnatural position of his head.[3] Notwithstanding the authoritative testimony of Sanson that this was a dislocation backwards, one cannot avoid the conclusion that it was either a unilateral subluxation, or perhaps a mere diastasis of the articulation, or else that it was an example of sprain of the muscles, and consequent contraction of one set, or paralysis of the opposing set of muscles. It is certain that it was not a complete luxation, nor, since there was no paralysis of the body below the point of injury, can it be properly made use of as an argument for non-interference where such paralysis does actually exist.

Let us see now what encouragement an attempt at reduction may offer, in a case which presents so little ground of hope where the reduction is not accomplished.

Dr. Spencer, of Ticonderoga, N. Y., relates that a man, æt. 50, fell backwards from a board fence, striking upon the superior and anterior portion of his head, dislocating the second from the third vertebra of the neck. His head was thrown back so far as to prevent his seeing his own body, and all below the injury was completely paralyzed. Repeated attempts were made to reduce the dislocation, "but the transverse processes had become so interlocked that every effort proved abortive," and he died forty-eight hours after the injury was received. Gaitskill also attempted reduction in a case of dislocation of the seventh

[1] Horner, Amer. Journ. Med. Sci., April, 1843, from Med. Exam.
[2] Purple, New York Journ. Med., May, 1853, p. 319.
[3] Sanson, Amer. Journ. Med. Sci., Feb. 1836, p. 514; from Gaz. des Hôpitaux.
[4] Spencer, Boston Med. and Surg. Journ., vol. x. No. 11.

cervical vertebra, but failed.[1] Boyer failed in two cases. It is related by Petit Radel, that a young patient at La Charité expired in the hands of the surgeons, upon such an attempt being made a few days after the accident;[2] and Dupuytren says "the reduction of these dislocations is very dangerous, and we have often known an individual perish from the compression or elongation of the spinal marrow which always attends these attempts."

Dr. Shuck, of Vienna, relates that a man, æt. 24, while engaged at his work on the fifth of Dec. 1838, twisted his head suddenly round, in consequence of one of his companions roaring into his ear, when he instantly felt something give way in his neck, and found it impossible to move his head. Next morning his head was turned to the right and bent down toward the shoulder. Every attempt to move his head caused great pain. He complained of weakness in his right arm, but all the other functions of his body were perfect. An attempt was immediately made to reduce the dislocation by lifting him by the head, but without success. On the 7th of Dec., the weakness and numbness of the right arm had increased, and the attempt to reduce the bones was renewed. The patient was laid horizontally upon a bed, and extension made from the chin and occiput while counter-extension was made from the shoulders. The force thus employed was gradually increased until the patient and assistant felt a snap as of two bones meeting, when it was found that the head was restored to its natural position, and the power of moving it had returned. The next day his arm was more powerless than before, and on the following day he had vertigo, but these symptoms soon yielded to copious bleedings, and he left the hospital cured on the 13th.[3]

Dr. Hickerman, of Ohio, has reported also in the *Ohio Medical Journal*, a case of dislocation of one of the cervical vertebræ, the original account of which I have not seen, but only an abridged statement published in the *Buffalo Medical Journal.* By exploring the pharynx a prominence was felt opposite the junction of the fourth and fifth cervical vertebræ; and the action of the heart was barely perceptible. Seizing the patient's head under his left arm, Dr. Hickerman in this manner made traction, while with the index finger of the right hand in the patients throat he made firm pressure obliquely upwards, backwards, and to the left; after continuing the pressure for about forty or fifty seconds, the part against which the finger was placed gradually, yet quickly, receded in the direction in which the pressure was made, and instantly, as quickly indeed as the act could be possibly executed, the patient opened her eyes, and natural respiration was established. She then also immediately became conscious of what was transpiring about her, and signified by signs, for she was yet unable to speak, that she had suffered pain in the epigastrium. Complete recovery took place.[4]

Schranth received under his care a patient who had a luxation of

[1] Gaitskill, London Repository, vol. xv. p. 282.
[2] Petit Radel, Note to Boyer Malad. Chir., vol. v. p. 118.
[3] Shuck, Amer. Journ. Med. Sci., July, 1841, p. 207.
[4] Hickerman, Buf. Med. Journ., vol. x. p. 702, April, 1855.

the "right transverse apophysis" of the fourth cervical vertebra, without lesion of the spinal marrow, which he reduced on the seventh day. The first attempt was unsuccessful; but the second, made with great caution, by the aid of four assistants, three of whom pulled the head upwards while the fourth pressed with his whole weight upon the shoulders, was completely successful. During the time that the traction was being made, the head was occasionally rotated slightly and moved laterally, and at the same moment the surgeon pushed firmly against the displaced apophysis. The reduction was attended with "various distinct crackings in the neck," which were loud enough to be heard. After some days of repose he resumed his occupation, no stiffness remaining in the movements of his neck.[1]

Dr. Edward Maxson, of Geneva, N. Y., was called on the 28th of Oct. 1856, to see a child about nine years old, who had met with a similar accident about forty hours before, namely, a dislocation of the right articulating apophysis of the fifth or sixth cervical vertebra, occasioned by suddenly turning her head around while at play. She at first complained only of pain and inability to straighten the neck; but whenever moved she became faint and irritable. A short time before the surgeon was called the mother had, in attempting to move her in bed, turned the face a little more to the left, when a severe convulsion immediately ensued. On examining the neck Dr. Maxson discovered the displacement of the transverse process. Having advised the parents of the danger necessarily incident to an attempt at replacement, and of the probable consequences of its being permitted to remain as it was, they consented that the trial should be made. "I grasped the head," says Dr. M., "with both hands, and proceeded according to Desault's method, only I first carried or turned the face very gently a little further toward the left shoulder, to, if possible, disengage the process; then lifting or extending the head, I turned the face very gently toward the right shoulder, when the difficulty was at once overcome, and she exclaimed: 'I can move my eyes.' Her countenance soon acquired a more natural appearance; the faintness passed off; she rested quietly through the night; had no return of the difficulty, and needed only an emollient anodyne to soothe the irritation and slight swelling which remained at the point of injury."[2]

Rust,[3] Wood, of New York,[4] and others, have seen and reported similar examples attended with like success.

So far the cases of successful reduction which we have described are examples of dislocation of only one of the articulating apophyses, and they are sufficiently numerous to establish the value of the practice. We have now to relate a case in itself unique, namely, a successful reduction of a dislocation of the fifth cervical vertebra, in which both apophyses appear to have been thrown forwards. It occurred in the practice of Dr. Daniel Ayres, of Brooklyn, N. Y., and

[1] Schranth, Amer. Journ. Med. Sci., May, 1848.
[2] Maxson, Buffalo Med. Journ., Jan. 1857, p. 479.
[3] Rust, Chelius, note by South,
[4] Wood, New York Journ. Med., Jan, 1857, p. 13.

will be best understood by a reproduction of his own published account of the case.

"E. K., the subject of this accident, was a laboring man, thirty years of age, tall and muscular, but not fat, with a neck longer than the average among men of equal height. On the evening of the 2d of October he became intoxicated, was brought home insensible, and did not recover from the combined effects of the shock and his libations until the following morning, when he was supposed by his wife to be laboring under cold and a stiff neck. She made some domestic applications to the affected part, and administered a dose of cathartic medicine. When it was thought sufficient time had elapsed without obtaining relief, he was seen by Dr. Potter, of this city, and afterwards by Dr. Cullen, both of whom recognized a condition which was not only very unusual, but one which they had never before observed. I was then requested to examine the case, which I did on the *ninth* day after the accident. With some assistance and great personal effort, he was able to get out of bed, moving very slowly and cautiously. Desiring to expectorate, he was obliged to get down on his hands and knees, which he accomplished with the same deliberation. When seated in a chair, the head was thrown back and permanently fixed; the face turned upwards with an anxious expression. The anterior portion of the neck, bulging forwards, was strongly convex, rendering the larynx very prominent. The integuments of this region were exceedingly tense and intolerant of pressure. The posterior portion of the neck exhibited a sharp, sudden angle at the junction of the fifth and sixth cervical vertebræ, around which the integuments lay in folds. It was difficult to reach the bottom of this angle even with strong pressure of the fingers, and of course the regular line formed by the projecting spinous processes was abruptly lost. He complained of intense and constant pain at this point, which was neither relieved nor aggravated by pressure. With difficulty he swallowed small quantities of liquid, pausing after each effort, and could not be induced to take solid food, since the first attempt to do so after the accident was followed by violent paroxysms of coughing and choking. His breathing was obstructed and somewhat labored, being unable fully to clear the bronchia of their secretion. This, however, seemed rather an effect of the tense condition of the soft parts of the neck, than the result of pressure upon the spinal cord, since he presented no evidence of paralysis, either of motion or sensation, in parts below the neck. The sterno-cleido-mastoid muscles of both sides were felt quite soft and relaxed.

"But one conclusion could be formed upon this state of facts, to wit: that the oblique processes of both sides were completely dislocated. The marked rigidity of the head seemed to preclude the probability of fracture through the vertebral bodies, and although the cartilage might be separated anteriorly, yet, the body not pressing backwards sufficiently to produce paralysis of the cord, it was hoped that the posterior vertebral ligament remained uninjured; it was, therefore, determined to make an effort at reduction on the following day. In addition to those originally connected with the case, I am under obligations to Drs. Ingraham, Turner, Palmedo, G. D. Ayres, and a number of other medical gentlemen who were present by invitation, all of whom confirmed the diagnosis, and rendered efficient services.

"The patient was placed upon a strong table in a recumbent position, with a pillow resting under the shoulders, the head being supported by the hand during the administration of chloroform, of which an ounce was given before anæsthesia ensued. Counter-extension being made by two folded sheets placed obliquely across the shoulders and properly held, the head was grasped by one hand placed under the chin, the other over the occiput, and by steadily and firmly drawing the head directly backwards, and then upwards, an attempt was made at reduction, but failed for want of sufficient power. Dr. Ingraham was then requested to place his hands immediately over my own in the same position as before, and steady traction was again made in the same direction. Our united strength was required in drawing the head backwards and upwards, to dislodge the superior oblique processes from their abnormal position. When this was felt to be yielding by Dr. Cullen (who kept one hand constantly at the seat of dislocation), Dr. Potter was directed to place his hands under our own, still in position, and assist in bringing the head forwards; at the same time the chest was depressed toward the table. The bones were distinctly felt to slip into their places; the line of the spine was instantly restored, the head and neck assuming their natural position and aspect. As soon as the patient became conscious, he expressed himself ignorant of what had taken place, but free from pain, and, in his own language, 'all right.' A bandage was arranged to support the head and keep it bent forwards. He had an anodyne for two nights following, after which no further treatment was necessary, and at the end of one week he had complete control over the movements of the head and neck. Beyond the debility and emaciation immediately dependent upon protracted fasting and loss of rest, he has experienced no uneasiness since the operation. His appetite is now good, and all the functions perform their duty normally. In a subsequent inquiry, to determine if possible the cause of the accident, he states that he distinctly recollects going into a store in Atlantic Street, near the ferry, and there having angry words with

Fig. 215.

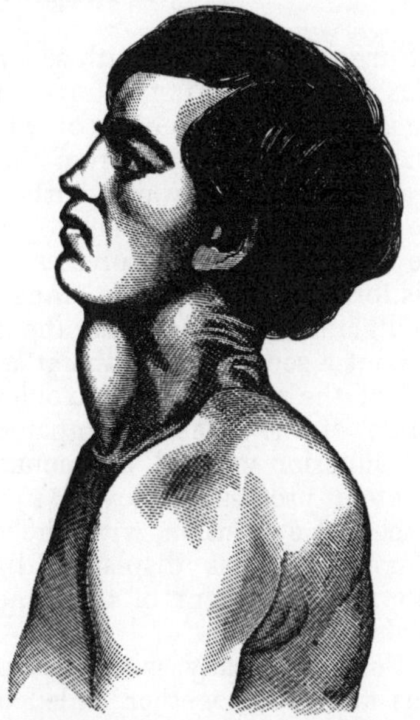

Ayres' case of bilateral dislocation of the fifth cervical vertebra.

an acquaintance; that he left the store and was proceeding up the street (which is here a rather steep ascent), when he was violently struck from behind, over the lower portion of the neck. He likewise remembers falling forwards and striking against some object, but does not know what it was, nor what took place until the following morning."[1]

§ 4. Dislocations of the Atlas.

Surgeons have met with several forms of displacement between the atlas and axis. First, a forced inclination forwards of the atlas upon the axis; in consequence of which the body or anterior arch of the atlas is made to recede from the odontoid process, and the transverse ligament glides upwards without breaking, so that the extremity of the odontoid process comes to occupy a position underneath or behind the ligament, and thus presses upon the cord. It is apparent also that this form of displacement cannot occur without a rupture of the vertical ligament which binds the transverse ligament to the axis, nor without a separation of the atlas from the axis posteriorly and a rupture of the posterior atlo-axoidean ligament. Second, a similar inclination of the atlas, accompanied with a rupture of the transverse and superior vertical ligaments, in consequence of which also the odontoid process is allowed to fall upon the cord. Third, the atlas in the same position, with the odontoid process broken at its base. Fourth, the atlas displaced directly forwards or backwards; and fifth, a displacement of only one articular process in a direction forwards.

We have already, when speaking of fractures of the atlas, or of the atlas and axis together, called attention to several examples of that form of the dislocation which is accompanied with a fracture of the odontoid process. The other forms of dislocation are characterized by so few symptoms peculiar to themselves, or which can be regarded as diagnostic and not already sufficiently studied in connection with other dislocations of the neck, that we shall not deem it necessary to do more than remind our readers that if permitted to remain unreduced a speedy and fatal issue is inevitable, and to point them to a couple of examples of recovery after reduction has been fortunately accomplished, for both of which I am indebted to Malgaigne. These may alone suffice to show that Dupuytren was in error when he declared that such accidents were wholly beyond the resources of our art.

An old man received upon his head a bundle of hay cast from the top of a wagon. He fell with his head bent forwards so that his chin touched the top of the sternum, and in this position it remained immovably fixed; all the other portions of his body preserved their natural functions. A surgeon, who was indeed the father of Malgaigne, being called, assured the patient that unless he could give him relief he would certainly die; but that inasmuch as the attempt might itself prove fatal, he ought at once to put in order his affairs. According-

[1] Ayres, New York Journ. Med., Jan. 1857, p. 9.

ingly the man partook of the sacrament; then the surgeon seated him upon the ground, and placing himself at his back with his knees resting upon his shoulders for the purpose of making counter-extension, and with a towel brought over his own shoulders and under the chin of the patient for extension, he proceeded to act upon the neck in the direction of the axis of the spine. The efforts were long and painful, but at last, while the head was lifted as far as possible, it was suddenly drawn backwards, and immediately it resumed its natural direction. Absolute quietude was enjoined, and the patient recovered in a short time and without any accident.

This patient was seen two years after by the younger Malgaigne, at which time no trace of the accident remained except an impossibility of turning the head to the right or to the left.

The other example is related by Ehrlich, but in this case the dislocation was backwards. A young man, æt. 16, while carrying a sack of flour up a ladder, fell backwards, and the sack falling over upon his face and head came to the ground before him. He was found lying with his head thrown back and to the right, the head resting upon the scapula of this side, but having so completely lost its "solidity" that by its own weight it would fall from one side to the other. On the front and left side of the neck there existed a prominence supposed to be formed by the atlas; the patient was unconscious; the pulse was scarcely perceptible, and the whole body was suffering under paralysis. Ehrlich directed the shoulders to be held by one assistant, and the head to be drawn upon by another, while he pressed with his own hands forcibly upon the displaced atlas from behind. After several fruitless attempts the reduction took place, accompanied with a sound distinctly audible to all of the assistants; the head resumed its position firmly, and the arms began to move. The head was afterwards maintained in place by a bandage. The cure proceeded rapidly, and after a time no trace of the injury remained but a disagreeable tension in the nape of the neck whenever he moved his head briskly to the one side or the other.[1]

§ 5. Dislocations of the Head upon the Atlas, or Occipito-Atloidean Dislocations.

Lassus, Palletta and Bouisson[2] have each reported one example of this dislocation. In neither case was the dislocation complete, but death occurred speedily in every instance. Dariste exhibited to the Anatomical Society of Paris, in 1838, a specimen of incomplete luxation of the occipito-atloid-articulation, with stretching of the transverse ligament. The patient from whom the specimen was taken having lived more than a year after the accident, when he died from a tubercle in the brain.[3]

[1] Malgaigne, Ehrlich, Malgaigne, op. cit., tom. ii. p. 334.

[2] Lassus, Palletta, Bouisson, Malgaigne, op. cit., p. 320.

[3] Dariste, Amer. Journ. Med. Sci., Nov. 1838, p. 237, from Archives Gén., May, 1838.

CHAPTER IV.

DISLOCATIONS OF THE RIBS.

THE ribs may be dislocated from the sternum, from the vertebræ, and from each other. Surgeons have also spoken of dislocations of the ribs from their cartilages, but these cases ought to be regarded as fractures of the cartilages, since there is no proper articulation at this point.

§ 1. DISLOCATIONS OF THE RIBS FROM THE VERTEBRÆ.

Examples of this dislocation have been mentioned by Ambrose Paré, Bransby Cooper, Alcock, Donne, Henkel, Kennedy, Buttet, and some others; but most of these reputed cases have not borne the test of a critical analysis, and while Vidal (de Cassis) is in doubt whether the claims of even one have been fully established, Boyer denies absolutely its possibility. We see no reason, however, to question the authenticity of several of these examples.

The case mentioned by Bransby Cooper, although very briefly narrated, leaves no room for doubt as to its real character. "Mr. Webster, surgeon at St. Albans, when examining the body of a patient who had died of fever, found the head of the seventh rib thrown upon the front of the corresponding vertebra, and there anchylosed. Upon inquiry, Mr. Webster learned that this gentleman, several years before, had been thrown from his horse across a gate, for which accident he had been subjected to the treatment usually followed in fractures of the ribs, and there is every reason to believe that it was at this time that the dislocation occurred."[1]

These accidents seem to have been generally occasioned by a fall or a blow upon the back, and the dislocation has been accompanied usually with a fracture of some other rib, or of the transverse or spinous processes of the corresponding vertebræ. The head of the rib has always been found to be displaced inwards. The lower ribs, including the false and floating, are those which have been most frequently displaced.

It would be difficult, if not impossible, during the life of the patient, to make a positive diagnosis, since the symptoms resemble so closely those which accompany a fracture of the rib near its posterior extremity. The nature of the accident producing the dislocation, the depression, mobility, and pain, are equally indicative of a fracture; while the failure to detect crepitus might easily be explained by the

[1] Webster, B. Cooper's ed. of Sir Astley Cooper, Amer. ed., p. 450.

thickness of the muscular walls at this point, or by the riding, or by other displacements of the broken fragments.

Chelius speaks of a peculiar "rustling," perceived when the body and ribs are moved by the surgeon or by the patient himself, and which is different from the sensation produced by emphysema or fracture.

The treatment ought to be the same which would be adopted in case the rib was broken. Replacement of the dislocated bone must be regarded as impossible; and it only remains that we insure quiet as far as possible in this portion of the chest, and combat the pain and inflammation by suitable remedies. The circular bandage, however, recommended in these cases by Sir Astley Cooper, could only be serviceable in dislocations of those ribs which have an attachment to the sternum; the floating ribs, which have been found dislocated quite as often as either of the others, could derive no support from circular pressure, or from any other mechanical contrivance.

§ 2. Dislocations of the Ribs from the Sternum.

Charles Bell observes: "A young man playing the dumb bells and throwing his arms behind him, feels something give way on the chest; and one of the cartilages of the ribs has started and stands prominent. To reduce it, we make the patient draw a full inspiration, and with the fingers knead the projecting cartilage into its place. We apply a compress and bandage, but the luxation is with difficulty retained."

Ravaton, Manzotti, and Monteggia, have each, according to Malgaigne, reported one example of traumatic dislocation; in all of which the cartilages were thrown forwards in advance of the sternum.

By pressure alone they have generally been replaced, the cartilage resuming its position suddenly and with a sound. The reduction may, nevertheless, be facilitated by bending the trunk backwards or by directing the patient to make a full inspiration.

To maintain the reduction has been found more difficult, and Sir Astley directs that "a long piece of wetted pasteboard should be placed in the course of three of the ribs and their cartilages, the injured rib being in the centre; this dries upon the chest, takes the exact form of the parts, prevents motion, and affords the same support as a splint upon a fractured limb. A flannel roller is to be applied over this splint, and a system of depletion pursued, to prevent inflammation of the thoracic viscera." Instead of the pasteboard, we might use either felt or gutta percha.

The patients spoken of by Ravaton and Manzotti were both cured in about one month.

Mr. Bransby Cooper says that a baker's boy applied for relief at Guy's Hospital, who was the subject of displacement of the cartilages of the fifth and sixth ribs from their junction with the sternum, produced partly by the constant action of the pectoral muscles in kneading bread, but principally by his defective constitution. Mr. Cooper stated to the boy the necessity of changing his occupation, and advised him to go into the country, but as he was unable to do so little hope was entertained of his recovery.[1]

§ 3. Dislocation of one Cartilage upon Another.

The cartilages of the sixth, seventh, and eighth ribs, at those points of their upper and lower margins which come in contact with each other, possess a true arthrodial articulation, being furnished with both ligaments and a synovial membrane. Sometimes, also, the same anatomical structure extends to the adjoining surfaces of the fifth and sixth ribs, as well as to the eighth and ninth.

This displacement, of which Boyer, Martin, and Malgaigne, have each reported one example, may take place when one falls upon his back, striking upon some projecting body, so that the chest is suddenly thrown forwards; in consequence of which the upper margin of the lower cartilage is depressed and entangled behind the lower margin of the upper. The inferior cartilage is, therefore, the one which is displaced rather than the superior, although this latter being made prominent by the pressure of the other from behind, seems alone to be displaced.

It is probable that the contraction of the pectoral and abdominal muscles has a chief agency in the production of these dislocations, and that they are not solely or directly due to the shock of the accident.

The treatment consists in pressing firmly upwards and backwards against the inferior margin of the upper, or overlapping rib, so as to disengage it from the lower, when by its own elasticity it will resume its natural position. The reduction might also be aided by a full inspiration.

CHAPTER V.

DISLOCATIONS OF THE CLAVICLE.

Of 23 dislocations of the clavicle observed by me, 5 belonged to the sternal end and 18 to the acromial. Of those belonging to the sternal end, 4 were dislocations forwards, and one was a dislocation upwards. I have never met with a dislocation backwards. Of the acromial dislocations, the whole number were dislocations upwards, or upwards and outwards.

[1] B. Cooper, ed. of Sir Astley Cooper, &c., op. cit., p. 447.

§ 1. Dislocation Forwards at the Sternal End.

Causes.—This accident is generally caused by a fall upon the point of the shoulder, in consequence of which the sternal end of the clavicle is driven forcibly inwards and forwards. It is probable, also, that the blow which produces the dislocation is received rather upon the anterior and outer face than exactly upon the extremity of the shoulder. A sudden effort of the muscles, as in the attempt to balance a weight upon the head, or to throw the shoulders backwards when under drill, has been known also to produce this dislocation. In one example it was occasioned by placing the knee against the spine and drawing the shoulders forcibly back. Various other accidents, the philosophy of whose agency is not so easily explained, are said to have produced the same result; but it is not improbable that in many of these cases, the precise manner in which the injury was received has not been correctly understood or reported.

Mr. Fergusson has once seen this displacement in a newly-born infant, which had happened during birth. It could be replaced with ease, but immediately slipped out again when left to itself. "Nothing was done; a new joint formed, and the child afterwards possessed as much power in the one arm as in the other."[1]

Symptoms.—The head of the bone, unless the person is exceedingly fat, or great swelling has supervened, can be distinctly felt and seen in front of the sternum; the corresponding shoulder falls a little back; the head inclining also sometimes to the same side; the movements of the arm are embarrassed, and accompanied almost always with an acute pain at the point of dislocation. The clavicular portion of the sterno-cleido-mastoid muscle presents an unusually sharp and projecting outline and a careful measurement indicates, if the dislocation is complete, a sensible approach of the acromion process toward the centre of the sternum. If now the surgeon places his knee against the spine, and draws the shoulders back, the projection of the clavicle in front diminishes or disappears; if he carries the shoulder up it descends; and if he depresses the shoulder, it ascends.

Fig. 216.

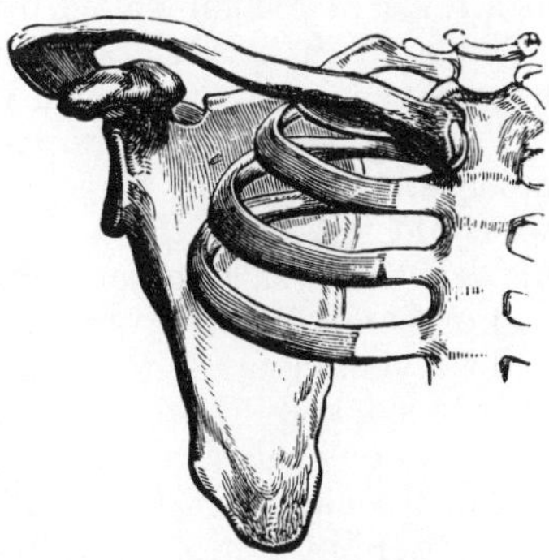

Dislocation of the sternal end forwards.

The simplicity and uniformity of the symptoms which usually characterize this accident will generally prevent the possibility of a mistake; but Pinel mentions the case of a man who having presented himself at one of the hospitals of Paris, suffering under this dislocation, the surgeon in chief thought it a tumor of the bone, and advised the application of a

[1] Fergusson, System of Practical Surgery., Amer. ed., 1853, p. 203.

plaster; and, on the other hand, a patient presented himself to Velpeau, who had been treated for a dislocation, when the bone was only expanded by disease.

I have myself also seen a fracture so near the sternal end of the bone as not to be easily distinguished from a dislocation.

Pathology.—In complete anterior luxation of the clavicle the capsular ligament suffers a complete disruption, and also the anterior with the posterior sterno-clavicular ligaments. The rhomboid and interclavicular ligaments suffer more or less according to the extent of the displacement. The interclavicular cartilage may retain its attachment to the sternum, or it may be carried forwards with the clavicle.

The head of the bone lies immediately underneath the skin and in front of the sternum; and generally it is found to have descended a little upon its anterior surface. Richerand saw a case in which the sternal extremity of the bone was placed three inches below the top of the sternum.

Wherever the bone lies it carries with it the clavicular fasciculus of the sterno-cleido-mastoid.

Treatment.—Not one of the four forward dislocations of the clavicle seen by me has been completely reduced, or if reduced they have not been retained in place. In the following example the reduction, although faithfully attempted, was never accomplished.

Mr. H., of Buffalo, æt. 45, was thrown by a horse, suffering at the same moment a fracture of the leg and a forward dislocation of the left clavicle at its sternal end.

Prof. James P. White, of this city, with whom I was in consultation, made several attempts to reduce the dislocation by placing the knee against the spine and pulling the shoulders forcibly back, and the same efforts were repeated by myself, but without accomplishing the reduction. We also endeavored to reduce it by pressing directly upon the projecting bone, and by placing a pad in the axilla, using the arm as a lever as recommended by Desault, but with no better result.

This patient was tolerably muscular, but while we were manipulating he was very much enfeebled by the shock of the accident.

Finding that it was impossible to reduce the dislocation by any moderate amount of force, and believing that if we were to succeed we could not retain the bone in place, and the more especially because his left side was so much bruised that he could not bear an axillary pad or bandages of any kind, we desisted from any further attempts.

Two years later I examined the shoulder and found the clavicle still unreduced, and its position unchanged. When he carries the shoulder forwards or backwards, there is a corresponding motion at the sternal end of the clavicle. The arm is not quite as strong as the other, and its freedom of motion is slightly impaired.

I have also in my museum the cast of a case of complete forward dislocation at this point; which accident occurred in a lad twelve years old, who had fallen into a cellar on the 20th of Aug. 1856. The late Dr. Lewis and Dr. Dayton, both excellent surgeons then residing in this city, had examined the arm, and dressings had been applied with a view to maintain the reduction; but on the fifth day after the accident I found the bone displaced; nor do I think reduction was ever afterwards maintained.

A lad was brought into the hospital, with a dislocation of the same character, on the 25th of Sept., 1858, who had been run over by a wagon on the same day. Dr. E. P. Smith, one of the surgeons of the hospital, attempted faithfully to reduce it, but was unable to do so. Five days after, I found the bone out and quite movable. All apparatus having been removed, we laid him upon his back in bed, and kept him in this position three weeks. He was then dismissed, with no change in the appearance of the bone, but he could move the arm as well as before the accident.

The fourth example of which I have spoken was only a partial luxation, and some doubts might be entertained as to whether it was not a pathologic condition; but after a careful examination of the patient, I have concluded that it was traumatic, or the result of some accident, such as a sudden and violent motion of the arm, and that in this way it had taken place without the knowledge of the patient. I found this man, John A. Frank, in my wards at the hospital. He was then fifty-nine years old, and he stated that the displacement occurred when he was ten years old; nor did he remember that it was the result of any injury; but only that one morning while tying on his cravat his attention was first called to it. The projection has since then neither increased nor diminished, nor has it ever been tender. The opposite clavicle is perfect.

Other surgeons have not met with, or at least they have not mentioned any cases in which the reduction of this dislocation was attended with difficulty, nor am I prepared to explain the difficulty which was experienced in my own (Mr. H.), and in Dr. E. P. Smith's case. Probably they ought to be regarded as exceptions to the general rule. But most surgeons have testified to the difficulty of retaining it in place when reduction has been fairly accomplished. Chelius says, "there commonly remains more or less deformity," and Malgaigne says that "it is difficult and rare to cure it without deformity."

Nevertheless Desault (or, rather, his pupil Bichat, who has published his lectures), who always speaks very confidently of his ability to retain either broken or dislocated bones in their places, says that he "almost always obtained complete success" with his apparatus. It is remarkable, however, that of the three examples furnished by Bichat to confirm this statement, all of which were treated by Desault himself, one recovered after a long time with a "very perceptible protuberance in front of the sternum," one with a "very slight protuberance," and in the other the "swelling was almost gone" on the twentieth day, and we are left in doubt as to whether the reduction was any more complete than in either of the other cases.[1] Richerand and Guersant succeeded no better with Desault's dressings.[2]

Other surgeons have made similar claims for their own forms of apparatus, but experience still continues to show that a complete retention of the dislocated bone is seldom to be expected.

[1] Desault on Fractures and Dislocations, by Xav. Bichat, Philada. ed., 1805, p. 53.

[2] Malgaigne, op. cit., tom. ii. p. 417.

Sir Astley Cooper recommends an apparatus, the construction and application of which are illustrated by the accompanying sketch (Fig. 217), the object of which is to draw the shoulders back, and at the same time, by the aid of two pads or cushions in the axillæ, to carry the shoulders outwards. The dressing is then completed by placing the arm in a sling. He advises, however, that in some way direct pressure should be made upon the projecting point of bone.

Fig. 217.

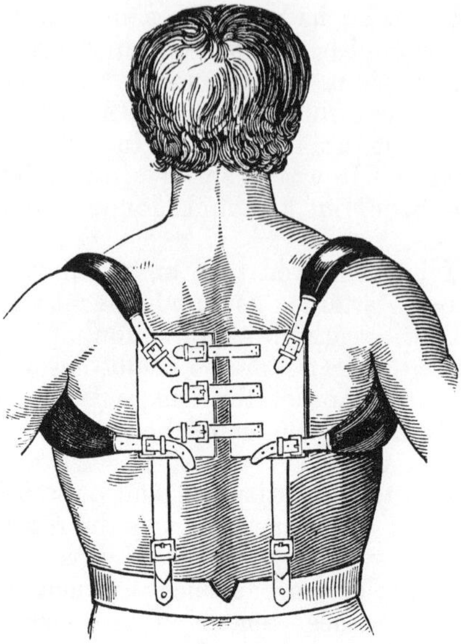

Sir Astley Cooper's apparatus for dislocated clavicle.

Velpeau objects to any plan which will draw the shoulders back; but, on the contrary, he thinks that the shoulders should be kept slightly forwards so as to diminish the tendency of the sternal end of the clavicle to escape in this direction.

Dr. Folts, of Boston, affirms that he has been able in one instance to maintain complete reduction with Bartlett's apparatus for broken clavicles.[1]

Until farther observations have determined the relative value of these and of many other processes, it will be well to adopt no fixed rule of action; but, having reduced the bone by either placing the knee upon the spine and drawing the shoulders back, or by making use of the humerus as a lever, we recommend that the surgeon shall seek to maintain it in place by such means as the experiment shall prove are most successful. Among these means, direct pressure upon the sternal end of the clavicle, the sling and perfect quietude of the muscles of the arm through the aid of bandages, are no doubt of the greatest importance, and can seldom be omitted. If then we find that a position of the shoulders more or less forwards or backwards best maintains the apposition, this position, whatever it is, ought to be continued.

In order to be successful, sufficient time must elapse for the torn ligaments to become firmly reunited, during which the reduction must be constant; since every time the bone escapes, the whole work of repair has to be recommenced as from the beginning. To this end at least four or six weeks are necessary, and sometimes the period must be lengthened far beyond these limits; so that it may often become a grave point of inquiry whether the long confinement of the limb will not entail more serious consequences than have ever been known to arise from leaving the bone displaced, which in no case yet reported has more than slightly impaired the functions of the arm.

[1] Folts, Boston Med. and Surg. Journ., vol. liii. p. 260.

§ 2. Dislocation of the Sternal End of the Clavicle Upwards.

Malgaigne has collected four undoubted examples of this dislocation, and I have been unable to find a report of any other except the very extraordinary case described by Dr. Rochester, of this city, at the September meeting of the Buffalo Medical Association, and which case, through the courtesy of Dr. Rochester, I was permitted to see several times.[1]

Jerry McAuliffe, æt. 44, on the 28th of August, 1858, while seated upon a load of wood, was caught under the bar of a gateway and violently crushed, the right shoulder being forced downwards and a little backwards. Dr. Rochester saw him very soon after the accident. On examination it was found that the sternal extremity of the right clavicle was thrown upwards so far as to rest upon the front of the thyroid cartilage, occasioning considerable pain, difficulty of respiration and loss of speech. Reduction was easily effected, and a retentive apparatus was immediately applied, consisting of a gutta-percha splint, moulded to the clavicle and ribs, and retained in place with adhesive plaster. Suitable bandages, a sling, &c., were also employed to maintain complete rest.

Notwithstanding all the care employed, the bone again became displaced, and when, nearly four months after the accident, this man came before the class of medical students at the Hospital of the Sisters of Charity, we found the sternal end of the clavicle carried upwards half an inch, and across toward the opposite side also about half an inch, and projecting somewhat in front. It was fixed in this position by ligaments which allowed it to move much more freely than natural, but which would not permit any great displacement. The corresponding shoulder was slightly depressed. McAuliffe said that he felt no inconvenience or abatement of strength in the arm except when he attempted to lift weights above his head.

The accident seems to have been produced in all the cases, so far as can be ascertained, by a force operating upon the end and top of the shoulder; in consequence of which the head of the clavicle is pushed and at the same time lifted, as it were, from its socket, tearing not only its capsule with the ligaments which immediately invest the capsule, but also in some instances the costo-clavicular ligament with some fibres of the subclavian muscle. The sternal end of the clavicle is found riding upon the top of the sternum, its head being placed between the sternal fasciculus of the sterno-cleido-mastoideus muscle, on the one hand, and the sterno-hyoideus muscle on the other. In one of the cases seen by Malgaigne the head had traversed in this direction completely the intra-clavicular space, and lay behind the sternal portion of the opposite sterno-cleido-mastoideus muscle.

The symptoms are a depression of the shoulder, with an elevation of the sternal end of the clavicle so as to increase sensibly the space between it and the first rib. The clavicle also encroaches more or

[1] Rochester, Buffalo Med. Journ., vol. xiv. p. 262.

less upon the súpra-sternal fossa, occasioning a corresponding diminution of the space between the end of the shoulder and the centre of the sternum. The sternal portion of one or both of the sterno-cleido-mastoidean muscles may also be seen raised and rendered tense by the pressure of the head of the bone from behind.

Reduction has been found easy, but Malgaigne thinks a perfect retention impossible, at least it does not seem to have been accomplished in any of the cases reported, although in most or all of them the remaining deformity was only slight. In no case did this trifling displacement seriously impair the functions of the arm.

The same appareil to which we shall give the preference in cases of dislocation upwards of the acromial end of the clavicle, at least with only such slight modifications as the peculiarities of the case will naturally suggest, will be suitable for this accident. The shoulder must be lifted by a sling, while the sternal end of the clavicle is pressed downwards by a pad and bandages; and all the muscles of the arm and chest, so far as is consistent with respiration and comfort, must be maintained in a state of perfect rest until the ligaments have become reunited.

§ 3. Dislocation of the Sternal End of the Clavicle Backwards.

The first case upon record of this kind of accident, caused by violence, was published by Pellieux in 1834, in the *Revue Médicale;* until which time its existence had been generally denied. In the *London and Edinburgh Journal of Medical Science* for October, 1841, several cases are mentioned.

Two forms of the accident have been described, one in which the head of the clavicle is driven backwards and a little downwards; and another in which it is displaced directly backwards, or backwards and a little upwards. In both of these classes, the end of the bone falls inwards toward the opposite clavicle, and occupies a space in the cellular tissue back of the sterno-hyoid and sterno-thyroid muscles, and in front of the œsophagus; the trachea, if reached at all, being probably thrust to the opposite side.

The examples in which it has been found below the top of the sternum are much the most numerous; indeed, it is probable that the other form is only a secondary displacement, occasioned by the action of the fibres of the sterno-cleido-mastoid muscle.

Causes.—Of the eleven examples mentioned by Malgaigne, four were occasioned by direct blows, and most of the remainder by crushing accidents, as by powerful lateral compression of the shoulders.

One of the cases produced by a direct blow, was accompanied with an external wound, and is the only instance of a compound dislocation of this kind upon record. The man was admitted into St. Thomas's Hospital in Sept. 1835, and, according to his own account, the sharp end of a pickaxe had been driven through the flesh against the bone, The sternal end of the clavicle was found to be displaced backwards. and, with the finger thrust into the wound on the front of the chest, it could be distinctly felt resting upon the side and front of the trachea, where it interfered somewhat with respiration and deglutition. He had a great desire to cough, with a sensation of pressure on his windpipe, which was greatly increased when his head was thrown back. There was also a slight emphysema in the region below the collar bone and over the top of the sternum. The shoulder having been brought back with straps attached to a back-board the bone readily resumed its place. The elbow was then brought forwards and bound to the side, and the wound being closed with adhesive plaster, he was put to bed with the shoulders much raised. No unfavorable symptoms followed, and in three weeks he left his bed. Three weeks later he left the hospital with the sternal end of the bone still falling a little backwards, and rather more movable than natural.[1]

The following example, related by Morel-Lavallée, will illustrate that class in which the dislocation results from an indirect blow, or from a crushing accident.

Lemoine, seventeen years old, had his right shoulder violently pressed against a wall by a carriage. He experienced at the moment some pain at the bottom of his neck, and a great sensation of suffocation, which lasted for more than a quarter of an hour. The dyspnœa gradually subsided, but the motion of the right arm not returning, he, on the eighth day after the accident, entered La Charité. On examination, the two shoulders were found to be on the same level, but the right one was nearer the mesial line. The internal extremity of the clavicle was half concealed behind the sternum. On depressing the shoulder, the inner end of the clavicle arose and disengaged itself from behind the sternum; but reduction was effected by elevating the shoulder, while at the same time it was carried outwards and backwards. Desault's bandage was then applied, but as it became loosened, Velpeau's was substituted, which kept the bone completely in position until the eighteenth day, when the patient was lost sight of.[2]

Symptoms.—The most constant symptoms are the absence of the head of the bone from its socket, and its complete or partial disappearance behind the sternum, an approach of the corresponding shoulder to the mesian line, an inclination of the head to the opposite side, elevation of the shoulder, pain at bottom of the neck, impairment of the motions of the arm, sometimes difficulty in respiration and in deglutition, partial arrest in the circulation of the arm from pressure upon the subclavian artery, and a slight projection of the acromial end of the clavicle, noticed twice by Morel-Lavallée.

It has not generally been found difficult to reduce this dislocation, nor, when reduced, is it so liable to again become displaced as are the dislocations forwards; yet in only a few instances has the restoration been so complete as not to leave some deformity.

In order to the reduction, the shoulder must be carried generally upwards, outwards, and backwards, and it may then be best maintained in position by laying the patient on his back upon an elevated

[1] South, note to Chelius's Surgery, Amer. ed., vol. ii. p. 218.

[2] Morel-Lavallée, Amer. Journ. Med. Sci., vol. xxix. p. 229, 1842; from Gaz. Méd.

cushion, as practised by Tyrrell in the case related by South. To this may be added such other measures, differing but little from those employed in other dislocations of the clavicle, as are necessary to insure complete rest to the muscles. Of course, no pads or bands across the clavicle can be of any service in this case.

As in the other cases of dislocation at this point, the patients have generally recovered nearly the full use of their arms, even in one or two instances in which the reduction has never been accomplished.

§ 4. Dislocation of the Acromial End of the Clavicle Upwards.

Of all the dislocations of the clavicle, this form is most frequent. I have met with it either as a partial or complete luxation eighteen times. The youngest subject was seven years of age, and the oldest sixty-three. All but one were males.

Causes.—It is produced generally by a fall upon the extremity of the shoulder. Twice the blow has been received rather upon the back than upon the extremity, and once it was occasioned by the fall of a board directly upon the top of the shoulder.

Symptoms.—When the dislocation is complete, the clavicle not only is lifted from its articular facet to the extent of the breadth of the bone, but it is pushed more or less outwards over the top of the acromion process; generally less than half an inch, but I have once seen it riding the process to the extent of three-quarters of an inch. In this last example, the case of James Moran, a strong, healthy laboring man, the clavicle was easily reduced, and it always went into place with a sensible click; but although every possible care was taken to retain it in place by bandages, compresses, an axillary pad and a sling, yet it was not accomplished, and on the third day he removed all the dressings, and refused to have them reapplied.

I have usually found the shoulder slightly depressed, and in one instance, where it is probable the deltoid muscle had suffered some injury, the elbow hung away from the body, and any attempts to lay it against the side produced an acute pain in the shoulder.[1] It has been noticed also, in most cases, that the clavicular portion of the trapezius muscle appeared lifted and tense, especially when the neck was straight.

Inability to raise the arm to a right angle with the body is a general but not constant symptom. In two instances where the displacement was only moderate, the patients were at first and for some time afterwards unable to lift the arm in any degree from the side. In one example, a lady sixty years of age had fallen upon her shoulder and produced a dislocation upwards, but she had not consulted a surgeon until she called upon me, five months after the accident. The clavicle was then raised from its socket about half an inch, but it could be easily pressed back to its place, the reduction being attended with a

[1] Report on Dislocations, by the author. Transac. of New York State Med. Soc., 1855, p. 19.

grating sensation, a circumstance which I have not noticed in any other instance. She was not even then able to raise her arm to her head, nor had she been able to do so since the accident occurred.

Fig. 218.

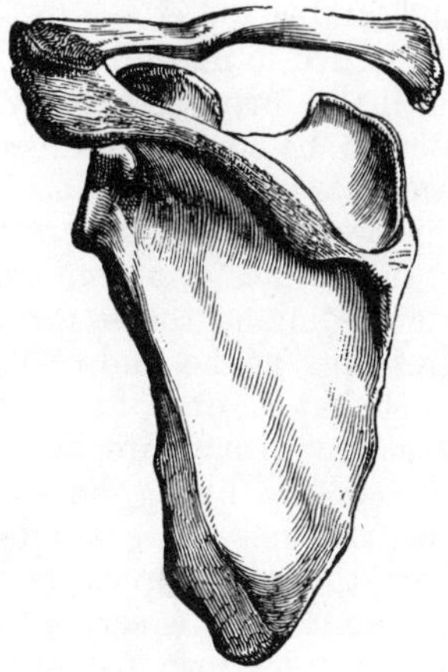

Dislocation of the acromial end of the clavicle, upwards and outwards.

In all the motions of the arm and shoulder, the clavicle is seen to move more freely than natural immediately under the skin, and these motions are usually attended with some pain at the point of dislocation.

This accident has been sometimes mistaken for a dislocation of the humerus, but unless the shoulder is already greatly swollen, the error is not likely to happen. If the point of the acromion process can be made out, it will be easy to determine, by sliding the finger along its spine, whether the clavicle is displaced or not, and by these means to settle the question of its complicity in the accident. The question as to whether the shoulder is dislocated or not may be more difficult of solution, as we shall hereafter have occasion again to observe.

Pathology.—Generally there exists simply a rupture of the capsule of the joint, and of the ligaments immediately investing the capsule, so that the clavicle rises from its socket only about half an inch, more or less, according to its diameter, and is carried outwards just sufficiently far to allow it to rest upon the upper margin of the acromial articulation. In at least thirteen of the cases seen by me, this has been the position of the acromial end of the clavicle, and for its complete reduction nothing more has been required than to press with moderate force upon the upper and outer end of the bone.

In three cases I have found the bone not only thus lifted in its socket, but also driven over upon the acromion from half to three-quarters of an inch; and in one instance, that of a gentleman, Mr. B., who was injured in a railroad accident, the acromial end of the clavicle was displaced outwards half an inch and backwards three-quarters of an inch, while the sternal end also was considerably lifted in its socket and slightly sent inwards. The head of the humerus fell forwards and the coracoid process was one inch nearer the sternum than the same process upon the opposite side. In such cases more or less of the fibres of the coraco-clavicular ligament must have suffered a disruption; indeed, without a rupture of its external fasciculus, which anatomists have called the trapezoid ligament, such a dislocation cannot take place.

Prognosis.—It is impossible for me to say what has been the precise result in all the cases which I have seen, but my notes furnish only one case of perfect retention after a complete dislocation at this point. David Thomas, aged about twenty-five years, fell sideways upon the ground, striking upon the extremity, and, as he thinks, a little upon the top of the shoulder. I found the clavicle dislocated upwards and outwards, so that it overlapped the acromion process half an inch. It was easily replaced, and having applied my own apparatus for broken collar bones, with the addition of a band across the shoulder and under the elbow to keep the clavicle down, I found that I had succeeded in retaining the bone in place. This dressing was continued until the forty-second day, when, on being removed, the clavicle was seen to be closely confined upon its articulation; and after a lapse of two years it still retains its position so completely that no difference can be detected between the opposite articulations.

In the case of Moran, already mentioned, whose clavicle overlapped the acromion process three-quarters of an inch, and who threw off the dressings at the end of three days, the same degree of displacement existed at the end of two years: the scapular end of the clavicle moving freely in every direction under the skin according as the arm was moved. In lifting, he says, the strength of his arm is undiminished until he raises the weight nearly to a level with his shoulders, and from this point upwards he can lift but little. For a laboring man it amounts to a serious maiming. I have seen the same loss of power in the arm to raise bodies above the head in at least two or three of the examples of less complete luxation, continuing after the lapse of several years; but in the majority of cases, although the bone does not remain reduced, the patients have recovered eventually the complete use of the arm in whatever position it may be placed.

Treatment.—When the bone simply rises upon its socket the reduction is always easily accomplished by pressing firmly upon its extremity with the fingers; but if, at the same time, it has been carried outwards, or outwards and backwards, the reduction is only accomplished by pulling the shoulders backwards, or by placing a pad in the axilla, using the arm as a lever, or by lifting the arm by the elbow and at the same time pressing the clavicle down; and it will sometimes require the application of all or several of these procedures at the same moment. In some cases the complete reduction has only been effected when the patient has been brought under the influence of an anæsthetic.

As to the maintenance of the bone in its socket for a length of time sufficient to insure a firm union of the broken tissues, this will be found always more difficult, and, in a great majority of cases, absolutely impossible. Nearly all surgeons who have written upon this subject have made the same observation; and if occasionally a new apparatus in the hands of a clever surgeon has seemed to promise better results, the same apparatus in the hands of other equally clever surgeons, and under circumstances equally favorable, has been found almost constantly to fail; and we have been compelled again to exercise anew our ingenuity, and to seek for new resources, or to abandon the effort in despair.

Only very lately a surgeon, Dr. Folts, of Boston, believed that he had found in Bartlett's apparatus for broken clavicles modified by the application of a shoulder-strap, the infallible remedy for this one of the many sad defects in our art. The most important part of this dressing, according to Dr. Folts, is the compress placed upon the upper and outer end of the clavicle, and the bandage or strap passed over the compress and under the point of the elbow to maintain it in position.[1]

Dr. Folts is no doubt correct in regarding this strap as an important if not the essential part of the apparatus; and it is surprising that by Sir Astley Cooper, as well as by many other experienced surgeons, its value should have been overlooked. The chief obstacle to the retention of the bone in place is the powerful action of the trapezius, which constantly tends to elevate the outer end of the bone. In some measure this may be resisted by elevating very forcibly the shoulder, or by inclining the head, but both of these positions are extremely fatiguing, and will not be long endured. The bandage or strap, adjusted in the manner which Dr. Folts has recommended, is the only means of counteracting the action of the trapezius, upon which any substantial reliance can be placed; but the principle has long been understood and practiced upon. Brasdor's tourniquet, or Petit's, secured by a strap brought under the point of the elbow, Boyer's double shoulder straps and Desault's third bandage, all aimed at the accomplishment of the same purpose; yet both Boyer and Desault found all these contrivances fail in a majority of cases. Mayor employed a dressing constructed with a strap to buckle over the dislocated clavicle (Fig. 219); but Nélaton has seen this apparatus fail, also, when applied in his own wards.

Fig. 219.

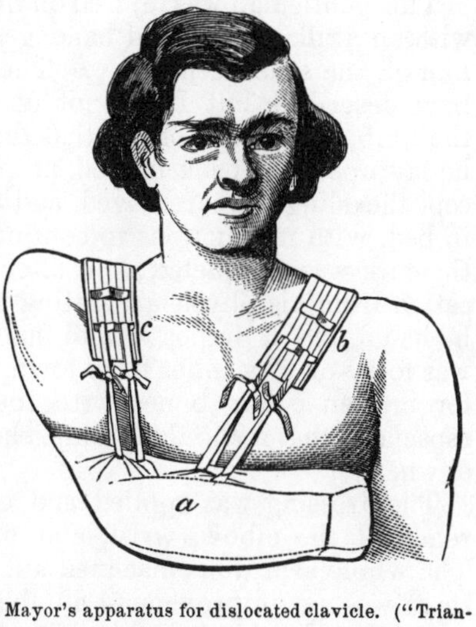

Mayor's apparatus for dislocated clavicle. ("Triangle cubito-bis-scapulaire.")

The experience of Dr. Folts at the time of his report did not extend beyond three cases, and the apparatus had been completely successful in only two of the three. Our own experience is sufficient to show that it will be found occasionally, but by no means constantly, successful. We have already mentioned one case in which we succeeded perfectly by this mode, but in several others which seemed equally favorable we have met with partial or complete failures.

The practical difficulties are, the sensibility and consequent inability sometimes of the point of the elbow to bear the requisite pressure, and the even greater sensibility of the skin over the top of the clavicle; the tendency of the bandage to slide off from the shoulder and also to become displaced from the end of the elbow; the

[1] Folts, Bost. Med. and Surg. Journ., vol. liii. p. 259.

gradual relaxation of the bandages, which, when existing even in the most inconsiderable degree, is sufficient sometimes to allow the bone to slip out from its shallow socket; the impossibility of fixing the scapula, upon whose immobility as well as upon the immobility of the clavicle the retention depends; and, finally, the great length of time requisite to unite firmly the ligaments and the capsule, if indeed they ever again become actually united.

The band can be prevented in some measure from sliding off from the clavicle by a counter-band attached to a collar upon the opposite shoulder, but not without causing some pain and giving rise to excoriations generally in the opposite axilla; and in a degree all the other difficulties may be met by patience and ingenuity, but unfortunately the smallest failure in any one of these numerous indications insures a defeat.

The axillary pad employed as a fulcrum upon which extension may be made is equally as dangerous here as in fractures, and I do not think it ought ever to be used for this purpose, but only as a means of moderate support and retention; indeed it would be well, perhaps, if it were discarded altogether.

The case of Mr. B., already quoted, with a dislocation outwards and backwards, affords not only an illustration of the inefficiency of either the shoulder-strap or the axillary pad in certain cases, but also, it seems to me, of the mischief which may result from their too diligent application; for I cannot persuade myself but that most of the maiming in this case was due to the apparatus rather than to the original accident.

This gentleman was injured on the 10th of November, 1855. A sling with an axillary pad and bandages was immediately applied. I saw him on the seventeenth day. The displacement was then such as I have described, but I did not observe any paralysis or emaciation of the limb. Having noticed that the clavicle fell into its socket when he lay upon his back in bed, at my suggestion all the dressings except the sling were removed, and the patient was laid upon his back in bed, with instructions to continue in this position if possible until the cure was completed; but after a few days I received a communication from his physician, stating that, owing to a troublesome cough, he had found it impossible to maintain this position. His residence was forty or fifty miles from town, and I sent him one of my dressings for broken collar bones with instructions as to its use; directing especially that a shoulder-strap should be used to keep the clavicle down.

The dressing was applied and continued six weeks, and on being removed, the elbow, wrist, and finger-joints were found to be stiff. The whole arm was emaciated and almost powerless. One year later there was no improvement in the condition of the arm; every joint from the shoulder down was almost completely anchylosed, the muscles were greatly wasted, and the hand trembled constantly.

These results, it seems to me, were due to too long and too tight bandaging of the arm, and especially to the pressure of the axillary pad. I do not state this positively, but this is my belief.

Is it worth while, then, to incur the dangers of too long confinement and of excessive bandaging for the purpose of attaining the always uncertain result of maintaining the bone in its socket? We certainly may be permitted to make the attempt within certain reasonable limits; and especially if the patient is a female and the avoidance of deformity is a point of serious consideration; but never without keeping constantly in mind the possibility of a permanent anchylosis and paralysis of the limb.

§ 5. Dislocation of the Acromial End of the Clavicle Downwards.

This form of dislocation is exceedingly rare, only three well-authenticated cases having been placed upon record, one of which was seen and dissected by Melle, in 1765, the second was met with by Fleury, in 1816, and the third is described by Tournel.

Cause.—So far as we can ascertain, it has been produced only by a force which has acted directly upon the top of the clavicle. In the case mentioned by Tournel, a horse had trod upon the shoulder, and in the example recorded by Melle, the accident occurred in a child six years old, from an attempt to support a great weight upon the top of the collar bone. In this last example the shoulder was dislocated also, and both dislocations had remained unreduced many years when the patient was seen by Melle.

This force acting directly upon the top of the clavicle would fail to dislocate the bone, except by first breaking down the coracoid process, if it did not happen sometimes that at the same moment the lower angle of the scapula was thrown outwards, in such a manner as to depress slightly the coracoid, and thus to permit the outer end of the clavicle to fall below the level of the acromion process.

Symptoms and Pathology.—This dislocation, whether it has been produced artificially upon the dead subject or accidentally upon the living, has always been found to be accompanied with a complete rupture of the acromio-clavicular ligaments not only, but also of the coraco-acromial and coraco-clavicular ligaments; the outer extremity of the bone resting between the acromion process and the capsule of the shoulder-joint, and a little posterior to the articulating facet which originally received the clavicle.

The superior angle of the scapula approaches the body slightly, and its inferior angle is thrown outwards. A marked depression exists at the point of dislocation, accompanied with a sharp pain, increased especially when an attempt is made to move the arm. The patient is unable to lift the arm voluntarily, but it can be moved pretty freely in the direction forwards and backwards by the hands of the surgeon: abduction is much more difficult.

Treatment.—Reduction is easily accomplished, at least in the only two examples upon the living subject in which the attempt has been made, it was effected promptly by drawing the shoulders gently outwards and backwards; nor has it been found any more difficult to maintain it in position when once replaced. When the scapula is restored to its natural position and its lower angle approaches again the side of the body, a reluxation becomes impossible; since the coracoid process now effectually prevents that descent of the clavicle upon which its displacement always depends. It is only necessary, therefore, to secure the scapula at its base and lower angle snugly to the body, by a broad band and compress, and all the indications of treatment are completely fulfilled.

§ 6. Dislocation of the Acromial End of the Clavicle under the Coracoid Process.

Pinjou met with one example of this singular dislocation,[1] and Godemer, of Mayenne, has recorded five more,[2] and these constitute the whole number which are at this day known to science.

Cause.—Age and a consequent relaxation of the ligaments seem to constitute a predisposing cause, since of the six recorded examples four were between the ages of sixty-seven and seventy-one, and the other two were adults. In all the cases, also, the dislocation was the result of a fall upon the shoulder.

The symptoms which have been said to characterize this accident are pain and a very marked depression at the point of displacement, with a corresponding projection of the acromion and coracoid processes; a rapid inclination outwards and downwards of the line of the clavicle, its outer extremity being felt in the axilla; the corresponding shoulder depressed and inclined forwards; freedom of motion in all directions except inwards and upwards; the lower angle of the scapula thrown outwards and backwards; to which Morel-Lavallé has added an actual increase of space between the acromion process and the sternum.

Treatment.—Godemer reduced all the examples which came under his notice easily by directing an assistant to pull the arm backwards and outwards while he himself seized upon the clavicle with his fingers and disengaged it from under the process; but Pinjou, after many efforts by the same method, failed completely, and the patient having left him, the clavicle was reduced the next day by an empiric. Vidal (de Cassis) recommends that instead of pulling the arm outwards, by which procedure the pectoralis major is made to antagonize the surgeon, the elbow shall be brought down to the side, and kept there by the left hand, while the right hand, placed in the axilla, shall pull the upper end of the humerus outwards, converting the arm into a lever of the third kind. This process, I confess, seems to be much the most rational.

Finally, having given the history of these cases as they have been reported, we shall scarcely have performed our duty as a faithful writer if we do not state frankly that we entertain a suspicion that both the gentlemen who have reported these curious examples have entertained us with fabulous or imaginary stories; and especially do these suspicions rest upon the cases reported by Godemer, who in five

[1] Pinjou, Journ. de Méd. de Lyon, Juillet, 1842, from Vidal (de Cassis).

[2] Godemer, Recueil des travaux de la Soc. Méd d'Indre et Loire, 1843, from Vidal.

years saw five cases, each presenting throughout the same class of symptoms, the same facility of reduction, accomplished by the same means, and always with the same perfect result.

If to these singular coincidences we add the fact that only one other surgeon has ever claimed to have met with the accident, and if we notice the actual anatomical difficulties which stand in the way of its occurrence, such especially as the complete occlusion of the subcoracoidean space by the tendons and muscles which pass from its extremity toward the chest and arm, we shall find a fair apology for some degree of scepticism.

CHAPTER VI.

DISLOCATIONS OF THE SHOULDER (HUMERUS AT ITS UPPER EXTREMITY).

Owing to the great exposure, and the peculiar anatomical structure of the shoulder-joint, its structure having reference mainly to freedom of motion rather than to firmness and security in the articulation, dislocations of the humerus are very common.

Writers have not been agreed as to the precise anatomical relations of these dislocations, nor as to the nomenclature. Velpeau, Malgaigne, Vidal (de Cassis), Skey, and Sir Astley Cooper, have each adopted explanations and classifications peculiar to themselves. With the arrangement established by this latter surgeon, English and American students are the most familiar; and believing that it is more simple, and quite as appropriate as either of the others, I shall adopt it as the basis of my own descriptions.

I shall have occasion, however, to dissent from the opinions and teachings of this distinguished surgeon, as to the exact seat and relations of the head of the humerus in some of these dislocations.

According to Sir Astley Cooper, there are three complete luxations of the shoulder, namely, downwards, forwards, and backwards.

§ 1. Dislocation of the Shoulder Downwards. (*Subglenoid.*)

This is usually called a dislocation into the axilla; the head of the bone resting rather upon the inner side of the inferior border of the scapula, near the base of that triangular surface which is found below the glenoid fossa.

Since in both the other complete dislocations of the shoulder, the head of the humerus, in order to escape from its socket, must be made to descend more or less downwards, we shall regard this dislocation as the type of all the others, and shall make it the subject of especial consideration as well as of reference when speaking of the other forms of dislocation.

Causes.—The most frequent causes of this accident are a fall from a height, in which the patient strikes upon the top of the shoulder, or a direct blow upon the same point. I have found the arm dislocated into the axilla by one or the other of these causes eight times. Three times it has been dislocated by a blow upon the outside of the arm *near* its upper end; three times by a fall upon the extended hand; once by a fall upon the elbow, and in this latter case the arm was probably carried away from the body at the moment of the receipt of the injury.

In all the above examples, the shoulder has been dislocated by the simple force of the blow, or with only slight aid from muscular action; but in a considerable number of cases the bone is displaced almost wholly by the action of the muscles, the arm having been previously violently abducted; and perhaps in some cases the capsule being torn before the resistance of the overstrained muscles has accomplished the displacement. Thus, in two instances I have known the dislocation to result from holding on to the reins after being thrown from a carriage; in the same number of cases the patients have fallen through a hatchway and been caught and suspended under the arms; once a woman met with this accident by holding on to a pump handle when she had slipped and fallen upon the ice. A few years since I examined the arm of a Swiss woman, Maria Norregan, who was then sixty-five years old, and whose humerus had been dislocated into the axilla seventeen years before, where it still remained. Her own account of the accident was, that she was returning from the Jura Mountains, near Neufchatel, with a load of hay upon her head. She had carried it a long way with her hands held upwards, without once stopping to rest, and when at length she threw down the load at her door, the right shoulder was dislocated. The arm became soon very painful, and swollen to the fingers' ends; but she was too remote from, and too poor, to employ a surgeon. A tailor, who used to do the minor surgery of the neighborhood, bled her three or four times, but the dislocation was not recognized until many months after.

A Mrs. Hunn informed me that when she was twenty-two years old she had a convulsion, and that her attendants, in trying to hold her upon her bed, actually pulled the shoulder out of joint. After the first accident the dislocation was not repeated for four years, but since then it had occurred from very slight causes many times. She was in the habit of reducing it herself by placing a ball in the axilla and using the arm as a lever.

Dr. Lehman reports the case of a sailor on board an American brig, who was subject to a dislocation into the axilla from very slight causes, and especially if he bent his body far over to raise anything. He could also, by pulling horizontally, remove the head of the bone from its socket. It was reduced easily, and he experienced no pain either in the reduction or dislocation, nor indeed, during the displacement.[1]

[1] Lehman, Amer. Journ. Med. Sci., vol. i. p. 242, 1828.

Pathology.—In this accident the head of the bone is made to press against the capsule below and immediately in front of the long head of the triceps, until the capsule gives way, and continuing to descend in the same direction it is finally arrested by the triangular surface of the inferior edge of the scapula immediately below the glenoid fossa. Owing to the pressure of the tendon of the triceps behind, it occupies a position also a little in advance of the centre of this triangle, or rather upon its anterior edge, so that it rests more or less upon the belly of the subscapularis muscle.

Fig. 220.

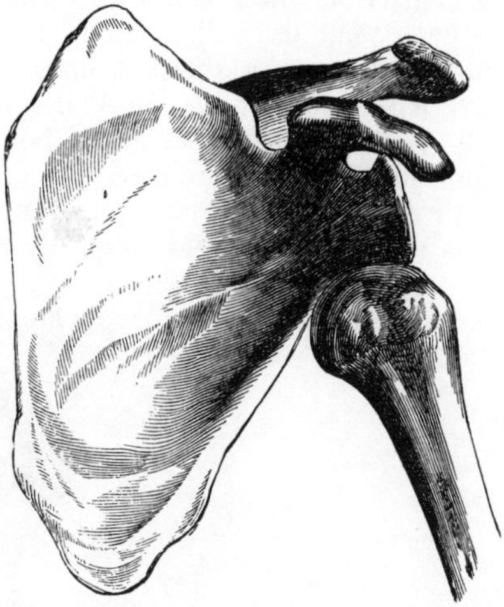

Dislocation of the shoulder downwards into the axilla. (Subglenoid.)

The capsule is generally torn quite extensively, especially below and in front; and, contrary to what has been affirmed by Sir Astley Cooper, the tendon of the long head of the biceps is often broken asunder or detached completely from its insertion; the supra-spinatus muscle is stretched or lacerated; the infra-spinatus, subscapularis and coraco-brachialis are put upon the stretch; the subscapularis being also sometimes completely torn from its attachment to the head of the humerus, and in either case, whether torn or merely compressed and stretched, the circumflex nerve, which runs along its lower margin, is subject to severe injury; the deltoid muscle is also placed in a condition of extreme tension; while the teres major and minor in this respect are subjected to but little change.

Symptoms.—A palpable depression immediately under the extremity of the acromion process, more distinct in children, in very old and in thin people, than in adults of middle life or than in fat or muscular people, but never absent completely, unless the shoulder is very much swollen; the elbow carried out from the body three or four inches, sometimes a little backwards, and the line of its axis directed toward the axilla; the outer surface of the arm presenting two planes inclined toward each other, and meeting at the point of insertion of the deltoid muscle; the head of the humerus felt in the axilla, particularly when the elbow is carried away from the body; numbness of the arm, accompanied generally with pain, especially when any attempt is made to press the elbow against the side; rigidity with inability to move the arm freely in any direction, but especially inwards; allowing, however, of pretty free passive motion, but not permitting the elbow to touch the body without great pain, which pain is occasioned mostly by the pressure of the humerus upon the axillary plexus; under no circumstances can the hand be placed upon the opposite shoulder while at the same moment the elbow touches the thorax; the head of the patient, and sometimes the whole body, inclined toward the injured arm; the arm lengthened from half an inch to an inch; a chafing or friction sound is not unfrequently present, especially if the bone has been some days dislocated; but Mr. Lawrence mentions a case in which there was a distinct crepitus, yet there was no fracture—Dr. Hays saw a similar case in Wills Hospital, Philadelphia, in a woman sixty years old, whose arm had been dislocated forwards eight weeks.[1] Other surgeons have related like examples, but it is probable that in all these cases there has been an exposure of the bone at or near the edge of the glenoid fossa, by the partial detachment of its liga-

Fig. 221.

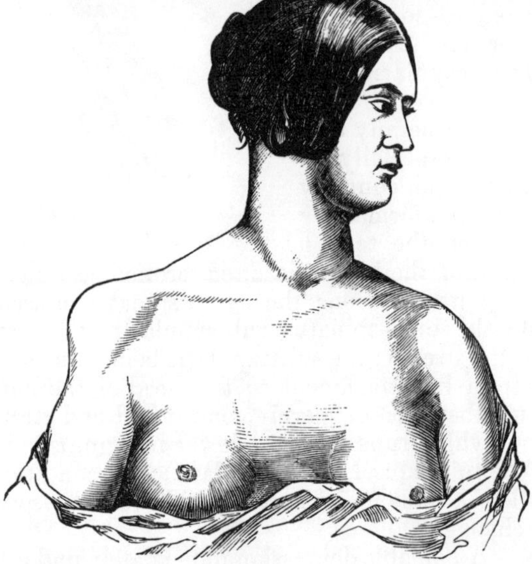

Dislocation of the shoulder downwards into the axilla. (Subglenoid).

mentous margin, or some portion of the head has become divested of its cartilaginous covering.

Decisive as these signs usually are of the true nature of the accident, cases will every now and then occur in which the diagnosis will be attended with great difficulty, and especially if a few hours have been permitted to elapse since the occurrence of the injury, so that considerable effusions of blood and of lymph may have taken place; while at a still later period, when the swelling has subsided, the diagnosis again becomes easy. "At this latter period," says Sir Astley Cooper, "it is that surgeons of the metropolis are usually consulted; and if we detect a dislocation which has been overlooked, it is our duty in candor to state to the patient that the difficulty of detecting the nature

[1] Lawrence, Hays, Amer. Journ. Med. Sci., vol. xxiv. p. 236, May, 1839.

of the accident is exceedingly diminished by the cessation of inflammation, and the absence of tumefaction."

It has never happened to me to have seen a case of dislocation into the axilla which was not easily recognized, nor have I met with any cases in the practice of other surgeons, but in my report to the New York State Medical Society, already referred to, I have related two cases which were not recognized by the patients themselves, and no surgeon was called until after several days or weeks, and three cases in which empirics having been employed they failed to detect the dislocation. Although, therefore, I am prepared to admit the justness of the observations made by Sir Astley Cooper, I think that if the case is seen within an hour or two after the accident, its nature may be generally determined promptly by the surgeon of ordinary experience; but upon this subject I have already spoken very fully in the chapter on fractures of the humerus; and from the examples and opinions which I have there presented it will be inferred that it is much more common to mistake a fracture for a dislocation, than a dislocation for a fracture, an observation which is equally as applicable to dislocations forwards as to the form of dislocation now under consideration.

Prognosis.—If the force which displaced the bone was not great, or if the shoulder-joint has not suffered any injury from the accident itself beyond the mere rupture of the capsule and a moderate straining of the muscles, and if the dislocation has been early and easily reduced, the patient is immediately after the reduction able to move the arm freely in all directions; very little swelling follows, and in a short time a perfect restoration of all the functions of the limb is accomplished.

It cannot, however, always be inferred from the degree of violence employed in the production of the dislocation, nor from the absence or presence of swelling, how much injury the tendons, muscles, and nerves have suffered, since the same causes produce greater lesions in one person than in another, and the amount of swelling may depend upon the accidental rupture of an unimportant bloodvessel, or upon some peculiarity in the constitution of the patient predisposing to serous, fibrous, or sanguineous effusions.

To whatever cause we may find occasion to attribute the result, it will nevertheless be observed that in a great majority of cases the limb is not restored to all its original strength and freedom of motion until after the lapse of some months; and the shoulder does not resume its perfect form and symmetry until a much later period: occasional pains, especially after exercise of the muscles, and in certain conditions of the weather, are present also at irregular intervals and for indefinite periods of time. Opposite and more favorable terminations must be regarded as exceptions to the rule.

Where the reduction has been made within a few hours, I have found the shoulder affected with muscular anchylosis with more or less weakness of the arm after a lapse of from a few days to one and two years.

A laborer, æt. 41, had dislocated his right shoulder into the axilla. Dr. H., an intelligent young surgeon, reduced the bone easily with his hands alone, while the patient was still unconscious from the shock of the injury. After six weeks he called upon me accompanied by his surgeon, thinking that it was not properly reduced because the arm was still painful, and he could not move it freely. The bone was, however, well in its socket. One year later I examined this man and found some anchylosis remaining in the shoulder-joint.

James Rogers, æt. 39, fell while running and struck upon his right shoulder. Dr. Eastman, Prof. of Anatomy in the Buffalo Medical College, reduced the dislocation four hours after the occurrence, in the following manner: The patient being seated in a chair, Dr. Eastman placed his knee in the axilla and manipulated, while one assistant supported the acromion process, and another pulled downwards upon the forearm. The time occupied in the reduction was about two minutes, and the bone finally resumed its position with a snap audible to all the persons in the room. For some months after, and at the period when I was invited to see him, the muscles about the shoulder were rigid, and the motions of the joint embarrassed; but at the end of two years, Dr. Eastman informed me that the joint had become free, and the arm as useful as before, except that he could not throw a stone.

In another case, a gentleman residing in an adjoining county, æt. 42, was thrown from his carriage, falling forwards upon his hands. The dislocation was reduced promptly by placing the heel in the axilla, and within fifteen minutes after it had occurred. Three months after this the patient consulted me on account of the immobility of the shoulder-joint, and because several surgeons had expressed a doubt whether it was properly reduced. The anchylosis was then so complete that the humerus could not be moved separately from the scapula, but there was no displacement. This gentleman again called upon me at the end of four years, and I then found the arm nearly restored to its original condition, but it was not quite so strong as before. He experienced also "curious" sensations in his arm and hand occasionally. The anchylosis had continued with very little improvement about two years, after which it had been gradually disappearing.

I need scarcely say that in those examples in which the reduction of the bone has been delayed beyond a few hours, or for several days or weeks, the continuance of the anchylosis has been more persistent; but in no case which has come under my observation, unless the bone still remained unreduced, has the anchylosis been permanent. For this reason I am disposed to think that muscular, rather than fibrous or ligamentous anchylosis, is the cause, generally, of the immobility of the joint. I have certainly never in any instance met with a true bony anchylosis as a consequence of a shoulder dislocation. The anchylosis in question seems to be a result simply of laceration, or more generally of a severe strain of the muscular fibres, resulting in inflammation and a contraction of these fibres; and its occurrence in any particular case may therefore be justly attributable either to the position of the bone when it is dislocated, to the force of the blow which has produced the dislocation, or to the violence applied in the attempts at reduction.

Paralysis and wasting of the muscles of the arm, either with or without muscular contraction and rigidity, are also observed in a certain number of cases. Especially has it been noticed that the deltoid muscle is liable to atrophy; and in their attempts to explain the frequency of its occurrence in this latter muscle, surgeons have generally referred to a probable rupture of the circumflex nerve, a circumstance which the autopsies show does occasionally take place; or to a mere stretching of this nerve; yet it is quite as fair to presume that in many cases it is due solely to the greater injury which the deltoid muscle has sustained by the unnatural position of the head of the bone during the continuance of the dislocation, for, with the exception of the supra-spinatus, it is placed more upon the stretch than any other. Nor is it improbable that in some cases it is due to the mere force of the blow which, having been received directly upon the top of the shoulder, has contused the muscle. In short, any of the causes which may determine in the deltoid inflammation and consequent rigidity, must finally result in desuetude and consequent atrophy.

In quite a number of cases my attention has been called to a remarkable fulness just in front of the head of the bone, which has continued sometimes for many months and even years after the reduction has been effected, the patients having in several cases applied to me to know whether this did not indicate that the bone was not in its socket, especially as it has been usually attended with some stiffness in the joint. Not unfrequently I have been told that surgeons who had noticed this fulness, thought the bone was not reduced; and in one instance I am informed that a jury returned a verdict against the surgeon, where there was no other evidence of malpractice than this fulness with some anchylosis, but which, in the opinion of these gentlemen, was conclusive evidence that the bone was not properly set. The deception is also often the more complete from the fact that there may exist a corresponding depression underneath the acromion process, behind.

It may be present where but little force has been used, either in the production of the dislocation, or in its reduction. I have seen it in a girl, only fourteen years of age, who had dislocated her left shoulder into the axilla, by a fall upon a slippery side-walk. I reduced the bone, assisted by Dr. George Burwell, of this city, within half an hour after the accident. Dr. Burwell held upon the acromion process while I lifted the arm to a right angle with the body, and pulled gently, and the reduction was at once accomplished; but we immediately noticed that the head of the bone seemed to press forwards in the socket so as to resemble what Sir Astley Cooper has described as a partial forward luxation. There was also a corresponding depression behind. Carrying the elbow back rendered the projection more decided, but bringing it forwards would not make it entirely disappear.

In other instances much more difficulty has been experienced and more force has been employed in the reduction. A man weighing two hundred pounds, and forty-one years of age, residing at Bath, in Steuben Co., fell from a load of hay in May, 1853, striking upon the top and front of the left shoulder. It was immediately ascertained that he had dislocated his arm into the axilla, and broken his leg. A young surgeon attempted within a few minutes to reduce the dislocation, but failed; and about two hours later it was reduced by another surgeon, with the aid of chloroform and Jarvis's adjuster. Four years after the accident had occurred, this gentleman came to me accompanied by the surgeon who had made the reduction, in consequence of its having been intimated by some medical men that it was not properly reduced. The arm was not as strong as the other; some anchylosis existed at the shoulder-joint; but especially it was noticed that there still remained a remarkable fulness in front as if the head of the bone was pressed forwards. By no manipulation or position could this fulness be made to disappear, yet the bone was plainly enough in its socket.

This phenomenon is probably due in some cases to a rupture of the supra-spinatus muscle, and the consequent preponderating action of the antagonizing muscles, or to the laceration of the capsule, but most often, I imagine, to a rupture or to a displacement of the long head of the biceps, a circumstance to which I shall more particularly allude under the subject of "partial dislocations."

Among the results of this dislocation must be placed a tendency to reluxation, which, although it may not often be made manifest by its actual occurrence, owing perhaps to the prudence of the surgeon, yet it does take place in a sufficient number of cases to establish its peculiar liability. Indeed, we need only consider how imperfect is the protection against this accident, when once the capsule has been torn, to appreciate this observation. Examples of spontaneous luxation, or of luxation of the shoulder from very trivial causes, after it has once been luxated, may be found in the experience of almost every surgeon. I have myself met with several persons who have had a second or third luxation from a slight cause, and in some instances, where the patients were subject to epilepsy, the luxations have occurred whenever the convulsions returned.

A gentleman residing in Toronto, Canada West, had a dislocation of the right shoulder into the axilla when he was quite a child, and the accident was renewed when twenty-nine years old by falling from a carriage head foremost, with his right arm extended and uplifted. Since then until he called upon me, a period of about six years, he has been constantly subject to the same dislocation; and he cannot raise his arm high above his shoulders without producing a sub-luxation, the head of the humerus resting upon the outer margin of the lower and anterior edge of the glenoid fossa, but by rotating the arm outwards it immediately resumes its place. I found the whole limb as fully developed, and he said it was quite as strong as the opposite limb.

I have already mentioned the case of Mrs. Hunn, whose arm had been dislocated more than twenty times in the last five years; and I remember a lad, Pat. Dolan, aged nineteen years, whose left arm was dislocated by falling from the mast-head of a vessel and hanging by his hand. No attempt was made to reduce it until fourteen hours after the accident, at which time it was set by two German doctors, but not until they had pulled upon it three hours. Four months after it was again dislocated by the slipping of an oar while he was rowing a boat. A surgeon having failed this time to bring it into place, I succeeded readily and without the aid of an anæsthetic, by pulling the arm directly upwards in the line of the body, while my foot was pressed upon the top of the scapula.

We have referred more than once to the occasional difficulty of diagnosis in this as well as in many other shoulder accidents; and I have alluded to five cases in which the dislocation was not recognized, but none of them had been seen by a surgeon. Other writers have, however, mentioned many examples of unreduced dislocations of the shoulder, for which surgeons of skill and experience were responsible. In other cases the dislocation has been clearly made out, but the surgeon has been unable to reduce the bone. It has been my fortune to succeed in several instances where others have made a fair trial and have failed, but the following case leaves me no opportunity to boast the superiority of my own skill above that of my *confrères*.

Mary Kanally, æt. 49, a large, fat, laboring woman, was admitted into the Buffalo Hospital of the Sisters of Charity, with a dislocation of the right humerus into the axilla, which had occurred twelve hours before. This is the same woman of whom I have before spoken as having produced the dislocation by a fall while holding upon the handle of a pump.

Drs. Lockwood and Baker, of this city, were first called, and attempted reduction. They made extension and counter-extension in every possible direction, and for a long time, but to no purpose. She was then sent to the hospital. Without attempting to describe minutely the various modes of extension and manipulation which I employed, I will briefly state that having placed her completely under the influence of chloroform, the manipulations were made assiduously during one hour without success. On the following morning she was bled freely from the opposite arm, and chloroform again administered; extension being made in the presence of Prof. Charles A. Lee and other gentlemen, with Jarvis's adjuster. After more than an hour the effort was again suspended. On the following day we made a third attempt; the patient being completely under the influence of chloroform, but with no better success. The chloroform produced a condition approaching apoplexy, and it was not again used. On the tenth day, assisted by Prof. James P. White and other surgeons, we applied the compound pulleys, moving the arm in various directions. Twice we thought the reduction was accomplished, but as often as we proceeded to examine it attentively we found it was not. If it did ever actually pass into the socket, it was immediately displaced.

The woman after this refused to submit to any further attempts, and she soon left the hospital, nor have I seen or heard from her since.

Sir Astley Cooper has thus described the appearances presented on dissection of a dislocation which had been long unreduced: "The head of the bone altered in its form; the surface toward the scapula being flattened. A complete capsular ligament surrounding the head of the os humeri. The glenoid cavity entirely filled by ligamentous matter, in which were suspended small portions of bone, which were of new formation, as no portion of the scapula or humerus was broken. A new cavity formed for the head of the os humeri on the inferior costa of the scapula (Fig. 222); but this was shallow, like that from which the bone had escaped."

Fig. 222.

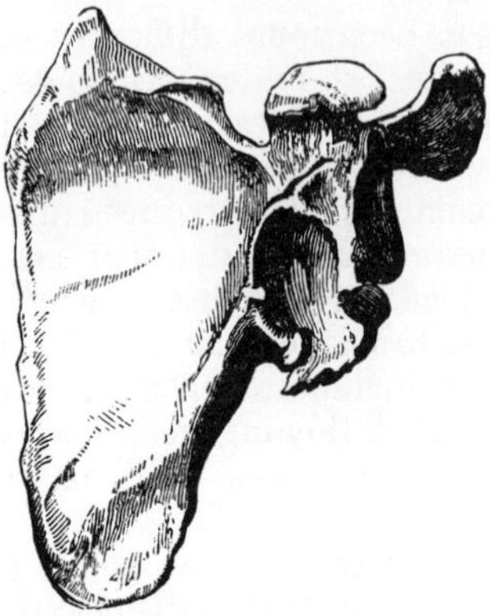

New socket, in an ancient luxation of the shoulder downwards. (From Sir A. Cooper.)

When the dislocation into the axilla remains unreduced, the consequences are always sufficiently grave, but they differ very much in degree, in character, and in persistence, according as the arm has remained a longer or shorter time unreduced, and according to the presence or absence of complications. These conditions will be best illustrated by a reference to examples.

Wm. S., a German, æt. 51, fell down a flight of steps while intoxicated, producing a dislocation of the left arm into the axilla. Eleven hours after the accident, he was received into the Buffalo Hospital of the Sisters of Charity. No attempt had been made to reduce the bone. The reduction was effected by myself with tolerable ease, by extending the arm perpendicularly above the head, while my foot pressed upon the top of the scapula. The head of the humerus could be plainly felt in the axilla approaching the socket, until it seemed to be directly over it, when, on lowering the arm, it was found to be reduced. After the reduction, the patient could not raise the arm more than eight inches from the body. The fingers, hand, and forearm were almost paralyzed. Three weeks later, when he left the hospital, his arm had improved, but he could not flex his fingers.

Mrs. G., æt. 70, fell down a flight of steps and dislocated her arm into the axilla. She did not suspect the nature of the injury, and no surgeon was called. I was consulted one week after the accident, at which time she was suffering great pain from the pressure of the head of the bone upon the axillary nerves. We first attempted to reduce the bone by resting the knee in the axilla while she was sitting, but without success. We then placed her in bed, and with my knee in the axilla, the acromion process being supported by the hands of an assistant, we restored the bone after a few moments, of pretty firm extension downwards and outwards. After the reduction she could not raise her arm, but the pain was much abated. One month later, the arm remained very weak. She could not raise it more than six inches toward her head, but I could raise it to a right angle with the body without causing pain. The whole hand felt numb, and was occasionally painful. The deltoid muscle was slightly atrophied. There was also a slight flatness under the acromion process behind, and on the outer side, with a corresponding fulness in front.

Mary Ann Hasler, æt. 47, was admitted to the hospital with a dislocation of the right humerus into the axilla. The arm had been dislocated three weeks in consequence of a fall upon the upper and outer part of the shoulder. An empiric, who saw it fifteen minutes after the fall, and when the arm was not swollen, said it was not dislocated. On the fifth day, a Catholic clergyman discovered that it was out, and attempted to reduce it, but was not successful. When she came under my notice, the arm was lengthened about one-quarter or one-half of an inch, and hung out from the body in a condition of almost complete paralysis. There was very little swelling about the shoulder or arm, and the head of the bone could be distinctly felt in the axilla. The patient being rendered partially insensible by chloroform, I placed my heel in the axilla, and by pulling moderately about thirty seconds in a direction slightly outwards from the line of the body, the bone was reduced. Seven days after the reduction, she left the hospital, the arm being yet quite useless, though not greatly swollen. There was also a striking fulness in front of the head of the bone.

Wm. Gardener, of Painted Post, N. Y., æt. 75, dislocated the right humerus into the axilla twenty years before I saw him by falling upon his hands with his arms extended. I found the arm weak and atrophied, so that he could raise it but slightly outwards from his side; he was unable to move it forwards much beyond the line of his body, but he could carry it back quite freely. The whole hand was in a condition of partial insensibility.

I have before mentioned the case of Maria Norrigan, the Swiss woman, whose arm had been dislocated downwards seventeen years. The deltoid muscle has become greatly wasted; the head of the bone can be felt obscurely in the axilla; the arm is shortened perceptibly; the elbow hangs freely against the side; the little and ring fingers are numb, and also one-half of the forearm; the whole hand and arm are weak and atrophied; she complains also occasionally of a troublesome sensation of formication over the arm and hand; she cannot straighten her fingers perfectly; the elbow may be raised from the side to a right angle with the body, but she cannot raise it herself more than one foot; she carries it back a little more freely than forwards.

In compound dislocations, the prognosis must always be regarded as exceedingly grave. In the only example which has come under my notice, the circumstances attending which I shall hereafter mention in the general chapter devoted to compound dislocations, the patient died from sloughing of the axillary artery. Mr. Scott has, however, reported a case, in a boy fourteen years of age, who recovered rapidly after the reduction was effected, and in thirteen months his arm was nearly as useful as before.[1]

Treatment.—The principles of treatment in this dislocation are very simple and easy to be comprehended. I speak now of recent uncomplicated cases of dislocation into the axilla; and, notwithstanding the various and sometimes almost contradictory views which surgeons have entertained as to the best and most rational modes of

[1] Scott, Amer. Journ. of Med. Sci., vol. xx. p. 515, Aug. 1837, from the London Lancet for March 4, 1837.

procedure, I continue to affirm that the laws which are to govern the reduction in a great majority of cases are established and indisputable.

Observe now the obvious anatomical facts, and then consider the inevitable inferences.

The capsule is torn, generally extensively, along the inner and lower margins of the socket. The head of the bone is lodged below and slightly in advance of its natural position, in consequence of which the points of origin and insertion of the deltoid muscle and the supra-spinatus are separated somewhat and their fibres rendered tense, insomuch that the arm is abducted and actually lengthened.

At first, and in the most simple cases, these are the only muscles which are in a state of extreme tension, but after the lapse of a few hours, or of a few days, nearly all the other muscles about the joint, most of which were originally only in a condition of moderate extension, and some of which were rather relaxed than extended, sympathize with those which are suffering the most, and a general contraction and rigidity ensue, increased also at the last by the supervention of inflammation and its consequences.

What, from these simple premises, must be the obvious practical deductions?

That in the simplest forms of the dislocation the most rational mode of reduction will be to elevate the arm sufficiently to relax the overstrained deltoid and supra-spinatus muscles, which bind the head of the bone in its new position, and to pull gently in the same direction, in order to overcome the moderate resistance offered by several other muscles, but whose tension cannot be relieved by the same manœuvre.

Failing in this, that we shall increase the relaxation of the first named muscles by pulling at a right angle with the body, or even directly upwards; and in the meanwhile, as we carry the arm more and more upwards we shall operate more powerfully against the resistance of the other muscles.

If in all these modifications of the same procedure, we keep the arm a little back of the axis of the body, we shall accomplish the indications the most perfectly.

Such are the conclusions which must be drawn from the anatomical, or, as Mr. Pott would call it, the "physiological" argument; and which assumes as its basis that the muscles constitute the sole or the main obstacle to the return of the bone to its socket. If any surgeon maintains that the premise is unsound, and that the restoration of the head of the bone is opposed by the untorn fibres of the capsule or by any other important circumstance than the action of the muscles (we speak of ordinary cases), we shall content ourselves by referring him again to the extensive laceration which this capsule generally suffers, and to the constrained and almost uniform position of the arm, as a sufficient reply to his objection.

It must not be forgotten that in all these modes of extension, for with all of them some slight degree of extension is found necessary, there must be afforded some point of resistance beyond the bone; and this it is really which has constituted one of the greatest impediments to reduction. It is not that the muscles are in such an extraordinary state of extension or rigidity that they must be operated against with great force; it is not that the margin of the glenoid fossa is an elevated barrier, like the margin of the acetabulum, over which the bone must be lifted before it can fall into its socket; but the explanation of the difficulty so often experienced in producing effective extension and counter-extension is to be sought for mainly in the fact that the scapula, upon which the humerus rests, is movable, being held to the body by little else than muscles, which, in fact, bind the scapula much less firmly to the body than the muscles of the shoulder now bind the scapula to the arm; while at the same time the scapula itself presents very few points against which a counter-extending force can be properly and efficiently applied.

Occasionally it will be only necessary to elevate the arm to an acute angle, or to a right angle with the body, when, the resistance of the deltoid and supra-spinatus being overcome, the bone will at once resume its place. In several instances which have come under my notice nothing more has been necessary; and where it can be done, the least possible pain and injury are inflicted. It is the method, therefore, which in all recent cases I have first tried and would wish to recommend. By it I have more than once succeeded when other and more violent efforts had failed.

At other times it will be necessary to add to this simple manipulation only a moderate degree of extension, such as the hands of the surgeon can make, without the application of direct counter-extension except what is effected by the weight and resistance of the body.

If, however, the bone refuses to move, we shall then be obliged to consider upon what point and by what means we can best apply a counter-extending force. Ample experience has taught me that the extremity of the acromion process is the only available point when we are making the extension in a line below a right angle, or in a line downwards more or less approaching the axis of the body. It has been supposed that the counter-extension could be made in the axilla against the inferior margin of the scapula; but several obstacles are presented to the successful application of force at this point. The axillary space is narrow and deep, so that even with the ingenious contrivance of placing first a ball of yarn in the axilla, and upon this the heel of the operator, it will be found exceedingly difficult to enter the axilla without at the same time pressing with considerable force against its muscular margins; but to press upon the pectoralis major and latissimus dorsi is to neutralize our own efforts. If, however, the heel or the ball does press fairly into the axilla, it will not find the scapula readily, but it must impinge first upon the head of the humerus, which is always a little to the inner side of the scapula. If it ever is made to reach actually the inferior border of the scapula, and I do not think it is, the effect must be still only to tilt the scapula upon itself by throwing back its lower angle, and not to separate the glenoid cavity or its upper and anterior margin from the head of the humerus.

Whatever success, therefore, may have attended this mode of practice, either in my own hands or in the hands of other surgeons, must be ascribed, not to the counter-extension thus effected, but simply to the operation of the heel as a wedge, which, by insinuating itself between the body and the head of the bone, has thrust it outwards and upwards into its socket; or to its having acted as a fulcrum upon which the humerus has operated as a lever.

It is to the extremity of the acromion process, then, that we must apply our counter-extension when we are employing this mode of extension. The fingers or hands of a faithful assistant may answer the purpose, or, having removed his boot, the operator may often press successfully with the ball of his foot, and the more he carries the arm outwards the more secure will be his seat upon the process; or we may adopt some of the contrivances for securing the process which have been suggested by other surgeons; such as a band crossing the shoulder, and made fast to a counter-band, which passes through the armpit and against the side of the body. Dr. Physick, of Philadelphia, reduced a dislocation in this way as early as the year 1790, in the case of a patient admitted to St. George's Hospital, in London, while he was a student of medicine, and he subsequently taught the same in his lectures. Physick directed that an assistant should press firmly against the process with the palm of his hand. Dorsey and Hays approve of the same method,[1] and perhaps a majority of American surgeons regard it favorably.

If we pull directly outwards, at a right angle with the body, we may still continue to press upon the acromion process with the foot; or we may perhaps trust to the method of making counter-extension first suggested by Nathan Smith, of New Haven.

Dr. Smith exclaims: "What surgeon of experience has not encountered the difficulty which almost always occurs in fixing the scapula?" and then proceeds to explain how difficult it has been found to hold securely even upon the acromion process by either the fingers of an assistant or the split band, and concludes by stating what seems to him the most effectual mode of rendering the scapula immobile, namely, to make the counter-extension from the opposite wrist. By this method the trapezii are provoked to contraction, and the scapula of the injured side is drawn firmly toward the spine and the opposite scapula. In illustration of the value of this procedure he relates the case of a gentleman who had suffered a dislocation of his left shoulder, and upon whom an unsuccessful attempt at reduction had already been made by a respectable surgeon. Dr. Smith being called, proceeded as follows: Two gentlemen made counter-extension from the opposite wrist, while Dr. Smith and Dr. Knapp made extension from the wrist of the injured side, at first pulling it downwards, but gradually raising it to the horizontal direction, and then gently depressing the wrist. On the effort being steadily continued for two or three minutes, the bone was observed to slip easily into its place. This gentleman subsequently informed Dr. Smith that this procedure gave him much less pain than that adopted by the first surgeon.[2]

[1] Physick, Amer. Journ. Med. Sci., vol. xix. p. 386, Feb. 1837. Dorsey's Elements of Surgery, vol. i. p 214. Philadelphia, 1813.

[2] Nathan Smith, Med. and Surg. Memoirs, 1831, p. 337.

But no position places the scapula so completely under our control as that in which the arm is carried directly upwards and the foot is placed upon the top of the scapula. By this method we may succeed generally when every other expedient has failed, yet it is painful, and I cannot but think that it increases the laceration of the capsule, and does sometimes serious injury to the muscles about the joint. La Mothe was the first to recommend this method,[1] but as early as the year 1764, Charles White, of Manchester, made fast a set of pulleys in the ceiling, and, placing a band around the wrist of the dislocated arm, he drew the patient up until the whole body was suspended. No pressure, however, was made upon the scapula from above, which is no doubt the most essential part of the process.[2] By La Mothe's plan, Jobert succeeded after twenty-three days when all the usual methods had failed.[3] Sometimes this procedure is modified by placing the hand of the operator against the top of the scapula, as is shown in the accompanying drawing.

Fig. 223.

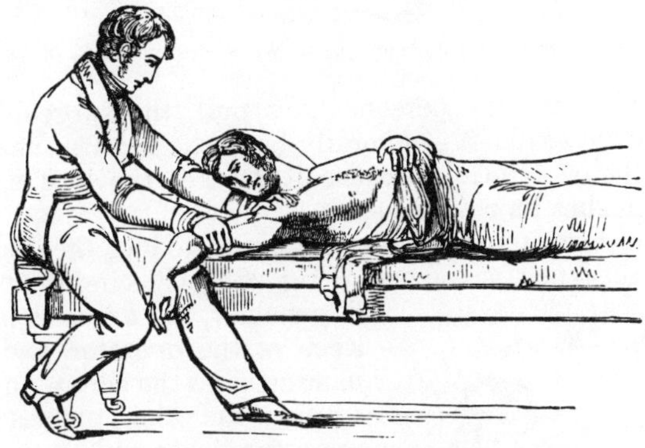

La Mothe's method, modified.

A gentle movement backwards or forwards, a slight rotation of the limb, or suddenly dropping the arm toward the body, diverting the attention of the patient, are little tricks of the operator, which now and then prove successful.

Sir Astley Cooper thus describes his method of applying the heel to the axilla (Fig. 224):—

"The patient should be placed in the recumbent posture upon a table or sofa, near to the edge of which he is to be brought; the surgeon then binds a wetted roller round the arm immediately above the elbow, upon which he ties a handkerchief; then he separates the patient's elbow from his side, and, with one foot resting upon the floor, he places the heel of his other foot in the axilla, receiving the head of the os humeri upon it, whilst he is himself in the sitting posture by the patient's side. He then draws the arm by means of the handkerchief, steadily, for three or four minutes, when, under

[1] La Mothe, Am. Journ. Med. Sci., vol. xix. p. 387, Nov. 1836, from Mélanges de Méd. et Chir., Paris, 1812.

[2] C. White, Ibid., from Med. Obs. and Inquiries, vol. ii. p. 273, London, 1764.

[3] Ibid., vol. xxiii. p. 237, Nov. 1838.

common circumstances, the head of the bone is easily replaced; but if more force be required, the handkerchief may be changed for a long

Fig. 224.

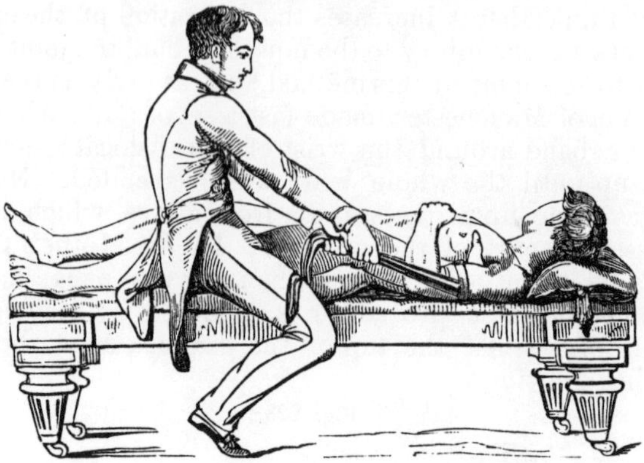

Sir Astley Cooper's method of applying extension with the heel in the axilla.

towel, by which several persons may pull, the surgeon's heel still remaining in the axilla. I generally bend the forearm nearly at right angles with the os humeri, because it relaxes the biceps, and consequently diminishes its resistance."

He was also accustomed in some cases to reduce the dislocation by substituting the knee for the heel. (Fig. 225.) Placing the patient upon a low chair, the axilla is laid over the knee of the operator, and while one hand steadies the acromion process and scapula, the other presses downwards upon the lower end of the humerus.

Fig. 225.

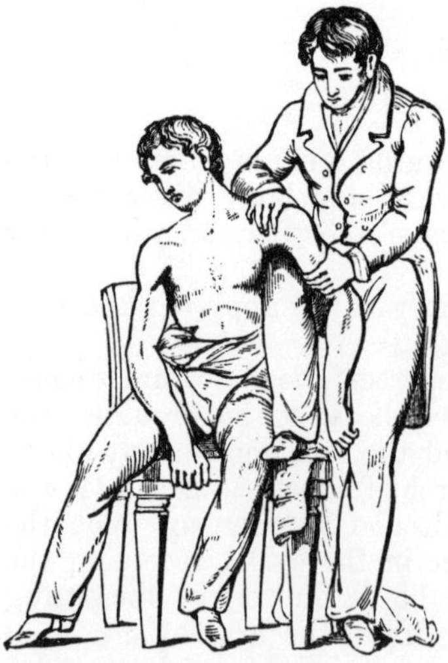

Sir Astley Cooper's method of operating with the knee in the axilla.

If some hours or days have elapsed since the occurrence of the dislocation, it will be necessary to resort to chloroform or ether for the purpose of paralyzing the muscles, as well as with the view of preventing pain, and it may be necessary, in addition, to resort to pulleys, or to some similar permanent mode of extension. The same measures also sometimes become necessary in very recent cases, especially in muscular subjects.

In employing the pulleys we generally operate not exactly in a line with the axis of the body, nor above a right angle, but between an angle of 45° and a right angle.

Mr. Skey has suggested a plan by which we may combine the principle of the heel in the axilla with the pulleys, but which plan would, in my judgment, be very much improved by a counter-extending force applied to the acromion process. I ought to say, however, that Mr. Skey prefers that the scapula should not be fixed, believing that the reduction is much more easily effected when the glenoid cavity is drawn downwards in the act of making the extension.

With all respect for the opinion of this distinguished surgeon, we cannot precisely agree with him, and while we would be disposed to recommend in some cases a trial of his method of applying the pulleys, we would at the same time, or certainly in the event of its failure, add the acromial support, and especially would we advise that the arm should be more abducted. The following is Mr. Skey's method, as described by himself:—

"There is no reason why, in very muscular subjects, or in old dislocations, the same principle may not be applied conjointly with the use of pulleys. For the purpose of retaining this admirable, because most efficient principle, I employ a well-padded iron knob, which may represent the heel, from which there extend laterally

Fig. 226.

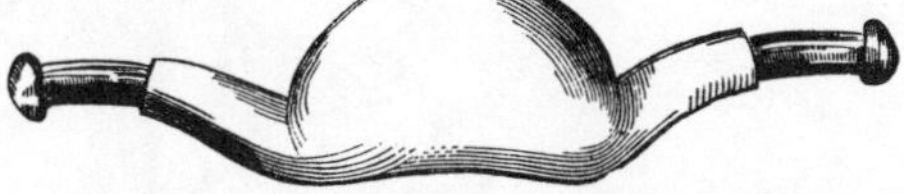

Iron knob employed by Skey, instead of the heel.

two strong straight branches of the same metal, each ending in a bulb or ring of about four inches in length, the office of which is designed to keep the margins of the axilla as free from pressure as possible." The iron knob is to be pressed well up into the axilla and attached to cords fastened to a staple; the patient lying upon his back or inclined a little to the opposite side. The arm is then to be drawn downwards by the pulleys, "as nearly as possible, parallel to, and in contact with the body."[1]

Fig. 227.

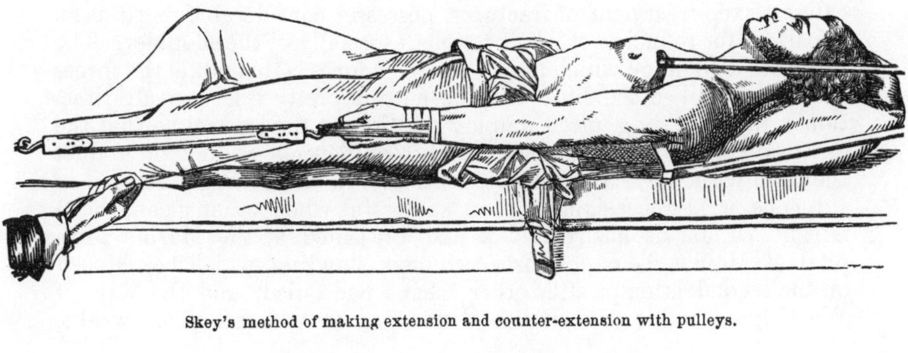

Skey's method of making extension and counter-extension with pulleys.

[1] Skey, Operative Surgery, Amer. ed., p. 93.

In this way Mr. Skey says that he has succeeded in reducing a great many dislocations, whether occurring in very muscular men, or after some days', or weeks', or even months' duration; and he thinks the plan especially applicable to cases which require long and persistent extension.

Mr. Skey and many other surgeons prefer to make the extension from the hand. I have succeeded as well, and it has seemed to be less painful to my patients, when I have followed the practice of Sir Astley, and made the extension from the arm. Sir Astley always made the extension more or less out from the line of the body, and generally almost at a right angle when using the pulleys, the scapula being made fast by "a girt buckled on the top of the acromion," or by a split cloth, as in the accompanying drawing.

Fig. 228.

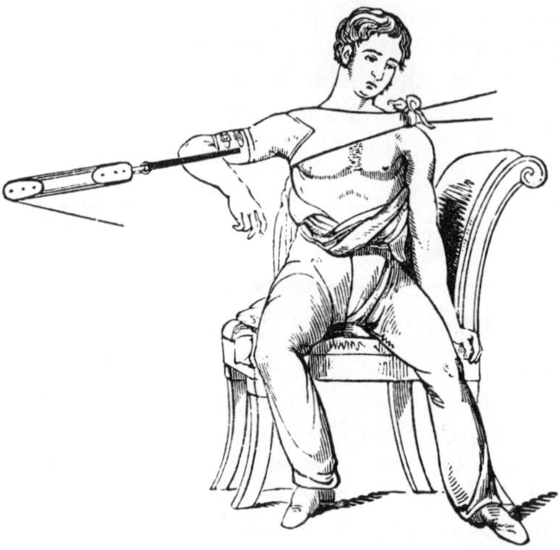

Sir Astley Cooper's mode of making extension with the pulleys.

The instrument invented by Dr. Jarvis, of Portland, Conn., called the adjuster, useless and even mischievous as we have found it in its application to the treatment of fractures, possesses considerable merit as an apparatus for reducing old dislocations, especially of the shoulder. The principal advantage which may be claimed for it is that while the forces are being applied the limb may be moved pretty freely in all directions; thus enabling us to employ rotation at the same time that the extension is made. We may also lift or depress, adduct or abduct the limb without relaxing the extension. In the hands of American surgeons, it has occasionally been successful when other means have failed. Dr. Jarvis has related a case presented at the Marine Hospital, at Mobile, Tenn., of forty-two days' standing, which he reduced on the second attempt after other means had failed,[1] and Dr. May, of Washington, reduced a similar dislocation at the end of six weeks,

[1] Boston Med. and Surg. Journ., vol. xxxix. p. 215.

by the same apparatus, without, however, having previously resorted to any other means.[1]

I have myself used the apparatus occasionally, both in my hospital and private practice, and can speak favorably of its operation.

Ancient Luxations.—Finally, I ought to speak somewhat more in detail of the manner of procedure, and of the principles involved in the reduction of old dislocations, or of dislocations requiring the interposition of mechanical appliances; especially with a view to the more complete exposition of my own practice in these cases.

If the dislocation is recent, but reduction is found impossible without the aid of mechanical apparatus, the difficulty will be understood to consist mainly, if not altogether, in the resistance offered by the muscles. If, in a few exceptional cases, the capsule, or an untorn tendon, or the margin of the glenoid fossa, present themselves as obstacles, they must still be considered as unusual and extraordinary impediments, the existence of which may be regarded rather as possible than probable.

Almost our sole purpose then, it will be understood, in all recent cases requiring mechanical appliances, and in some ancient cases, is to overcome the contraction of the muscles.

We prefer always to place the patient upon a mattress laid upon the floor; two silk handkerchiefs, or two pieces of a cotton roller, are then laid along the radial and ulnar sides of the humerus, and over the middle of these, immediately above the condyles, a wetted roller is applied, its end being made fast with a needle and thread rather than with a pin. The upper ends of the longitudinal strips, or of the handkerchiefs, are now turned down and tied to the opposite ends, thus converting them both into lateral loops. For the purpose of making counter-extension, a sheet is passed around the body under the axilla, and made fast to a staple; while an intelligent assistant is to manage the scapula with his naked hands, either by pulling with his fingers placed under the process, or by pushing with the palm of his hand and ball of his thumb. The pulleys, secured to a staple exactly opposite to that which holds the counter-extending band, are made ready, but not for the present attached to the arm.

As soon as the patient is placed completely under the influence of an anæsthetic, the operator is ready to proceed with the reduction. It is my maxim never to attempt to accomplish by complicated and violent measures, what may be done as well by more simple and gentle means. I think it proper, therefore, to make several attempts at reduction by manipulation alone, aided now by the anæsthetic, the extending and counter-extending bands, &c., before resorting to the pulleys. Seating himself upon the mattress, with his boots drawn, the surgeon should bend the forearm to a right angle with the arm, and planting one heel in the axilla, with one hand he should seize upon the loops at the elbow, and with the other steady the hand and forearm of the patient, while he proceeds to make firm traction for a few seconds in the line of the body, or only a little out from this

[1] Boston Med. and Surg. Journ., vol. xxxv. p. 454.

line. Failing in this, he may direct the assistant to seize upon the scapula, and make counter-extension; still not succeeding, he may change his foot from the axilla to the acromion process and pull directly outwards at a right angle with the body, or he may swing himself gradually around until he comes to be above the head of the patient, and the foot presses firmly upon the top of the scapula; now descending again in the same direction, he will very probably find the limb reduced, or capable of being reduced easily, by operating upon it as a lever by laying it across the body while at the same moment it is rotated slightly outwards.

If still the reduction is not accomplished, the pulleys must at once be put in requisition. The sheet passed around the chest and fastened to a staple, is only a means of supporting the body and rendering it more steady; as a means of counter-extension its value is inconsiderable. To make fast the scapula we must still rely mainly upon the naked hands of strong men or upon a strap drawn firmly across the process and held in place by an assistant.

It must be constantly borne in mind that we intend to conquer the muscles by fatiguing them, and that this cannot be done by a force suddenly applied, however great it may be, but only by gentle, steady, and long-continued extension. The muscles when attacked openly and vigorously, resist, and will suffer laceration rather than yield, while on the other hand, an insidious but persevering approach seldom fails to end in their defeat. The forearm is again flexed, and the arm carried out to a right angle with the body, the pulleys secured to the loops, and the assistant takes hold upon the process, while the surgeon draws gently upon the rope attached to the pulleys; as soon as everything is moderately tense, he is to desist for a few moments. Again the rope is drawn upon gently, and again the progress of the extension is suspended. In this way the operator is to proceed during half an hour, or two hours, as the nature of the case may demand; occasionally rotating the humerus, and occasionally lifting its head toward the socket. Meanwhile, it is understood that the principal counter-extension is made by the assistants, who must relieve each other at the acromion process. The sheet in the axilla, or rather against the side of the chest, has some value in this respect when the arm is at a right angle with the body, but in itself it cannot control the scapula, only as it holds the body to which the scapula is attached. Much, therefore, as we may regret the inconvenience of making counter-extension by hands alone, experience and anatomy alike must teach that here it is the only mode. If these dislocations are reduced often by other methods, as no doubt they are, then it is only an evidence that in these examples little or no counter-extension was necessary.

Sometimes the dislocation is not reduced when the extension is given up, but if then a resort is promptly made to some one of the simple methods already described, while the muscles are still exhausted, it very often happens that the reduction is easily accomplished.

It will be prudent in all cases in order to prevent a reluxation, whether the dislocation is recent or ancient, as soon as its reduction is effected, to place the arm in a sling and secure the elbow to the side by a few turns of a roller. I do not think the axillary pad necessary, and I am afraid it has sometimes done as much mischief as the dislocation itself.

The following examples will illustrate the variety of expedients to which we are obliged sometimes to resort before our efforts prove successful:—

Thomas Leeding, of Niagara Co., N. Y., æt. 52, a laborer and a muscular man, dislocated his right arm into the axilla by jumping from the cars when they were in full motion. The blow was received upon the shoulder. An intelligent country surgeon, assisted by several other persons, attempted reduction within an hour after the accident, but failed, and as the patient had some distance to travel, he was not brought under my notice until eighteen hours had elapsed. We first administered chloroform, and then while an assistant held firmly upon the acromion process, I pulled in the line of the body, then outwards, and finally upwards, but to no purpose. Having then applied Jarvis's "adjuster," and after the arm had been kept extended at a right angle with the body fifteen minutes, we removed the apparatus and found the bone in its place.

John Harrington, of this city, æt. 50, a very large and powerful man, fell while intoxicated, and dislocated his left humerus into the axilla. No surgeon was called until the tenth day, when he first consulted Dr. Dudley, who at once brought him to me. Without delay we applied the pulleys, and placing the arm at a right angle with the body we made extension fifteen minutes; occasionally also rotating the arm. We then removed the pulleys, and while an assistant held upon the acromion process, with my heel in the axilla I made extension in the line of the axis of the body, then outwards, and finally upwards with my foot upon the top of the scapula. I next seated my patient in a chair, and drew his arm and axilla forcibly over my knee. The bone was not yet reduced; I therefore bled him twenty-four ounces, or until partial syncope was induced, and proceeded to repeat most of these processes, but with no better result. At this moment I determined to use sulphuric ether, which had just been introduced as an anæsthetic, and while he was completely under its influence the pulleys were again applied and the extension continued for some time, and until the rope broke. He was then again placed in a chair, and the axilla brought over my knee, when in a moment the reduction was accomplished.

John Bowles, of Buffalo, aged 45 years, an Irish laborer, tolerably muscular, but spare. Bowles fell down a flight of stairs, and dislocated his left humerus into the axilla. The shoulder became much swollen, and was very painful, but he did not suspect a dislocation, and did not consult a surgeon. Eight weeks after the accident he applied to me. There were present the usual signs of this dislocation, but the arm was by careful measurement one inch and a half longer than the other.

The reduction was accomplished on the same day, in presence of Drs. Lee, Webster, Coventry, Ford, and Jewett. The time occupied in the reduction was about two hours. An attempt was first made with the heel in the axilla and with violent rotation and extension. The same plan was repeated with the aid of ether, which was administered freely. Jarvis's adjuster was now applied, with no result, except that either in consequence of the force employed by the adjuster, or in consequence of the free use of ether, or of both, he became convulsed violently, which was accompanied by frothing at the mouth, and other grave symptoms. The adjuster was removed, and the exhibition of ether discontinued. As soon as the convulsions ceased, and before consciousness had returned, extension, rotation, &c., were again made by hands. Finally, after all extension was relinquished, placing my knee in the axilla I reduced the bone by a very slight rotary action upon the arm. The bone was at once plainly in its socket, but the unusual length of the limb continued, being one inch and a half longer, though it could be shortened to the same length as the other by lifting the elbow. A pad was placed in the axilla, and the arm secured with a sling and roller. The next day the arm remained in place, but it was now only one inch longer than the other. At the end of a fortnight it was only three-quarters of an inch longer, and could be reduced to the same length by lifting; the pain and swelling about the shoulder, which never were great, were subsiding, and the patient was dismissed.

However skilfully our efforts may be directed, they will be found occasionally to fail; either owing to adhesions which have taken place, between the head of the bone, or rather its capsule, and the adjacent tendons, muscles, etc., to some extraordinary position of the head and neck of the bone in its relation to ligamentous or tendinous structures, to a filling up of the glenoid fossa, or to some other cause not fully explained. Such failures have happened not only in the hands of ignorant and unskilful surgeons destitute of appliances, but also in the hands of those who are the most expert, and who are the most completely provided with all the necessary apparatus. Indeed, if the truth were known, it would probably be found that the number of failures has been greater than the successes. The records of surgery, however, furnish a great many examples of ancient dislocations of the humerus reduced after periods ranging from one month to six, or even longer. Dieffenbach has been able to accomplish the reduction of a forward dislocation after two years, but not until he had cut the tendons of the pectoralis major, latissimus dorsi, teres major, and teres minor, and had divided the ligaments surrounding the new joint.[1]

It would be unjust to the young surgeon not to call especial attention to the numerous examples of serious and even fatal accidents which have followed upon the attempts to reduce ancient luxations at this joint. My friend, George C. Blackman, of Cincinnati, a distinguished surgeon, having recently met with one of these unfortunate accidents in his own practice, has had the candor to make a public statement of the case and of the circumstances which attended it. In

[1] Dieffenbach, Bost. Med. and Surg. Journ., vol. xxii. p. 382, from Medicin. Zeitung.

a letter to the editor of the *Western Lancet*, published in the November number for 1856, he writes as follows:—

"About the 10th ult., aided by yourself, I succeeded in reducing by manipulation, without the pulleys, a dislocation into the axilla, of eighty days' standing. The reduction was accomplished in a very few minutes, under the influence of chloroform and ether, and the next morning the patient left for the country, in a comfortable condition. Since that I have received no tidings from him. Encouraged by the result in this case, another patient, himself a physician, a tall, athletic man, and about fifty years of age, decided to submit to the same manipulation, although his arm had been dislocated for about sixteen weeks. The dislocation was downwards and inwards, and about the tenth week an unsuccessful attempt, by another surgeon, had been made with the pulleys, to which the force of six men was applied for two and a half hours. The patient being under the influence of chloroform and ether, aided by yourself, Drs. Fries, Cary, Graham, and Kauffman, I commenced my manipulations, adducting, rotating, abducting, and elevating the arm. These efforts had been made for about ten minutes, and the least possible violence employed, when a tumefaction appeared in the pectoral region, which in a few minutes attained considerable size. Supposing that the axillary artery was ruptured, as no pulse could be felt at the wrist, a ligature was immediately applied to the vessel at the upper part of its course. The operation was performed about 10 o'clock A. M., and compression of the pectoral region made by means of a sponge and broad roller. On removing this the next morning, the tumefaction had nearly disappeared. The patient continued comfortable, and about nine days after the application of the ligature, I was compelled to leave the city on a professional visit to Indiana. I left on Friday afternoon and returned on Monday morning, at which time I learned that my patient had died on Sunday morning, from hemorrhage at the seat of ligature. Two physicians, his most intimate friends, lodged in the same house with him, but before they reached his bedside the quantity of blood lost was so great that he sank exhausted in about two hours from the first and only attack of hemorrhage. Previous to my departure for Indiana, I had suggested to the physicians in charge, the importance of having compressed sponge at hand, to be used in any emergency of the kind, but this was not used by the attendant; instead of applying pressure instantaneously, he went in search of the physicians, who, at that early hour in the morning, were in bed. The time thus lost unquestionably led to the fatal catastrophe.

"I might refer you to numerous instances of success in the reduction of old dislocations—from two to six months' standing—which have occurred since the days of Wiseman, but I propose to notice only the accidents by which some of these attempts have occasionally been followed. One of the earliest recorded, so far as we have been able to learn, is the case reported by Desault.[1]

"During the effort of this surgeon to reduce an old dislocation, suddenly a considerable '*tumeur aerienne*' appeared below the clavicle,

[1] Desault, Journ. de Chir., t. iv. p. 301.

which Desault attributed to the '*degagement de l'air amassé entre les cellules rompues du tissu cellulaire!*' In a few days this tumor entirely subsided under the influence of '*astringents et une compression méthodique.*' Whether it was the result of a disengagement of air from the lacerated cells of the cellular membrane, as supposed by Desault, or of a rupture of bloodvessels, we leave the reader to determine.

"It is somewhat singular that Desault should have met with two cases of this extraordinary phenomenon. Pelletan's explanation, in our opinion, throws some light on this subject. In an attempt to reduce a luxation of four months' standing, the same kind of '*tumeur aerienne*' appeared. It was opened, and the hemorrhage from the torn artery was fatal.[1]

"Malgaigne states that he is acquainted but with a single instance of an 'emphysème véritable' following a reduction, and that is the one reported by Flaubert, in his *Mém. sur plusieurs cas de luxations dans lesquels les efforts pour la réduction ont été suivis d'accidents graves*, which appeared in the *Répertoire d'Anat. et de Phys.*, 1827. The patient, a female, æt. 70, screamed violently during the operation, and Malgaigne is disposed to believe that the emphysema was independent of the luxation, or the reduction.

"Malgaigne, himself, attempted reduction in a case of sixty-eight days' standing, but was forced to discontinue his efforts in consequence of the sudden appearance of a tumefaction in the axilla, and on the shoulder. Ice was applied, and in the course of a few hours the swelling was arrested, and by the twenty-second day, the blood which he thinks came from ruptured muscular branches, was completely absorbed.[2]

"A case occurred to Flaubert, in which, besides the tumefaction, the pulse could not be felt at the wrist. The hand was cold, insensible, and immovable. The next day, however, the pulse returned to the wrist, and in the course of twenty-six days the effused blood was absorbed. Froriep lost a patient from a rupture of the axillary vein, which proved fatal in an hour and a half after the operation. The reader may find in the comprehensive treatise of Malgaigne, details of cases in which the axillary artery was ruptured. We pass over those observed by Verduc, Petit, Platner, Delpech, and that referred to by Sir Charles Bell, in his *Operative Surgery*. The late Dr. John C. Warren tied the subclavian to arrest the progress of an enormous aneurismal tumor in the axilla, the result of the reduction of a recent dislocation, and of supposed pressure of the operator's boot. In this instance the coats of the artery were so contused that sloughing took place during a fit of coughing, five days after the accident.[3] In 1824, M. Leudet lost a patient at the hospital at Rouen. The dislocation was of only eleven days' standing, and was complicated with a fracture of the margin of the glenoid cavity, as in the two fatal cases which occurred in the practice of Prof. Gibson, of Philadelphia. The latter cases are too familiar to every surgical student to require par-

[1] Pelletan, Chir. Clin., t. ii. p. 951.
[2] Malgaigne, op. cit., p. 150.
[3] Warren, Amer. Journ. Med. Sci., vol. xi., N. S., 1846.

ticular mention in this place. Prof. Gibson, in connection with the report of the above cases, gives briefly the details of a fatal operation by David, of Rouen. The luxation had existed several months, and great force was employed in the reduction. This resulted in an inflammation, mortification, and death. Some years since, Lisfranc attempted the reduction in a case of four months' standing. He succeeded; but on visiting the patient an hour afterwards he was found dead. His death was attributed to cerebral congestion, as the autopsy showed the axillary artery, veins, and nerves uninjured.[1] In the same volume, MM. Lenoir and Larrey refer to cases in which they had met with lesion of the brachial plexus, giving rise to paralysis, and yet these were recent cases, and the reduction was most readily accomplished. But I will not multiply cases of this kind; those already related will suffice, in the minds of many, to answer the question—At what period of time after a dislocation of the shoulder, is an attempt at reduction justifiable? When Prof. Gibson lost his first patient, he wrote that 'should a case, similar in external appearance to that of James Scofield again occur, I shall feel justified in adopting a similar course.'[2] When he had lost his second patient (John Langton), he expressed his views as follows: 'The conclusions which I am now prepared to draw are directly the reverse of what I have stated in some of the foregoing pages; I am now disposed to condemn, in the most unqualified terms, all attempts at the restoration of ancient luxations of the humerus and other bones—except in cases where the patient is remarkably thin and debilitated, and where there has been little or no inflammation at the time or subsequent to the displacement.' At a meeting of the *Société de Chirurgie* of Paris, July 3, 1850, M. Maisonneuve reported a case in which, after M. Velpeau had failed, he succeeded in reducing a luxation of the shoulder of twelve weeks' standing, and elated with this triumph over the veteran of La Charité, he asserts there are but few cases in which, with the aid of chloroform, we may not succeed. '*Quelles resistances y a-t-il a vaincre ici, en effet?*' he asks. '*Il n'y a presque pas d'engrenage; les muscles sont neutralisés par le chloroforme; il ne reste donc que des adherences fibreuses: l'on pourra presque toujours les surmonter, ou les rompre.*'[3] But these fibrous adhesions are not the only obstacles to overcome: where the tissues surrounding the head have become consolidated by inflammation, the axillary vessels and nerves must be in danger of laceration. Perhaps, however, as M. Maisonneuve suggests, this accident may be avoided by '*extensions préparatoires*,' as in the attempts to restore contracted limbs to the natural shape."

Norris has reported three cases of ancient dislocation into the axilla, treated at the Pennsylvania Hospital; one, of four weeks' standing, was reduced in thirty seconds by the aid of the pulleys; the second, which had existed seven weeks, was reduced by the same means in about one hour; and the third, dislocated ten weeks, was left unreduced after extension and counter-extension had been made for an hour. In the second case, however, suppuration occurred in or about

[1] Lisfranc, Bul. de la Soc. Chir., t. i. p. 718.
[2] Gibson, Elements of Surg., vol. i. p. 824, 4th ed.
[3] Maisonneuve, Bul. de la Soc. Chir., t. i. p. 716.

the joint, and, on the tenth day, the abscess was opened, giving exit to a large amount of pus. He left the hospital with the parts about the shoulder still much hardened and stiff.[1]

Dislocation, with Fracture of the Humerus near its Upper End.

We have thus far omitted to speak of the treatment of dislocations of the humerus accompanied with fracture near its upper end. The older writers, almost without an exception, agreed in declaring the reduction of these dislocations impossible, until the fracture had united. And, so late as the year 1828, we have the report of a case treated in this manner by a surgeon in Massachusetts. Dr. Warren, of Boston, himself reduced the dislocation at the end of four weeks, when the fracture was found to have united.[2]

But, whatever difficulty surgeons may have experienced before the introduction of anæsthetics, it is quite certain that at the present day such delay is no longer necessary, at least in a great majority of cases. In order to the reduction, even extension and counter-extension are rendered unnecessary, provided the muscular system is thoroughly relaxed, for, by simply pressing firmly the head of the bone toward the socket, the reduction has often been speedily accomplished.

Richet reports an example of this kind in a man sixty-eight years of age, in whom the dislocation was complicated with a fracture of the neck of the humerus. The attempt was not made until the fourth day, when it proved successful without extension. The fracture was afterwards adjusted and consolidated so that he recovered the complete use of his arm.[3]

At a meeting of the New York Academy of Medicine in May, 1855, Dr. Watson reported a case of fracture of the humerus near its head, complicated with a dislocation into the axilla. The patient was a robust man, past the middle age, and had received the injury by a blow on the shoulder from a steam engine. He was very much prostrated at the time of being admitted into the hospital, and the examination was not made until the following morning. The arm was then found lying close to the side, but in other respects it presented the usual signs of a dislocation. Ether was immediately administered; and while extension and counter-extension were applied, and a sweeping motion given to the arm, drawing it from the body, firm pressure with the fingers was made in the axilla, forcing the head toward the socket, and the bone slipped into its position.[4]

In the *Transactions of the American Medical Association*, I have reported a case of supposed dislocation accompanied with a fracture, which I succeeded in reducing on the eighth day.[5]

Many other examples have been recorded by other surgeons in

[1] Norris, Amer. Journ. Med. Sci., vol. xxxi. p. 24.

[2] Boston Med. and Surg. Journ., No. i., 1828; also, Amer. Journ. Med. Sci., vol. ii. p. 233.

[3] Richet, Amer. Journ. Med. Sci., vol. xii., new ser., p. 293, from Bulletin de Thérap.

[4] Watson, Amer. Journ. Med. Sci., vol. xvi., new ser., p. 383.

[5] Op. cit., vol. ix. p. 93.

which the reduction has been accomplished immediately, and without much difficulty, by simple pressure upon the head of the bone, while the patient was under the influence of an anæsthetic, and without the aid of extension; indeed, it is quite doubtful whether extension in these cases is of any service. If, however, the surgeon were to fail by pressure alone, it would be proper to employ extension and manipulation;[1] in the event of a failure by these means, the case ought to be treated as a fracture, and the earliest period after the union of the fragments should be seized upon to accomplish the reduction of the dislocation. The frequent success of the older surgeons by this method is sufficient to warrant the attempt.

The treatment of compound dislocations of this joint will be considered in a separate chapter devoted to the general consideration of compound dislocations of all the joints connected with the long bones.

§ 2. Dislocation of the Humerus Forwards. (*Subcoracoid and Subclavicular.*)

Causes.—The causes of this dislocation are the same with those which produce dislocation downwards into the axilla, except that it is more likely to occur in a fall upon the elbow or upon the hand when the line of the axis of the arm and forearm is thrown behind the body. If it is the result of a direct blow, the impulse has usually been received rather upon the back than upon the outer side of the head of the humerus; or the upper end of the bone having been originally thrown directly downwards upon the inferior edge of the scapula, may have been made to assume the position forwards beneath the pectoral muscle, in consequence of the peculiar action of the muscles, or of the position of the arm in an attempt to rise. By this latter mode of explanation the dislocation forwards is consecutive only upon a dislocation downwards.

In several instances which have come under my notice the dislocation has been due to muscular action alone. In one example the dislocation occurred frequently in consequence of epileptic convulsions. This was in the person of a lad, æt. 18, of a slender frame and feeble muscles. When the dislocation had taken place, he was frequently able to reduce it himself; sometimes he was obliged to call upon a surgeon, and at other times he left it out a day or two, or until it became reduced spontaneously. This spontaneous reduction generally took place at night, during sleep. At the time he called upon me the bone had been out two days, and he could not reduce it. I administered chloroform, and then made repeated and prolonged efforts to reduce it, adopting all the usual modes of manipulation, but without resorting to mechanical appliances. The father now refused to allow me to proceed, and he was taken home with the bone unreduced. The following day he called at my office, to say that during the night, while

[1] Hartshorne, Case reduced by Manipulation, Amer. Journ. Med. Sci., Jan. 1855, pp. 273–4, from Med. Examiner.

asleep, and, he thinks, while turning over in bed, the bone suddenly resumed its place.

Pathology.—Omitting for the present to speak of partial luxations, the existence of which, as a form of traumatic dislocation, we are prepared to question, we shall proceed at once to describe the anatomical relations and the various lesions which generally accompany a complete luxation forwards.

Of these we shall observe two principal varieties, differing mainly in the degree or extent of the displacement.

Thus, we may find the head of the humerus resting beneath the coracoid process (Fig. 229), having the conjoined tendon of the short head of the biceps and of the coraco-brachialis lying upon its anterior surface, while its posterior and outer surface rests upon the venter of the scapula in front of the glenoid fossa; in which position it has usually thrust up, to a greater or less extent, the belly of the subscapular muscle.

Fig. 229.

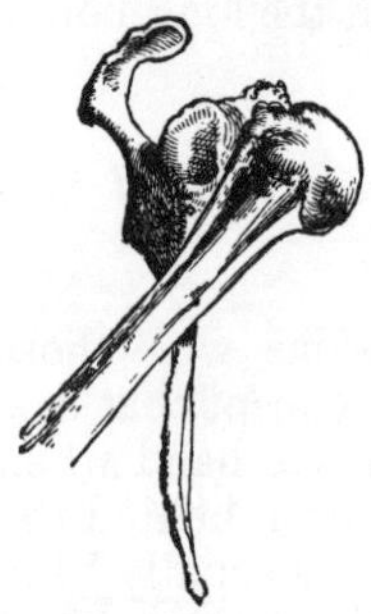

Subcoracoid dislocation.

Sir Astley Cooper, Fergusson, and others, when mentioning this form of dislocation, call it a "dislocation into the axilla;" by Boyer it is called a "primary luxation forwards." Dr. Wood, of New York, has reported an example, accompanied with a fracture of the neck of the humerus, which he has named "dislocation under the subscapularis muscle." The drawing which accompanies the report, made from the autopsy, sufficiently shows that it was a dislocation of the same character which we are now describing.[1] And Dr. Parker, of the same city, has called attention to a similar case, an account of which was first given in Reese's edition of Cooper's *Surgical Dictionary*. The head of the humerus reposed in the "subscapular fossa."[2] By Malgaigne, Vidal (de Cassis), and others, this is called a subcoracoid dislocation, a term which, as being more distinctive and appropriate than either of the others, I shall choose to adopt.

Fig. 230.

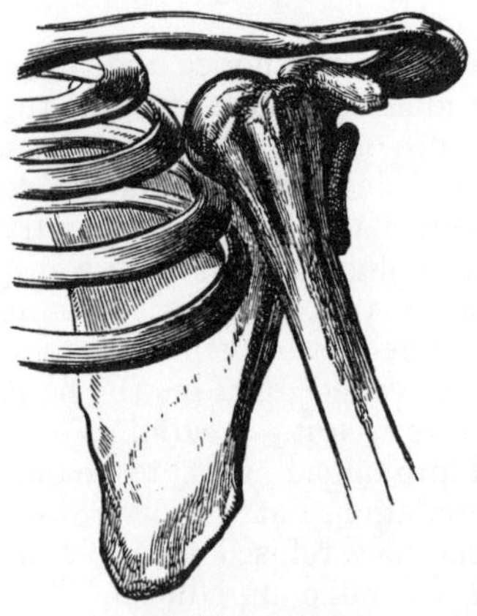

Subclavicular dislocation.

In the second variety (Fig. 230), the head, having escaped from underneath the coracoid process, is made to approach nearer to the sternum, so as to apply itself more or less closely to the inferior edge of the clavicle. In which case the head and neck will be placed behind both the pectoralis major and minor, and also behind the short head of the biceps and coraco-brachi-

[1] Wood, New York Journ. of Med., May, 1850, p. 282.
[2] Parker, New York Journ. of Med., March, 1852, p. 187.

alis; or between these several muscles on the one hand, and the serratus magnus, covering the second and third ribs, on the other hand.

It is in this latter position that the head of the humerus is usually found, and upon the appearances which accompany this more advanced form of dislocation writers have generally based their descriptions, diagnosis, treatment, &c., of forward luxations.

In either form of the accident, the deltoid, with the supra- and infraspinatus, is greatly stretched, and the two latter sometimes torn; the subscapularis is displaced upwards and backwards, while its tendon is in some instances completely wrenched from the head of the humerus. Mr. Erichsen has seen the lesser tubercle itself completely broken off in two examples of this accident which he has been permitted to examine after death.[1] Occasionally the axillary nerves are carried forwards with the head of the bone; and in this case the pain produced by their being thus pressed upon is even greater than in dislocations into the axilla.

In this accident, as in dislocation downwards, the long head of the biceps is sometimes broken; the circumflex nerve may be contused or ruptured, and the capsule is generally torn very extensively.

Symptoms.—If the dislocation is subclavicular (Fig. 230), a depression exists under the outer end of the acromion process, extending also un-

Fig. 231.

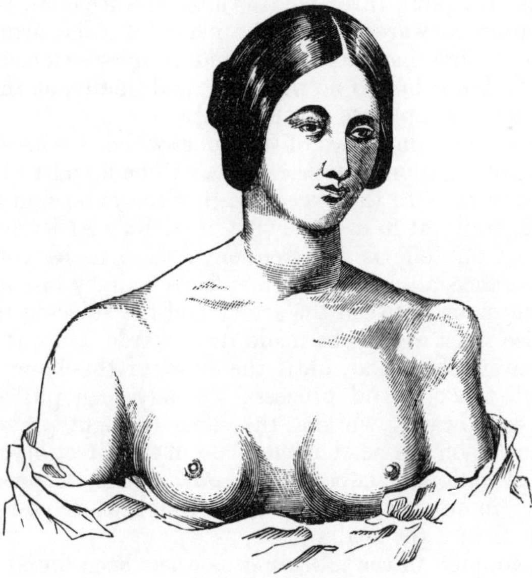

Subcoracoid luxation.

derneath its posterior margin; the elbow hangs away from the body, and a little backwards; the axis of the limb is much changed, being

[1] Erichsen, Science and Art of Surgery, 2d Amer. ed., p. 250.

thrown inwards in the direction of the middle of the clavicle, the whole body inclining moderately to the same side; there is also more or less inability to move the arm, especially in a direction forwards or outwards; a fulness is seen underneath the clavicle, and to the sternal side of the coracoid process, occasioned by the head of the humerus; the head moving with the shaft. To these we may add the common sign of all dislocations of the humerus, mentioned by Dugas, viz: the impossibility of placing the hand upon the opposite shoulder while at the same moment the elbow is made to touch the front of the chest.

If the dislocation is forwards, but subcoracoid (Fig. 231), the head of the bone will be found below this process and deep in the anterior margin of the axillary fossa. It cannot, therefore, be so distinctly felt; but the other signs are the same as in the dislocation forwards under the clavicle.

Prognosis.—While on the one hand experience has shown that the axillary nerves and artery are less liable to suffer serious and permanent injury than in dislocation downwards, and that the capsule, with the tendinous, and muscular tissues about the joint, are no more liable to laceration, on the other hand, the difficulty of reduction has been often increased, and consequently a larger number of examples, in proportion to the actual number which occur, have been left unreduced.

Dr. Norris relates a case which the surgeon who was first called supposed to be a mere contusion, but which, on being admitted to the Pennsylvania Hospital, three months after the accident, was found to be a dislocation forwards under the clavicle. The arm was almost useless. Dr. Norris made extension and counter-extension with pulleys nearly an hour, but to no purpose; and finally, at the request of the patient, the attempt was given over.[1]

Treatment.—The same rules of treatment which we have established in relation to dislocations into the axilla will be found to be applicable to this dislocation, with the exception that the extension will have to be made, generally at first, somewhat in a line backwards from the body, and that our efforts will frequently have to be continued with more perseverance, although with less fear of injury in consequence of supposed adhesions between the artery and the adjacent tissues. The extension also must always be made downwards and outwards, if the dislocation is subclavicular, until the head of the bone has escaped from beneath the coracoid process; we may then pull directly outwards or even upwards, while at the same moment pressure is made with the hand upon the head of the bone in the direction of the socket.

If the dislocation is subcoracoid, our modes of procedure need scarcely vary in any respect from those which we have recommended for dislocations into the axilla.

The plan adopted in the following case has been found sufficient in several examples of subcoracoid dislocation.

Mr. McA., of Buffalo, æt. 73, moderately muscular, fell through a trap-door, striking upon his right elbow and dislocating the humerus forwards. Within two hours after the accident I found the head of

[1] Norris, Amer. Journn. Med. Sci., vol. xxv. p. 279.

the bone resting under the coracoid process, where it could be distinctly felt and seen. There was a marked depression under the acromion process, and the arm was carried out from the body and slightly back. He had not suffered much pain. The patient was seated in a chair, and while Dr. Lemon, who was at that time my pupil, supported the acromion process, I pushed the head of the humerus outwards toward the socket, with my left hand, while with my right I pulled gently upon the arm in the direction of the axis of the body. After about twenty seconds it slid suddenly into its place with an audible snap.

Simple manipulation alone will also be found sufficient in many cases of subclavicular dislocation.

A German, Simeon Grennas, æt. 21, fell upon an icy side-walk and dislocated his right humerus under the clavicle. We found him about an hour after the accident sitting with his head inclined to his right side, and supporting his elbow with his left hand. A marked depression existed under the outer end of the acromion process, and instead of the usual fulness there was a flatness under the process behind. The elbow was carried out from the body and very slightly backwards. While Dr. Boardman supported the acromion process I lifted the elbow from the side, carrying it first upwards and backwards, and then forwards, making thus a short detour with the arm, and when the manœuvre was nearly completed the bone slid into its socket with a slight snap. No extension was used, and no more force was employed than was sufficient to lift and rotate the arm. He was not at the time of the reduction faint, nor were his muscles relaxed from any other cause.

More than once I have accomplished the reduction by extension made directly upwards, as in the following example.

A gentleman, forty-five years of age, had his left shoulder dislocated forwards under the clavicle in a railroad collision on the 8th of October, 1858. A young surgeon had been making extension in various ways for half an hour, when, by placing my foot upon the top of the scapula and drawing the arm directly upwards, I accomplished the reduction immediately and without much effort. Six months after the accident, I found the deltoid muscle considerably wasted, and he was still unable to raise his arm to a right angle with the body.

I have in this way also reduced a dislocation which had existed seventeen days, the nature of the accident having been misunderstood by the attending surgeon. The man was twenty-three years old, and quite muscular. The dislocation had been produced by a severe blow received directly upon the shoulder, and the arm was still considerably swollen and very tender. The reduction was accomplished in a few seconds while the patient was under the influence of chloroform, but by my hands alone, aided only by the pressure of the foot upon the top of the scapula.

In December, 1857, Dr. White, of this city, and myself reduced a subclavicular dislocation of the right shoulder, which had existed sixty days, in a man sixty-eight years of age. The surgeon who first saw the man thought it was only a sprain or a severe bruise. When he came to Buffalo, the whole limb was enormously swollen, and neither

Dr. White nor myself had much expectation of accomplishing a reduction without a resort to pulleys and anæsthetics. He was, however, placed upon the floor, and after extension made for about half an hour, during which time we had pulled the arm in various directions, upwards, outwards, and downwards, I at last succeeded while my heel was placed in the axilla, and while the limb was undergoing a slight rotation. No anæsthetic was employed.

These several cases are mentioned that the surgeon may understand how impossible it is always to establish absolute and invariable rules of procedure which shall be applicable to every accident of this character. The method which will succeed readily in one case may fail completely in another, although belonging to the same class, and not apparently differing in its anatomical relations. Before relinquishing the attempt, we ought to have put in requisition all the expedients which the experience of other surgeons has shown to be worthy of a trial.

§ 3. Dislocation of the Humerus Backwards. (*Subspinous.*)

This form of dislocation has been seldom met with. Only two cases, according to Sir Astley Cooper, occurred in Guy's Hospital in thirty-eight years; but in the last edition of Sir Astley Cooper's treatise on *Fractures and Dislocations*, edited by Bransby Cooper, nine cases are mentioned.[1] Sedillot,[2] Malgaigne, Desclaux,[3] Van Buren,[4] W. Parker,[5] Lepelletier,[6] Trowbridge,[7] Physick, and Snyder,[8] have each seen one example.[9]

Causes.—One of the patients mentioned in Mr. Cooper's book had his shoulder dislocated backwards in an epileptic convulsion; one had fallen upon his shoulder; another met with the accident while pushing a person violently with the arm elevated; and a fourth, seen by Mr. Coley, "was pulled down by a calf which he was driving, a cord having been tied to one of the calf's legs, and being held fast by the man's hand." Of the manner in which the other cases were produced no precise account is given. Desclaux's patient fell from a height with his arm in front of him. In the case seen by Dr. Parker, of New York, a woman, æt. 60, had fallen forwards and struck upon the outside of her elbow, arm, and shoulder. No attempt was made to reduce it until the fourteenth day, she not having for some time called the attention of any surgeon to its condition. Trowbridge's patient was thrown from a horse, striking on the palm of his hand.

Pathology.—Mr. Cooper has given us a careful account of the dissection in the case of Mr. Complin, already alluded to, whose arm had been dislocated by muscular spasm. This gentleman was fifty-two

[1] A. Cooper, op. cit., p. 352, etc.

[2] Sedillot, Amer. Journ. of Med. Sci., vol. xiii. p. 551, Feb. 1834.

[3] Desclaux, New York Journ. of Med., Nov. 1851, p. 109, from Revue Médicale.

[4] Van Buren, ibid., Nov. 1851, p. 110. [5] Parker, ibid., March, 1852, p. 186.

[6] Lepelletier, Amer. Journ. Med. Sci., vol. xvi. p. 526, from Arch. Gén., Nov. 1834.

[7] Trowbridge, Bost. Med. and Surg. Journ., vol. xxvii. p. 99. [8] Gibson's Surgery.

[9] Examples have also been seen by Dupuytren, Arnolt, Best, Levacher, Berard, Fizeau, Velpeau, Fergusson and Kirkbride. New York Journ. Med., March, 1852, p. 193.

years of age, and had been subject to epileptic fits, in one of which the shoulder was dislocated. Many attempts were made to reduce it, but although it seemed to be easily drawn into its socket by extension merely, yet, as soon as the force ceased, the head of the bone slipped again upon the dorsum scapulæ, and in this situation it was finally permitted to remain until his death, which did not take place until five years after. In the mean time, he was able to move the limb but very slightly, so that his arm was almost useless.

Mr. Cooper, to whom the arm was sent after death, found the head of the bone resting under the spine of the scapula, and against the posterior edge of the glenoid fossa, where it had formed a slight depression, and the head itself had become somewhat changed in form by absorption. The tendon of the subscapularis muscle and the internal portion of the capsular ligament were torn at the point where the muscle was inserted, but the greater portion of the capsule remained, having been pressed back by the head of the bone. The supra-spinatus was stretched, while the infra-spinatus and teres minor were relaxed. The long head of the biceps was elongated but not ruptured. The glenoid fossa was rough and irregular upon its surface, the cartilage being absorbed.

The fact that the bone would not remain in place when reduced, was explained by the rupture of the subscapularis, and the consequent loss of antagonism to the action of the infra-spinatus and teres minor.[1]

Fig. 232.

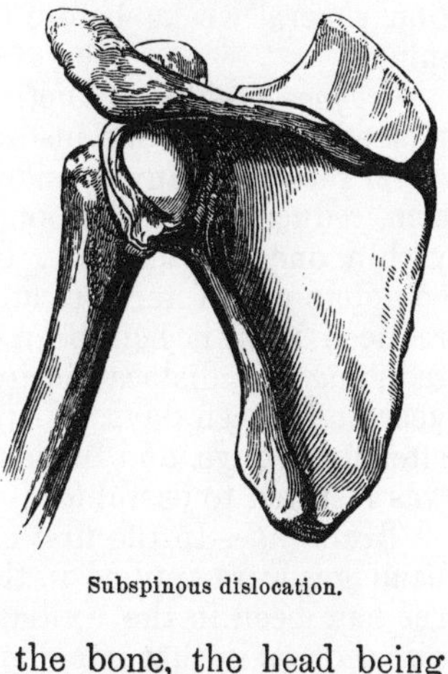

Subspinous dislocation.

The accompanying drawing is a copy of that furnished by Mr. Cooper to illustrate the position occupied by the bone.

I ought to mention that this case has been regarded by Vidal (de Cassis), Malgaigne, and others, as only subacromial, and as a variety of the dislocation backwards, differing from that in which the head of the bone occupies a position underneath the spine. But as I can see no difference except in the degree or extent of the displacement, I prefer not to regard the distinction made by these surgeons.

Symptoms.—The signs of this accident are, a projection under the spine of the scapula, produced by the head of the bone, the head being obedient to the motions of the arm; a corresponding depression in front and under the outer extremity of the acromion process; a wide space between the head of the bone and the coracoid process, into which the fingers may be pushed deeply; the axis of the shaft of the humerus directed upwards and outwards toward a point posterior to the glenoid fossa; the arm laid against the side of the body, and carried forwards across the chest; the humerus rotated inwards, unless

[1] Sir A. Cooper, op. cit., p. 354.

the subscapularis muscle is torn; immobility, but the motions of the arm are not generally so much impaired as in either of the other dislocations; and finally, as in all other dislocations of the humerus, the hand cannot be laid upon the opposite shoulder while the elbow touches the side or front of the chest. In Parker's case the elbow was thrown outwards, although the arm was carried very much across the chest. Desclaux's patient held his hand upon his head, with his arm horizontally across his body.

Usually the diagnosis will be easily made, but Sir Astley relates one case in which, on the morning following the accident, a surgeon was unable to discover the dislocation, and on the seventeenth day Bransby Cooper failed to make the diagnosis; nor indeed, on the twenty-third day did Sir Astley himself determine that it was a dislocation, until he had unexpectedly reduced it while manipulating upon the arm. In a second example, Sir Astley at first believed it to be a fracture, but a more careful examination showed it to be a dislocation backwards. In this instance the limb could not be rotated outwards, as the subscapularis was not torn, and continued to offer resistance when the arm was moved in this direction; he was also suffering much more pain than did the other patients, owing, as Sir Astley thinks, to pressure upon the articular nerves. In the case of Mr. Collinson, also mentioned by Mr. Cooper, a surgeon who saw the patient immediately after the accident, failed to discover the true nature of the injury; and Trowbridge's patient had suffered a dislocation several weeks before the nature of the accident was fully determined.

Prognosis.—The reduction has always been sooner or later accomplished, except in one instance; in this case we have seen that the arm never recovered any considerable degree of usefulness. Mr. Collinson's arm, reduced on the second day, was restored to all of its functions within one month. Dr. Parker's patient had nearly recovered the complete use of her arm at the end of four weeks, although it was not reduced until it had been out fourteen days. Sedillot succeeded in reducing the dislocation in the case of his patient, at the end of one year and fifteen days. Lepelletier after forty-five days. Trowbridge after forty days, and in this latter case, we are informed that the arm was restored to usefulness.

Treatment.—In the first case mentioned by Sir Astley Cooper, "the bandages were applied in the same manner as if the head of the humerus had been in the axilla, and the extension was made in the same direction as in that accident" (downwards and a little outwards). In less than five minutes the bone slipped into its socket with a loud snap. The second case was treated successfully in the same way. Mr. Dunn also having failed to reduce by pulling upwards, finally succeeded by pulling at the wrist downwards and forwards, while an assistant pushed the head of the bone toward the socket; the heel was not placed in the axilla, which Mr. Bransby Cooper thinks would have only retarded the reduction. Mr. Key also failed to accomplish reduction while carrying the arm upwards and backwards, but when the patient had become faint, by placing the heel in the axilla and pulling downwards a minute or two, the bone was reduced. Vidal (de Cassis) recommends the same plan, namely, that we shall pull in the direction in which we find the limb; Trowbridge employed the pulleys successfully, the extension being made downwards and forwards; while Dr. Parker succeeded equally well with his patient, by "pulling the arm outwards, downwards, and slightly forwards." Counter-extension was at the same time made by a sheet in the axilla, and the head of the humerus was pushed toward the socket by the hand. In Mr. Collinson's case, the scapula was supported by a towel, while "gradual extension of the limb was made directly outwards, and then the arm being moved slowly forwards, the head of the bone was distinctly heard to snap into its socket." The time occupied was not more than two or three minutes. Sir Astley, however, seems to give the preference to the method which succeeded so happily in the case of Mr. G., while he was still manipulating with a view to determine the character of the accident. "I readily reduced the bone," he remarks, "by raising the hand and arm, and by turning the hand backwards behind the head." In one other instance, having failed to reduce it by slight extension outwards, he raised the arm perpendicularly, and at the same time forced it backwards behind the patient's head, and the reduction was promptly effected.

After the reduction, a compress should be placed against the head of the bone, and underneath the spine of the scapula, and this should be secured in its place by several turns of a roller. The forearm ought also to be placed in a sling, with the elbow thrown a little back of the centre of the body, so as to direct the head of the humerus forwards.

§ 4. Partial Dislocations of the Humerus.

Sir Astley Cooper has related in his treatise two cases of supposed incomplete luxation of the head of the humerus forwards; and in confirmation of his views he has added an account of the appearances presented on dissection in the body of a subject brought into the rooms of St. Thomas's Hospital. Bransby Cooper, in his edition of the same work, furnishes the report of a similar case which came under the observation of Mr. Douglas, of Glasgow. Hargrave and Dupuytren have each reported one example of this species of dislocation, in which its existence was said to be confirmed by dissection.

Petit, Duverney, Chopart, Sedillot, Miller, Gibson, Malgaigne, and many others have admitted its possibility; Malgaigne, however, only admits its existence when the capsule remains entire.

Without intending to examine very much at length the value of these opinions, I shall content myself with declaring that the existence of this, or of any other form of partial luxation of the shoulder-joint, as a traumatic accident, has not up to this moment been fairly established; and that the anatomical structure of the joint renders its occurrence exceedingly improbable, if not absolutely impossible.

The only example mentioned by Sir Astley Cooper, in which a dissection was made, showed that the long head of the biceps had been ruptured, and that the capsule was torn, while the head of the humerus was resting under the coracoid process. We shall have no difficulty, therefore, in assigning it to its proper place as a complete, sub-coracoid dislocation. In Mr. Hargrave's case, also, the tendon of the biceps was torn; while Dupuytren omits to mention what was the actual fact in relation to this tendon in the case seen by him, but it is distinctly stated that the head of the bone rested upon the ribs. Mr. Hargrave seems, therefore, to have described a case of rupture of the long head of the biceps, and it is probable that Dupuytren, who knew nothing of the previous history of the subject, has given us a faithful account of a pathological dislocation, a result of disease, and not of a direct injury.

If the head of the humerus is driven from its socket by violence, and remains thus displaced, it is, we assume, a complete luxation; since it is only by having placed the semi-diameter of the head of the bone outside of the margin of the glenoid fossa that it can be made for one moment to retain its abnormal position. To accomplish this amount of displacement upwards, or upwards and forwards, or directly forwards, the acromion or the coracoid processes must be broken. While its occurrence in any other direction must involve at least a most extraordinary extension, if not an actual laceration of the capsule. If we admit with Malgaigne that occasionally the capsule has been found capable of such extraordinary extension without actual rupture, we still are unwilling to regard this as a fair example of a partial dislocation, since the head of the bone no longer moves in its socket, being at no point in actual contact with the articular surface of the glenoid fossa. It is essentially a complete dislocation, according to all the admitted definitions of this term.

It is quite probable that a majority of these accidents were examples of rupture or of displacement of the tendon of the long head of the biceps, the effect of which, as Mr. John G. Smith,[1] and Mr. Soden[2] have shown by a number of dissections, is to allow the head of the humerus to be drawn upwards and forwards in its socket, until it is arrested by the two processes, and by the coraco-acromial ligament. Says Mr. Soden: "To enable the bone to maintain its equilibrium, it is necessary that the capsular muscles should exactly counterbalance each other; and as there is no muscle from the ribs to the humerus to antagonize the upper capsular muscles" (that is, to draw the head of the humerus downwards), "it is suggested that

Fig. 233.

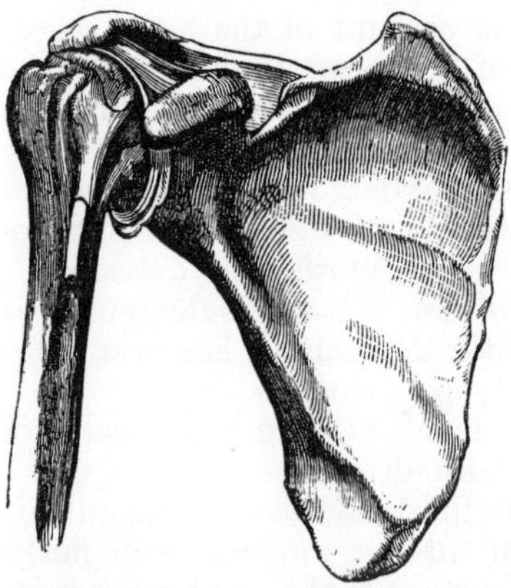

Displacement of the long head of the biceps.

[1] Amer. Journ. Med. Sci., vol. xvi. p. 219, May, 1835, from Lond. Med. Gaz.
[2] Ibid., vol. xxix. p. 480, from Lond. Med. Gaz., July, 1841.

this office is performed by the singular course of the long tendon of the biceps, which, by passing over the head of the bone, when the muscle is put in action, tends to throw the head downwards and backwards; it follows, therefore, that the tendon being removed, the head of the bone would rise upwards and forwards."

The drawing (Fig. 233) represents the case of displacement of the tendon of the biceps seen by Mr. Soden, and of which he had been permitted to make a dissection.[1]

I have myself frequently observed, and I have before, when speaking of the prognosis or results of dislocations, called attention to the fact, that the head of the humerus sometimes remains for a long time after the reduction has been effected slightly advanced in its socket, so as to lead to a suspicion that it is not properly reduced. While I am writing, two additional illustrations have come under my notice, in one of which the patient, a lad of about fourteen years of age, had been subjected to the pulleys during four consecutive hours to accomplish a more complete reduction.

The same thing, also, has been noticed by me occasionally where the shoulder had been subjected to a violent wrench, but no actual dislocation had ever occurred. In either case the explanation is probably the same, the long head of the biceps has been broken or displaced. I mean to say that in this circumstance we may find a sufficient and perhaps the most frequent explanation; yet it is quite probable that in a considerable number of cases, the laceration of the capsule, and the action of the muscles, are alone concerned in the production of this phenomenon.

Alfred Mercer, of Syracuse, N. Y., in a very interesting paper on this same subject, relates several examples of forward displacement after injuries to the shoulder-joint, one of which as being exceedingly pertinent I shall take the liberty of quoting.

"Mrs. B., a well developed woman, of full habit, aged fifty-six, seven years since was thrown from a carriage, dislocating her right shoulder, which was reduced a short time after the accident, but the shoulder was painful, and tender to the touch, and almost useless for months after. She could carry the arm forwards and backwards, but could not raise it from the side, or carry the hand behind her, or raise it to her head, for fourteen months. She has gradually gained better use of her arm, but now, July, 1858, she cannot raise the elbow from the side more than half way to a horizontal position without assistance, but with assistance, the arm may be carried into any position without pain or resistance. Measurement shows no appreciable difference in the size or length of the arm, or size of the shoulder; but the point of the shoulder is still tender to the touch, is prominent in front, and correspondingly flattened behind. The head of the humerus appears to rest against the outside of the coracoid process, but the fulness of habit obscures the diagnosis, compared with the other cases. Several doctors, at different times, have examined the shoulder; some have said it was not properly reduced, and advised a suit for malpractice.

[1] Pirrie's System of Surg., Amer. ed., p. 255; also, Sir Astley Cooper, edited by Bransby Cooper, Amer. ed., p. 363.

"I examined the shoulder again in November last; it presented the same general appearance, although the patient was much thinner in flesh from recent sickness. Some six weeks previous to this examination, in a sudden and thoughtless effort to raise the arm above the head, the muscles unexpectedly obeyed the will; since which time she has had perfect use of it, though the deformity still remains. She thinks she felt or heard a snap when the arm went up, but it was followed by no pain, soreness, or swelling."[1]

There can be no doubt, we think, that in this case at least, the the deformity and maiming were due in a great measure to a displacement of the long head of the biceps.

CHAPTER VII.

DISLOCATIONS OF THE HEAD OF THE RADIUS.

I HAVE met with eighteen examples of dislocation of the head of the radius; of which, fourteen were dislocated forwards and only four backwards: or, rejecting those cases which were complicated with fracture, I have recorded eight cases of simple forward luxation, and two of simple backward luxation. My experience, therefore, does not correspond with the experience of Boyer, Velpeau, Vidal (de Cassis), Chelius, B. Cooper, Guthrie, Gibson, and some others, who declare that the dislocation backwards is the more frequent of the two. Indeed, I ought to say of both of the examples of backward luxation of the radius which have come under my notice, and which I have marked as simple, that they were ancient luxations, and I am not entirely certain, therefore, that they had not been originally complicated with a fracture, although at the time of my examination they presented no such evidence.

§ 1. Dislocation of the Head of the Radius Forwards.

Causes.—A fall upon the elbow, the blow being received directly upon the posterior face of the head of the radius; a fall upon the hand with the forearm extended and pronated; extreme pronation of the forearm; or, according to Denucé, a blow upon the inside of the elbow, which is equivalent to a violent adduction of the forearm.

In children, and especially in those of a strumous habit, whose ligaments are feeble, a subluxation forwards, or even a complete luxation, is occasionally produced by being lifted suddenly from the floor

[1] Mercer, Buffalo Med. Journ., vol. xiv. p. 641, April, 1859.

by the hand or by an attempt to sustain the child when he is about to fall. I have seen several examples of this latter form of the accident produced in this way. Batchelder,[1] Sylvester,[2] Goyrand,[3] and many other surgeons have mentioned similar cases.

Dr. Krackowitzer related to the New York Academy, in 1856, a case of complete dislocation forwards, produced, as was supposed, in the act of turning the child in delivery. The arm was ecchymosed, and the dislocation was very distinct.[4]

Pathological Anatomy.—The head of the radius is carried forwards upon the humerus, and sometimes a little inwards or outwards; the anterior and external lateral ligaments, with the annular, are generally more or less broken. Sometimes the anterior and external lateral are alone broken, the annular ligament being then sufficiently stretched to allow of the complete dislocation; or the anterior and annular having given way, the external lateral may remain intact.

Fig. 234.

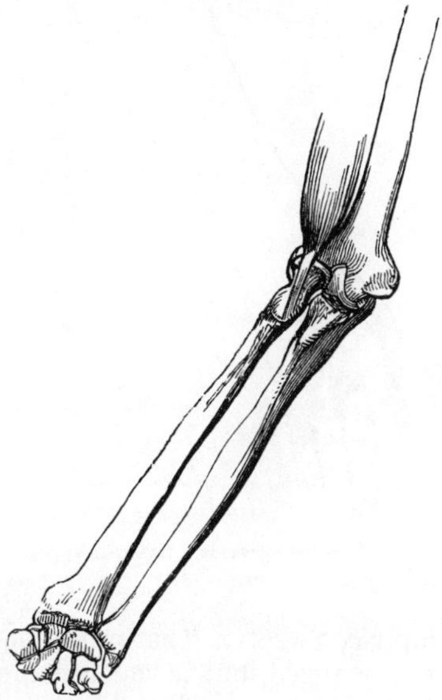

Head of radius forwards. Anatomical relations.

Symptoms.—The head of the radius can in general be distinctly felt in its new situation, rotating under the finger when the hand is pronated and supinated; we may sometimes also recognize a depression corresponding to its natural situation, behind and below the little head of the humerus. The external border of the forearm is slightly shortened, and the arm inclines unnaturally outwards. The tendon of the biceps is relaxed. The forearm is generally pronated, sometimes it is in a position midway between supination and pronation, but I have never seen it supinated. I have particularly noticed this fact in my report made to the New York State Medical Society in 1855, and Denucé, who has also examined these cases carefully, affirms that it is seldom supinated, notwithstanding the general statements of surgeons to the contrary.

The arm is usually a little flexed, and cannot be perfectly extended without causing pain; nor can it be flexed much, if at all, beyond a right angle, owing to the impediment offered by the humerus, against which the head of the radius now impinges.

Prognosis.—Denucé says, "The reduction is often impossible, more frequently still, difficult to maintain." In proof of which he refers to

[1] New York Journ. Med., May, 1856, p. 333.
[2] Amer. Journ. Med. Sci., vol. xxxi. p. 206, Jan. 1843.
[3] Ibid., vol. xxxii. p. 228, July, 1843.
[4] Krackowitzer, New York Journ. Med., March, 1856, p. 262.

the observations of Danyau and Robert. In the case of recent luxation related by Robert, it was found impossible to maintain a reduction which he thought he had several times accomplished, and he believed that the difficulty consisted in a portion of the torn annular ligament having become entangled between the head of the radius and the condyle of the humerus.[1]

Fig. 235.

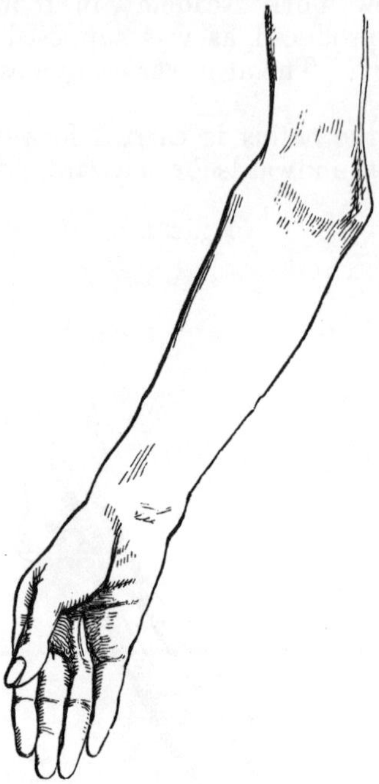

Head of radius forwards. External appearance of limb.

Sir Astley Cooper was unable to accomplish the reduction in two recent cases; and of the six cases which came under his immediate observation, only two were ever reduced. In Bransby Cooper's edition of Sir Astley's work, other similar examples of non-reduction are related.

Malgaigne says that in a collection of twenty-five cases which he has made, the accident was unrecognized or neglected in six, and ineffectual efforts at reduction had been made in eleven; so that only eight of the whole number were reduced.

I have myself met with five of these simple dislocations which were not reduced, two of which, however, had not been recognized, and no attempts at reduction had ever been made; one had been treated by an empiric, Sweet, a "natural bone-setter," but without success; one had been reduced, but it had become reluxated, and in the remaining example I was myself unable to reduce the dislocation on the seventh day.

The following are brief notes of four of these cases:—

A young man, æt. 23, presented himself at my office, upon whom the accident had occurred about one year before. The surgeon who was first called did not recognize the dislocation, and no attempt had ever been made to replace the bones. The forearm was forcibly pronated and could not be supinated, but he could extend it completely, and flex it somewhat beyond a right angle. It was strong, and nearly as useful as before.

H. H. B., æt. 6; dislocation produced by a fall upon the elbow. The surgeon who was called did not detect the nature of the injury. Eighteen years after, I found the head of the radius lying in front of the old socket, having formed a new socket in which it moved freely. From the elbow to the hand the arm inclined outwards, or to the

[1] Mémoire sur les Luxations du Coude, par Paul Denucé. Paris, 1854.

radial side; pronation and supination were perfect. He could flex the arm to an acute angle, but not so completely as the other. The arm was as strong as the other, but it was frequently hurt by lifting.

Ira E. Irish, æt. 12. "Sweet" was at first employed, but failed to reduce it. Thirty-nine years after, when Mr. Irish was fifty-one years old, I examined the arm. He could not flex the forearm upon the arm beyond a right angle; and when the attempt was made, the radius struck against the humerus. Complete supination was impossible. The arm was as strong as the other except in raising a weight above his head. Occasionally he was annoyed with slight pains in this limb.

Urias Lett, a colored barber of Buffalo, aged forty-eight years, was thrown from a carriage, producing a dislocation of the right radius, and severely bruising the elbow-joint. He drove a couple of spirited horses several miles after the accident, and did not see Dr. K., a highly accomplished young surgeon, until six hours had elapsed. The elbow was then much swollen and exquisitely tender, and Lett would not permit much if any examination, to enable Dr. K. to determine his condition. The Dr. applied simple dressings, and the next day requested me to see him. The whole arm was then swollen and tender, and very little examination was admissible. The dressings were, therefore, not completely removed, but only laid open sufficiently to enable us to see the joint. We suspected a forward luxation of the head of the radius, but could not positively determine the point—the patient not permitting any kind or degree of manipulation. We decided, therefore, to wait a few days, until the inflammation had somewhat abated, and then, if the existence of a dislocation was ascertained, to attempt its reduction. On the seventh day the swelling had measurably subsided, and the diagnosis became satisfactory. We immediately placed him under the complete influence of chloroform, and made long continued and violent efforts at reduction, but without success. Severe inflammation again followed these efforts, and Lett would never consent to another trial. After four years, I find the bone still out. He can flex the forearm upon the arm almost as far as he can the opposite limb; he can carry it nearly to his mouth; the head of the radius sliding off upon the outer face of the humerus, and not resting plumply against it; indeed, the radius seems to have been gradually pushed outwards as well as forwards. The hand is forcibly pronated, and cannot be supinated. The attempt to supine produces a click in the neighborhood of the head of the radius, as if it struck against a bone. The arm is as strong as the other, and not wasted. He has constantly pursued his occupation as a barber, after only a few weeks confinement.

If the dislocation is accompanied with a fracture of the ulna, unless the fracture is transverse or incomplete, reduction is not generally accomplished. When speaking of fractures of the shaft of the ulna, I have related several examples illustrative of this remark. Norris has made the same observation.[1] I have, however, three times met with this accident thus complicated in children, in the treatment of which a much better result has been obtained. In the first example, a lad

[1] Norris, Amer. Journ. Med. Sci., vol. xxxi. p. 21.

aged nine years had broken the ulna in its upper third and dislocated the radius forwards. Dr. White, of this city, and myself were in immediate attendance. Both the fracture and dislocation were easily reduced, and in a few weeks the limb was sound and perfect, except that a slight fulness remained in front of the head of the radius, and this continued for several years. In the second example, a lad of the same age as the other, was treated by Dr. Austin Flint and myself. We reduced both the fracture and the dislocation by extending the arm from the wrist, while at the same moment pressure was made upon the head of the radius from before backwards. A right-angled splint was applied and continued during a period of four weeks, being removed daily for the purpose of giving to the joint gentle, passive motion, &c. After this the arm was permitted to straighten gradually, and at the end of a month more, the joint was moving freely, and with no degree of displacement at the point of fracture or dislocation.

It is quite probable that in each of the above cases the separation was not complete, although crepitus was distinct, and the displacement of the broken ends was very marked. In the following case the fracture was certainly incomplete:—

Elizabeth Carmody, æt. 4, was brought to me, August 6, 1851, with a fracture of the ulna, two inches below its upper end, the fragments being inclined backwards, while the radius was dislocated forwards. Both bones were easily replaced, and the functions of the arm were soon completely restored.[1]

Where the restoration has been promptly effected and maintained steadily, the motions of the joint are soon restored; but in one case the head of the radius has been found to play very freely and loosely after the lapse of two years, and in others it has remained slightly prominent in front, as if it was a little in advance of its socket.

Treatment.—Extension and counter-extension should be made in the direction in which we already find the limb, namely, with the forearm slightly bent upon the arm, while at the same moment the surgeon should seize the elbow with his hands, and press the head of the radius back with his two thumbs.

Other methods will often succeed; but by this we relax the biceps, and put the parts in the best position to accomplish the reduction easily and promptly. Sir Astley directed to supine the forearm while the extension was being made from the hand, but Denucé prefers that the forearm should be in a position of pronation.

After the reduction is effected it is never safe to straighten the arm completely at once, nor indeed for some weeks; not until the ligaments have been sufficiently restored to resist the action of the biceps. The arm must therefore be flexed and placed in a sling, or, if the radius is disposed to become reluxated, a right-angled splint ought to be placed upon the back of the arm and forearm, and, by the aid of a compress and roller, an attempt should be made to retain it in place.

Nor will it be found safe at any period to compel the arm by force

[1] This case was erroneously reported to the N. Y. State Medical Society as an example of fracture of the radius, with dislocation.

to resume the straight position, since this bone, when it has once been dislocated, will for a long time be liable to luxation.

A boy, aged about four years, was presented at my clinic by his father, having a forward dislocation of the head of the radius. The dislocation still existed after several months. The father's purpose in bringing the child was to ascertain whether he could not claim damages for malpractice. The account which he gave was as follows: The surgeon called it a dislocation forwards, and pretended to reduce it. A right-angled splint was applied, with a roller. At the end of three weeks the father removed the splint, but did not discover anything out of place. Finding, however, that the elbow was stiff, he took measures to straighten it forcibly. In a few days he discovered the head of the bone out of place, and so it has remained ever since.

I explained to him that there was much reason to suppose that the surgeon had properly reduced the dislocation, and that he had himself reproduced the accident, by straightening the arm, through the action of the biceps upon the upper end of the radius. The father declined any further surgical interference, and no prosecution has followed.

Dr. Batchelder, of New York, in a very excellent paper on dislocations of the head of the radius, describes a method of reduction suggested to him first by Dr. Goodhue, of Chester, Vermont, and which he has himself found more successful than any other method; indeed, he says it never fails, yet he does not inform us in precisely how many cases he has made the trial. The plan suggested by Dr. Goodhue consists essentially in first making extension from the hand, and pressing at the same time downwards and backwards upon the head of the radius until it has descended to a level with the articulating surface of the humerus. As soon as this is accomplished, the forearm is to be suddenly flexed upon the arm in such a direction as that the hand shall pass outside of the shoulder; at the same moment, also, the pressure must be continued vigorously upon the head of the radius.[1]

§ 2. Dislocation of the Head of the Radius Backwards.

Denucé has collected fourteen examples of this luxation; but Malgaigne, who rejects a portion of these cases, and adds one or two more, admits only twelve. In addition to those mentioned by these two writers, I have found recorded, or incidentally noticed, one by May,[2] one by Bransby Cooper,[3] one by Lawrence,[4] one by Liston,[5] two by Case,[6] two by Gibson,[7] one by Parker,[8] three by Markoe,[9] and to these

[1] Goodhue, New York Journ. of Med., May, 1856, p. 333.

[2] May, Sir Astley Cooper on Dislocations, &c., by B. Cooper, op. cit., p. 403.

[3] B. Cooper, ibid., p. 404.

[4] Lawrence, Pirrie's System of Surgery, p. 259.

[5] Liston, Practical Surgery, p. 88.

[6] Case, Amer. Journ. of Med. Sci., vol. vi. p. 254, from 11th No. of Provincial Med. Gazette.

[7] Gibson, Institutes and Practice of Surgery, 6th ed., vol. i. p. 379.

[8] Parker, New York Journ. of Med., March, 1852, p. 188.

[9] Markoe, ibid., May, 1855, p. 382.

my own observations have added four more, in all twenty-eight supposed examples.

Of the examples brought under my own notice I have already in the preceding section affirmed that two of them were accompanied with fracture, and I am not entirely certain but that they all were. Markoe, of New York, whom we have mentioned as having reported three cases, found in each case a fracture of the internal condyle of the humerus, and, after an examination of a number of the reported examples, he does not find any evidence that this dislocation ever occurs as a simple uncomplicated accident. I am unable to complete the critical analysis which Dr. Markoe has undertaken; yet I confess that, so far as I have been able to do so, the testimony strongly confirms his conclusions. While I am prepared to admit the possibility of the luxation without either a fracture of the lower end of the humerus or of the ulna, I have found no written account of any case, nor have I seen an example, which was absolutely conclusive.

The example reported by Parker as having occurred in the practice of N. K. Freeman, of New York, is one of the few which seems to admit of but very little doubt.

In July, 1850, Dr. Freeman was called to see a gentleman, æt. 37, who was seriously injured by jumping from the railroad cars while they were in motion, and found a backward luxation of the head of the radius of the right arm. "The symptoms," says Dr. Freeman, "were marked; the hand and forearm were prone, and the attempt to place them in the supine position caused great pain; while the head of the radius formed a considerable projection posterior to the external condyle of the humerus, where the cavity on its extremity could be distinctly felt. Assisted by Dr. Walsh, of Fordham, who firmly grasped the humerus, I was enabled to reduce it by extending the forearm and flexing it upon the arm, at the same time pronating the hand, and pressing forwards the head of the radius with my thumb. After the reduction was effected, I requested Dr. Walsh to examine it; when, upon slight extension being made upon the forearm, with supination of the hand, the bone was again dislocated. I immediately reduced it in the same manner as before, and directed the patient to keep the forearm flexed and the hand prone, and, laying it upon a pillow, apply cold water. He complained of severe pain for two days, which gradually subsided, and on the fourth day he was able to move and extend the forearm."

Causes.—A direct blow upon the front and upper part of the radius; a fall upon the elbow, or upon the hand; a violent effort to supine the forearm while it is grasped and held firmly in a state of pronation; probably, also, sometimes it is occasioned by a twisting of the arm in machinery, &c.

Pathological Anatomy.—In the only example of which a dissection has been made, reported by Sir Astley Cooper, "the coronary ligament was found to be torn through at its forepart, and the oblique had given way. The capsular ligament was partially torn, and the head would have receded much more, had it not been supported by the fascia which extends over the muscles of the forearm." The head of the radius was thrown behind the external condyle of the humerus, and rather to the outer side. This was an ancient luxation found in the dissecting-room of St. Thomas's Hospital, and the accompanying drawing is copied from the sketch made at the time.

Fig. 236.

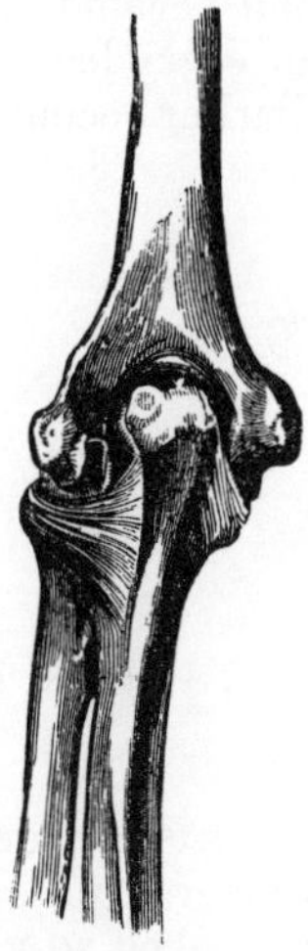

Dislocation of the head of the radius backwards.

If the luxation is not complete, as occasionally happens with children, the annular ligament may not be torn.

Symptoms.—The head of the bone is felt rotating behind the outer condyle, and a depression exists corresponding to its original position. The forearm is slightly flexed and prone; and the whole arm is deflected outwards from the elbow downwards; flexion and extension are difficult, while supination is impossible.

Treatment.—Most surgeons have agreed that while extension and counter-extension are being made, the forearm should be forcibly supinated. At the same time, also, the head of the radius must be strongly pushed forwards. Martin recommends to extend forcibly, and then suddenly flex the arm, in a manner very similar to the plan recommended by Batchelder in dislocations forwards. In Dr. Freeman's case, just quoted, the reduction was effected while the forearm was prone, and supination seemed to throw it again out of place.

According to Markoe, where the accident is complicated with a fracture of the inner condyle, when the reduction is accomplished the arm should be placed in a position about ten degrees less than a right angle, and supported by a splint with bandages, &c.

If the dislocation is simple, however, I can see no objections to its being nearly or quite extended, since in this dislocation the action of the biceps would only tend to retain the head of the radius in place.

§ 3. Dislocation of the Head of the Radius Outwards.

Denucé has collected four examples of this accident, unaccompanied with a fracture, and he proceeds to speak of it as a distinct form of dislocation. In two of the examples, however, mentioned by him, it was consecutive upon a forward luxation, and I have several times seen the head of the radius very much inclined outwards in what are properly termed forward dislocations. For these reasons it is not very plain to me that we ought to consider this even as a distinct form of primary dislocation, but rather as a consecutive luxation, or at least as only a modification of the forward or backward luxation. Indeed, I think the radius never will be found thrown directly outwards, but always in a direction inclining forwards or backwards.

Parker, of New York, mentions a case which came under his notice, in a child four years old, who six weeks before, had fallen down stairs "backwardly, with the right arm twisted behind the back, in such a position that the whole weight of her body came upon her arm." No attempt was ever made to reduce the bone, and the head of the radius continued to project externally. By pressure it was easily reduced, but became immediately displaced when the forearm was either flexed or extended. The motions of the joint were completely restored. Dr. Parker recommended no treatment.[1]

CHAPTER VIII.

DISLOCATIONS OF THE UPPER END OF THE ULNA BACKWARDS.

THIS accident, the existence of which as a simple luxation, is rendered probable by a certain number of cases, has nevertheless been described so variously and often indefinitely, that it is impossible to declare its history, except in a few points, with any degree of accuracy. No doubt many of the cases which have been reported were examples only of a subluxation of both radius and ulna backwards. In other cases the radius or the external condyle of the humerus being broken, the ulna has been actually displaced, not only backwards but upwards; indeed it is very certain that without either a luxation of the radius, or a fracture with displacement of the external condyle of the humerus, or a fracture or bending of the radius, an upward displacement of the ulna, to the degree represented by the reporters of these cases, could never have occurred. The example mentioned by Sir Astley Cooper, and of which a dissection was made, is plainly a case of subluxation of both bones; or if the luxation of the ulna may be regarded as having been complete, the head of the radius was also displaced more or less upwards from its original socket, a new socket, Sir Astley himself informs us, having been formed for its reception, upon the external condyle. But this is the only example, the actual condition of which has been proven by an autopsy.

Nevertheless it seems possible that a simple luxation, or subluxation of the ulna backwards, may occur without either of the above mentioned complications, and that, to the extent of a few lines, it may be made to pass upwards upon the back of the humerus, by the falling of the forearm to the ulnar side; in which case the character of the accident would probably be recognized by the projection of the olecranon process, while the head of the radius might be felt moving in its socket—by the partial flexion and complete pronation of the forearm, and by the general immobility of the joint.

[1] Parker, New York Journ. Med., March, 1852, p. 189.

Its reduction ought to be accomplished easily by the same measures which have been found successful in reducing a dislocation of both bones backwards.

Fig. 237.

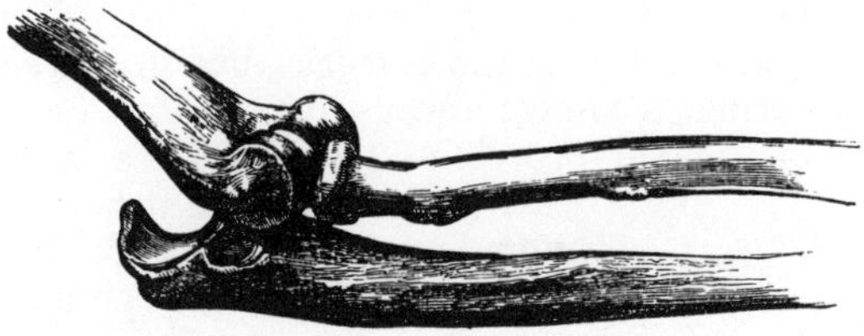

Dislocation of the upper end of the ulna backwards.

Pirrie says that in a case occurring in the practice of Mr. Gosset, in which the coronoid process rested on the internal condyle, and the pain on bending the arm was insupportable, owing, it was supposed, to the pressure of the coronoid process against the ulnar nerve, "reduction was accomplished by extension and counter-extension applied by two persons pulling in opposite directions, and by the pressure of the olecranon process downwards and outwards, while the forearm was suddenly flexed."[1]

CHAPTER IX.

DISLOCATIONS OF THE RADIUS AND ULNA (FORE-ARM AT THE ELBOW-JOINT.)

THE radius and ulna may be dislocated at the elbow-joint, backwards; laterally, that is, either inwards, or outwards; and forwards.

§ 1. DISLOCATIONS OF THE RADIUS AND ULNA BACKWARDS.

Causes.—In thirty-three cases observed by me, the average age is about nineteen years; the youngest being four years old, and the oldest fifty-three. Nineteen of this number occurred in children under fourteen years of age.

Generally the dislocation has been produced by a fall upon the palm of the hand, as when in running a person has fallen forwards with the forearm extended in front of the body, or he may have fallen from a height; once I have known it produced by a blow received upon the back and lower part of the humerus.

[1] Gosset, Pirrie's Surg., Amer. ed., p. 259.

It is said also to be produced occasionally by twisting the forearm violently, as when the limb has been caught and wrenched about by machinery, by a blow upon the front and upper part of the forearm, and by forced flexion.

Pathology.—The radius and ulna are not only carried backwards behind the articulating surface of the humerus, but they are also, through the action of the triceps, almost always drawn more or less upwards, so that often the coronoid process of the ulna rests in the olecranon fossa. In some cases it has been known to mount even higher, while in others it is arrested short of this point. The radius still retaining its relative position to the ulna, lies upon the back of the humerus, or rather upon the posterior margin of its articulating surface.

Fig. 238.

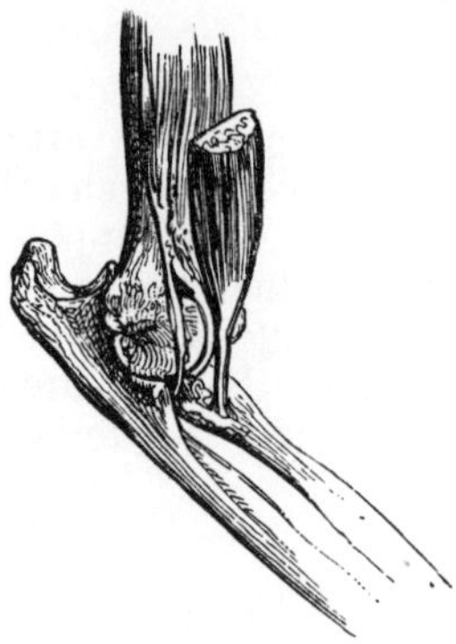

Dislocation of the radius and ulna backwards.

The anterior and two lateral ligaments are generally more or less completely torn asunder; but the posterior ligament and the annular do not usually suffer disruption.

The biceps muscle is drawn over the lower articulating surface of the humerus, but is in a condition of only moderate tension, while the brachialis anticus is forcibly stretched or even torn.

The median nerve is also pressed upon in front by the humerus, and the ulnar is occasionally painfully stretched over the projecting extremity of the ulna from behind.

Symptoms.—Sir Astley Cooper does not mention particularly the position of the arm as to flexion or extension, except to say that "the flexion of the joint is in a great degree lost;" nor, in his original work, published in London in 1823, is there any illustration accompanying the text to indicate in what position he had usually seen the limb; but in the later editions, edited by Mr. Bransby Cooper, is found a drawing which represents the forearm at a right angle with the arm. It is very certain that Sir Astley never sanctioned this error by anything which he had written or communicated to others. It is very certain, I say, because the fact that it seldom, if ever, occupies this position could not have escaped the notice of one whose experience was so large, and whose habits of observation were generally so accurate. The truth is that it is almost constantly found only slightly flexed, or forming an angle in front of about 120°.

This fact is especially noticed in my records twenty-one times, and if it had ever been found in any other position it would certainly have been stated. Once, where the dislocation was accompanied with a fracture of the outer condyle of the humerus, the arm was at first straight, a position in which it is said to be found occasionally with children, but never in any instance have I found it flexed to a right angle; yet I will not deny that such unusual phenomena are possible;

indeed, it is certain that they have occasionally been presented, but they must be regarded as only exceptional, and as by no means diagnostic of this accident.

Sir Astley Cooper and Miller declare that in this dislocation the forearm is usually supine; Pirrie says: "The hand is between pronation and supination, but more inclined to the latter;" Desault thinks it is sometimes in supination and sometimes in pronation; Denucé concludes that it will occupy that position, whatever it may be, in which the force of the blow has thrown it; while by most surgical writers no allusion is made to the position of the forearm in reference to pronation or supination. For myself, I can only say that I have found the forearm and hand constantly in a position of moderate, but positive, pronation, and I am compelled to regard it, therefore, as one of the usual signs of a backward dislocation of these bones.

The limb can be neither flexed nor extended without force, and such motion is almost always accompanied with pain. It is, however, possible in most cases to give to the arm a slight lateral motion, such as does not belong to it in its natural condition.

In front and deep in the fold of the elbow is felt the lower end of the humerus, forming a hard, broad, and somewhat irregular projection, over which the integuments and muscles are swollen, and tender to pressure. Behind, the head of the radius may be felt, when not much tumefaction exists, rotating or moving under the finger when the forearm is supinated and pronated; while the olecranon process projects strongly backwards and upwards. If now we flex the arm slightly, this projection of the olecranon process will be sensibly increased; but if an attempt is made to straighten the arm, it will be diminished, the reverse of what we have seen to happen in cases of fracture of the lower end of the humerus (at the base of the condyles). This circumstance becomes, therefore, an important diagnostic mark between these two accidents.

The relation of the olecranon process also to the condyles is changed, and the upper end of this process, instead of being a little below the internal condyle, as it would be naturally when the arm is slightly flexed, is found generally carried upwards toward the shoulder, from half an inch to one inch or more above the condyle.

Measuring from the internal condyle to the styloid process of the ulna, the arm is shortened; the same result will be obtained also by measuring from the acromion process, to either of the styloid processes; while from the acromion process to the condyle, the length will be the same in both arms.

The signs which have now been enumerated will be sufficient to enable us to make the diagnosis promptly in the great majority of cases, but if considerable swelling has already taken place, the diagnosis may be rendered exceedingly difficult, if not impossible; and in such cases we should confine the patient at once to his bed, and proceed to reduce the tumefaction by cool water lotions as rapidly as possible, examining the limb carefully from day to day in order that we may seize the earliest opportunity to ascertain its actual condition and apply the proper remedy.

In relation to the difficulty of diagnosis in certain examples of this accident, and under certain circumstances, Mr. Skey, in his *Operative Surgery*, has made some very judicious remarks.

"Severe injuries of the elbow-joint, whether in the form of fracture, dislocation, or a compound of the two, are frequently followed, at a short interval, by swelling of a formidable kind, in which it is impossible, but by the aid of a perfect intimacy with the anatomical structure of the joint, to detect the relations of one part with another; but even under this difficulty, the two points in question are readily distinguishable. In such forms of swelling, the arm, including the length of six inches both above and below the joint, may be involved in the extravasation, and this swelling may distend the arm to a circumference of one-third beyond its natural size. In such circumstances, in which it is impossible to determine with any certainty whether any, or what bones are broken, or whether or not dislocated, the difficulty of the case should at once be stated to the friends of the patient."

Prognosis.—If the luxation is recent, reduction is in general easily effected, but if considerable time has elapsed, the reduction is often accomplished with difficulty. As to the probability of its reluxation, I have already spoken when considering the subject of fractures of the coronoid process. Unless this process is broken, it is not likely to occur except where some violence has again been applied. It has happened to me, however, to find these bones unreduced in several instances. In some of these examples surgeons recognized the accident and supposed that they had accomplished reduction, while in others the dislocation was mistaken for a fracture.

A lad, W. F., twelve years old, residing in this county, was brought to me six weeks after the accident had occurred. The surgeon who was first called declared it to be a dislocation, and told the parents he had reduced it; but the dislocation was now complete, and the arm immovably fixed in its abnormal position.

On the tenth of May, 1850, J. P., of Canada West, æt. 25, was thrown from a load of hay, striking upon his left hand, and producing a dislocation backwards of both bones at the elbow-joint. A Canadian surgeon, who saw the patient within three hours, recognized the dislocation, and by pulling the arm straight forwards he supposed he had reduced it; the patient also thought he felt the bones slip into place. No attempt was made subsequently to flex the arm, and it was immediately dressed with a straight splint laid along the palmar surface. On the sixth day it was found to be unreduced, and the surgeon again attempted to reduce it as before, and thought he had succeeded. The same splint was reapplied. At about the end of six weeks three surgeons, residing in Canada also, placed the patient under the complete influence of chloroform, and attempted the reduction. They first made extension for half an hour in a straight line, then five men seized upon the arm and forearm, bending it with great force to a right angle. It was now believed that the ulna was reduced, but not the radius. Four days after, the attempt was renewed. Three months after the accident the young man called upon me, and I found the arm nearly straight, with almost complete anchylosis at the elbow-joint

Both the radius and ulna were displaced backwards, but not upwards. The arm was of the same length with the other, and the relation of the condyles to the olecranon was so manifest, that the absence of the usual displacement upwards was easily determined. I was unwilling to make any further attempts at reduction, not believing that I should succeed after so much time had elapsed, and after so many ineffectual attempts had been made by clever surgeons.

In the following examples the dislocation was supposed to have been a fracture of the lower end of the humerus.

A man, residing in Pittsfield, Mass., dislocated his left arm by falling from a horse. The surgeon who was called regarded it as a fracture at the base of the condyles, and treated it accordingly. Ten weeks after, the error was discovered and an attempt was made to reduce it, but without success. A second attempt was also made with the same result.

The patient was brought to me eight months after the accident with the bones still unreduced. The forearm hung at a very obtuse angle with the arm, and there was very slight motion at the elbow-joint. I discouraged any further attempts at reduction.

Mr. W., of Alleghany Co., N. Y., æt. 43, fell from a load of hay striking upon his left arm, Feb. 16, 1853. Four hours after he was seen by a young, but very intelligent surgeon, who thought the humerus was broken just above the condyles. After eight weeks, the fact that it was a dislocation having become apparent, three surgeons, well known to me as men of large experience, attempted its reduction, aided by pulleys and chloroform. The patient was also bled and nauseated with antimony. The efforts were protracted through many hours, and frequently varied. A second attempt made by these same gentlemen a few days after was equally unsuccessful.

On the ninth week Mr. W. came to me, and I placed him at once in the Buffalo Hospital of the Sisters of Charity, where, assisted by my friend, Prof. Moore, of Rochester, I renewed the attempts at reduction. The patient was placed under the influence of chloroform, and during a great portion of the time occupied the pulleys were in use. The elbow was pulled upon, twisted, flexed and extended until there seemed to be neither adhesions, nor ligaments, nor capsule to prevent the reduction. We could move the joint in every direction, even laterally, as well as forwards and backwards. Still the bones would not return to their sockets. Section of the triceps seemed to be the only remaining expedient, but the injury already done to the joint was so great that we did not deem it prudent to prosecute the attempt any further. We had occupied two hours in the various procedures. Violent inflammation supervened, but he was able to return home in about two weeks. Two years after, I learned that the arm still remained unreduced, and nearly anchylosed; the whole limb was also much atrophied and very weak.

John Sharkie, æt. 53, fell on the 4th of Aug., 1854. A botanic doctor, who saw him on the same day, and a regular physician, who saw him on the third day, thought he had broken his arm. About six weeks after this he came under the charge of an almshouse doctor, who "rebroke" it, supposing it to be a fracture; and two months later he "broke" it again, but as the arm was not improved by these operations he finally urged the poor fellow to submit to amputation; and it was in reference to this last proposition that Sharkie consulted me. I found the radius and ulna dislocated backwards and upwards one inch; the arm perfectly straight and the elbow anchylosed; no pronation or supination. I did not think it prudent to make any attempt to reduce it, but assured him that if let alone it would ultimately be quite useful in many ways, and that he should never think of having it cut off.

In three or four instances, also, the accident has been overlooked by the patient himself, or by some empiric, no surgeon having been called to see the case until after the lapse of several days or weeks.

In general, when the reduction has been effected promptly, the patients have recovered the complete use of the elbow-joint within a few weeks; but many exceptions have from time to time come under my notice.

A lad eight years old was brought to me, whose arm had been dislocated six months before, and the reduction of which had been accomplished easily and promptly by Sir Astley Cooper's method. At this time the arm was bent to a right angle, and quite stiff at the elbow-joint. Four years later I learned that the stiffness still continued in a great measure, with only slight improvement.

Fig. 239.

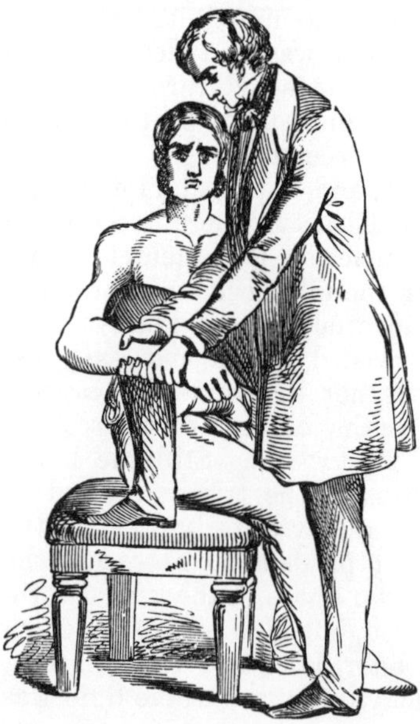

Reduction with the knee in the bend of the elbow.

Treatment.—Sir Astley Cooper thus describes his own method of reducing this dislocation (Fig. 239): "The patient is made to sit upon a chair, and the surgeon, placing his knee on the inner side of the elbow-joint, in the bend of the arm, takes hold of the patient's wrist, and bends the arm. At the same time he presses on the radius and ulna with his knee, so as to separate them from the os humeri, and thus the coronoid process is thrown from the posterior fossa of the humerus; and whilst this pressure is supported by the knee, the arm is to be forcibly but slowly bent, and the reduction is soon effected."

The same practice has been recommended by Erichsen, Gibson, Samuel Cooper, and others. The plan recommended by Dorsey is nearly identical with that just described, only that, instead of the knee, he advises that the surgeon "interlock his fingers in front of the arm, just above the elbow, and draw it backwards."

On the other hand, Liston and Miller recommend, as a better mode of proceeding, that the patient shall be seated upon a chair, and that the arm and forearm shall be pulled directly backwards, so as to relax as completely as possible the triceps muscle while counter-extension is made against the scapula.

Skey says: "Extension of the forearm should be made from the hand or wrist in a straight direction downwards, as if for the purpose of simply elongating the arm."

Pirrie prefers that an assistant shall grasp the forearm near its middle, instead of the wrist, and pull the arm straight forwards, while at the same moment the surgeon seizes upon the olecranon process with the fingers of one hand, and, placing the palm of the other against the front and upper part of the forearm, pulls forcibly backwards, so as to draw out the coronoid process from the olecranon fossa.

For myself, having generally practised the method recommended by Sir Astley, and having usually succeeded in the first attempt and with the employment of only moderate force, I confess that my predilections are in its favor; yet I am not entirely certain but that an equal experience with either of the other modes recommended might have changed these convictions. The truth is, I think, that in recent cases very little force is generally requisite to accomplish the reduction, and that it is not very material which of these several modes we adopt; but in case of a failure by one mode, we ought immediately and without hesitation to resort to another, as the following case of failure by flexion will illustrate:—

A lad, æt. 11, fell in a gymnasium from a height of six feet, striking probably upon his hand. I saw him within twenty minutes, and found the arm in the usual position. I attempted immediately to reduce it by Sir Astley's method, but, after a fair yet unsuccessful trial, I extended the forearm upon the arm until it was nearly straight, and then, with only moderate force, drew it promptly into place.

If we still continue to encounter difficulties, the patient ought at once to be placed under the influence of an anæsthetic, and, if necessary, the pulleys should be employed.

When the reduction is accomplished, which is indicated generally by the sudden slipping of the bones and by the restoration of the natural form to the elbow-joint, the surgeon, in order to confirm his opinion, must flex the forearm upon the arm to a right angle. If the bones are in place, and there is not much swelling, this can generally be done without causing much, if any, pain; but if it cannot be done, this fact furnishes presumptive evidence that the reduction is not effected. In one instance, however, of recent luxation, this rule has not held good. A girl, æt. 10, fell from a tree upon her hand. I was in attendance within half an hour, and found the usual signs characterizing this accident. Reduction was accomplished readily by pulling at the hand moderately, with the forearm flexed, while my left hand pressed back the lower part of the humerus. After the reduction it was found impossible to flex the arm to a right angle without causing severe pain, and it became necessary, after placing it in a sling, to allow the hand to drop very low beside the body. A good deal of inflammation followed; but in a few weeks the arm was well, only that for a period of two years or more the elbow remained very tender.

On the other hand, an omission to apply this rule has often led the surgeon to believe the reduction accomplished when it was not. Very recently this same thing has happened to myself, and as it is the only instance in which I have omitted to adopt this test, and the only one also in which I have left a bone unreduced which I believed to have been reduced, it will be proper to state the case and its results more fully.

A lad, æt. 11, fell from a fence on the 22d of December, 1858, and dislocated both bones backwards. I saw him within two hours from the occurrence of the accident. The elbow was already considerably swollen and quite tender, but the signs of dislocation were very manifest. Seizing the wrist with one hand, and placing my knee against the front and lower part of the humerus, I pulled steadily for some time, and with much more force than is usually necessary, until at length two distinct and successive snaps were felt, such as one often feels when the two bones resume their sockets. Relinquishing my grasp, it was observed by myself and the parents that the deformity had disappeared. The reduction seemed to be complete, and so I announced. I then requested the lad to permit me to bend the elbow, and place it in a sling, but this he peremptorily refused to do, and ran away from me, nor would any arguments or entreaties persuade him to allow me again to touch it. I reassured the parents and child, however, that all was right, and left the house. During several successive days I saw the little patient, but although the arm remained swollen and very tender, I did not suspect the cause until the ninth day; and on the tenth day, having placed him under the influence of chloroform, the reduction was easily and satisfactorily accomplished. The recovery has been slow. At the end of six weeks I found the motions of the elbow-joint not completely restored, and the forefinger was partially paralyzed; but from this condition it has gradually recovered, and two months later the functions of the arm and hand were completely restored.

The mistake in this instance was the more mortifying because I had just seen a case in a lad only a little older, in which another surgeon had committed the same error, and after the lapse of twelve or fourteen days I had myself made the reduction; and I was fully awake, therefore, to the possibility of the mistake.

The circumstance of the diminution and apparent disappearance of the deformity, and the sensation of a double click, can only be explained by assuming that originally the coronoid process was resting in the olecranon fossa, and that by manipulation the bones had been removed nearer their sockets, yet not actually reduced. The swelling, also, rendered more difficult a diagnosis which, now, nothing but the flexion of the forearm could have determined positively.

If much time has elapsed since the occurrence of the dislocation the reduction is accomplished with difficulty, if, indeed, it can be reduced at all. There are many cases upon record, however, in which surgeons have been successful after the lapse of many weeks, or even months. Boyer thought it was not possible to effect the reduction after four or six weeks; but Capelletti, of Trieste, succeeded after seventy days;[1] Sir Astley Cooper at three months;[2] Malgaigne after three months and twenty-one days.[3] Roux succeeded in the case of a young man, twenty-two years of age, whose elbow had been dislocated five months.[4] Blackman, of Cincinnati, informs me that he has reduced a lateral luxation after five months. Brainard, of Chicago, reduced a dislocated elbow in a boy of nineteen years, after five months and thirteen days. In this case the surgeon who had first seen the patient supposed that he had reduced the dislocation.[5] Gorre, Gerdy, and Drake, succeeded in four cases after six months;[6] and finally, Starch claims to have been successful after two years and one month.[7] To which enumeration Denucé has added seventeen other examples, said to have been reduced at various periods, ranging from one month to one hundred and fourteen days.[8]

Nevertheless the fact is in the main as stated by Boyer; and if so many cases can be found in which surgeons have succeeded at a later period, they are not probably in the proportion of one to ten as compared with the failures; but the failures have not received the same publicity. Nor indeed have all the severe accidents, such as violent inflammation, suppuration, gangrene, and even death, been faithfully declared. Denucé says he has been able to trace out five or six examples in which, although the arm was reduced, grave accidents resulted, and Velpeau's patient actually died in consequence.

Dixi Crosby, of New Hampshire, has treated two cases of ancient dislocation of the forearm backwards, by bending the elbow forcibly so as to break the olecranon process, after which the reduction was easily accomplished by extension. R. D. Mussey, of Cincinnati, has succeeded once in the same manner. In all these examples the elbow was restored to a very useful amount of motion.[9]

The dislocation being reduced, it may be a matter of prudence sometimes to apply a right-angled splint, first carefully padded, to the palmar surface of the arm and forearm; remembering, however, that considerable swelling will soon occur, and that it ought not therefore to be bandaged to the limb very tightly. At least once a day it should be removed, and the arm examined; and in very few cases can it be necessary or judicious to continue its application beyond one week. At the same time if there is any especial tendency in the radius to become displaced backwards, owing to a rupture of its annular ligament, this must be prevented, if possible, by a compress and bandage. Some surgeons regard these precautions as necessary in all cases, but I have seldom employed any splint or bandage whatever, nor have I ever had reason to regret this omission.

Finally, we are to place the arm in a sling, and adopt such measures

1 Cappelletti, Am. Journ. Med., vol. xix., from Annal. Univ. de Méd. for Oct. 1835.
2 Sir Astley Cooper, On Dislocations and Fractures, Amer. ed., p. 388.
3 Malgaigne, Am. Journ. Med. Sci., vol. xxiii. p. 238, from Revue Méd., Dec. 1837.
4 Roux, Amer. Journ. Med. Sci., vol. xvi. p. 526, from Archives Gén , Dec. 1834.
5 Brainard, Illinois and Indiana Med. Journ., 1847.
6 Mémoire sur les luxations du coude, par Paul Denucé, Paris, 1854, pp. 86, 87.
7 Denucé, op. cit., p. 87.
8 Op. cit.
9 Crosby, Mussey, Trans. Amer. Med. Assoc., vol. iii. p. 357.

as are calculated at first to reduce the inflammation; and at a very early day we ought to begin to move the elbow-joint, in order to prevent anchylosis.

§ 2. Dislocation of the Radius and Ulna Outwards (to the Radial Side.)

The large majority of outward dislocations of the forearm are incomplete; indeed, only nine examples of a complete dislocation have been collected by Denucé including two seen by himself. Malgaigne has since added two more, making in all eleven cases. All these examples have occurred in the practice of French surgeons. So far as I am able to discover, no American or English surgeon has ever reported a single example.

Incomplete dislocations must therefore in this case be regarded as typical; but even these are by no means frequent.

Causes.—A careful examination of a large number of recorded examples, and of those which have come under my own eye, renders it certain that a majority of these accidents result from a blow received directly upon the inner side of the forearm or upon the outer side of the humerus, or from the action of two forces pressing in an opposite direction. Of course these forces must act upon the bones somewhere in the neighborhood of the elbow-joint. Occasionally it has been produced by a fall upon the hand; sometimes by a violent twist of the arm, as when the hand is caught in machinery; and in other cases it has been found consecutive upon a dislocation backwards, being produced in the attempts made to accomplish reduction of this latter form of dislocation.

Fig. 240.

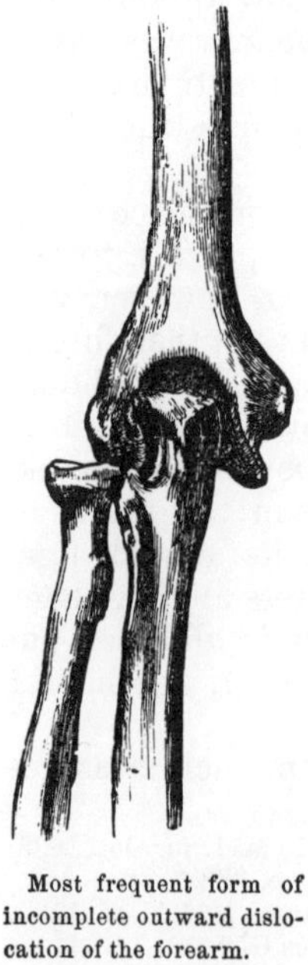

Most frequent form of incomplete outward dislocation of the forearm.

Pathology.—In most of the examples of simple, incomplete outward luxation of the forearm, the great sigmoid cavity of the ulna still embraces the lower end of the humerus, but instead of reposing upon the trochlea, it is carried outwards half an inch or more so as to rest its central crest upon the depression which separates the condyle from the trochlea. (Fig. 240.) If the annular ligament remains unbroken the radius is displaced in the same direction and to the same extent, its head resting against and directly below the epicondyle.

Occasionally, however, where the violence has been greater, the central crest of the great sigmoid cavity rests fairly upon the condyle, or upon the articulating surface of the humerus where the head of the radius was formerly applied, and the dislocation approaches more nearly to the character of a complete luxation. At the same time, owing perhaps to the resistance afforded by the skin, or some of the ligaments, the head of the radius may be thrown either forwards or backwards so as to be out of line with the ulna. Such a displacement generally implies a rupture of the annular ligament.

We have now only to suppose the action of a more considerable force in the same direction to render the dislocation complete; in which case the upper end of the radius is sometimes thrown completely forwards, and its head may even be found resting in front of the ulna, occasioning an extreme pronation of the forearm and hand.

The anconeus and brachialis anticus are the only muscles in either of these dislocations whose fibres are generally much disturbed; the biceps and triceps being only made to traverse the articulation a little more obliquely.

Denucé, Malgaigne, A. Cooper, and others have preferred to speak of the dislocation backwards and outwards as a distinct form or species of dislocation. I prefer to regard it as only a variety of the outward luxation, since it may, and no doubt often does, occur consecutively upon a simple incomplete outward dislocation; and if the dislocation outward is complete, the bones of the forearm can scarcely fail to be drawn more or less upwards. Sometimes also it has been consecutive upon a simple backward dislocation, or upon unsuccessful attempts at reduction where the form of dislocation was originally backwards; yet as it does not so naturally follow upon a complete backward dislocation as upon a complete outward luxation, I find sufficient reason for studying its mechanism in this place.

The beak of the olecranon process not only, but a large portion of the body of this process now lies above and behind the condyle; the brachialis anticus becomes more stretched if not actually torn, and the biceps is laid against the articulating surface of the humerus; but the triceps becomes again relaxed, as in simple dislocation backwards and upwards.

In all these dislocations the capsular ligaments are more or less extensively torn, but the principal arteries and nerves do not generally suffer greatly if at all.

Symptoms.—The forearm is usually flexed to about the same angle at which we have found it in dislocations backwards, sometimes it is demi-flexed, and it is also forcibly pronated. The elbow-joint is immovable. The most striking diagnostic sign, however, consists in the unnatural form of the elbow-joint, which is so remarkable as not to be easily misunderstood. The internal condyle of the humerus (epitrochlea) projects strongly to the inner side, leaving a deep depression below; while upon the outer side the head of the radius, with its cup-like extremity, can be distinctly felt, and made to rotate outside of its socket. The olecranon process, driven from its fossa, projects more or less posteriorly, and even the fossa itself may sometimes be plainly felt.

A girl, twelve years old, had fallen upon the inside of her elbow, producing a dislocation outwards of the forearm. I saw her within half an hour. The forearm was bent upon the arm about fifteen degrees, and immovably fixed. The head of the radius could be distinctly felt external to, and a little in front of the outer condyle, while the olecranon process of the ulna, which rested upon the back and outer surface of the humerus, was less distinctly felt than in the opposite arm. The inner condyle projected sharply to the inside, and the olecranon fossa was plainly felt with the fingers. The child was suffering very little pain.

Seizing the wrist with my right hand and the lower end of the humerus with the left, and making moderate extension in these opposite directions, the bones easily, and after only a moment's effort, resumed their places. Her recovery was rapid and complete.

If the dislocation is complete the position of the arm is usually the same, but the pronation of the hand is greater, and the projection of the inner condyle more striking.

If now the bones by a continuance of the original force, or by the action of the triceps, are drawn upwards also, the arm becomes a little more flexed, and the olecranon process more prominent, while the length of the whole limb is sensibly diminished.

Prognosis.—In recent cases of incomplete outward luxation, and where no complications exist, the reduction is generally easily effected; and M. Thierry claims to have reduced an outward and backward luxation after eight months. A patient of whom Debruyn has spoken was not so fortunate. On the 16th of April, 1841, a lad, æt. 18, fell upon the palm of his hand and dislocated both bones outwards and backwards; on the following morning a surgeon attempted to reduce the dislocation, and the attempt was repeated on the next day by another surgeon; but on the day following this last attempt, gangrene ensued in consequence of the great violence employed by the surgeons, and although the limb was amputated the patient died. The autopsy showed that both the brachial artery and the median nerve were torn asunder, and that the tendons of the biceps and brachialis anticus were slipped behind the outer condyle, probably having been thrown into this position during the violent twistings to which the arm had been subjected.[1]

I have seen three examples of dislocation upwards and outwards which the medical attendants had failed to reduce. The first was in the case of a lad, Wm. Kinkaid, fourteen years old, who had fallen from a wagon and struck upon the palm of his left hand. The surgeon who was immediately called made extension, and supposed that the reduction was accomplished. The lad was brought to me a few months after the accident. The arm was slightly flexed, and neither prone nor supine. There existed only a slight motion at the elbow-joint. I did not think it worth while to make any attempt at reduction. Several years after this, in the month of February, 1859, I had an opportunity of examining the arm again. He had now recovered considerable motion in the joint, but he could not tie his cravat. Pronation and supination were perfect.

In the second example, a lady, æt. 33, had fallen upon the inside of her elbow, and reduction not having been accomplished, I found her,

[1] Denucé, op. cit., p. 103.

nine weeks after the accident, with scarcely any motion at the elbow-joint, and complaining of a numbness in the forearm and hand.

The third instance of unreduced dislocation I will relate more at length.

Francis Banfield, aged twenty-two years, a resident of Alleghany County, N. Y., on the 31st of September, 1857, fell from the sweep of a threshing machine to the ground, a distance of about five feet, striking upon the palm of his hand, his arm being extended in front of him. On rising he found his arm forcibly flexed and abducted. He straightened it without difficulty, and it assumed the position it now occupies. A physician was called and saw the patient an hour and a half after the accident, who pronounced it a case of dislocation of the radius and ulna, and made efforts at reduction, which he continued from 8½ A. M. until 2 P. M., a period of five and a half hours, to no purpose, when he abandoned the attempt. During the attempt at reduction, the extension was made at times with the arm flexed, and at others extended. At 9 P. M., another physician was called, who made efforts at reduction until 3 A. M., upwards of six hours, at which time he also abandoned the attempt. On the third day another physician, the patient being under the influence of ether, made efforts at reduction for twenty minutes, when he pronounced it in place, and applied a bandage. From the patient's account the arm was swollen to such an extent as to render this point difficult to determine. On the fifth day the first physician was called, and believing that he discovered a grating, pronounced it a fracture of the external condyle.

Four months after the accident, when the patient applied to me, the limb presented the following appearances: "The forearm extended upon the arm; looking at the limb along its radial margin we notice a gentle outward inclination of the forearm from the elbow down, but by manipulation this may be greatly increased; the power of pronation and supination is not affected; the inner condyle projects an inch to the ulnar side; the head of the radius, completely removed from its socket, projects to an equal extent on the radial side. The top of the olcranon process is an inch higher than the top of the inner condyle, so that the radius and ulna are carried upwards as well as outwards."

I believe that the external condyle was not broken, as in that case, the arm would be *permanently* deflected outwards to a much greater extent. For although this arm may be deflected outwards by the surgeon to an angle of 135°, still the degree of mobility which exists would be adverse to the supposition of its being a fracture of the external condyle. The condyles also can be plainly felt in their natural situations, which would not be the case, if a fracture of the external condyle existed. The patient was advised not to submit to any further attempts at reduction.

Treatment.—In relation to the treatment of these accidents we have little to add to what has already been said of the treatment of dislocations backwards. The reduction, if effected at all, has generally been accomplished by moderate extension, or by extension combined with lateral pressure. If the head of the radius is in front of the humerus, or of the ulna, the hand should be first supined, and then the extension should be applied. In some cases the reduction has been effected by placing the knee in the bend of the elbow and flexing the forearm, while the surgeon was making extension from the hand.

§ 3. Dislocation of the Radius and Ulna Inwards (to the Ulnar Side).

This form of dislocation is much more rare than the dislocation outwards, a fact which may perhaps find a sufficient explanation in the peculiar form of the trochlea, the inner half of which rises much higher than the outer, forming thus an elevated inclined plane, over which the articulating surface of the ulna must rise before the dislocation can occur.

Like the opposite dislocation, the typical form of the accident is that in which the displacement is incomplete; indeed, no example of a complete inward dislocation has, we think, been yet recorded.

Causes.—A fall upon the hand or forearm, a blow upon the radial side of the forearm near its upper end, or upon the ulnar side of the arm, near its lower end, a violent wrenching of the limb, are among the causes which may occasion this dislocation.

Pathology.—The ridge which divides antero-posteriorly the greater sigmoid cavity of the ulna, having been driven over the elevated inner margin of the trochlea, falls down upon the epitrochlea, so as, in some sense, to embrace it instead of the trochlea; while the head of the radius passes inwards also, and is made to occupy the trochlea, from which the ulna has escaped. Generally the head of the radius is found in the same line with the ulna (Fig. 241), but it may suffer a subluxation and be found a little in advance of the ulna, or possibly a little in the rear.

Fig. 241.

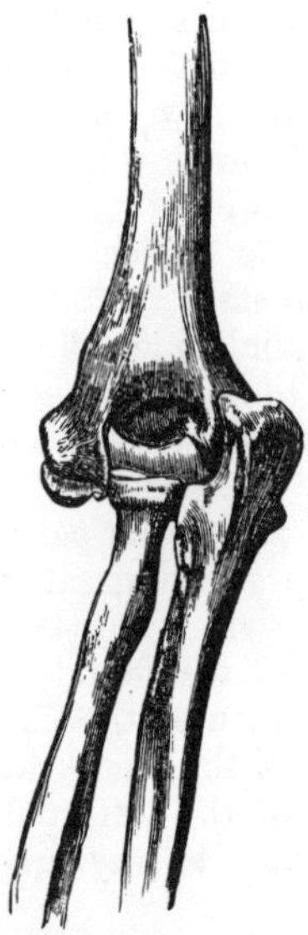

Most frequent form of incomplete inward dislocation of the forearm.

I choose also to regard the dislocation inwards and upwards as only a variety of the dislocation inwards; in which form of the accident the coronoid process of the ulna is thrust upwards above the epicondyle, and the head of the radius occupies the olecranon fossa, or rests upon the back of the humerus somewhere in this vicinity.

In addition to the injury suffered by the ligaments and muscles, the ulnar nerve in both varieties of inward dislocation is peculiarly liable to contusion, in consequence of its being crushed between the olecranon process and the epitrochlea.

Symptoms.—If the dislocation is only inwards, the olecranon process can be felt projecting upon the inner side, and completely concealing the epicondyle; while the head of the radius, having abandoned its socket, may be felt indistinctly in the bend of the arm. The external condyle (epicondyle) is remarkably prominent. The forearm is generally more or less flexed, and the hand forcibly pronated. The natural outward deflection of the forearm is also lost, or it may be even inclined slightly inwards. This phenomenon is explained by the position of the epicondyle, upon which the greater sigmoid cavity now rests, allowing the ulna to overlap a little upon the humerus; rendering the forearm actually somewhat shorter along its ulnar margin, although the head of the radius may still occupy the summit of the trochlea.

If the bones are displaced upwards as well as inwards, a considerable shortening is declared, and the head of the radius may now be felt behind the trochlea, or over the olecranon fossa. In three of the four examples seen by Malgaigne, all of them ancient, the forearm was in a state of supination. Other surgeons have met with cases in which the forearm was supine, but they must be considered as exceptions to the rule.

Prognosis.—Malgaigne was unable to reduce the dislocation in a recent case of incomplete internal dislocation, which came under his own notice. Triquet succeeded in a child seven years old, on the fifteenth day, after many trials; but the movements of the elbow-joint were never restored. Debruyn succeeded on the fifth day, but not without difficulty; and in the only remaining example which has been put upon record, the precise character of the accident having been determined by Velpeau, reduction was easily accomplished, and on the eighth day the patient was dismissed.[1]

Of the four examples of inward and backward luxation seen by Malgaigne, not one was ever reduced; but as the history of them all is not complete, it is by no means to be inferred that reduction could not have been easily accomplished, at least in some of them, at the first. Nor, with such imperfect details before us, can we understand fully what complications may have existed, such as would perhaps render these exceptional, rather than illustrative examples.

One of these patients had a completely anchylosed elbow at the end of two years, but pronation and supination were preserved. In the case of another, however, even flexion and extension were as perfect as in the normal condition.

Treatment.—The indications of treatment are the same as in dislocations outwards, with only such slight modifications as the judgment of every surgeon must naturally suggest. I prefer to employ by way of illustration the example diagnosticated by Velpeau.

On the 10th of May, 1848, Alexandrine Guyot, æt. 22, entered the Hospital of La Charité, with an incomplete inward dislocation of the forearm which had just occurred. The hand and forearm were in a state of forced pronation, half-flexed, and the whole limb from the elbow downwards was deflected inwards. There were present also all the other usual signs of this dislocation, and Velpeau had no doubt as to its true character.

In order to accomplish reduction, one assistant made counter-extension upon the arm, while a second made direct extension upon the forearm. At first the tractions were made in the direction of the fore-

[1] Denucé, op. cit., pp. 154–156.

arm (flexed and prone), but gradually the arm was straightened and supinated. Then the surgeon, seizing with one hand the superior extremity of the forearm, and with the other the inferior extremity of the arm, acted forcibly upon the two portions in opposite directions, and immediately the reduction was effected with a noise.[1]

§ 4. Dislocation of the Radius and Ulna Forwards.

Sir Astley Cooper, Vidal (de Cassis), and others have denied that this dislocation was possible without a fracture of the olecranon process; but Monin, Prior, Velpeau, and Denucé have each reported one example, so that its existence may now be considered as established. Nevertheless, it is only as a result of very violent and extraordinary accidents, by which the forearm is forcibly flexed, or greatly extended, or twisted, or in some other unusual and indirect way the olecranon is placed in front of the humerus.

The following is a summary of the facts in Velpeau's case. Alexandrine Carelli, æt. 23, was knocked down by a carriage, on the first of July, 1848, the wheel passing over the right arm. The arm was found in a right-angled position, and it could neither be flexed nor extended; the forearm was strongly supinated; the projecting angle usually made by the olecranon process was replaced by the irregular extremity of the humerus; the forearm was shortened upon the arm; the head of the radius resting in the coronoid fossa, and the olecranon process being also carried upwards, and a little outwards. Reduction was easily accomplished, and the patient left on the nineteenth day, with only a slight remaining stiffness in the joint.[2]

Chapel has reported a case of dislocation forwards and outwards which he readily reduced soon after it occurred, while Colson, Leva and Guyot have each reported one example of *sub*-luxation forwards, in which the extremity of the olecranon process has been found resting upon the extremity of the humeral trochlea.[3]

Treatment.—If the dislocation is complete and the forearm is shortened and flexed upon the arm, the reduction should be first attempted by violent flexion, or by flexion combined with extension from the wrist and counter-extension from the lower portion of the humerus. If the dislocation is incomplete, and the forearm is extended upon the arm, the reduction may be readily accomplished by extension alone, or by moderate flexion.

[1] Denucé, op. cit., p. 155. [2] Ibid., p. 110. [3] Ibid., p. 120.

CHAPTER X.

DISLOCATIONS OF THE WRIST (RADIO-CARPAL ARTICULATION).

REGARDED as an accident of not unusual occurrence by Hippocrates, J. L. Petit, Duverney, Boyer, and by most if not all the older writers, its frequency began to be questioned by Pouteau, and finally its existence was almost absolutely denied by Dupuytren, who remarks: "I have for a long time publicly taught that fractures of the carpal end of the radius are extremely common; that I had always found these supposed dislocations of the wrist turn out to be fractures; and that in spite of all which has been said upon the subject, I have never met with, or heard of, one single well authenticated and convincing case of the dislocation in question." Dupuytren subsequently declared that he would not positively deny the possibility of the accident, yet that "it must at least be admitted that the áccident is an extremely rare one." Wishing to explain this infrequency, he says: "In examining the structure of the soft parts, one cannot fail to perceive that it is not the ligaments which prevent the displacement of the articular surface forwards, but that this effect is especially due to the multitude of flexor tendons, deprived as they are at this point of all the fleshy parts, and reduced to the simple fibrous tissue which composes them. These tendons are bound together beneath the anterior annular ligament of the wrist; and thus offer so efficient a resistance that severe falls are insufficient to tear them through; the hand is forced into a state of extreme tension, and the tendons are firmly applied on the anterior part of the radio-carpal articulation. If the extension is still further augmented, the wrist-joint is yet more closely clasped by these parts, and their power of resistance is incalculable; I am convinced that a force equivalent to one thousand pounds weight would be inadequate to overcome it; and the known power of the tendo Achillis is sufficient to prove that this computation is not exaggerated.

"The risk of dislocation backwards by a fall on the dorsal surface of the hand is equally precluded by the tendons of the extensor muscles. Their arrangement and relations at the back of the joint are similar; it is true they are not quite so strong; but we must admit that their power of resistance is very considerable, when we take into consideration how they are inclosed in sheaths as they cross beneath the posterior annular ligament of the wrist. I have not alluded to the ulna, for it has really little or nothing to do with these movements, as it does not articulate (directly) with the hand.

"To sum up, then, the extreme rarity of dislocation forwards or backwards is owing to the obstacles opposed by the flexor and extensor tendons."

The opinion of such a writer as Dupuytren, whose experience was very great, and who described only what he had seen, is always entitled to profound respect; yet it has been the practice of nearly all who have made any reference to his opinions in this matter to speak of them lightly, and not a few have falsely represented him as saying that such a dislocation was "impossible." The fact is, that surgeons do still constantly mistake fractures of the lower end of the radius for dislocations, as my own personal observation can attest; and notwithstanding examples have been reported by René, Marjolin, Padieu, Cruveilhier, Voillemier, Boinet, Malgaigne, Scoutetten, Bransby Cooper, Fergusson, W. Parker, and others, yet the whole number of cases for which the distinction is claimed is, to this day, so inconsiderable as only to establish the value and accuracy of Dupuytren's opinion that the "accident is an extremely rare one." But it is, perhaps, most remarkable that while very few of these supposed examples have been verified by an autopsy, in every instance in which the autopsy has been made, the dislocation has been found to be complicated with a fracture, generally of the lower extremity of the radius or of the styloid apophysis of the ulna.

The existence of a complication, however, does not render the accident any the less a dislocation, although it may render the diagnosis more difficult, and modify somewhat the indications of treatment. A knowledge of the fact also that such complications have always been observed in the autopsy may leave us in doubt as to what is the natural history of a simple, uncomplicated dislocation, if, indeed, it does not warrant a suspicion that such a case never occurs. We shall, nevertheless, after a careful analysis of the cases as they have been reported, and by a consideration of the anatomy of this articulation, be able to determine with some degree of accuracy, perhaps, what are, or what ought to be the usual causes, signs, treatment, &c., of these accidents.

Partial luxations have also been frequently described by surgeons. I have never met with an example, but the following case, related to me by the patient himself, I believe to have been a case in point.

Lewis C., of Buffalo, æt. 18, by a fall upon his hand, broke the left forearm below the middle, and at the same time, as he affirms, partially dislocated the carpal bones backwards. Dr. Spaulding, of Williamsville, N. Y., who is now dead, took charge of the limb, and pronounced it a fracture with partial dislocation, and for more than a year after the accident, the bones had a tendency to become displaced in the same direction. Whenever he attempted to lift even the weight of half a pound, with his hand supine and his forearm extended horizontally, the lower end of the radius would spring suddenly forwards, and all power in the arm would be lost. When this happened, as it did quite often, he always reduced the bones himself, by simply pushing upon them in the direction of the articulation.

Fourteen years after the accident, I examined the arm and found it in all respects perfect, except that the forearm was shortened about one-third of an inch, which shortening was due, no doubt, to the overlapping of the broken bones.

§ 1. Dislocations of the Carpal Bones Backwards.

Causes.—The same casualty, namely, a fall upon the palm of the hand, which, as we have elsewhere noticed, produces frequently a fracture of the lower end of the radius, occasionally a dislocation of the radius and ulna backwards, at the elbow-joint, may also, it is believed, occasion sometimes a dislocation of the carpal bones backwards. In several of the cases reported, this cause has been assigned; but in the only example of simple dislocation which has ever come under my notice, and which I have every reason to believe was a simple dislocation unaccompanied with a fracture, the carpal bones were thrown back by a fall upon the back of the hand. The following is a brief account of the case:—

The Rev. Stephen Porter, of Geneva, N. Y., æt. 75, while walking with his son after dark, and holding in his right hand a satchel, slipped and fell. In the effort to save himself, and still retaining his grasp upon the satchel, his right hand struck the side-walk flexed, and in such a way as that the whole force of the fall was received upon the back of the hand and wrist, thus throwing the hand into a state of extreme flexion. In less than twenty minutes he was at my house. No swelling had yet occurred, and the moment I looked at the wrist I said to him, "You have broken your arm;" so much did it resemble a fracture of the lower end of the radius. A farther examination led me to a different conclusion. The palmar surface of the wrist presented an abrupt rising near the radio-carpal articulation, the summit of which was on the same plane and continuous with the bones of the forearm, and a corresponding elevation existed upon the dorsal surface terminating in the carpal bones and hand; the hand was slightly inclined backwards, but the fingers were moderately flexed upon the palm. To this extent the accident bore the features of a fracture of the radius; but the hand did not fall to the radial side; the projections upon the palmar and dorsal surfaces were more abrupt than I had ever seen in a case of fracture, and which, if it were a fracture, would imply that the broken extremities had been driven off from each other completely; the most salient angles of these projections were abrupt, but not sharp or ragged; the styloid apophyses could be distinctly felt, and I was not only able to determine that they were not broken, but by observing their relations to the palmar and dorsal eminences, it was easy to see that these latter corresponded to the situation of the articulation.

In addition to these evidences that I had to deal with a dislocation, and not a fracture, we had the testimony furnished by the reduction, which was not made, however, until by every possible means the diagnosis was definitely settled. Seizing the hand of the gentleman with my own hand, palm to palm, and making moderate but steady extension in a straight line, the bones suddenly resumed their places with the usual sensation or sound accompanying reductions. There was no grating, or chafing, or crushing, nor was the reduction accomplished gradually, but suddenly. To test still further the accuracy of the diagnosis, I now pressed forcibly upon the wrist from before back, but without producing any degree of displacement, nor could any crepitus still be detected. No splint was applied, and on the following morning Mr. Porter preached from one of the pulpits in this city, only retaining his arm in a sling.

Sixteen months after the accident, Sept. 15, 1858, this gentleman again called upon me and I found the arm perfect in all respects, except that it was not quite as strong as before, the lower extremity of the ulna was preternaturally movable, and occasionally he felt a sudden slipping in the radio-carpal articulation.

Pathological Anatomy.—In the examples of compound or complicated dislocations, which alone have been exposed by dissections, the posterior and lateral ligaments have been found extensively torn, as also frequently the anterior ligament, with or without separation of the radial or ulnar apophyses; the extensor muscles torn up from the lower part of the forearm and displaced; the first row of the carpal bones lying underneath the tendons, and upon the bones of the forearm, sometimes having been carried directly upwards, sometimes upwards and a little inwards, and at other times upwards and outwards; the arteries and nerves have occasionally escaped serious injury, but more often they have been displaced, bruised, or torn asunder.

Such are, briefly, the pathological circumstances which may be supposed to exist, in a lesser or greater degree, in nearly all cases of simple dislocations.

Fig. 242.

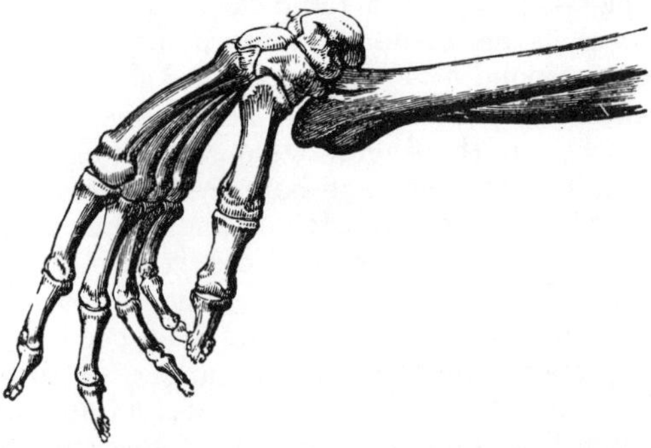

Dislocation of the carpal bones backwards. (From Fergusson.)

In compound dislocations, however, the muscles, or rather the tendons, are twisted, torn, and thrust aside, producing very extensive lesions among the deeper structures of the forearm and hand before the integuments can be made to yield.

On the 2d of May, 1852, Silas Usher, æt. 54, had his right arm caught between the bumpers of two cars, bruising the hand and dislocating the carpal bones backwards, the radius and ulna being thrown forwards and pushed completely through the skin into the palm of the hand. Most of the flexor tendons had been merely thrust aside, but one or two were torn asunder; the median nerve was torn off, but the radial and ulnar nerves were apparently uninjured, and there was no fracture. The patient being a temperate man, in perfect health, and the bones having been easily replaced by moderate extension, it was determined to make an effort to save the arm. The limb was therefore laid on a carefully padded splint, and cool water lotions diligently applied. Phlegmonous erysipelas began to develop itself on the third day; and on the ninth, gangrene having attacked the limb, I amputated a little above the middle of the humerus. On the fourteenth day hemorrhage occurred suddenly from the stump, and when I reached him he was pulseless and dying.

The result demonstrated the error of the attempt to save the limb without resection of the lower ends of the bones of the forearm.

Symptoms.—The usual signs have already been sufficiently stated in the example which we have given. The most important diagnostic marks are found in the abruptness of the angles formed by the projecting bones; the relation of these prominences to the styloid apophyses; in the total absence of crepitus; and in the reduction, which is accomplished easily, suddenly, and with a characteristic sensation. If a fracture complicates the accident, crepitus may also be present. It should be remembered, moreover, that when the styloid process of the radius is broken, if the hand is moved backwards and forwards this process will move also, which might lead to the supposition that the radius was broken higher up, and that it was not a dislocation at all.

Fig. 243.

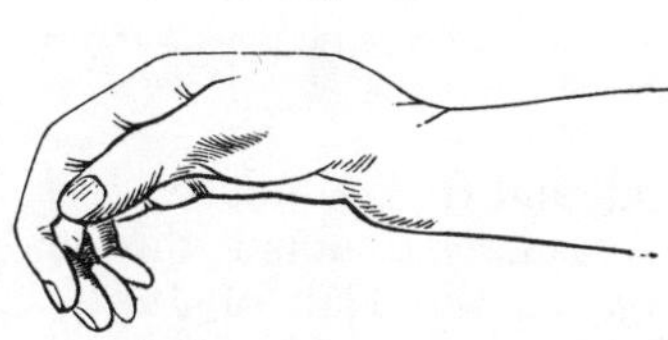

Dislocation of the carpal bones backwards. (From Skey.)

Prognosis.—In compound dislocations the prognosis is exceeding grave, unless the surgeon determines to resort to amputation, or, what is generally much preferable, to resection. In dislocations complicated with fracture of the posterior edge of the articulating surface of the radius ("Barton's fracture"[1]), some difficulty may be experienced in retaining the bones in place; but when this fracture does not exist, the posterior margin of the articulation, considerably elevated above its anterior margin, constitutes a sufficient protection against a reluxation in that direction. In all cases, also, complicated with fracture, even of an apophysis, intense inflammation and swelling are likely to follow, and the danger of a permanent anchylosis is greatly increased.

Treatment.—Extension in a straight line has generally been found sufficient to accomplish the reduction; to which may be added a slight rocking or lateral motion, if necessary.

The reduction may be effected also by pressing the hand backwards, while the surgeon pushes the carpus downwards from behind and above, in the direction of the articulation.

[1] Philadelphia Medical Examiner, 1838.

Unless a tendency to displacement exists, no splints or bandages of any kind ought to be applied, but it should be treated by rest and cool water lotions until all danger from inflammation has passed.

§ 2. Dislocations of the Carpal Bones Forwards.

The causes, mechanism, symptoms, pathology, treatment, &c., of this accident resemble in so many points those of the preceding dislocation, with only the differences necessarily due to a change in the direction of the bones, that I find it not worth while to do more than to relate one single example contained in Bransby Cooper's edition of Sir Astley's work on *Fractures and Dislocations*. The case did not come under the observation of Mr. Cooper himself, but was related to him by Mr. Haydon, a surgeon residing in London. It is especially interesting as furnishing an example of a dislocation of both wrists at the same moment, and from similar causes, but in opposite directions.

Fig. 244.

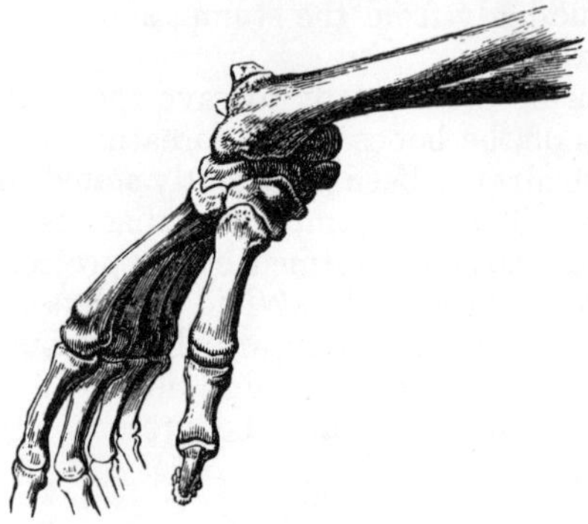

Dislocation of the carpal bones forwards. (From Fergusson.)

A lad, aged about thirteen years, was thrown violently from a horse on the 11th of June, 1840, striking upon the palms of both hands and upon his forehead. The left carpus was found to be dislocated backwards, the radius lying in front and upon the scaphoides and trapezium. The right carpus was dislocated forwards, the radius and ulna projecting posteriorly, and the bones of the carpus forming an "irregular knotty tumor, terminating abruptly" anteriorly.

A very careful examination was made to determine what parts came in contact with the resisting force, but, although the palms of both hands were extensively bruised, there was not the slightest bruise on the back of either hand. Nor were the gentlemen present able to find any evidence whatever that the dislocation was accompanied with a fracture. "Moreover," says Mr. Haydon, "we were strengthened in our opinion that this was a case of dislocation, unattended with any fracture, because the dislocations appeared so perfect; the two tumors in each member so distinct; the reduction so complete; the strength of the parts after reduction so great; and, lastly, by the very trifling pain felt after reduction, for within an hour after, the

Fig. 245.

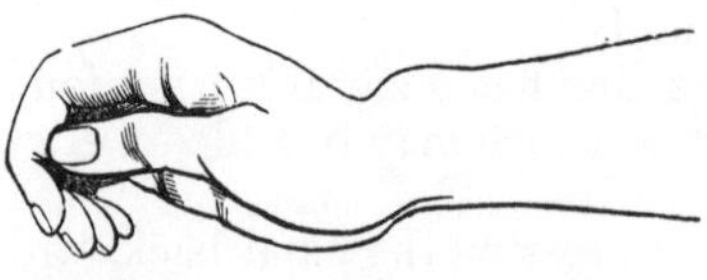

Dislocation of the carpal bones forwards. (From Skey.)

patient could rotate the hand and supinate it when prone—this could not, we believe, have been done had there existed a fracture."

CHAPTER XI.

DISLOCATIONS OF THE LOWER END OF THE ULNA (INFERIOR RADIO-ULNAR ARTICULATION).

IN connection with fractures of the lower end of the radius this accident is not very uncommon. I have myself met with it under these circumstances several times; but without a fracture it is quite rare. Dupuytren met with but two cases in his long and extensive practice. Sir Astley Cooper does not record a single instance, and many surgeons affirm that they have never seen the dislocation in question.

§ 1. DISLOCATIONS OF THE LOWER END OF THE ULNA BACKWARDS.

To the eleven or twelve examples collected and referred to by Malgaigne, I am only able to add one case of ancient luxation seen by myself.

Causes.—Duges mentions the case of a little girl in whom the accident occurred in both arms, but at different periods, by being lifted by the hands. One of the patients seen by Desault, a child five years old, had the ulna dislocated backwards by extension accompanied with forced pronation, and in another example cited by him forced pronation alone, as in wringing wet clothes, was found to have been sufficient. In Hurteaux's case the patient had fallen upon her wrist.

Pathological Anatomy.—Rupture of the synovial membrane (sacciform ligament), and also of the ligament which binds the ulna to the cuneiform bone: the little head or lower extremity of the ulna abandoning its socket in the radius, and being thrown backwards, or in some cases backwards and outwards so as to cross obliquely the lower end of the radius; or it may incline inwards as well as backwards.

Several examples are mentioned also in which the end of the bone has been thrust completely through the integuments.

Prognosis.—In recent cases the reduction has generally been accomplished without difficulty, and in only three or four instances has the bone become spontaneously displaced.

Loder reduced the ulna after eight weeks, and Rognetta after sixty days. In the example to which I have already referred as having been seen by myself, the dislocation had existed twenty years, the accident having occurred in Ireland when the person was fifteen years old. When I examined the arm, July 21, 1850, the right ulna projected backwards and a little outwards, about half an inch. He said he had been lame with it for several years, but the motions of the wrist-joint were now completely restored, and both pronation and supination were perfect.

Symptoms.—The hand is usually fixed in a position midway between supination and pronation. Boyer, however, found the hand in a state of extreme pronation. The extremity of the ulna is felt and seen distinctly upon the back of the wrist, prominent and movable; and the styloid process is no longer in a line with the metacarpal bone of the little finger; the fingers, hand and forearm are slightly flexed.

Treatment.—The reduction may be accomplished by holding firmly upon the radius and at the same moment pushing the ulna forcibly toward its socket; or by simply supinating the hand strongly. Some cases demand also extension with counter-extension.

Generally the bone has been found to remain in its place without assistance, yet in three or four of the examples upon record the constant tendency to displacement when the pressure was removed, has rendered it necessary to employ splints and compresses.

§ 2. Dislocation of the Lower End of the Ulna Forwards.

The dislocation forwards is said by Malgaigne to be more rare than the dislocation backwards. In addition to the nine cases collected by him, I have been able to add one reported by Parker, of Liverpool; leaving, therefore, a difference of only three or four in favor of the luxation backwards; and not sufficient, I think, to warrant any positive conclusions as to the relative frequency of the two accidents.

While the dislocation backwards is usually caused by violent pronation of the hand, this dislocation is most often occasioned by violent supination. The hand is therefore generally found to be supinated forcibly, and the projection formed by the end of the bone is seen upon the front of the wrist instead of the back.

By pushing the ulna toward its socket while an attempt is made to flex the hand, or by extension, supination, &c., it is made to resume its position readily. In the case reported by Parker, however, the reduction was effected only while the hand was prone.

Parker's case, already referred to, is thus related:—

"John Dalton, aged forty, applied to the hospital Aug. 9th, 1841, under the following circumstances:—

"States that he is a carter, and falling down, the shaft of the cart fell upon his hand and forearm, in such a way as to supinate them forcibly. He complains of pain in the left wrist. The forearm is supinated, and cannot be pronated, the attempt causing much suffering. The wrist-joint can be flexed or extended without much pain. On looking at the back of the wrist, the appearance is characteristic; the natural prominence of the ulna is wanting; an evident depression exists, as if the lower end of the ulna had been dissected out; it can be traced, however, on a plane anterior to the radius, its button-like head being distinctly felt under the flexor tendons. Several ineffectual and very painful attempts were made to accomplish the reduction, by pushing the head of the ulna into its natural situation. This was at last effected by seizing the hand to make extension (counter-extension being made at the elbow), then forcibly pronating the hand, at the same time pressing backwards the dislocated head of the bone with the fingers of the left hand. After persevering for a short time, the bone was felt to assume its natural position, the wrist acquired its usual appearance, and the ordinary movements of the joint could be readily performed. There was no tendency to re-dislocation, and the man was dismissed with directions to keep the joint quiet, and to foment it. He attended as an out patient for two or three days, after which, complaining of nothing but a little weakness in the part, a bandage was applied, and ordered to be worn for a short time."[1]

CHAPTER XII.

DISLOCATIONS OF THE CARPAL BONES (AMONG THEMSELVES).

Bound together on all sides by strong ligaments, and enjoying only a very limited degree of motion among themselves, the carpal bones seldom become displaced except in gunshot wounds, or in connection with extensive lacerations and fractures of the neighboring parts. Simple dislocations, or rather sub-luxations of these bones do, however, occasionally take place, but so far as we have been able to ascertain, only in one direction, namely, backwards.

The bones of the carpus, which are said occasionally to have suffered simple backward subluxation, are the os magnum, cuneiforme, unciforme, and pisiforme.

Richerand, the editor of Boyer's Lectures, says that he once met with a subluxation of the os magnum backwards, of which he has given us the following account: "Mrs. B., in a labor pain, seized violently the edge of her mattress, and squeezed it forcibly, turning her wrist forwards; she instantly heard a slight crack, and felt some pain, to which her other sufferings did not allow her to attend. Fifteen days afterwards, happily delivered, and recovered by the care of Professor Baudelocque, she showed her left hand to this celebrated accoucheur, and expressed her disquietude about the tumor which appeared on it, especially when much bent. I was called to visit the

[1] Parker, Amer. Journ. Med. Sci., April, 1843, p. 470; from Lond. and Edin. Month. Journ. Med. Sci., Dec. 1842.

lady. I found that this hard circumscribed tumor, which disappeared almost totally by extending the hand, was formed by the head of the os magnum, luxated backwards; I replaced it entirely by extending the hand, and making gentle pressure on it. As the affection did not impede the motion of the part, as the tumor disappeared on extending the hand, and as it would have been even little apparent in any state of the hand had Mrs. B. been more in flesh, I advised her not to be uneasy about it, and to apply no remedy to it."[1]

Richerand adds also that Boyer and Chopart had each met with the same dislocation.

Bransby Cooper saw the os magnum displaced backwards in a stout, muscular young man by a fall upon the back of the hand when in extreme flexion. The hand remained slightly bent, and the projection of the os magnum was very distinct. Reduction was attempted by extending the whole hand, at the same time making pressure upon the displaced bone; this not succeeding, extension was made from the middle and forefingers only, while pressure was kept up on the os magnum, when suddenly the bone resumed its natural position. On flexing the hand, however, the dislocation was immediately reproduced; and it became necessary to apply a compress and splint. For several days after, he was in the habit of pushing it out by flexing the hand, in order that the young men at Guy's Hospital might see its reduction; which was always easily accomplished by simply pushing upon it.

Sir Astley says that both the os magnum and cuneiforme are sometimes thrown a little backwards, from simple relaxation of the ligaments, producing a great degree of weakness so as to render the hand useless unless the wrist be supported; and he mentions the case of a young lady in whom the os magnum was thus displaced and who was obliged to give up her music in consequence; for when she wished to use her hand she was compelled to wear two short splints, made fast to the back and forepart of the hand and forearm. Another lady whose hand was weak from a similar cause, wore for the purpose of giving it strength, a strong steel chain bracelet, clasped very tightly around the wrist.[2]

Gras has described a dislocation of the pisiform bone,[3] and Fergusson says he has known an example in which this bone was detached from its lower connections by the action of the flexor carpi-ulnaris.[4] Little benefit, he thinks, can be expected from any attempts to keep it in place when it is dislocated, nor is its displacement of much consequence. Erichsen thinks he has seen a dislocation of the os lunare produced by a fall upon the hand when forcibly flexed. By extension and pressure it was easily replaced, but when the hand was flexed the dislocation was immediately reproduced.[5]

Notwithstanding that Sir Astley, Miller, and others have taught that the cuneiform bone is liable to displacement, and South has

[1] Richerand, Boyer's Lectures on Diseases of Bones, Amer. ed., 1805, p. 261.
[2] Sir A. Cooper, op. cit., p. 435. [3] Note to Chelius by South, op. cit., p. 234.
[4] Fergusson, op. cit., p. 190.
[5] Erichsen, Science and Art of Surg., Amer. ed., 1859, p. 259.

affirmed the same of the unciform, I have found no account of an example of simple dislocation of single carpal bones except in the cases of the os magnum, pisiformis, and lunare, as above mentioned.

Maisonneuve has reported an example of simple dislocation, without wound of the integuments, at the middle carpal articulation. A man had fallen forty feet, and was carried dying to the Hôtel Dieu. The symptoms were almost precisely those of a dislocation of both rows of the carpal bones backwards. The reduction was not accomplished during life, but after death a simple effort of traction was sufficient to replace the bones. The dissection showed that the bones of the second row were almost completely separated from those of the first, upon which they were overlapped backwards. A small fragment of both the scaphoides and cuneiform remained attached to the second row, but with this exception, the separation was complete.[1]

CHAPTER XIII.

DISLOCATION OF THE METACARPAL BONES (AT THE CARPO-METACARPAL ARTICULATIONS).

THE metacarpal bone of the thumb may be dislocated either backwards or forwards. The former is the most frequent; and it is produced generally by a fall upon the thumb, which throws it into a state of extreme flexion; it has also been occasioned by a force acting in an opposite direction, as when a flash of powder is exploded in the palm of the hand, or a blow is received upon the extremity and volar aspect of the last phalanx.

The dislocation may be partial or complete. In the few examples of partial dislocation which have been recorded, the position of the finger has been either moderately flexed or straight, and the signs of the accident have been occasionally so obscure as to have led to an error in the diagnosis, and the luxation has remained unreduced. When the dislocation is recognized, reduction is in most cases easily accomplished by pressure, combined with extension; after which it is sometimes necessary to apply a splint to maintain the apposition. If the reduction is not accomplished the joint is permanently maimed.

Complete backward luxations are more frequent than incomplete, and are produced by the same class of causes; generally by a fall upon the palmar surface of the thumb.

The symptoms are sufficiently clear, although the position of the thumb is not always the same. It has been found perfectly straight, without any inclination either way, or flexed more or less, with the

[1] Maisonneuve, Malgaigne, op. cit., from Mém. de la Soc. de Chirurg., t. ii.

metacarpal bone also inclined inwards toward the palm. The motions of the joint are interrupted, and the proximal extremity of the metacarpal bone riding upon the back of the trapezium, projects sensibly in this direction, and the trapezium is also felt unusually prominent under the thenar eminence. The overlapping varies from a line or two to three-quarters of an inch. In the patient mentioned by Bourguet, the head of the metacarpal bone almost reached the styloid process of the radius.

The reduction is to be effected by extension alone, or by extension with moderate pressure.

In two of the examples reported, although the reduction was accomplished very easily, the dislocation was reproduced when the extension ceased, and it became necessary to apply splints. Malgaigne did not observe in the case seen by him, any such tendency to displacement.

In the case of Bourguet's patient the reduction was never accomplished, although the attempt was made on the second day by a surgeon, and repeated after about two months by Bourguet himself.

Fergusson, who has met with several of these dislocations, says that he has seen even a splint and roller fail of keeping the bones in place; and he recommends, for the purpose of security, that the splint should extend some distance upon the forearm.

Sir Astley Cooper says that in the cases of this accident which he has seen the metacarpal bone of the thumb has been thrown inwards, between the trapezium and the root of the metacarpal bone supporting the forefinger; forming a protuberance toward the palm of the hand; the thumb has been bent backwards, and adduction was impossible.

This distinguished surgeon cites no examples, nor are we able to find upon record an instance of complete inward dislocation of this bone, such as Sir Astley has described.

Vidal (de Cassis) believes that he has met with a partial forward dislocation, which he reduced readily, but the patient having removed the retentive means, the dislocation was reproduced and the bone was not again replaced.[1]

Malgaigne has collected only three examples of a dislocation of either of the other metacarpal bones. One, observed by Bourguet, was a dislocation forwards of the metacarpal bone of the index finger, having been caused by a great force applied to the back of the phalanx near the carpus. Reduction was effected by extension and pressure, the bone resuming its place insensibly and not suddenly. With the aid of splints it was retained in position, and the cure was perfect. The second, seen by Roux, was a backward luxation at the carpo-metacarpal articulation of the second, or great finger, produced by an explosion in a mine. By pressure made directly upon the projecting bone he was unable to reduce it, but by uniting pressure with extension from the finger, he succeeded readily. After the reduction was effected, it was noticed that when the hand was straightened the bone became reluxated, but that it was easily kept in place when the hand was flexed. The third example (occurring in the same joint), men-

[1] Vidal (de Cassis), Traité de Pathologié Externe, etc., 3d Paris ed,, t. ii. p. 564.

tioned by Malgaigne, occasioned by a fall upon the clenched hand, was probably incomplete, and Malgaigne is not quite certain that it was not a fracture.

In April, 1849, Stephen Peterson, æt. 24, was admitted into the Buffalo Hospital of the Sisters of Charity, with a partial dislocation backwards of the proximal ends of the metacarpal bones of the index and great fingers of the right hand; produced, as he affirms, by striking a man with his clenched fist, about one year previous. He says that he called upon a surgeon immediately, but he was unable to keep the bones in place. The projection was very manifest at the time of my examination, and the hand had never recovered the power of grasping bodies firmly.

During the same year I found in the hospital a precisely similar case, in the person of Francis M'Coit, æt. 32, a sailor, which had occurred four years before, in consequence of a blow given with his fist. The same bones were partially displaced backwards, and remained unreduced. This man had also consulted a surgeon soon after the injury was received.

In both of the above examples I instituted a careful examination to determine whether it was not the bones of the carpus thus displaced; but the result was conclusive as to the nature of the accident, and I have obtained casts of both in order to illustrate partial dislocations of the metacarpal bones.

CHAPTER XIV.

DISLOCATIONS OF THE FIRST PHALANGES OF THE THUMB AND FINGERS (AT THE METACARPO-PHALANGEAL ARTICULATIONS).

§ 1. Dislocations of the First Phalanx of the Thumb Backwards.

This bone may be dislocated backwards or forwards, but most frequently the dislocation is backwards.

The backward dislocation is occasioned generally by a fall or blow upon the distal end and palmar surface of the thumb; the proximal extremity of the first phalanx sliding back upon the distal extremity of the metacarpal bone, and standing off from it at nearly a right angle, the last being again flexed upon the first phalanx at about a right angle also; meanwhile the distal end of the metacarpal bone is seen projecting strongly in the palm of the hand. (Fig. 246.)

These are the usual signs which characterize this accident, and they are always sufficiently diagnostic. In a few cases, however, the phalanges have been found extended upon the metacarpal bone in almost a straight line, indicating, we presume, some extraordinary lesion of the tendons or muscles.

Fig. 246.

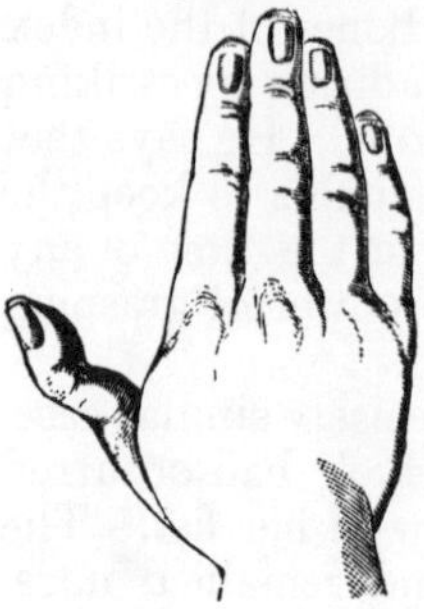

Dislocation of the first phalanx of the thumb backwards.

The reduction is sometimes, in recent cases, accomplished with great ease; as the following examples will illustrate.

A servant girl, æt. 25, fell down a flight of steps Nov. 15, 1850, striking upon the inside of her right hand and thumb. When I saw her, only a few minutes afterwards, I found the first phalanx standing back almost at a right angle with the metacarpal bone, and the second phalanx also flexed to a right angle with the first. Assisted by my pupil, Mr. Boardman, the reduction was effected in about twenty seconds, by bending the first phalanx farther back, and at the same moment pressing the proximal end of this phalanx forwards in the direction of the joint. Without employing great force, the reduction took place suddenly and with a snap. Very little swelling followed, and in three weeks she was able to use her needle without inconvenience.

Michael Wolf, æt. 35, fell from a height causing a fracture of his left arm, and a dislocation of his right thumb backwards. I saw him within two hours after the accident. The thumb was much swollen, and its position the same as in the case just described. Although Wolf was a strong, muscular man, the reduction was accomplished in a few seconds by applying over the last phalanx the Indian toy called a "puzzle," and making extension in a straight line, while an assistant made counter-extension from the hand and wrist. The use of the joint was soon completely restored.

Examples, however, are constantly occurring, which are only reduced after long continued and painful efforts, or which, indeed, completely exhaust the patience and baffle the skill of the most experienced surgeons.

Mary J. S., æt. 23, fell upon her right hand with her fingers and thumb extended, in Sept. 1853, and dislocated this bone backwards. A young surgeon attempted to reduce the dislocation half an hour after the accident, by the same manœuvre adopted by myself successfully in the case of the servant girl; only that he made extension upon the last phalanx at the same moment. The surgeon believes that the bone was reduced, but one week later he found it displaced, and, as he believes, reduced it again. The same thing occurred a third time.

Six months after this the girl consulted me to ascertain what could be done for her relief. The thumb occupied the usual position, and admitted of no motion except at the carpo-metacarpal articulation.

It is quite probable that the dislocation was never reduced, an error which, if it did occur, might easily be excused, when we remember that from the first the thumb was greatly swollen.

In May, 1848, having been called to see G. H., who had attempted suicide by cutting his throat, my attention was arrested by the appearance of his left thumb, and which I found to be occasioned by an ancient dislocation of the first phalanx backwards. The accident had occurred, he afterwards told me, twelve years before, in consequence of a fall while wrestling. A very respectable country surgeon was called, and made three separate attempts to reduce it, but failed.

The several bones of the thumb occupied their usual positions, that is to say, the positions which they usually occupy in this dislocation, yet notwithstanding the almost complete anchylosis of the phalangeal articulations, and the awkward encroachment of the distal end of the metacarpal bone upon the palm, the hand was quite useful.

On the 25th of July, 1857, Catherine Ernst was brought to me by her parents having a dislocation of the first phalanx of the right hand, which had already existed some days, and upon which several unsuccessful attempts at reduction had been made. The dislocation was backwards, but the phalanges, instead of standing at a right angle with each other and with the metacarpal bone, as is usually the case, were in a straight line with each other and parallel with the metacarpal bone. Whether this phenomenon existed from the first, or was due to the efforts already made at reduction, I could not determine, but the same thing has been noticed occasionally by other surgeons. The first phalanx, moreover, instead of being placed directly behind the metacarpal bone, occupied a position upon its back a little to the radial side of the centre.

During quite half an hour I made continued and varied attempts to reduce the bone, by extension, by forced dorsal flexion, and by pressing the upper end of the first phalanx in the direction of the joint while pressure was made against its lower end so as to bring it into dorsal flexion, and finally by calling to my aid the "puzzle" and chloroform, but all to no purpose.

One week later I repeated these efforts, and with no better success. The parents peremptorily refused to allow me to cut the lateral ligaments or flexor tendons, so the bone remains unreduced.

Surgical writers have recorded, from time to time, a great many similar cases, and it is asserted upon the authority of Bromfield, quoted by Hey, that the extending force has been increased to such an amount as to tear off the last phalanx without having succeeded in reducing the first; but while surgeons have united in their testimony as to the exceeding obstinacy of a large proportion of these dislocations, they are far from being agreed as to the source of the difficulty.

Sir Astley Cooper finds a sufficient explanation in the six short and powerful muscles which are inserted into the first and last phalanx, and especially in the flexors.[1] Hey believes the resistance to be in the lateral ligaments between which the lower end of the metacarpal bone escapes and becomes imprisoned. Ballingall, Malgaigne, Erich-

[1] Lawrie, of Glasgow, says that Sir Astley in a conversation with him declared that the "sesamoid bones" were the sources of the difficulty. See Amer. Journn. Med. Sci., vol. xxii. p. 230, with observations and experiments by Lawrie.

sen, and Vidal (de Cassis) think the metacarpal bone is locked between the two heads of the flexor brevis, or rather between the opposing sets of muscles which centre in the sesamoid bones, as a button is fastened into a button-hole. Pailloux, Lawrie, Michel, Leva, Blechy, and Roser affirm that the anterior ligament being torn from one of its attachments falls between the joint surfaces and interposes an effectual obstacle to reduction. Dupuytren ascribes the difficulty to the altered relations of the lateral ligaments, which are naturally parallel to the axis of the metacarpal bone, but which are now placed at a right angle; to the spasm of the muscles, and to the shortness of the member, in consequence of which the force of extension has to be applied very near to the seat of the dislocation. Lisfranc found in an ancient luxation the tendon of the long flexor so displaced inwards and entangled behind the extremity of the bone as to prevent reduction. Deville discovered in an autopsy a similar displacement of this tendon outwards.

The modes of reduction practiced and recommended by these different surgeons are as diversified and irreconcilable as their views of the mechanism and pathological anatomy of the accident.

Sir Astley Cooper recommends that extension shall be made by bending the thumb toward the palm of the hand, to relax the flexor muscles as much as possible; and then, by fastening a clove hitch (Fig. 247), upon the first phalanx, previously covered with a piece of soft leather, the extension is to be continued, only inclining the thumb a little inwards toward the palm of the hand. If these means fail after having been continued a considerable length of time, he advises that a weight shall be suspended to the thumb, passing over a pulley. (Fig. 248.) Finally, in the event of the failure of this method also, Sir Astley thought that no further attempts should be made, and especially that no operation for the division of parts was justifiable.

Fig. 247.

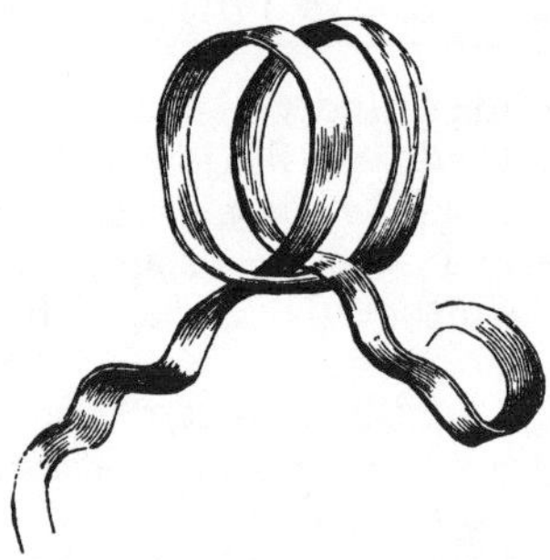

Clove hitch.

Lizars and Pirrie adopt the views of Sir Astley with little or no qualification.

Charles Bell proposed flexing the joint, employing also at the same time pressure; and in obstinate cases he advised subcutaneous section of the lateral ligaments with a small knife, a method which has since been practiced successfully by Liston, Reinhardt, Gibson, of Philadelphia, Parker, of New York, and others. Syme and Lizars justify the practice in certain cases. Hey declared that neither extension nor flexion was useful, but that the bones could be best brought into place by pressure alone.

Roser, from his experiments upon the cadaver, concludes that the dislocated phalanx must first be bent forcibly backwards, or into the position termed by some writers dorsal flexion, so as to throw the head of the phalanx forwards upon the articulating surface of the

Fig. 248.

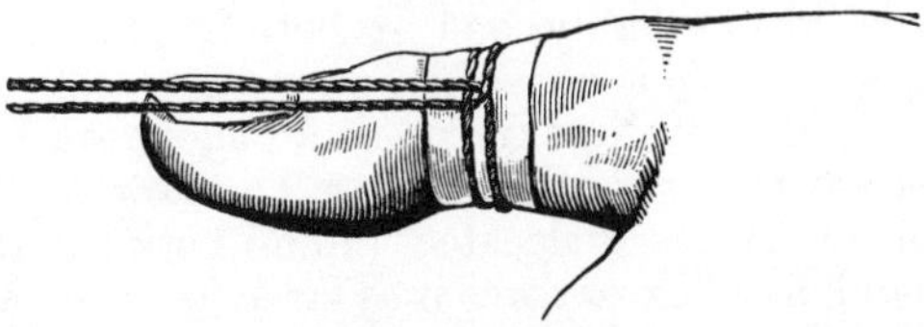

Sir Astley Cooper's method of reducing dislocations of the thumb, with pulleys.

metacarpal bone. Parker, of New York, in his notes to the American edition of Samuel Cooper's work, recommends the same procedure.

Vidal (de Cassis) recommends also that the extension should be made first backwards, so as to increase the displacement of the first phalanx in this direction, and to throw forwards its articular surface in the direction of the articular surface of the metacarpal bone.

This method, namely, dorsal flexion as the first and most essential part of the manœuvre, seems to have met with more general approval than any other, and the following observations, made by the venerable Reuben D. Mussey, of Cincinnati, illustrate the general practice among American surgeons at this day.

"I tilt the dislocated phalanx up until it stands upon its articulating end, place both forefingers so as to hold it in that position, and at the same time press against the distal extremity of the metacarpal bone, make firm pressure with the thumbs against the base of the dislocated phalanx, and slide it into its place, which can generally be accomplished with ease.

"More than twenty-five years ago, the chairman of this committee, from attention to the mechanism of the metacarpo-phalangeal joint of the thumb, convinced himself that the principal impediment to the reduction of the first phalanx from backward displacement is the short flexor of the thumb, between the two portions of which (lying close together where they are fastened to the sesamoid bones) the head of the metacarpal bone has been thrust, the contracted part or neck of this bone lying firmly grasped by them. Fifteen years ago, a case occurred of this dislocation which he could not reduce in the ordinary way. A subcutaneous division of one of the heads of this muscle was made with an iris knife, and the reduction was accomplished with the greatest ease.

"Last year, another case occurred in which we failed of reduction by Dr. Crosby's method, which we believe to be the best, and the subcutaneous division of both heads of the muscle was made, and the reduction instantly effected. The punctures were covered with collodion, and the thumb supported by a splint. As the patient was intemperate, entire abstinence from liquor and the adoption of a light diet were enjoined. Neither pain nor inflammation followed, and a month afterwards the joint had free motion. After the intemperate and irregular habits were resumed, the joint in a few weeks was found anchylosed. In these cases, the knife, in the subcutaneous operation, was carried down to the metacarpal bone, so far behind its head as to preclude the possibility of mistaking the lateral ligaments for the muscles. These ligaments are very short and inserted close to the articular surfaces, and are probably, one or both, ruptured in this dislocation."[1]

Dr. J. P. Batchelder, of New York, in a paper read before the New York Medical Association in 1856, says: "The surgeon should take the metacarpal portion of the dislocated thumb between the thumb and finger of one hand, and flex or force it as far as may be into the palm of the hand, for the purpose of relaxing the muscles connected with the proximal end of the phalanx, particularly the flexor brevis pollicis. He should then apply the end of the thumb of this hand against the displaced extremity of the dislocated phalanx, for the purpose of forcing it downwards, and at the same time grasp the displaced thumb with his other hand, and move it forcibly backwards and forwards, as in strongly forced flexion and extension, the pressure against the upper extremity of the first phalanx being kept up. In this way the dislocated bone may be made to descend, so as to be almost or quite on a line with the articulating surface of the metacarpal bone, when the thumb may be forcibly flexed, and, if it be not reduced, as forcibly extended, and brought backwards to a right angle with the metacarpal bone, when, if the downward pressure, with the thumb placed as before directed for that purpose, has been continued (which thumb, by maintaining its position, acts as a fulcrum, as well as by its pressure), the bone will slip into its place, and the reduction be effected in less time than has been spent in describing the process."[2]

Six successful cases of treatment by this method are mentioned in the *American Journal of Medical Sciences* for April, 1858; one by Rickard, one by Morgan, two by Cutter, and two by Crosby.

By those who have regarded extension as an important element in the reduction, various instruments have been devised for the purpose of obtaining a secure hold upon the dislocated member. Sir Astley Cooper, as we have already seen, recommended the sailor's clove hitch;[3] Lawrie advises that the thumb shall be thrust into the open handle of a large door key;[4] Charrière and Luër, of Paris, have each invented forceps, so constructed with fenestra and straps, as that when the blades are closed the member is held very firmly in its grasp. Richard J. Levis, of Philadelphia, recommends "a thin strip of hard wood, about ten inches in length, and one inch, or rather more, in width. (Fig. 249.) One end of the piece is perforated with six or eight holes. The opposite end is partly cut away, forming a projecting pin, and leaving a shoulder on each side of it. Toward this end of the strip, a sort of handle shape is given to it, so as to insure a secure grasp to the operator. Two pieces of strong tape or other material, about one yard in length, are prepared. One of these is passed through the holes at the

[1] Mussey, Trans. Amer. Med. Assoc., vol. iii. 1850, p. 357.
[2] Batchelder, New York Journ. Med., May, 1856, p. 340.
[3] Op. cit., p. 561; also Bost. Med. and Surg. Journ., Oct. 1, 1857.
[4] Lawrie, Am. Journ. Med. Sci., vol. xxii. p. 229.

end of the strip, leaving a loop on one side. The other tape is passed through another pair of holes, according as it may be a thumb or finger

Fig. 249.

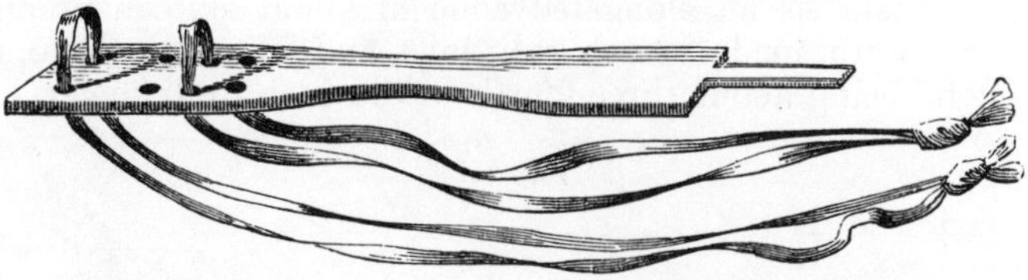

Levis's instrument for reduction of dislocations of fingers or the thumb.

to which it is to be applied, or varied to suit the length of the finger, leaving a similar loop. If a dislocated thumb is to be acted on, the second tapes should be passed through the holes nearest the first. The ends of each separate tape are then tied together.

"To apply this apparatus, the finger is passed through the loops. (Fig. 250). The loop nearest the first joint is then tightened by drawing on the tape, which is then brought along the strip to the opposite end, across one of the shoulders, and secured by winding it firmly around

Fig. 250.

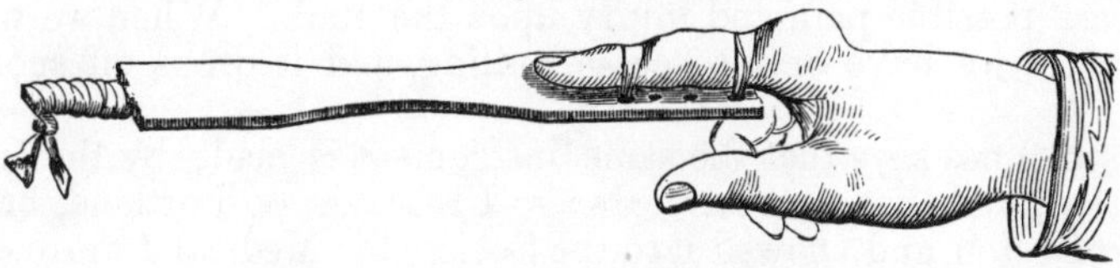

Levis's instrument applied to the first finger.

the projecting pin. The other tape is tightened in a like manner, crossing the other shoulder, and winding around the pin in an opposite direction, when, for security, the ends of the tapes are finally tied together."[1]

This apparatus enables the operator to apply both extension and flexion or leverage in any direction. The proximal end of the phalanx may be lifted, or even rotated so as to allow one side of the bone to approach the socket before the other.

Malgaigne describes an apparatus invented by Kirchoff, which is very similar to, yet not quite so complete, as this of Levis.

In the April number of the *Buffalo Medical Journal*, for 1847, I have described an instrument, or rather a toy, in my possession, which I suggested might be useful for the purpose of making extension upon dislocated fingers; and which, as will be seen by a reference to one of the cases already reported in this chapter, I have since applied successfully. It is made by the Indians in this vicinity, and may always be obtained during the watering season, at the Indian toy

[1] Levis, Amer. Journ. Med. Sci., Jan. 1857, p. 62.

shops at Niagara Falls. The Indians call it a "puzzle" (Fig. 251), and know no other use for it than to fasten it upon the thumb or finger of some victim, and then pull him about until he begs to be released.

The "puzzle" is an elongated cone of about sixteen or eighteen inches in length, made of ash splittings, and braided; the open end of the cone being about three-fourths of an inch in diameter, and the

Fig. 251.

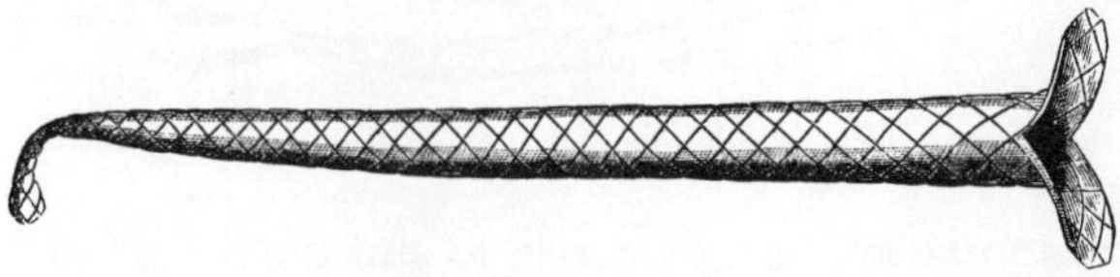

Indian "puzzle," employed for the reduction of dislocations in small joints.

opposite end terminating in a braided cord. When applied to the finger, it is slipped on lightly, forming a cap to the extremity, and to half the length of the finger, but on traction being made from the opposite end, it fastens itself to the limb with a most uncompromising grasp. If constructed of appropriate size and of suitable materials, it becomes the more securely fastened in proportion as the extension is increased; yet, applying itself equally to all the surfaces, it inflicts the least possible pain and injury upon the limb. When we wish to remove it, we have only to cease pulling, and it drops off spontaneously.

Dr. Holmes says that the same instrument is made by the Indians of Maine, and that several years ago Dr. Davis, of Portland, brought one to Boston, and showed it to the Society for Medical Improvement, suggesting that it might be used in the same manner which I have recommended.[1]

Finally, in some compound dislocations it would be better not to attempt the reduction of the dislocation until resection has been practiced. Samuel Cooper relates a case in which the reduction was followed by inflammation and death within a week after the accident, and Norris, of Philadelphia, mentions an instance which came under his observation, where violent inflammation and tetanus followed the reduction.[2] Roux, Evans, Wardrop, Gooch, Sir Astley Cooper, and many other surgeons, have practiced resection successfully in these accidents, and have added their testimony in favor of this mode of procedure.

§ 2. Dislocations of the First Phalanx of the Thumb forwards.

Up to the present moment, I have met with but two examples of this dislocation, while the backward dislocation has been seen by me five times.

[1] Trans. Amer. Med. Assoc., vol. i. p. 267.
[2] Norris, Amer. Journ. Med. Sci., vol. xxxi. p. 16.

Horace Kneeland, of Rochester, N. Y., æt. 24, dislocated the first phalanx of the right thumb forwards, by striking a man with his clenched fist; the force of the blow being received upon the back of the second joint of the thumb. The dislocation had existed three days when he called upon me, and in the meanwhile several attempts had been made to reduce the bone by simple extension. The first phalanx was in front of the metacarpal bone, and in the same plane; but the last phalanx was slightly inclined backwards. The hand was already swollen and quite painful.

Seizing the dislocated thumb in the palm of my right hand, with my fingers resting upon the back of the patient's hand, I forced the two phalanges into flexion by firm and steady pressure continued for a few seconds, when suddenly the bones resumed their places, and all deformity disappeared.

Intense inflammation resulted, followed, after a few days, by suppuration under the palmar fascia; and in the end the thumb was almost completely anchylosed.[1]

On the 24th of April, 1855, J. M. Booth, of Buffalo, æt. 19, called at my office, having a dislocation forwards of the first phalanx, occasioned about half an hour before by being thrown from a horse. The last two phalanges were neither flexed nor extended, but straight, and parallel with the metacarpal bone.

By the same manœuvre adopted in the preceding case, but with only very moderate force, the dislocation was promptly reduced.

The usual causes of this accident are, falls or blows upon the thumb while it is flexed; and the symptoms which characterize it are, in general, such as we have seen in the two examples which have just been given. The metacarpal bone projects posteriorly, and the first phalanx produces a corresponding projection toward the palm; the two phalanges are extended upon each other, and parallel with the metacarpal bones. Nélaton saw a case in which the first phalanx was flexed about 45°; and in several examples it has been observed to be slightly rotated inwards.

In the few examples of this accident which have been reported, the reduction was easily accomplished; or, at least, we may say that the difficulties in the way of reduction were not so great as they are usually found to be in dislocations backwards. Malgaigne has been able to collect but four undoubted examples, all of which were reduced; and Lenoir was able to effect the reduction by moderate measures, after the bone had been dislocated thirty-eight days.

Lombard, after the trial of other plans, finally succeeded by reversing the phalanx. Employing, as we have before termed it, "dorsal flexion," with extension and lateral motion; but in all, or nearly all the other examples, the reduction has been effected by flexing the thumb forcibly toward the palm; the reverse of the method which we have seen preferred, especially by American surgeons, in dislocations backwards. My own experience also authorizes me to recommend this plan.

[1] Trans. N. Y. State Med. Soc., 1855, p. 73.

§ 3. Dislocations of the First Phalanx of the Fingers.

The index and little fingers, owing to their exposed situations, are most liable to these dislocations. I have met with two examples of traumatic dislocations of these joints, one of which was a forward, and the other a backward luxation, and both had occurred in the index finger.

James Nesbitt, of Buffalo, æt. 11, dislocated the index finger of the right hand, backwards, by a fall down a flight of stairs. On the same day, Feb. 11, 1851, he called upon me, and I found the finger neither flexed nor extended, but straight and immovable. The projections occasioned by the ends of the two bones were very marked, and such as to render an error in the diagnosis impossible. Reduction was accomplished with great ease, by reversing the finger and employing moderate extension, while at the same time the proximal extremity of the first phalanx was pushed toward the distal end of the metacarpal bone. In short, the process was the same as that which we have recommended in dislocations of the thumb backwards.

Fig. 252.

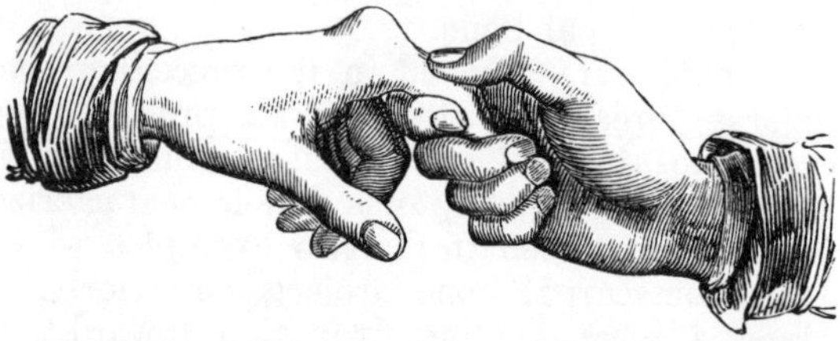

Backward dislocation of first phalanx. Reduction by extension.

In the example of dislocation forwards, occasioned by a blow from a hard ball, received upon the end of the finger, the first phalanx was in a position of extreme extension, and the second moderately flexed. Reduction was effected with great ease by extension in a straight line. But if the surgeon were to experience difficulty in the reduction, it would no doubt be advisable to resort to the method of extreme flexion.

In one instance, I have seen nearly all the fingers of the left hand, and the thumb of the right dislocated backwards, by the contraction of the cicatrix after a severe burn.

CHAPTER XV.

DISLOCATIONS OF THE SECOND AND THIRD PHALANGES OF THE THUMB AND FINGERS.

NOTWITHSTANDING slight differences in the form of the articulations between the thumb and fingers, and in the size and situation of the bones which compose the phalanges of the fingers, we are disposed, contrary to the practice of some other writers upon this subject, to consider all the dislocations to which these several joints are liable, under one section. Nor, indeed, after the attention which we have given to the dislocations at the metacarpo-phalangeal articulations, do we find much to add in relation to these accidents; since in almost every point of view in which they may be considered, they have so much in common.

The last phalanx of the thumb is, of all the phalanges, most liable to dislocation, and this generally takes place backwards. Very frequently, also, it is accompanied with such a laceration as to render it compound. The dislocated phalanx is usually reversed in the backward dislocation, and straight, or nearly so, in the forward dislocation.

Reduction may be accomplished easily by forced dorsal flexion, in the case of the backward luxation, and by forced palmar flexion, in the case of the forward dislocation.

In the winter of 1848, a young man was brought into my clinic, who had met with a forward subluxation of this phalanx about one month before. He had fallen upon the end of his thumb, and as the accident was followed by a good deal of inflammation and swelling, he did not notice the displacement until some time afterwards. The proximal end of the last phalanx projected two or three lines toward the palm; the finger was straight, and this joint anchylosed. I did not think the chance of restoring and maintaining the bone in position sufficient to warrant any interference, and he was dismissed with an assurance that after a few months it would occasion him no great inconvenience.

On the 2d of March, 1851, Thomas Burton, aged about twenty-two years, by a fall dislocated the second phalanx of the middle finger of the right hand, backwards. The force of the concussion was received upon the extremity of the finger. Nine hours after the accident I found the bones unreduced; the finger nearly straight, or with only slight flexion of the second phalanx upon the first; the third phalanx forcibly straightened upon the second; all the joints rigid; finger very painful and somewhat swollen.

By moderate extension alone, applied for a few seconds, the reduction was accomplished.

Fig. 253.

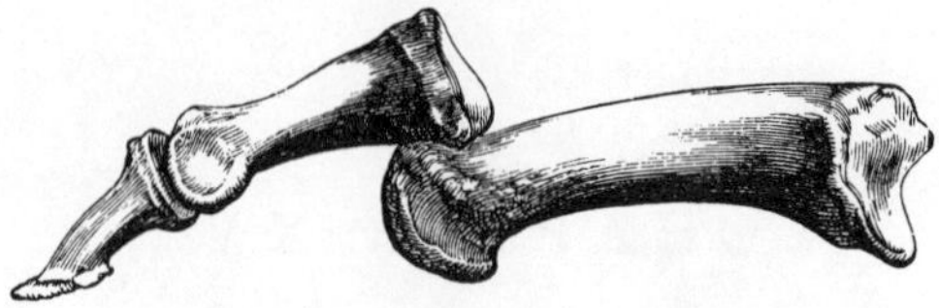

Dislocation of the second phalanx backwards.

James Cooper, of this city, æt. 23, came to me on Sunday morning the 14th of Dec., 1851, to obtain counsel in relation to his finger which had been dislocated the day before, but which he had himself reduced by simple extension made in a straight line. His own account of it was, that he fell upon a slippery side-walk, striking upon the end of his ring finger in such a way that it seemed to double under him. On examination, he found the second bone dislocated inwards, or to the ulnar side, completely, the end of the first phalanx forming a broad projection upon the opposite side; the last two phalanges fell over toward the middle finger, but they were neither flexed nor extended. Seizing upon the end of the finger with his right hand and pulling forcibly, he promptly reduced the dislocation himself.

The bones were now completely in place, but the joints were swollen, tender, and quite stiff.

In Sept., 1851, by the politeness of Dr. Briggs, the attending surgeon, I was permited to see in the hospital of the New York State Prison, at Auburn, a forward dislocation of the second phalanx of the little finger of the left hand, unreduced. This man was at the date of my examination forty-one years old, and the dislocation had existed eighteen years; having been occasioned by a fall. A surgeon in Greene Co., N. Y., had attempted to reduce it soon after the dislocation occurred, but had failed. The joint was nearly anchylosed, yet the finger was quite as useful for all ordinary purposes as before.

Fig. 254.

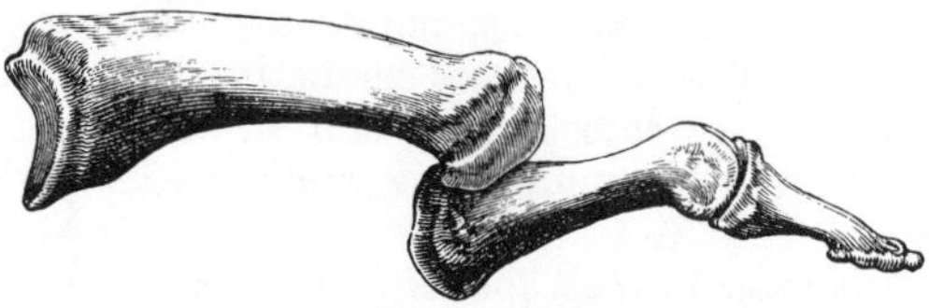

Dislocation of the second phalanx forwards.

Dislocation of the last phalanx is frequently occasioned in the game of base ball, by the ball being received upon the extremity of the finger.

A young man who was studying medicine, and a private pupil of mine, in attempting to catch a very hard ball, received it upon the extremity of the middle finger of the left hand, dislocating the last phalanx forwards. Twenty minutes after the accident, I found the distal extremity of the second phalanx projecting backwards through the skin, the tendon of the extensor muscle being torn completely off from its point of attachment to the last phalanx. The last phalanx was in a position of slight dorsal flexion, or extreme extension.

Seizing upon the extremity of the finger, I attempted to reduce the dislocation by direct traction, aided by pressure upon the exposed end of the second phalanx, but I was unable to succeed until I brought the last phalanx into a position of palmar flexion.

A slight disposition to reluxation was manifested, and a gutta-percha splint was therefore applied; and to prevent inflammation, the young man was directed to keep it moistened with cool water lotions. Only a moderate amount of inflammation followed, and in a few weeks the cure was complete.

Such accidents, attended with laceration of the integuments, frequently demand amputation, or at least resection of the projecting bone, but we think Mr. Miller is scarcely right when he says that compound dislocations of the fingers almost always are of such severity as to demand amputation.

CHAPTER XVI.

DISLOCATIONS OF THE THIGH (COXO-FEMORAL).

THE femur is especially liable to dislocation in four directions, namely, upwards and backwards upon the dorsum ilii, upwards and backwards into the ischiatic notch, downwards and forwards into the foramen thyroideum, and upwards and forwards upon the pubes.

Dislocations are occasionally met with which cannot be arranged properly under either of these divisions; indeed, it is scarcely necessary to say that the head of the bone may be thrown in almost every direction from its socket, upwards, downwards, inwards, and outwards, or in either of the diagonals between these lines; and that while in a vast majority of cases, it will assume one of the positions first named, it may in a few exceptional examples fall short of, or much exceed the limits assigned in this division. Thus, we shall have occasion hereafter to mention examples of dislocation directly upwards, in which the head of the bone will be found resting upon the fossa between the upper margin of the acetabulum and the anterior, inferior spinous process of the ilium, or still higher between the anterior superior and the anterior inferior spinous processes, or a little to the one side or to the other of these points. Examples will be shown of dislocations directly downwards, in which the head of the femur will rest upon the notch between the lower margin of the acetabulum and the tuber ischii, or still lower, and actually below the tuberosity, or downwards and backwards below the spine of the ischium, into the lower or lesser sacro-sciatic notch. The head may be thrust across the foramen thyroideum, and be only arrested in the perineum upon the ramus, or even beyond the ramus of the ischium and pubes; it may lodge upon the anterior surface of the body of the pubes, as well as upon its superior edge; and finally, it may rest against the posterior margin of the acetabulum instead of rising upon the dorsum, or it may only mount upon its margin, in either of the directions named.

In regard to frequency, the four principal dislocations occur in the order in which we have mentioned them; thus, of 104 dislocations of the hip which I have taken the pains to collate, excluding the anomalous or extraordinary dislocations, and which my intelligent pupil, Mr. Frank Hodge, has carefully analyzed, 55 were upon the dorsum ilii, 28 into the great ischiatic notch, 13 upon the foramen thyroideum, and 8 upon the pubes. Chelius and Samuel Cooper have, however, reversed the order of the last two varieties, arranging dislocations upon the pubes, in the order of frequency, before dislocations into the foramen thyroideum.

Coxo-femoral dislocations may occur at any period of life; one example is mentioned, in the *Gazette Médicale*, of a recent dislocation upon the dorsum ilii, in a child eighteen months old.[1] Mr. Kirby has reported, in the *Dublin Medical Press* for October 26, 1842, a case of recent dislocation in the same direction, in a child of three years,[2] and Dr. Buchanan has seen another, at the same age, in a little girl; the dislocation being into the ischiatic notch.[3] Mr. Image communicated to the Suffolk branch of the Provincial Medical and Surgical Association, the case of a boy, three and a half years old, with a dislocation upon the dorsum ilii. It had existed twelve days when he was admitted to the Suffolk Hospital in May, 1847. Mr. Image, in reporting this case to the Society, remarked that he had been induced to lay it before them, "in consequence of a charge having been urged against a neighboring surgeon, of pretending to reduce a dislocation of the femur on the dorsum ilii, in a child only four years old, that child being a pauper, and chargeable to the parish. It was agreed and proved by authorities that no such case was recorded, and therefore had not occurred, and that seven years old was the earliest period at which this accident had taken place."[4]

J. M. Litten, of Austin, Texas, reports a case of dislocation upon the dorsum ilii, in a girl four years old, which he reduced by manipulation.[5]

Dr. J. C. Warren, of Boston, met with an incomplete dislocation toward the foramen thyroideum, in a child six years old, which, having been displaced eight or ten weeks, he was unable to reduce.[6]

[1] New York Journ. Med., Nov. 1850, p. 416.
[2] Amer. Journ. Med. Sci., vol. xxxi. p. 207, Jan. 1843.
[3] Lond. Med.-Chir. Rev., Dec. 1828, p. 251.
[4] New York Journ. Med., Sept. 1848, p. 281.
[5] Ibid., March, 1852, p. 259.
[6] Boston Med. and Surg. Journ., vol. xxiv. p. 220.

Sir Astley Cooper mentions a case in a girl seven years old.[1] I have myself met with two dislocations upon the dorsum ilii, which occurred at ten years, and one into the foramen thyroideum.[2] Norris reports a case at eleven years,[3] and Gibson at twelve.[4] On the other hand, Gauthier has seen a dislocation of the hip in a woman eighty-six years of age.[5] The large majority, however, occur between the fifteenth and forty-fifth years of life. From an analysis of eighty-four cases, we have obtained the following results:—

Under 15 years	15 cases
15 to 30 "	32 "
30 to 45 "	29 "
45 to 60 "	7 "
60 to 85 "	1 case

The youngest being two years and one month, the oldest sixty-two years, and the average being a fraction less than thirty-four.

They are much more frequent in men than in women; owing, probably, to the greater exposure of the former to the accidents from which these dislocations usually result, and possibly, also, in some measure, to certain peculiarities in the form and structure of the neck of the femur in the male. Of one hundred and fifteen cases collected by me, one hundred and four were in males and eleven in females. Dr. J. K. Rodgers, of New York, mentioned, however, at a meeting of the New York Kappa Lambda Society, that he had seen and reduced four dislocations of the femur upon the dorsum ilii in females, and that a fifth case had recently come to his knowledge in the New York city hospital.[6]

Gibson mentions an example of dislocation of both thighs at the same moment.[7]

§ 1. Dislocations Upwards and Backwards on the Dorsum Ilii.

Syn.—"Upwards on the dorsum ilii;" Sir A. Cooper, Miller, Pirrie. "Upwards and outwards;" Boyer, Dupuytren. "Upwards and backwards upon the back of the hip bone;" Chelius. "Iliac;" Gerdy, Vidal (de Cassis), Malgaigne.

Causes.—Generally they are occasioned by some violence which forces the thigh into a state of extreme adduction, or of adduction united with rotation inwards; and especially when at the same moment the head of the femur is driven upwards and backwards. Thus, a dislocation upon the dorsum may result from a fall from a height, when the force of the concussion is received upon the outside of the knee; the thigh being thus converted into a lever of the first kind, whose long arm is outside of the margin of the acetabulum; or the disloca-

[1] A. Coop. on Disloc., Amer. ed., p. 83, case 27.
[2] Buf. Med. Journ., vol. viii. p. 6. Trans. New York State Med. Soc., 1855. My Report on Disloc.
[3] Amer. Journ. Med. Sci., Feb. 1839, p. 296. [4] Gibson's Surg., vol. i. p. 389.
[5] Gauthier, Malgaigne, op. cit., p. 805.
[6] J. K. Rodgers, New York Journ. Med., July, 1839, vol. i. First ser. p. 220.
[7] Gibson's Surg., vol. i. p. 385. Sixth ed.

tion may be occasioned by a fall upon the foot or knee, while the limb is adducted, by which the head of the femur will be at the same moment driven upwards and outwards from its socket. The accident is equally liable to result from the fall of a heavy weight, such as a mass of earth, upon the back of the pelvis when the body is much bent forwards.

The following case presents an extraordinary example of this form of dislocation, produced by a force acting upon the thigh as a lever of the first kind.

B.,of Rochester, N. Y., æt. 10, fell, in Feb. 1841, from the top of the high bank just below the Genesee Falls, at Rochester, a distance of about one hundred feet. Before he reached the bottom of the precipice, he struck upon an oblique plane of ice, from which he slid gradually down upon the surface of the river, which was then completely frozen over. He did not lose his consciousness in the descent, nor after his arrest upon the river, but began immediately to call for assistance. He remembers very well that when he struck the glacier, the concussion was received upon the right side of the right knee, and a mark of contusion at this point confirmed his statement. Dr. Ellwood, of Rochester, assisted by myself, reduced the dislocation within one hour after its occurrence. We employed pulleys, but the reduction was accomplished easily in about two minutes, and without the application of much force; the bone resuming its place with an audible snap. His recovery was rapid and complete.[1]

Pathological Anatomy.—The capsule is lacerated more or less extensively, but especially in its posterior half; the round ligament is ruptured; some of the small external rotator muscles are generally stretched or torn completely asunder, the glutæus maximus, medius, and minimus are pushed upwards and folded upon each other, the head of the femur resting upon or within the fibres of the deeper muscles; the triceps adductor is put upon the stretch.

Fig. 255.

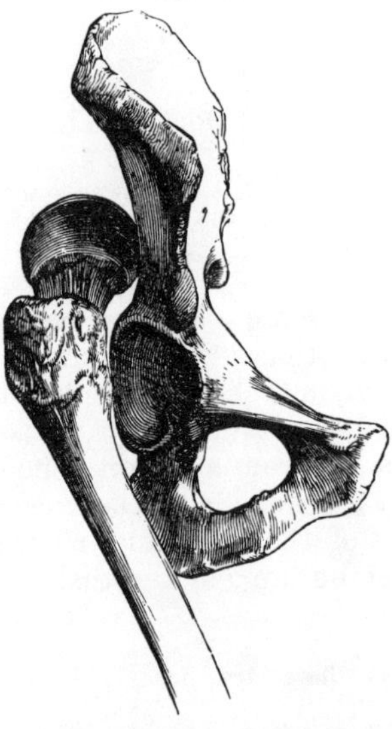

Dislocation upon the dorsum ilii.

Surgeons have not been agreed as to the cause of the great difficulty which has usually been experienced in the reduction of this and of all other forms of coxo-femoral dislocations. While some have ascribed it alone to the resistance of the muscles, others have with equal confidence, ascribed the opposition to an entanglement of the head and neck of the bone in the rent capsule; and still others believe that the impediment ought to be looked for sometimes in the muscles and sometimes in the capsule, or in both at the same moment.

Sir Astley Cooper thought that the capsular ligament was generally too much torn to offer any impediment

[1] Trans. New York State Med. Soc., 1855, p. 76. My Report on Dislocations.

to reduction, and he refers to some dissections in confirmation of this opinion. Nathan Smith affirmed that the chief obstacle to reduction by extension was to be found in the resistance offered by the gluteii muscles, which, although at first relaxed, would soon become tense under the stimulus of the extension, and which, in order that the bone might resume its position, must actually be stretched considerably beyond their normal length. W. W. Reid declares that the sole resistance is at first in the abductors and rotators, but that finally the psoas magnus, iliacus internus, and triceps adductor become tense where the pulleys are employed.

Dr. Fenner, of New Orleans, gives the particulars of a dissection of the hip of a man admitted into the Charity Hospital, who died from injuries received by the bursting of a steamboat boiler. His condition being considered hopeless, no attempt was made to reduce the dislocation. The limb was shortened one inch and a half, and the toes turned inwards. Extensive ecchymosis existed. On raising the glutæus maximus and medius, the naked head of the femur was found lying on the dorsum ilii with the ligamentum teres hanging to it, but partially torn off. Portions of the obturator externus, pyriformis, and gemelli were ruptured and lacerated. The capsule was torn through one-half of its extent.

Dr. Fenner now proceeded to cut away the muscles, and when all the external muscles about the joint had been removed the thigh could not be brought down; the iliacus internus and psoas magnus were then severed, which permitted it to descend a little, but the head could not be replaced; the triceps adductor was then divided without effect. The ilio-femoral ligament was found tensely stretched. All the muscles between the pelvis and the thigh were then severed, and still it was impossible to reduce the dislocation; the head of the femur could not be forced back through the rent in the capsule from which it had escaped; and it was not until the opening was enlarged from one-half to three-quarters of an inch, that the reduction was accomplished.

Dr. Fenner infers that the capsule possesses sufficient elasticity to allow the smooth head of the femur to pass out through a lacerated opening which might at once contract, so as to offer considerable resistance to its return, and that occasionally this is the true explanation of the difficulty in reduction.[1] Dr. Gunn, of Ann Arbor, Michigan, after repeated experiments made upon the dead body, concludes that the muscles offer no impediment whatever to the reduction, and that the "untorn portion of the capsular ligament, by binding down the head of the dislocated bone, prevents its ready return over the edge of the acetabulum to its place in the socket."[2] Dr. Moore, of Rochester, who has often repeated the same experiments upon the cadaver, declares also that in attempting to reduce the femur by extension alone he has constantly observed that the untorn portion of the capsule offered the main resistance, and that reduction could not be accomplished until this was more completely broken up;[3] while Markoe, of New York,

[1] New York Journ. Med., Sept. 1848, p. 268; from New Orleans Med. and Surg. Journ., July, 1848.

[2] Ibid., Nov. 1853, p. 423 et seq.

[3] Ibid., July, 1855, p. 69.

attributes the resistance to both the muscles and the capsule, but chiefly to the action of the former, especially the rotators.[1]

The conclusion to which we ought to arrive seems to be that in some cases, the capsule being completely, or almost completely torn away, the muscles offer the only resistance; and that according to the exact position of the limb or degree of displacement, one or another set of muscular fibres will oppose the reduction; and in other cases, the muscles being paralyzed by the shock, or by anæsthetics, the partially torn capsule, into which the head of the bone is received as in a button-hole, prevents its free return into its socket.

Symptoms.—Sir Astley Cooper affirmed that the limb was sometimes found shortened in this dislocation, to the extent of three inches. Liston, B. Cooper, Gibson, and others repeat the affirmation. Chelius places the extreme of shortening at two and a half inches, Miller at two inches, while Malgaigne declares that he has never seen the limb shortened more than half an inch, and that in some cases it is not shortened at all, and the very opposite opinions entertained by other surgeons, he attributes to errors in the measurement. I am certain, however, that Malgaigne has fallen into some error, and that, while the average shortening is about one inch or one inch and a half, it does occasionally reach three inches.

Fig. 256.

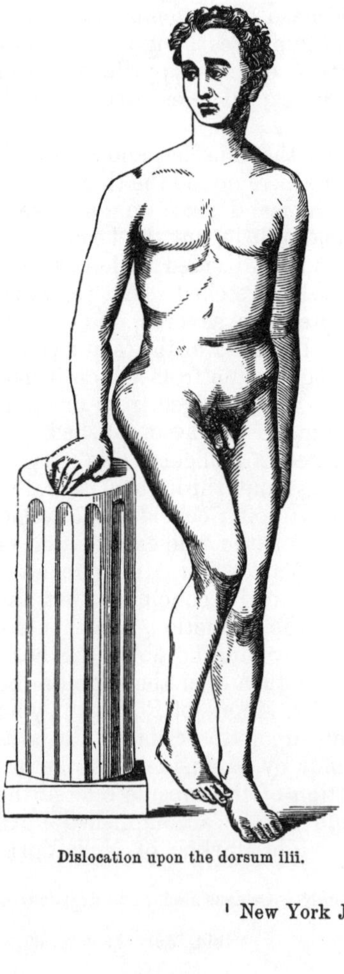

Dislocation upon the dorsum ilii.

The thigh is rotated inwards, adducted and slightly flexed upon the pelvis. The great toe of the dislocated limb, when the patient stands erect (and in this position the examination ought if possible to be made), rests upon the instep of the foot of the sound limb, and the knee touches the opposite thigh near the upper margin of the patella. It must not be supposed, however, that the position of the limb is in all cases precisely such as we have described. Indeed the degree of rotation, adduction, flexion &c., will vary according as the head of the femur is more or less displaced, the capsule more or less torn, or as it may be torn in its upper or lower margins, as the muscles may be ac-

[1] New York Journal Med., Jan. 1855.

tually rent asunder or only put upon the stretch, and perhaps also according to the amount of injury and consequent relaxation which they may have sustained from the shock. The thigh can be easily flexed; adduction is more difficult, but abduction is almost impossible, except to a very limited extent: the body of the patient is a little bent forwards; the roundness of the hip is lost in consequence of the relaxation of the gluteii muscles; the trochanter major is depressed, and approaches the anterior superior spinous process of the ilium, and if the patient is not fat, and swelling has not already taken place, the head of the femur may be felt in its new position rotating under the hand when the limb is turned inwards or outwards, but especially may it be felt when, by flexing or extending the limb, the head is made to move downwards and upwards, upon the dorsum ilii.

As we have already said, this examination ought to be made, if possible, in the erect posture; after which, it will be well to place the patient alternately upon his back, upon his sound side, and upon his belly, until the diagnosis is rendered complete.

The differential diagnosis between dislocation upon the dorsum ilii and a fracture of the neck of the femur may be briefly stated as follows.

In fracture, we may expect to find crepitus; the limb is in most cases mobile; the toes are generally turned out; the limb is shortened moderately or not at all; the patient is sometimes able to walk for a short distance; fractures of the neck of the femur generally occur in advanced life.

In dislocation, crepitus is not often present, and only when a fracture coexists; the limb is immobile, or nearly so; the toes are turned in; the limb is shortened more; the patient is unable to bear the weight of his body upon his foot for one moment. Skey, however, says he has seen a patient with a recent dislocation, who walked one-quarter of a mile, to the hospital. I do not think any other similar case is upon record. Dislocations of the femur generally occur in middle life.

I have been frequently told by persons who have called upon me with children suffering under hip-disease, that they had been informed the hip was out, and they expected me to reduce it. In two or three instances they have blamed their surgeons very much, because they had not detected the accident at the time of its occurrence. Norris, of Philadelphia, mentions an extraordinary example of this kind, as having been presented at the Pennsylvania Hospital, and which ought to serve as a sufficient warning to prevent similar mistakes in future. A lad, twelve years old, was brought to the hospital from a neighboring State, who a short time previous had been suddenly attacked with lameness in his right limb, and which, by his friends was attributed to some injury received in play. Two physicians, who had been called to see the boy, pronounced him to be laboring under dislocation of the hip, and had made two strong efforts with the pulleys, to reduce it; but after causing great suffering they gave up all hopes of ever replacing the bone, and sent him to Philadelphia. The symptoms were plainly those of hip-joint disease in its early stage. The attitude was that assumed by those laboring under this affection; the leg seemed lengthened, but a careful measurement showed that it was of the same length with the other; the buttock was flattened and the motions of the joint tolerably free but painful.[1]

If the supposed dislocation occurs in a child, or in a person under ten years of age, we ought to take especial pains to ascertain that it is not a separation of the epiphysis, of which accident we have mentioned some examples when speaking of fractures of the neck of the femur.

Prognosis.—Boyer says the limb remains always weaker than the other, the round ligament never uniting completely; and that inflammation of the cartilages and synovial glands may ensue, ending in caries of the joint. Such results have, indeed, been occasionally met with, nor are examples wanting in which more rapid inflammation, resulting in the formation of acute abscesses, has followed, but these are only rare accidents. In the large majority of cases the patients recover speedily, and in the course of a few weeks, or months at most, the limb seems to be as sound and as useful as before.

Examples of non-reduction, however, from an error of diagnosis, or what is more pertinent to our present purpose, from a failure to accomplish the reduction where the attempt has been made, are numerous. Fortunately, Mr. Chelius, the author of a most excellent "*System of Surgery*," to which we have already had frequent occasion to refer, has sufficient reputation, the world over, to enable him to bear a portion of these failures, without injury to himself or to the profession which he so eminently adorns. We shall therefore make no apology for reporting the following unsuccessful attempt to reduce a dislocation of the hip in which Mr. Chelius himself was the operator.

On the 11th of June, 1851, John Mauren, a German, æt. 19, called at my office and related as follows: "When ten years old, I fell from a tree, a height of six feet, and dislocated my left hip. I was then living twelve miles from Heidelberg, and I was immediately taken there, but I did not see Mr. Chelius until the next morning. He took me to the University, and before the medical class attempted to reduce it, but he could not. During several weeks following, he tried six times, using pulleys, &c., but he could never succeed."

On examination I found the limb shortened two inches, the head of the femur lying upon the dorsum ilii; the knee was turned in, but the toes were inclined a little outwards. He was able to walk rapidly, of course with a manifest halt, yet without pain and discomfort.

Treatment.—Regarding dislocations of the femur upon the dorsum ilii as the type of all the coxo-femoral dislocations, the remarks which we shall make under this section may be considered applicable with only certain qualifications to all the others.

We shall arrange the various methods of reduction which have been employed by surgeons under two principal heads, namely, manipulation and extension. It is not possible, however, to classify rigidly the different procedures, so as to bring them under these two simple divisions without some violence; since neither manipulation nor ex-

[1] Norris, Amer. Journ. Med. Sci., vol. xxv. p. 280.

tension has usually been employed alone, but almost always some degree of extension has been recommended in connection with the manipulation; if not in the first instance, at least in the event of the failure of manipulation alone; while, on the other hand, extension is seldom if ever practiced without manipulation. We intend then to imply by these designations respectively, that either manipulation or extension has constituted the prevailing feature in the treatment.

Reduction by manipulation dates from the earliest records of our science. Says Hippocrates: "In some the thigh is reduced with no preparation, with slight extension directed by the hands, and with slight movement; and in some the reduction is effected by bending the limb at the joint, and making rotation."[1]

Richard Wiseman, who wrote in 1676, speaks as follows: "If the thigh-bone be luxated inwards, and the patient young and of a tender constitution, it may be reduced by the hand of the chirurgeon, viz: he must lay one hand on the thigh, and the other on the patient's leg, and having somewhat extended it toward the sound leg, he must suddenly force the knee up toward the belly, and press back the head of the femur into its acetabulum, and it will knap in. For there is no need of so great extension in this kind of luxation; for the most considerable muscles being upon the stretch, the bowing of the knee as aforesaid reduceth it; yet in rough bodies it may require stronger extension."[2]

Richard Boulton repeated, in 1713, almost the same instructions, affirming that this plan was applicable especially to dislocations inwards, in the case of "young and tender children."[3]

In 1742 Daniel Turner declared that he had reduced three dislocations of the hip, one of which was a backward dislocation, by a method combining extension with manipulation, but alone "by the strength of the arm or without any other instrument." Extension and counter-extension being made by assistants, and "as soon as the surgeon perceives the bone moving out," says Turner, "let him take his opportunity, giving order to the extenders below suddenly to lift up the patient's thigh toward his belly, pressing with his hands, either to the right or left, as the situation of the same requires, and therewith force back its head toward the acetabulum, whereunto it will, flipping over the tip of the cartilage, snap sometimes with a loud noise."[4]

Thomas Anderson, surgeon of Leith, in Scotland, was called, in Sept. 1772, to see a man who had dislocated his left femur into the foramen thyroideum. When he arrived four other surgeons were present, and prepared to use the pulleys, which they did in his presence several times, but to no purpose. After examining the limb carefully, "I was convinced," says Mr. Anderson, "that attempting the reduction in the common method, with the thigh extended, was im-

[1] Works of Hippocrates, Syd. ed., vol. ii. p. 643.

[2] Eight Chirurgical Treatises. By Richard Wiseman, Serjeant-Chirurgeon to King Charles II. London, 1676. Book vii. chap. viii.

[3] A System of Rational and Practical Surgery. By Richard Bovlton. London, 1713, p. 346.

[4] The Art of Surgery, by Daniel Turner, London, 1742, vol. ii. p. 339.

proper, as the muscles were all put on the stretch, the action of which is, perhaps, sufficient to overbalance any extension we can apply. But by bringing the thigh to near a right angle with the trunk, by which the muscles would be greatly relaxed, I imagined that the reduction might more readily take place, and with much less extension.

"When I made this examination, he was lying on a table on his back. I raised the thigh to about a right angle with the trunk, and, with my right hand at the ham, laid hold of the thigh, and made what extension I could. From this trial I found I could dislodge the head of the bone. At the same time that I did this, with my left hand at the head and inside of the thigh, I pressed it toward the acetabulum, while my right gave the femur a little circular turn, so as to bring the rotula inwards to its natural situation; and, on the second attempt, it went in with a snap observable to the gentlemen standing around, but more so to the poor man, who instantly cried out he was well and free from pain. His knees could then be brought together; the legs were of the same length, and the foot in its natural situation. The knees were kept together for some time, with a roller, to confine the motion of the thigh; and in three weeks he was at his work, without the least stiffness in the joint."

Subsequently Mr. Anderson reduced by a similar method a dislocation upon the dorsum ilii in a child eight years old, and which had been out nineteen days.[1]

Says Pouteau, in a memoir on dislocations of the thigh upwards and outwards: "We observe then, first, that the thigh ought to be flexed to a right angle with the body during the extension and counter-extension; second, that we ought to rotate the thigh from within outwards, when the extension appears to be sufficient; third, that this position puts into relaxation, as much as possible, the triceps and gluteal muscles which oppose the chief resistance to the extension, thus saving the patient from excessive pain; fourth, that the flexion of the thigh places the head of the bone in the best position for a return to the cotyloid cavity during extension; fifth, that feeble extension suffices for the reduction, because all of the muscles of the thigh are relaxed."[2]

On the 7th of Jan. 1811, Dr. Philip Syng Physick, of Philadelphia, reduced an outward dislocation of the hip, after extension had failed, by flexing the thigh to a right angle with the body, and then giving to the limb "an outward circular sweep.[3]

So early as 1815, and perhaps much earlier, Nathan Smith, Prof. of Surgery in the New Haven Medical College, taught that the only correct mode of reducing a dislocation upon the ilium was to flex the leg upon the thigh, the thigh upon the pelvis, and then to carry the limb diagonally to the opposite side, from whence it was to be brought outwards and downwards;[4] and in 1824, Dr. Smith, being under oath,

[1] Anderson. Medical Commentaries, Edinburgh, 1776, vol. ii. pp. 261–4.

[2] Vidal (de Cassis); from Œuvres posthumes de Pouteau, Paris, 1783.

[3] Physick, Dorsey's Surg., 1813, vi. p. 242. Mem. of Nathan Smith, 1831, p. 172. Phelps' paper, in Trans. New York State Med. Soc., 1856, p. 169.

[4] Trans. N. Y. St. Med. Soc., 1854, p. 55.

affirmed as follows: "I do not think that the mechanical powers, such as the wheel and axle, or the pulleys, are necessary to reduce a dislocated hip, or any other dislocation." He further adds that he once reduced a dislocation upon the dorsum ilii after he had pulled in every direction but the right, "by carrying the knee toward the patient's face."[1] Subsequently the son of Dr. Smith, Nathan R. Smith, the present distinguished teacher of surgery in the medical college at Baltimore, gave a more full account of his father's method, illustrating his views of the pathology of these dislocations, and the mechanism of their reduction by several drawings. It must be noticed, however, that Dr. Nathan Smith left no written explanation of his views and practice, except that which is to be found in the affidavit already quoted, and that the account published by his son is from memory, and it is given as follows: "The patient being prepared for the operation by whatever means may be deemed necessary, may be placed in an attitude convenient for the operation, with the body securely fixed, by placing him in the horizontal posture, on a narrow table covered with blankets, and on the sound side. To the table his body should be firmly fixed, and this can be conveniently done by folding a sheet several times, lengthways—then applying the middle of the broad band thus made to the inner and upper part of the sound thigh—carrying its extremities under the table, crossing them beneath it, and then carrying them obliquely up and crossing them firmly over the trunk, above the injured hip. The ends may then be secured beneath the table. To support the trunk the more firmly, a pillow may be placed on each side of it upon the table, and be included in the bandage. Should the operator design to employ any degree of extension, a counter-extending band may be placed in the perineum, and carried up to the extremity of the table, be fixed to some more firm body, or held by the hands of assistants.

"The operator now standing on the side to which the patient's back presents, grasps the knee of the dislocated member with his right hand (if the left femur be dislocated—*vice versa*, if the right), and the ankle with the left. The first effort which he makes is to flex the leg upon the thigh, in order to make the leg a lever with which he may operate on the thigh-bone. The next movement is a gentle rotation of the thigh outwards, by inclining the foot toward the ground, and rotating the knee outwards. Next the thigh is to be *slightly* abducted by pressing the knee directly outwards. Lastly, the surgeon freely flexes the thigh upon the pelvis by thrusting the knee upwards toward the face of the patient, *and at the same moment the abduction is to be increased.*

"Professor N. Smith regarded the free flexion of the thigh upon the pelvis as a very important part of the compound movement. He believed that it threw the head of the bone downwards, behind the acetabulum, where the margin of the cup is less prominent, and over which, therefore, the adductor muscles would drag it with less difficulty into its place.

[1] Report of the Trial of an Action for Malpractice. Lowell *v.* Faxon and Hawks, Machias, Maine, 1824; also Buf. Med. Journ., vol. xiii. p. 515.

"The operator may slightly vary these movements, as he increases them, so as to give some degree of rocking motion to the head of the os femoris, which will thereby be disengaged with the more facility from its confined situation among the muscles."[1]

Fig. 257.

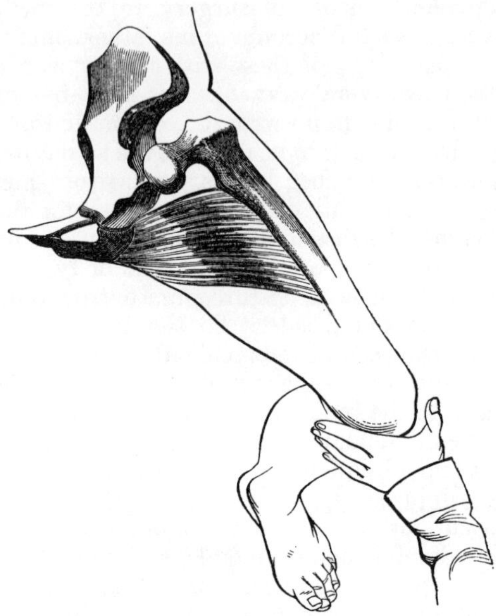

Nathan Smith's method of reduction by manipulation. (From Smith's "Memoirs.")

Dr. Luke Howe, of Boston, who was a pupil of Nathan Smith's, gives the following account of the method practiced by him successfully, about the year 1820, and which method he says, was recommended by his preceptor: "The patient was permitted to lie on his back on the bed where I found him, the knee of the luxated limb turned in and over the other. I raised the knee in the direction it inclined to take, which was toward the breast of the opposite side, till the descent of the head of the bone gave an inclination of the knee outwards, when I made use of the leg, being at right angle with the thigh, as a lever to rotate the latter and turn the head of it inwards. It then readily returned to its socket, with an audible snap. During this operation, the two assistants who had been placed to make the lateral extension and counter-extension, if ultimately required, were directed to draw moderately at their towels. How much of the success of the operation is to be imputed to their extension, and the rotation of the thigh by the leg, I am unable to determine; but as Dr. Smith succeeded without the aid of either, and as the head of the

[1] Medical and Surgical Memoirs, by Nathan Smith, late Prof. of Surgery, &c., in Yale College. Edited by Nathan R. Smith, Prof. of Surgery in Univ. of Maryland. Baltimore, 1831, pp. 163–182.

femur seemed to descend by an easy and natural process, I am inclined to believe that all that is necessary in such cases, is to elevate the knee, when the ilium, the muscles attached to it, and perhaps the ligaments, become the natural fulcrum, over which the thigh, as a lever, acts to bring the head down and inwards into the socket."[1]

Kluge, in 1825, combined moderate extension with manipulation, by flexing both the leg and thigh, while at the same moment the thigh was abducted and the knee rotated inwards.[2] Wathman, in 1826, directed that in this dislocation the limb should be seized by the knee and ankle and slowly lifted forwards until it came to a right angle with the long axis of the body; when, if the outward "self-twisting of the thigh" occurs, "which cannot be prevented by fast holding," the movement of the head of the bone is declared, and it will only remain for the surgeon to let down the thigh gradually upon the bed so that the two limbs will come side by side, and the reduction will be accomplished.[3]

Rust recommended also, in 1826, a similar plan, combining moderate extension by the hands, with flexion and abduction of the thigh.[4]

Colombat, whose opinions date from 1830, suggested that the patient should lay himself forwards upon a bed or a table no higher than his hips, with the sound leg and foot resting upon the floor, and that then the surgeon seizing the foot with one hand, so as to flex the leg, should, with the other hand, exercise a moderate degree of extension, and at the same time move the limb to the right or to the left, backwards and forwards, in order to disengage the head of the femur; and, finally, that he should communicate to the thigh a sudden movement of circular rotation, either from within outwards, or from without inwards, as the surgeon might choose.[5]

Collin states that, in 1833, he had reduced four dislocations of the hip by a method very similar to this recommended by Colombat.[6]

Dr. William Ingalls, of Chelsea, Mass., reduced a compound dislocation of the femur, in which the head of the bone rested upon the pubes, after an unsuccessful attempt had been made to reduce it by extension. "An assistant, taking the ankle of the dislocated limb in his right hand, and placing his left in the ham, bent the leg at right angles upon the thigh, and the thigh upon the pelvis, then lifting with a power little more than sufficient to elevate the whole limb, he carried it to its greatest state of abduction, at the same time rotating the femur inwards while Dr. Ingalls passed his thumb through the wound, and pressing upon the head of the femur, directed it toward the acetabulum. At this moment he directed the limb to be forced toward its fellow, by which the reduction was effected with the greatest possible ease and elegance."[7]

Similar methods of reduction, with only such slight variations as scarcely deserve a special notice, have been suggested and practiced

[1] Howe, Boston Med. and Surg. Journ., vol. xxii. p. 249, May, 1840.
[2] Chelius's Surg., by South, Amer. ed., vol. ii. p. 241. [3] Ibid., p. 240.
[4] Ibid., p. 241, note by South. [5] Malgaigne, op. cit., vol. ii. p. 825.
[6] Malgaigne, op. cit., p. 823.
[7] Ingalls, Bransby Cooper's ed. of Sir Astley's English ed , 1842, and Amer. ed., 1852.

from time to time by Palletta, in 1818;[1] Desprez, in 1835;[2] Vial, in 1841;[3] Fischer, Mahr, and Clarke, in 1849.[4]

In 1851, Dr. W. W. Reid, of Rochester, N. Y., published an account of the method practiced by himself successfully in three cases of dislocation upon the dorsum ilii, the first of which dated from the year 1844. His method, as applied to a dislocation upon the dorsum ilii, consists in "flexing the leg upon the thigh, carrying the thigh over the sound one, upwards over the pelvis as high as the umbilicus, and then abducting and rotating it."[5]

Dr. Markoe, of New York, adopts the same procedure, except that when the limb has been sufficiently flexed and abducted, he directs that the limb shall be gradually brought down, and he affirms that it is during this last manœuvre that he has usually found the bone resume its place in the socket.[6]

Reduction by extension dates from a period equally early with reduction by manipulation. Hippocrates recommended, when other and gentler means had failed, to make extension and counter-extension; the extending bands being made fast above the knee and above the ankle, so as to distribute the points of pressure; and the counter-extending bands being secured around the chest under the armpits, and also, if thought necessary, in the perineum of the sound side.

Fig. 258.

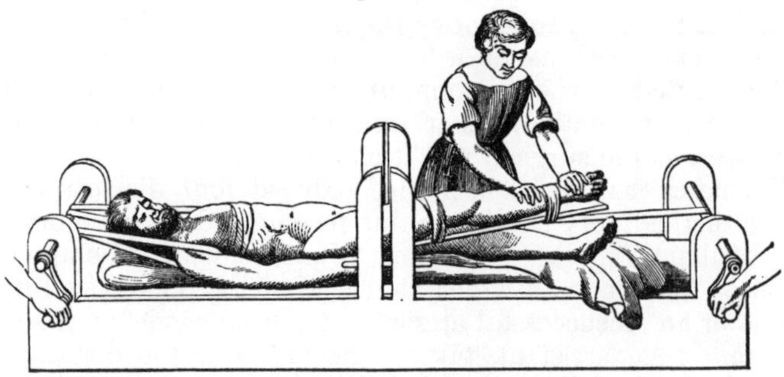

Hippocrates's mode of reducing dislocations of the hip by extension.

Among the methods recommended and practiced by Hippocrates, was sitting across the upper round of a ladder with a weight attached to the thigh of the dislocated limb; or suspending the patient from a sort of gallows with the head downwards, and if the weight of the patient's own body proved insufficient, the surgeon might add his also; a method which Hippocrates characterizes as "a good, proper, and natural mode of reduction, and one which has something of display in it, if any one takes delight in such ostentatious modes of procedure."[7]

1 Chelius's Surg.; note by South. 2 Malgaigne. 3 Ibid.
4 Dublin Med. Press, Dec. 3, 1851. New York Journ. Med., March, 1852.
5 Reid, Buf. Med. Journ., vol. vii., August, 1851, pp. 129–143.
6 Markoe, New York Journ. Med., Jan. 1855.
7 Works of Hippocrates, Syd. ed., London, vol. ii. p. 641.

With various modifications as to the position of the limb, and as to the points upon which the extending and counter-extending forces are to be applied, and with differently constructed appliances, surgeons have continued to employ extension down to this day.

The great majority have regarded flexion of the thigh as essential to success; some holding the limb only slightly flexed, and others insisting that the flexion should be increased to a right angle with the body.

The French surgeons, including Boyer and Vidal (de Cassis), prefer generally to apply the extending bands to the feet, in order that the muscles of the thigh may not be stimulated to contraction by the pressure of the bandages. Mr. Skey adopts the same method.

Sir Astley Cooper, Samuel Cooper, B. Cooper, Fergusson, Miller, Pirrie, Erichsen, and the English surgeons generally, make fast the lacq above the knee. J. L. Petit and Duverney, among the French, and Dorsey, Gibson, with most of the American surgeons, recommend the same, but Gerdy seeks to multiply the points of application, and for this purpose secures the extending band to the whole length of the leg, and to a small portion of the thigh above the knee.

The counter-extending bands are now almost universally made to operate against the perineum of the dislocated limb, but Roux, following the practice of Hippocrates, places it in the perineum of the sound limb. Gibson recommends the same practice.

Lizars recommends that sometimes the reduction should be attempted by simply placing the heel in the perineum and making the extension with the hands, very much as Sir Astley Cooper advises us to proceed in dislocations of the humerus. Morgan and Cock, of Guy's Hospital, have reduced six cases of dislocation of the hip-joint by placing the foot between the thighs, so that it pressed against the upper part of the dislocated bone, and thrust it away from the pelvis; extension and rotation of the limb being made at the same time by assistants.[1] Three of these were examples of dislocation upon the dorsum ilii, two upon the pubes, and one into the foramen thyroideum; and most of them had occurred in weak or elderly persons.

Ambrose Paré was among the first to recommend the use of pulleys for the reduction of dislocations. Most surgeons since his day have employed them for the purpose of making the extension more energetic and steady, and that it might be longer continued. Sir Astley Cooper's plan of procedure is as follows:—

The patient having been bled freely and the muscles still farther relaxed by nauseating doses of antimony and by the hot bath, he is to be placed on his back upon a table of convenient height between two staples; a strong padded leathern girth or perineal band, constructed so as to receive the thigh and to press at the same moment against the perineum and the outer surface of the pelvis, is then applied and made fast to one of the staples situated behind the patient in the direction of the axis of the limb. A wetted linen roller is next to be tightly applied just above the knee, and upon this a leathern strap is to be buckled,

[1] Cock and Morgan, Chelius, op. cit., vol. ii. p. 242, note by South.

having two short straps with rings at right angles with the circular part; or instead of this, a round towel made in the knot called the clove-hitch. The knee is to be slightly bent, but not quite to a right angle, and brought across the opposite thigh a little above the knee. The pulleys being now attached, the extension is to be commenced.

Fig. 259.

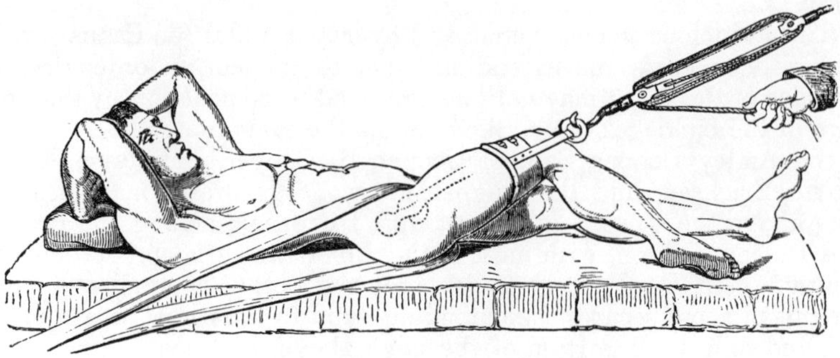

Reduction of a dislocation on the dorsum ilii, by pulleys.

A very simple and efficient mode of making the extension, if one has not the pulleys, is to employ for this purpose a small rope, the ends being tied together and the rope being then doubled upon itself once or twice, so as to make four or eight parallel cords. The opposite ends of this bundle of ropes being made fast to the limb and the staple, the extension is made by thrusting a stick through its centre

Fig. 260.

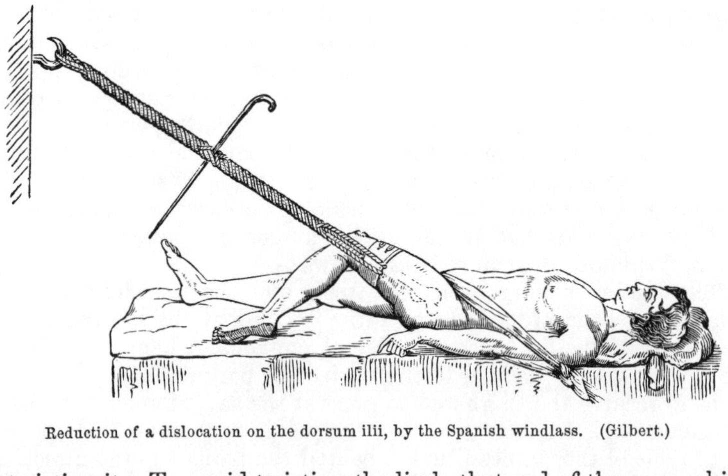

Reduction of a dislocation on the dorsum ilii, by the Spanish windlass. (Gilbert.)

and twisting it. To avoid twisting the limb, that end of the rope which is attached to the patient may play in a swivel.

I have several times had occasion to resort to this plan; and indeed it has been for some time known and practiced among surgeons in this country,[1] having been first, according to Prof. Gilbert, introduced by Fahnestock, of Pittsburg, Pa.

Jarvis's adjuster, to which I have already made allusion when speaking of dislocations of the humerus, has been often used with success in dislocations of the hip as well as in dislocations of the shoulder.[2] Its power is equal to that of the pulleys, while the direction of the force can be varied with much greater ease. The most serious objections to the instrument as employed for the reduction of dislocations, are its complexity and its expensiveness.

Fig. 261.

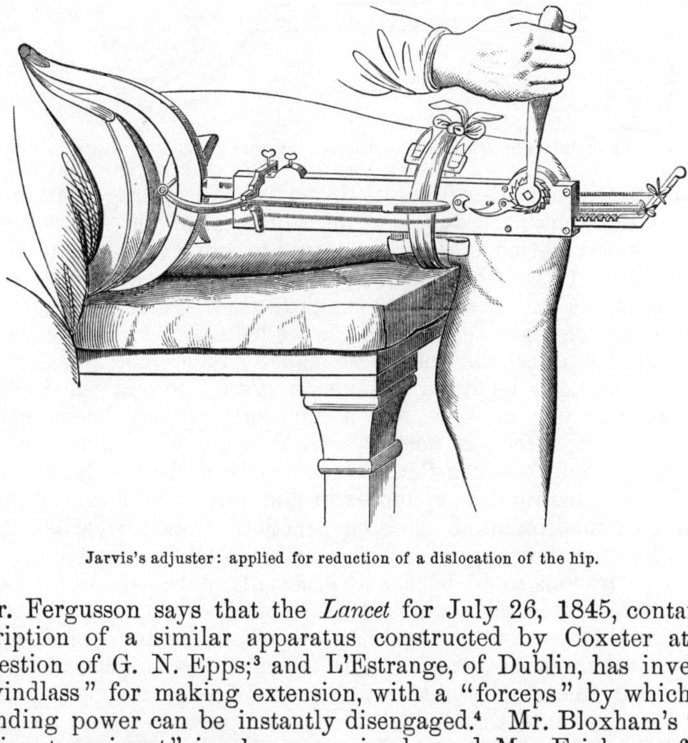

Jarvis's adjuster: applied for reduction of a dislocation of the hip.

Mr. Fergusson says that the *Lancet* for July 26, 1845, contains a description of a similar apparatus constructed by Coxeter at the suggestion of G. N. Epps;[3] and L'Estrange, of Dublin, has invented a "windlass" for making extension, with a "forceps" by which the extending power can be instantly disengaged.[4] Mr. Bloxham's "dislocation tourniquet" is also very simple, and Mr. Erichsen affirms that by it "any amount of extending force that may be required can be readily set up and maintained."[5] Sedillot, a French surgeon, has suggested that when pulleys are used, we should measure the exact power employed in the reduction, by an ingeniously contrived apparatus

[1] Gilbert, of Philadelphia. Note to Pirrie's Surg.; also Am. Journ. Med. Sci., vol. xxxv. April, 1845.

[2] Crandall, Bost. Med. and Surg. Journ., vol. xxxix. p. 77; Atlee, Trans. Amer. Med. Assoc., vol. iii. 1850, p. 357.

[3] Fergusson, 4th Amer. ed., p. 200.

[4] Ibid., p. 198.

[5] Erichsen, Amer. ed., 1859, p. 242.

called the dynamometer.[1] Such an instrument might occasionally be useful in preventing the application of excessive force, especially when the patient is under the influence of an anæsthetic.

Fig. 262.

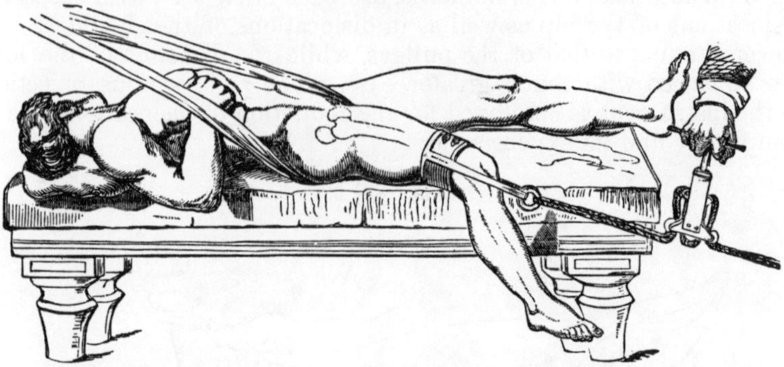

Bloxham's "dislocation tourniquet," applied for reduction of a dislocation on the pubes.

Finally, without attempting to determine the precise relative value of these different procedures, all of which claim for themselves the testimony of experience, we are prepared to admit that no one of them is without merit, and that each may in certain cases possess advantages over the others. Precisely what the cases are to which each individual method may be especially applicable, we believe it would be impossible to declare unless the cases were actually before us; and even then it would probably be found difficult to say which was the best until a fair trial of one or more, and a final success, had determined the question. The time has not yet arrived in which we may institute a rigid comparison between the relative merits of the two leading plans of reduction, manipulation, and extension, for while it is true that reduction by manipulation has been practiced from the earliest day, it is equally true that extension has been generally preferred and practiced by surgeons in all ages, and especially since Sir Astley Cooper gave his admirable instructions upon the method of applying extension and counter-extension. Indeed it was not until Dr. Reid, of Rochester, again called the attention of the profession to this subject, illustrating his views by the results of several successful experiments and by ingenious arguments, that reduction by manipulation could be said to have been fairly introduced as an established method of practice; a large majority of all the cases upon record of reduction by manipulation having been reported since the year 1851, the period of Dr. Reid's first communication to the *Buffalo Medical Journal*.

The following summary of a paper prepared by myself, with the view of determining, if possible, the relative value of the two methods, and exhibiting an analysis of sixty-four cases in which manipulation was employed, will enable the reader to form some estimate of the difficulty in which this subject is involved; and if it does not actually

[1] Amer. Journ. Med. Sci., vol. xv. p. 530.

decide a moot-point, it will at least demonstrate that the method by manipulation is not without its hazards.[1]

Of forty-one cases in which the fact is stated, twenty-eight were reduced on the first attempt, seven on the second, four on the third, and two on the seventh. In seven examples the head of the femur has been thrown from one position to another upon the pelvis, travelling from the dorsum of the ilium to the ischiatic notch, and from thence to the foramen ovale; or directly from the dorsum to the foramen, and back again; or in other directions, according to the character of the original dislocation; in some instances these changes being made as often as seven times in succession. In the majority of cases no evil consequences seem to have followed upon these changes of position. One of my own cases will especially serve to show with what impunity sometimes these changes may be made.

John Caswell, æt. 28, was admitted to the Buffalo Hospital of the Sisters of Charity on the 13th of January, 1858, with a dislocation of the left femur upon the dorsum ilii, which had occurred six days before. His own account of the accident was that he was standing at the bottom of a well, bent forwards until his body was at a right angle with his thighs, when a bucket holding five hundred pounds of earth fell upon his back and hips. No attempt had been made to reduce the dislocation. Five times in succession manipulation made by myself failed, leaving the head of the bone each time upon the dorsum ilii; the sixth attempt, made with the addition of moderate extension by the hands, threw the head into the foramen thyroideum. By reversing the movements, it was easily replaced upon the dorsum ilii. The seventh trial was made in the same manner, except that when I supposed the head of the bone to be opposite the lower margin of the socket I did not permit the limb to turn either outwards or inwards, but while lifting at the knee with my hands, with sufficient power to raise his hips from the table, I brought the limb down gradually to a line parallel with the opposite, and thus finally the reduction was accomplished. No pain or inflammation followed, and in two weeks he left the hospital; but whether he was able to walk or not at that time, I am unable to say.[2]

In Markoe's paper, published in the *New York Journal* for January, 1855, several similar cases are reported, in which the results have been equally fortunate; but the case mentioned as having been under the care of Dr. Post, of the New York Hospital, had a more serious termination. This patient, John Kelly, æt. 21, had a dislocation into the ischiatic notch, and on the same day the reduction was attempted by manipulation. On the first trial the head of the bone was thrown into the foramen ovale; and, after having been moved backwards and forwards between these two points several times, it was finally carried directly from the foramen ovale into the socket by manual extension applied in the ordinary way, but without pulleys. "In this case," says

[1] Reduction of Dislocation of the Femur by Manipulation. By the Author. Buffalo Medical Journal, Nov. 1857; Feb., March, June, 1859. With tables constructed by my very intelligent pupil, Lucien Damainville.

[2] Buffalo Medical Journal, vol. xiii. p. 682.

Markoe, "the cure was very slow, and he left the hospital with some degree of pain and swelling about the joint. I learned that an abscess formed in or about the joint, which was opened, and when I saw him, a year after, there was every appearance of seated morbus coxarius."

In Case 14, of Markoe's paper, the thigh was broken at the neck after manipulation had been employed, but while extension was being made by the hands, united with "a lifting outwards." Whether the fracture was due to the extension, or to the manipulation, seems not to be clearly determined. The dislocation had existed seven weeks when this attempt at reduction was made.

So far as I am able to say, these are all the examples in which a serious injury has been, with any propriety, charged to the manipulation.

Assisted by my pupil, Mr. Hodge, I have also succeeded in collecting sixty-two cases of attempts at reduction by extension; a great majority of which, we find, were reduced in the first trials; but five cases of recent dislocation were not reduced until after several attempts had been made.

In five cases the femur was broken. The first occurred in St. Thomas's Hospital, London. Ben. Whittenburg, æt. 40, was admitted Nov. 4, 1827, with a dislocation into the ischiatic notch, of twenty-two weeks' duration. After bleeding, &c., had been practiced, an attempt was made to reduce the bone by pulleys, in which the reporter professes to believe they were successful, but on the following day it was plainly enough not in place. Mr. Travers again resorted to extension, and while extension was kept up and the assistants were rotating the limb outwards, the neck of the femur gave way.[1] Malgaigne mentions a case in which, while he was himself directing the operation, the thigh was broken through its lower third. He was attempting to reduce the bone by extension, but it was not until he gave the signal for rotation outwards, that the bone gave way.[2] Gibson says that Dr. Physick, at the Pennsylvania Hospital, while engaged in reducing a dislocated thigh by the pulleys, broke the femur in consequence of exerting too much force upon it in a lateral direction by an additional pulley; and that a similar accident is supposed to have happened to Drs. Harris and Randolph in the same hospital, in the year 1838, while using the pulleys upon a boy twelve years of age; for during extension and counter-extension, at the moment of rotating the limb, and of drawing it forcibly outwards by a towel, a sudden crack was heard.[3]

The fifth case is related by Sir Astley Cooper, as having occurred at the Brighton Hospital, under the care of Mr. Gwynne; the dislocation was upon the dorsum ilii, and was supposed to have existed about one month. The neck of the femur was broken in the first attempt at reduction, and while the surgeon was making extension, with gentle rotation.[4]

Sir Astley says, "There are plenty of cases upon record, of fatal abscesses from violent attempts at the reduction of dislocated hips." We

[1] London Med.-Chir. Rev., Nov. 1828, p. 239.
[2] Malgaigne, op. cit., vol. ii. pp. 146 and 830.
[3] Gibson's Surgery, sixth ed., vol. i. p. 389.
[4] Sir Astley Cooper on Disloc., &c., Amer. ed., p. 88.

presume that this remark has reference to attempts at reduction by extension, since in his day, this was almost the only mode in use among surgeons. He adds, moreover, that Mr. Skey has mentioned, in the *Lancet*,[1] a fatal case of phlebitis following protracted extension of the hip.

Malgaigne has collected no less than eight similar examples, with several more in which serious consequences and even death followed promptly upon violent attempts at reduction by mechanical means.[2]

The head of the bone has been repeatedly thrown from the dorsum ilii into the ischiatic notch, and B. Cooper mentions a case in which the bone was carried from the foramen ovale into the ischiatic notch, from which latter position it could not afterwards be changed.[3]

As to the relative chances of failure by the two methods, the testimony of the recorded cases is equally unsatisfactory. Of the failures by extension, the experience of almost every surgeon, the journals and the treatises furnish a sufficient number of examples; while among the sixty-four cases of attempts at reduction by manipulation collected by me, and excepting the cases in which the bone was broken, only two were positive failures. It is somewhat remarkable, however, that these two cases occurred in the experience of the New York City Hospital; and that they are taken from a total of fifteen, this being the whole number which had been treated by this method at the date of these observations, in the New York Hospital. One had existed one month, and after repeated trials by manipulation and frequent changes of position, it was finally reduced by pulleys. The other, a dislocation into the ischiatic notch, had existed only a few hours. At least seven or eight trials were made to accomplish the reduction by manipulation, but without success. The first attempt by extension failed also, but in the second attempt the femur was kept at a right angle with the body, and the bone was soon brought into its socket.[4]

We have in these two examples, not only a record of failure by manipulation, but an equal record of success by extension; while, on the other hand, we find in an analysis of the sixty-four cases, sixteen triumphs of manipulation over extension.

We must not omit to say, in order that the reader may form a just estimate of the value of these statistics, that the great majority, especially of the cases treated by manipulation, have occurred in private practice, and it is unnecessary to say that such statistics do not furnish the most reliable basis for conclusions. As a general rule, unsuccessful cases are not published by private practitioners, but successful cases are pretty certain to be made known; while, on the other hand, a series of cases furnished by any single hospital will generally be found to have given both unsuccessful and successful cases. The writer has heard lately of a complete failure to reduce by manipulation in a recent luxation of the hip, after repeated efforts on several successive days, and where skilful surgeons were in attendance; but it is believed that no account of the result has been published.

[1] Op. cit., vol. i. p. 767, 1840–41. Cooper on Disloc., p. 69.
[2] Malgaigne, op. cit., vol. ii. p. 164 et seq.
[3] Sir Astley Cooper on Disloc. By Bransby Cooper, Amer. ed., p. 96.
[4] Van Buren, New York Med. Times, Jan. 1856, p. 126.

We have already called attention to the fact, that in the New York City Hospital, two of the fifteen cases reported were failures; a circumstance of remarkable significance, especially when we consider the skill of the several gentlemen who were the operators in these cases; and it plainly renders a new series of statistics necessary, drawn solely from the experience of one or more similar large establishments, before we shall be prepared to decide positively upon the relative value of the two procedures.

Nevertheless, we shall not hesitate to express our present convictions upon this subject, reserving to ourselves the right of a change of opinion whenever the proofs shall warrant it.

Manipulation, owing to the great power which may be brought to bear upon the neck and head of the bone through the action of the shaft of the femur as a lever, is most liable to throw the head of the bone into new positions, and consequently most liable to rupture the various soft tissues about the joint, to produce inflammation, suppuration, and caries. For the same reason it is most liable, also, to fracture the neck of the femur. It is not certain in our mind but that, when the principles which control the reduction are more completely understood, these evils may be lessened; yet we can scarcely persuade ourselves that by any future observations, the state of the question will ever be greatly changed. We cannot but think, also, that some conclusions ought to be drawn from the circumstance that, since the time of Hippocrates to the present day, manipulation has been occasionally recommended and successful examples reported; the reduction being accomplished in most instances by processes identical, or nearly so, with those now adopted; yet generally the writers appear to have been ignorant of what had been done before, and indeed, they have generally avowed their belief that the method suggested by themselves was altogether new and original. Possibly, this slowness to establish, and total inability to sustain and perpetuate a reputation, was not the fault of the method, and had no relation to its failures. Until within a few years, the number of surgical books, and especially of medical journals, was comparatively very small, so that valuable truths often died with their discoverers, or were known and remembered only by a few; but it is possible, also, that it has a deeper significance, and that it implies some defect in the procedure, or serious danger, in consequence of which it has from time to time lapsed into desuetude and finally into complete oblivion.

The rules which the author would give for the employment of manipulation are very simple.

The patient being laid on his back upon a mattress, the surgeon, assuming that it is a dislocation upon the dorsum ilii, should seize the foot with one hand and the other he should place under the knee; then, flexing the leg upon the thigh, the knee is to be carefully lifted toward the face of the patient, until it meets with some resistance; it must then be moved outwards and slightly rotated in the same direction until resistance is again encountered, when it must be gradually brought downwards again to the bed. We do not know that the whole process could be expressed in simpler or more intelligible terms, than to say, that the limb should follow constantly its own inclinations.

All writers have united in the necessity of flexion; and, indeed, with very few exceptions, the advocates of extension have insisted upon carrying the dislocated limb more or less across the sound one; they have also been nearly unanimous in their statements that the thigh should then be abducted and finally brought down. Nathan Smith has added the injunction to rotate the shaft of the femur outwards, and to press gently upon the inside of the knee while the thigh is being flexed upon the body, so as to compel the head of the bone to hug the outer margin of the acetabulum and to prevent its falling into the ischiatic notch; a suggestion which has been erroneously interpreted by some writers to mean that he would carry up the limb abducted, a thing which is simply impossible until the reduction is accomplished. In adopting this practice, however, we must not forget the danger which we incur when the limb is completely flexed, and the head of the femur is below the edge of the acetabulum, of throwing it over into the foramen ovale. Dr. Nathan Smith has also noticed the advantage which sometimes may be gained by giving to the limb at this moment a slight rocking motion.

These movements of the limb, with perhaps other slight modifications, such as lifting the knee moderately when the bone refuses to mount over the margin of the acetabulum, pressing with the hand upon the head of the bone, &c., are all which have been usually practiced in successful manipulation.

We repeat, however, that as a general rule, the knee must be carried only in those directions which offer no resistance, and these will be found almost always to be the same; the knee of the dislocated femur hanging over the sound one will be made easily to ascend to about a right angle with the body, we can then carry it outwards a short distance, probably not more than four or five degrees; at this moment, frequently the thigh will begin to rotate outwards of itself, and with considerable force, or as Wathman says, "a self-twisting of the thigh occurs which cannot be prevented by fast holding." When this action takes place the reduction is immediately accomplished; and it is in fact at this moment, before the limb begins to descend, that the bone most frequently resumes its socket. If it does not, then as soon as the limb begins to fall the reduction occurs; generally with a loud snap. It is pretty certain that this manipulation is to fail if the knee has descended more than a few inches without the reduction having taken place; and it will be better to repeat the manœuvre at once, rather than to bring the limb completely down..

Generally anæsthetics ought not to be employed, since the operation, if successful, is not usually painful, and we need that the patient should preserve his consciousness in order to admonish us when we are using improper violence. It is probable, also, that the action of certain muscles sometimes affords material assistance in the reduction. If, however, the patient is very sensitive, or the parts about the joint are very tender, or manipulation without anæsthetics has failed, then certainly these agents may be properly and advantageously employed.

If we propose to attempt reduction by extension, it is no longer necessary to resort to the lancet, antimony, and the hot bath, as preliminary measures, since the muscles can be at once overcome by the much more certain and more powerful agents, chloroform, ether, &c.

The patient is therefore to be placed at once upon a bed of suitable height, reclining on his back, but partly over upon the sound side. Observing now the line of the axis of the dislocated thigh, one strong staple is to be secured into the wall upon one side of the room, and another upon the opposite side, both of which shall correspond as nearly as possible with the line of the shaft of the femur. The staple in front of the body will be higher than the bed, and the staple behind will be, in the same proportion, lower than the bed. The limb being stripped, two pieces of strong factory cloth, each about four inches wide and two feet long, should be laid parallel with and on each side of the limb; the centre of each strip being about opposite that portion of the thigh which is just above the two condyles. Over the centre of these strips, above the condyles and patella, a strong roller, three inches wide and at least three yards long, previously wetted in water, is to be turned as tightly as it can be drawn until the whole roller is exhausted; the extremity of the roller being made fast with a needle and thread rather than with pins. The upper ends of the side strips are then to be brought down and tied to the lower ends, forming thus two lateral loops upon which one of the hooks of the compound pulleys is to be made fast, while the other hook is secured to the front staple in the wall. Instead of these rollers we may employ, if we choose, a leathern thigh belt. (Fig. 263.) For the purpose of counter-extension, a sheet is folded diagonally, and its centre being applied to the perineum of the dislocated limb, the ends are tied firmly into the back staple. To prevent the body from moving laterally, under the action of the pulleys, one assistant should be seated upon the bed, with his back against

Fig. 263.

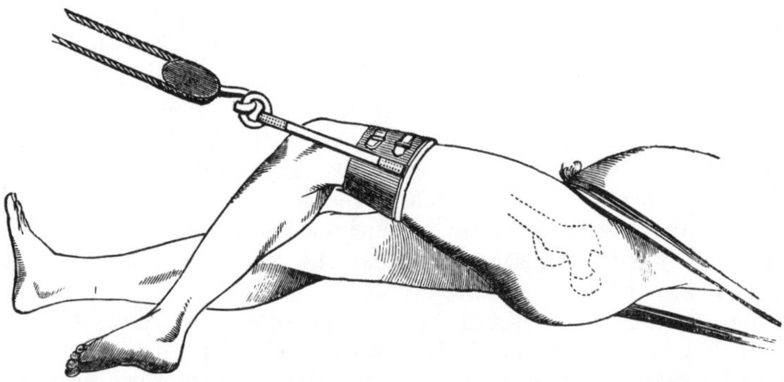

Reduction of dislocation upwards and backwards upon the dorsum ilii, by the pulleys and thigh belt.

the side and back of the patient, and his right arm thrown over the body; it is well also to station another beside the sound limb, so as to retain it also in its place upon the bed. Underneath the upper part of the dislocated limb a strong and broad bandage should be placed, of sufficient length to tie over the neck of the surgeon when he is standing about half bent over the body of the patient.

Everything being arranged, and all portions of the apparatus having been sufficiently tested to make sure that nothing will give way during the operation, the anæsthetic is to be administered, and as the patient falls gradually under its influence, the action of the pulleys should commence, and be slowly but steadily increased, a third assistant managing the rope, so as to leave the surgeon unembarrassed, and able to direct his whole attention to the position of the trochanter major and of the head of the femur. In order to this, he should place one hand upon each of these prominences, and watch carefully their descent.

The length of time which will be required to bring down the limb must differ greatly in different persons, according to the peculiar circumstances of the case, and the condition, age, &c., of the patient; but it must never be forgotten that a slow and steady action is much more effective than rapid and irregular tractions, and it is in this especially, rather than in the relative amount of power, that the pulleys possess always so great an advantage over the hands.

When the surgeon finds that the head of the bone has nearly or quite reached the socket, if it does not take its place spontaneously, he may place his neck in the noose which passes underneath the thigh, and lift upwards, in order to raise the trochanter major, and thus enable the head to rotate toward the acetabulum. It is in this part of the manœuvre, and especially when at the same moment one of the assistants, after bending the leg upon the thigh so as to make of it a lever, has rotated the thigh outwards, that the fracture of the neck has generally taken place; and we cannot be too cautious, therefore, particularly in old persons, not to bear very strongly upon the noose, nor to permit the assistant to rotate outwards with great force.

If the bone does not enter the socket, we may increase or diminish the flexion, or suddenly release the tension, or, in fine, again resort to manipulation alone.

When the reduction is accomplished, the patient should be laid upon his back, with the knees resting over a pillow, and tied together lightly with a towel or a strip of cotton cloth. In order also the more certainly to prevent a reluxation, the thigh of the dislocated limb should be gently rotated outwards, by which the head will be pressed forwards against the anterior portion of the capsule.

Such an accident, however, as a recurrence of the dislocation, in the case of the femur, is exceedingly rare; and I should have deemed it altogether impossible, except as the result of considerable violence again applied, had not at least two examples been reported to us upon very excellent authority. Malgaigne says he has himself seen an example of reluxation upon the dorsum ilii, occasioned by an untimely movement;[1] and Verneuil has seen, six days after the reduction of a dislocation upon the ischiatic notch, the dislocation reproduced by a sudden effort of the patient to sit up.[2]

[1] Malgaigne, op. cit., tom. ii. p. 830. [2] Ibid., p. 840.

Of course, in these remarks we mean to except those cases in which the upper margin of the acetabulum is broken off, and the head of the femur has consequently lost its natural support in this direction.

Sir Astley Cooper mentions the case of a man who could throw out the head of the thigh-bone from the acetabulum at pleasure, and reduce it with equal facility. A similar case is alluded to by Samuel Cooper,[1] and another is related in an inaugural essay by Dr. Lewis, of North Carolina, who graduated at the University of Pennsylvania in 1841.[2]

These are only examples of extraordinary relaxation and extension of the capsular ligament.

§ 2. Dislocations Upwards and Backwards into the Great Ischiatic Notch.

Syn.—"Upwards and backwards into the ischiatic notch;" Sir A. Cooper. "Upwards and backwards into the great sacro-sciatic notch;" Lizars. "Backwards into the sacro-sciatic foramen;" S. Cooper. "Backwards into the ischiatic notch;" Liston, B. Cooper, Miller, Pirrie, Erichsen, Skey, Gibson. "Downwards and outwards on the os ischium;" Boyer, Dorsey. "Backwards and downwards into the ischiatic notch;" Chelius, Petit, Duverney. "Upon the ischium;" Bertrandi. "Sacro-sciatic;" Gerdy. "Ischiatic;" Malgaigne.

Boyer considers this dislocation as only secondary upon a dislocation upon the dorsum ilii; but it is very certain that it often occurs as a primary accident. Not unfrequently, also, what was primarily a dislocation into the ischiatic notch, becomes subsequently a dislocation upon the dorsum ilii.

Fig. 264.

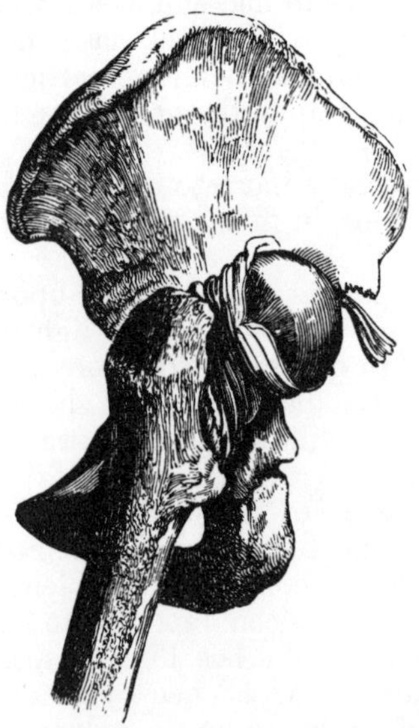

Dislocation upwards and backwards into the great ischiatic notch. (From A. Cooper.)

Causes.—A fall upon the foot or knee, when the limb is very much in advance of the body; or the fall of a heavy weight upon the back and pelvis when the thigh is nearly, or quite at a right angle with the body. Indeed the causes are very similar to those which produce dislocations upon the dorsum ilii, except that it is necessary to suppose the limb in a position more nearly at a right angle with the trunk, at the moment in which the force is applied.

Pathological Anatomy.—Mr. Syme, who dissected the body of a man recently dead, whose thigh had been dislocated into the ischiatic notch, found the glutæus maximus nearly torn asunder, the head of the femur

[1] S. Cooper's First Lines, vol. ii. p. 386, Amer. ed., 1844.
[2] Gibson's Surgery, vol. i. p. 387, 6th ed.

being imbedded in its substance; the glutæus minimus, the pyriformis, and the gemellus superior lacerated; the capsular ligament extensively torn close to the edge of the acetabulum, and the round ligament completely separated from the femur. The head of the femur was lying in the great ischiatic notch, upon the gemelli and the sacro-sciatic nerve, behind the acetabulum and a little above it; being situated between the upper margin of the notch, and the great sacro-sciatic ligaments.[1] Figure 264 is a representation of this specimen.

Fig. 265.

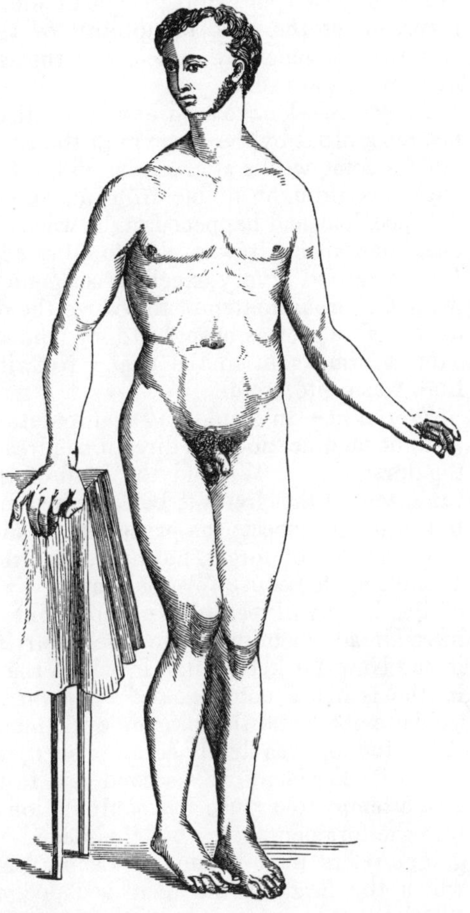

Dislocation upwards and backwards, into the great ischiatic notch.

Symptoms.—The position of the limb is in some cases nearly the same as in certain dislocations upon the dorsum. It is shortened usually about a half an inch, the thigh being flexed upon the body, adducted and rotated inwards; but the flexion is usually less than in dislocations upon the dorsum, while on the other hand, it is sometimes much greater. Generally it is such that when the patient is standing the end of the great toe of the dislocated limb touches the ball of the great toe of the sound limb. The head of the femur may also often be distinctly felt in its new position, especially when the limb is moved upwards or downwards. The trochanter major is approximated toward the anterior superior spinous process of the ilium.

Sir Astley Cooper remarks that this dislocation is the most difficult to detect and to reduce, and Mr. Syme mentions a case in which the nature of the accident was overlooked by himself, and the thigh was not reduced until the thirteenth day;[2] and subse-

[1] Amer. Journn. Med. Sci., vol. xxxii. p. 460.
[2] Ibid., vol. xviii. p. 242.

quently Mr. Syme has called attention to what he considers as one of the most important diagnostic marks; indeed, he says it is never absent, nor is it ever met with in any other injury of the hip-joint, "whether dislocation, fracture, or bruise;" this is "an arched form of the lumbar part of the spine, which cannot be straightened so long as the thigh is straight, or on a line with the patient's trunk. When the limb is raised or bent upwards upon the pelvis, the back rests flat upon the bed; but so soon as the limb is allowed to descend, the back becomes arched as before;"[1] but in addition to this valuable sign, the inversion of the toes, immobility of the limb, and the absence of crepitus, are generally sufficient in themselves to distinguish it from a fracture of the neck.

Prognosis.—I have seen one dislocation of this character which was not recognized by the surgeon at the time of the receipt of the injury, nor for some weeks afterwards. This was in a lad twelve years old, who was brought to me from an adjacent county in August, 1847. The accident had happened eight weeks before. His limb was shortened one inch; it was also forcibly adducted and rotated inwards. Dr. Colegrove, a very excellent surgeon, practicing near the city, had made a thorough attempt to reduce the dislocation with pulleys a few days before he was brought to me, and I did not deem it advisable to subject him again to the trial. Notwithstanding the dislocation his limb was quite useful.

Treatment.—In employing manipulation, we may follow, with only a slight modification, the directions already given in dislocations upon the dorsum ilii. We find the head of the femur lower, consequently the extent of the circuit to be described in the manœuvre is diminished, but in other respects the processes are identical.

We must not forget, however, that there is especial danger while attempting to reduce this dislocation by manipulation that the head of the bone will be thrown across into the foramen thyroideum. I have already mentioned one case occurring under the care of Dr. Post in the New York Hospital, in which the head of the femur, originally in the ischiatic notch, passed backwards and forwards between the ischiatic notch and the foramen ovale many times, and which, although the reduction was finally accomplished, was followed by morbus coxarius. Parker mentions a second case in the same paper,[2] in which his first attempt to reduce by manipulation carried the head of the bone into the foramen ovale; but the second attempt was successful. Malgaigne refers to a patient of Lenoir's, and to another of his own, in which the head of the bone was lodged under the margin of the acetabulum during the attempts at reduction.[3]

On the 23d of March, 1855, Charles McCormick, æt. 21, a laborer on the "State Line Railroad," was caught between two cars, with his back resting against one car, and his right knee against the other, the right thigh being raised to a right angle with his body. As the cars came

[1] Amer. Journ. of Med. Sci., Oct. 1843, p. 461, from Lond. and Edinb. Month. Journ., July, 1843.

[2] Markoe's Paper, N. Y. Journ. of Med., Jan. 1855.

[3] Malgaigne, op. cit., tom. ii. p. 839.

together he felt a "cracking" at his hip-joint, and found himself immediately unable to walk or stand.

Two hours after the accident, assisted by my son Theodore, and Austin Flint, Jr., I examined the limb carefully, and made arrangements for the reduction with the pulleys, in case the attempt by manipulation should fail.

The patient lying upon his back, I seized the right leg and thigh with my hands, the leg being moderately flexed upon the thigh, and carried the knee slowly up toward the belly, until it had approached within twelve or fifteen inches, when noticing a slight resistance to further progress in this direction, I carried the knee across the body outwards, until I again encountered a slight resistance, and immediately I began to allow the limb to descend. At this moment a sudden slip or snap occurred near the joint, and I supposed reduction was accomplished; but, on bringing the limb down completely, I found it was still in the ischiatic notch. I think the head had slipped off from the lower lip of the acetabulum, after having been gradually lifted upon it.

Without delay, I commenced to repeat the manipulation, and in precisely the same manner. Again, at the same point, when the limb was just beginning to descend, a much more distinct sensation of slipping was felt, and on dropping the limb it was found to be in place and in form, with all its mobility completely restored.

No anæsthetic was employed, and no person supported the body or interfered in any way to assist in the reduction. No outcry was made by the patient, yet he informed me that the manipulation hurt him considerably. The amount of force employed by myself was just sufficient to lift the limb, and the time occupied in the whole procedure was only a few seconds.

After the reduction he remained upon his back, in bed, eleven days, in pursuance of my instructions. At the end of this time he began to walk about, but was unable to resume work until after eight weeks or more. It is probable that he could have walked immediately after the reduction, without much, if any inconvenience, so trivial was the inflammation which resulted from the accident. He never complained of pain, but only of a slight soreness back of the trochanter major, near the head of the bone. This soreness continued several weeks, and was especially present when he bent forwards. After the lapse of four months, when I last saw him, he occasionally felt a pain at this point in stooping, but the motions of the joint were free; he walked rapidly and without halt.

If the reduction is attempted by extension, we ought to remember that the head of the bone lies more behind than above the socket, and that it is not requisite to carry it downwards so much as forwards; and especially that it must mount over the most elevated margin of the socket, in order to resume its position. The extension ought, therefore, to be made at an angle of 45°; and if this is not alone sufficient, the head of the bone should be lifted by a jack-towel upwards and in the direction of the socket. Bransby Cooper thought that the limb should be flexed quite to a right angle whilst the extension was being made; but this can only be necessary when the head of the bone is dislocated directly backwards.

Fig. 266.

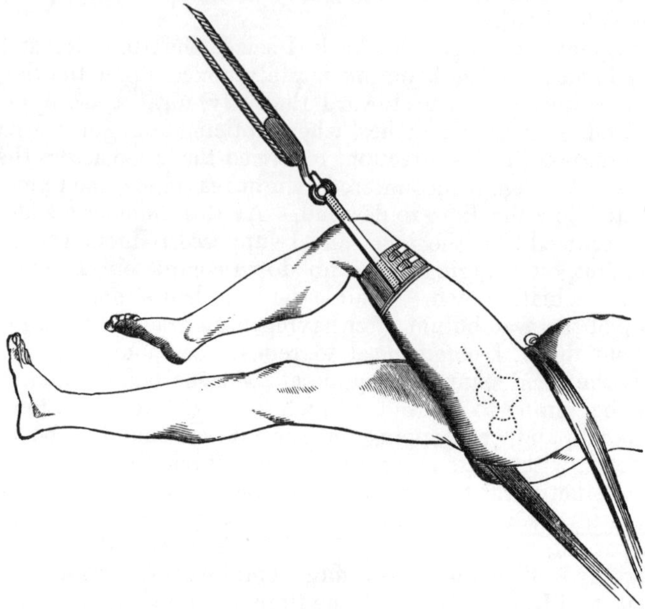

Reduction of dislocation upwards and backwards into the great ischiatic notch, by extension.

Care must be taken that the counter-extending band does not slide off from the pelvis, toward the upper part of the thigh, as it is constantly disposed to do, when the limb is so much flexed. This disposition may be restrained in some measure, by attaching to the counter-extending band another band which shall pass off from the first at a right angle, and embrace the pelvis upon the opposite or sound side.

Dr. Annan, of Baltimore, believes that the great difficulty which surgeons have experienced in their attempts to reduce this dislocation, has arisen from this malposition of the counter-extending band; and, as he has been unable to prevent its sliding off from the pelvis where the method of Sir Astley Cooper has been tried, he suggests the following plan: The patient is to be placed upon his face on a table; the pelvis secured by a band passing around it, and going off laterally at right angles from the sound side, to be fastened to a post or a ring fixed in the wall; another band is to be put around the upper part of the thigh of the injured limb, which should be given to the assistants, or attached to the pulleys, in case they are to be employed; this band also acting at a right angle with the axis of the body, but in the opposite direction, so as to antagonize the band which acts upon the pelvis. The extending band, made fast in the usual manner, above the knee, is then to be tightened, but only sufficiently to prevent the head of the bone from ascending. The ankle of the dislocated limb should now be laid hold of, and adducted, or drawn over the back of the sound limb; "which," says Dr. Annan, "will force the head of the bone out of the notch, and make it describe the segment of a circle, and pass a little downwards in the direction of the acetabulum. Care must be taken," he adds, "that the extending band is sufficiently tightened, and that it does not yield, otherwise the drawing of the leg across the other will only move the head of the bone in the notch, as if it was a joint. If lateral extension only was employed in this case, the head of the femur would be drawn out of the notch, but it would ascend upon the dorsum of the ilium, above the acetabulum. Whereas, by simply drawing the limb laterally as much as is required to make the extending band serve as a fulcrum, and then using the leg as a lever, the head of the bone is not only forced inwards, but is moved downwards, and must necessarily pass into the socket."[1]

Lente relates a case under the care of Dr. Hoffman, in the New York City Hospital, in which, when the extension was suddenly relaxed by cutting the cord, and the thigh, at the same instant, was abducted and rotated outwards, the head of the femur left the ischiatic notch and rose upon the dorsum ilii, assuming a position directly above the acetabulum, and below the anterior superior spinous process; and from which position it was subsequently, with great difficulty, returned to the socket.[2]

§ 3. Dislocations Downwards and Forwards into the Foramen Thyroideum.

Syn.—"Downwards into the foramen ovale;" Sir A. Cooper. "Downwards into the obturator foramen;" Lizars. "Downwards and forwards into the foramen obturatorium;" B. Cooper. "Inwards and downwards into the oval hole;" Chelius. "Downwards and forwards into the foramen ovale;" Pirrie. "Downwards and inwards;" Boyer. "Sub-pubic;" Gerdy. "Ischio-pubic;" Malgaigne.

Causes.—In order to produce this dislocation the limb must be, at the moment of the receipt of the injury, in a position of abduction. Perhaps most often it is occasioned by the fall of a heavy weight upon the back of the pelvis when the body is bent and the thighs spread asunder.

Pathological Anatomy.—The capsule gives way upon the inner side especially; the round ligament is torn from its attachment, and the head of the femur pressing forwards and downwards, finds a lodgement upon the obturator externus muscle, over the foramen thyroideum.

Symptoms.—The thigh is lengthened from one to two inches, greatly abducted and flexed, the body being also bent forwards or flexed upon the thigh. The dislocated limb is advanced before the other, and the

[1] Annan, Amer. Journ. Med. Sci., vol. xix. p. 382, Feb. 1837.

[2] Lente New York Journ. Med., Nov. 1850, p. 314.

toes generally point directly forwards, but they may incline either outwards or inwards. The hip is flattened; the trochanter major is

Fig. 267.

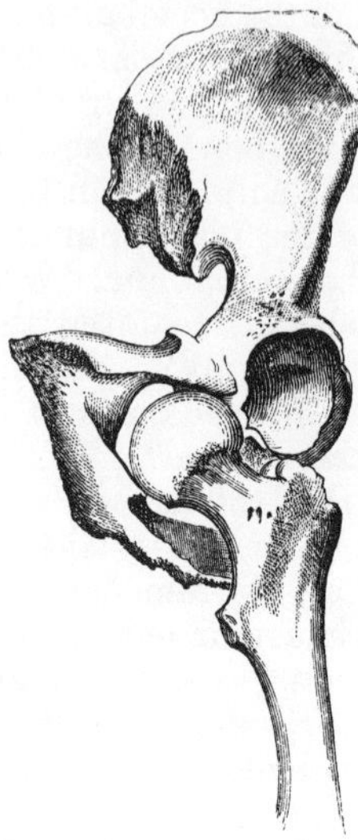

Dislocation downwards and forwards into the foramen thyroideum.

Fig. 268.

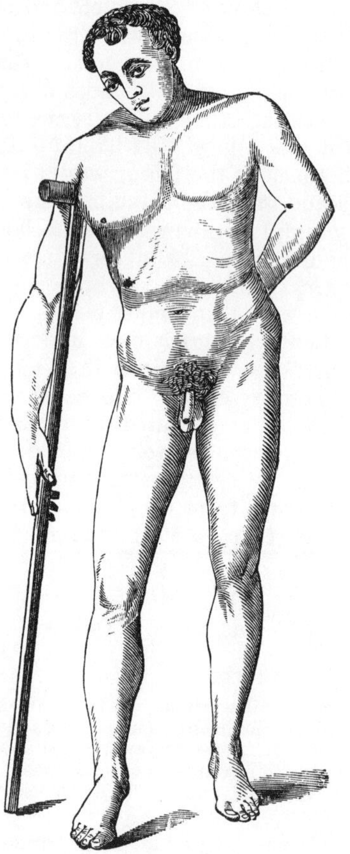

Dislocation downwards and forwards into the foramen thyroideum.

less prominent than upon the opposite side; and the head of the bone may sometimes be felt in its new position. The lengthening of the limb alone is sufficient to distinguish this accident from a fracture of the neck.

Treatment.—It is pretty certain that in the following example there was a spontaneous reduction, or rather I ought to say, an accidental reduction of a dislocated femur from the thyroid foramen. Perhaps it was only an example of a partial luxation; of which species of forward luxation I shall hereafter relate another case as having come under my own notice.

Jacob Lower, æt. 10, fell from a tree, a height of about twelve feet, to the ground. It is not known how he struck. He became immediately quite faint, and when he had partly recovered, he attempted to get up, but could not. He said his leg was broken, and cried out lustily whenever it was moved. The father arrived in about an hour, and found him still lying on his back where he had fallen, with his right leg carried away from the other and turned outwards. He lifted him up to place him in a small hand-wagon, which was long enough for his body, but only one foot and a half in width. Finding that his right leg was so much abducted as to prevent his being laid in so narrow a space, he seized upon it, and with some force pressed the knee inwards across the opposite leg, when suddenly it resumed its position with a loud snap like a "cannon." I use the language of the father. On the following day I examined the limb carefully and found its motions free. He was, however, vomiting the contents of his stomach, and passing blood from the bladder quite freely. The vomiting soon ceased, but the hemorrhage from the bladder continued three or four days. On the ninth day he walked out, and on the twelfth he was seen climbing upon the top of a house. I saw him again after the lapse of a year, and found that he was still complaining of an occasional soreness in the region of the hip-joint.

If we attempt to reduce by manipulation, it will be necessary to follow the same rule which we have stated as applicable to dislocations backwards, namely, to carry the limb only in those directions in which it is found to move easily. Instead, therefore, of holding the leg in a position of adduction while the thigh is flexed upon the abdomen, it will be necessary to carry it up abducted; and when the further progress of the knee toward the belly is arrested, the limb must be moved inwards, and finally brought down adducted. When the knee is about opposite the pubes, or a little lower in its descent, the femur should be gently rotated inwards for the purpose of directing the head toward the acetabulum. The reduction may also be sometimes facilitated by giving to the shaft of the femur a slight rocking motion when it is about to enter the socket; and also by pressing with the hand against the head of the bone, or by lifting at the limb moderately.

In one of the examples recorded by Markoe (Case 8), the reduction was accomplished in the second attempt, by rotating the thigh inwards just as the thigh had descended below a right angle with the body, in the manner which we have above directed; but in a second example (Case 9), a similar manœuvre carried the head across into the ischiatic notch, while the reduction was finally accomplished by rotating the thigh outwards, and at the same moment adducting the limb strongly in a direction which carried the knee behind the other one. Markoe concludes that the latter mode is preferable, because it will throw the head of the bone a little upwards as well as outwards; in which direction it will find a more gently inclined plane toward the socket. He admits, however, that both methods may accomplish the same result. But I am quite certain that the method by rotation of the shaft of the femur inwards is in general most likely to succeed. In this way also, I think, both W. H. Van Buren, of New York,[1] and R. L. Brodie, of the U. S. Army, were successful;[2] but it is especially worthy of notice that Anderson, so long ago as 1772, in the case already quoted, when we were considering the history of reduction by manipulation, practiced successfully almost precisely the same method. In one example mentioned by Markoe (Case 7), it is pretty evident

[1] W. H. Van Buren, New York Med. Times, Jan. 1856, p. 127.

[2] R. L. Brodie, Memphis Med. Recorder, Sept. 1857, p. 90; from Charleston Med. Rev.

that the head of the femur was thrown into the ischiatic notch, by having flexed the thigh too much, so that "the knee touched the thorax." Indeed, it is questionable whether it will be best ever to bring the thigh much, if at all, above a right angle with the body, since any further flexion can only throw the head below the acetabulum, when in fact it is already too low.

July 21, 1858, Nathaniel Smith, a painter by trade, æt. 33, fell from the second story window of the city post-office, upon a stone pavement, striking, as he believes, upon the inside of his right knee. I saw him within an hour, and found the right tibia partially dislocated outwards, the corresponding patella dislocated completely outwards, and the right femur in the foramen thyroideum. His thigh was forcibly abducted; slightly rotated outwards, and lengthened, by measurement made from the pelvis to the ankle, one inch and a half. The distance from the anterior superior spinous process to the fold of the groin was ten inches, but upon the sound side it was only eight and a half. The head of the femur could be distinctly felt in front, just under the pubes.

Having administered chloroform, I first reduced the tibia and the patella, then seizing the thigh and leg, I flexed the thigh upon the body, carrying the limb upwards abducted until it was nearly or quite at a right angle with the body, then inclining the knee slightly inwards, I brought it down again, and when the thigh had nearly reached the bed, it fell into its socket with a dull flapping sensation. In every step of the procedure I followed the inclination of the limb. The recovery was rapid and complete.

Sir Astley Cooper says that this dislocation is in general reduced

Fig. 269.

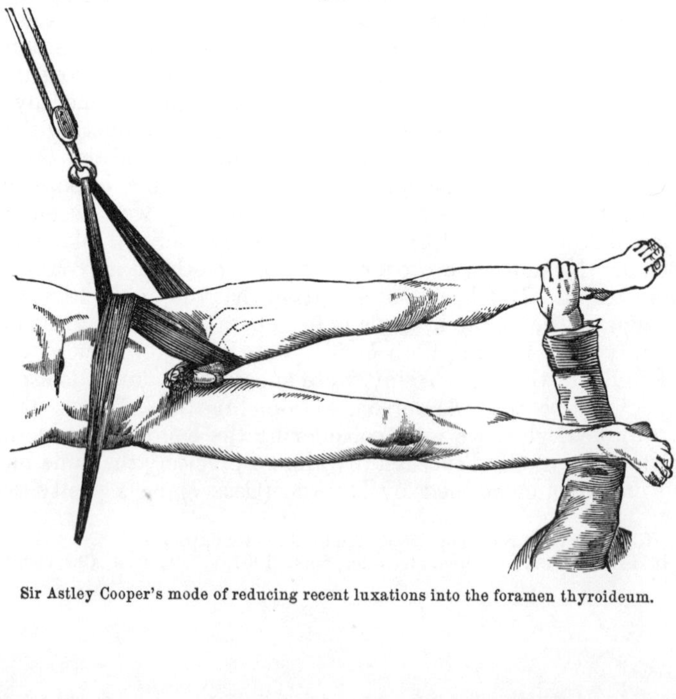

Sir Astley Cooper's mode of reducing recent luxations into the foramen thyroideum.

very easily by the aid of pulleys; at least if the accident is recent. He advises that the patient shall be placed upon his back with his thighs separated as far as possible. The pulleys are to be made fast to a band drawn through the perineum of the dislocated limb, in a direction upwards and outwards; while a counter-band is to be passed around the pelvis through the band attached to the pulleys, and secured to a staple, or delivered to assistants placed upon the sound side of the body. When everything is arranged, the pulleys should be acted upon until the head of the femur is felt moving from the foramen ovale; at this moment the surgeon must pass his hand behind the sound limb, and seizing upon the ankle of the dislocated limb, adduct it forcibly, thus converting the limb into a lever of the first order.

If the dislocation has existed some time, he recommends that this procedure shall be varied by placing the patient upon his sound side instead of his back, and attaching the pulleys perpendicularly over the body. Sir Astley especially cautions us not to flex the thigh during these manœuvres, lest we force the head of the bone backwards into the ischiatic notch, from whence he affirms that it cannot afterwards be returned to its socket; but the experience of surgeons has since shown that this latter statement is incorrect, and that it may, in some cases, be afterwards reduced, although it has fallen into the ischiatic notch. Mr. Liston says that this accident happened to himself while attempting to reduce a dislocation of only a few hours' standing, in a young and powerful man, but he had no difficulty in returning it to its first position.[1]

Brainard, of Chicago, reduced a dislocation of that form of which we are now speaking, after both the compound pulleys and Jarvis's adjuster had failed, by placing between the thighs a piece of wood wrapped about with several layers of a wadded quilt, and making use of this as a fulcrum upon which the thigh operated as a lever. The legs were simply pressed together, care being taken to keep the knees straight.[2]

After the reduction is accomplished, the patient should be laid upon his back in bed, but instead of rotating the limb outwards, as we have advised after a dislocation upon the dorsum ilii, or into the ischiatic notch, it should be gently rotated inwards, and the knees thus bound together.

§ 4. Dislocations Upwards and Forwards upon the Pubes.

Syn.—"Upwards and forwards on the horizontal branch of the share-bone;" Chelius. "Forwards upon the pubes;" Pirrie. "On the body of the pubes, below the spine and transverse part of the bone;" Skey. "Sur-pubic;" Gerdy. "Ilio-pubic;" Malgaigne.

Causes.—This accident is generally occasioned by a fall upon the foot when the leg is thrown backwards behind the centre of gravity; as in a fall from the back end of a wagon, the foot being instinctively thrown backwards in order to save the head; or it may happen to a person

[1] Practical Surg., Amer. ed., p. 93.
[2] Brainard, North Western Med. and Surg. Journ., 1852.

who, while walking, suddenly puts one foot into a hole, in consequence of which the pelvis advances but the leg and upper part of the body incline forcibly backwards. Occasionally it has resulted from a fall upon the back of the pelvis, or from a severe blow received upon the same part. A patient was admitted under the care of Dr. Ure, into St. Mary's Hospital, London, with a dislocation upon the pubes, occasioned by swimming. His account of it was, that, when in the act of "striking out" he felt a catch in the right groin which he thought was cramp, and that he was able to walk after the accident, but with a good deal of difficulty. The examination proved that he had a dislocation upon the pubes, which Dr. Ure easily reduced.[1]

Pathological Anatomy.—Sir Astley Cooper dissected the hip of a person whose thigh had been dislocated upon the pubes for some time, the true nature of the accident not having been at first recognized. The acetabulum was partly filled by bone, and partly occupied by the trochanter major, both of which were much altered in their form. The capsular ligament was extensively torn and the ligamentum teres broken off completely. The head and neck of the femur had torn up Poupart's ligament, so as to penetrate between it and the pubes, and lay underneath the iliacus internus and psoas muscles; the anterior crural nerve was lying upon these muscles, over the neck of the femur. The head and neck were flattened and otherwise much changed in form. Upon the pubes a socket was formed for the neck of the thigh-bone, the head being above the level of the pubes. The femoral artery and vein were to the inner side. This specimen is still preserved in St. Thomas's Hospital, Fig. 270.

Fig. 270.

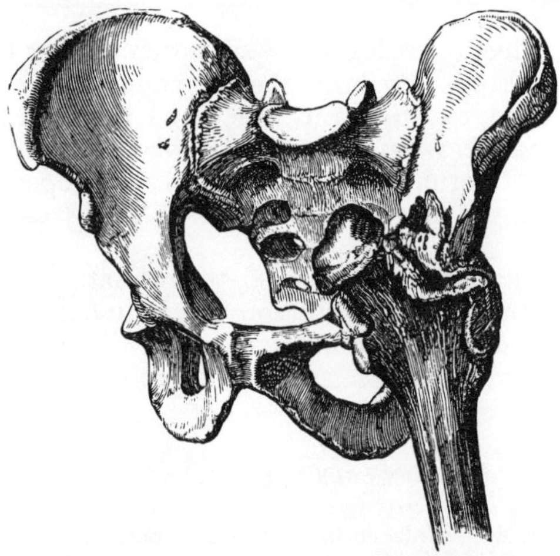

Specimen of dislocation upon the pubes, in St. Thomas's Hospital. (From Sir A. Cooper.)

In many cases, however, the head of the bone does not rise so far upon the pubes, but rests either upon its upper or its anterior margin.

[1] Medical News and Library, vol. xvi. p. 1; from Lond. Lancet, Nov. 7, 1857.

Symptoms.—The thigh is shortened, abducted, flexed slightly, rarely extended, and rotated outwards. (Fig. 271.) The trochanter major is lost, or nearly so, while the head of the bone may be generally felt like a round ball, lying upon or in front of the body of the pubes to the outside of the femoral artery and vein. Larrey saw a patient in whom the femur was placed nearly at a right angle with the body; and Physick once met with a dislocation upon the pubes "directly before the acetabulum," in which the limb was not at all shortened, but, on the contrary, a very little lengthened.[1] Other surgeons have occasionally seen similar examples.

Fig. 271.

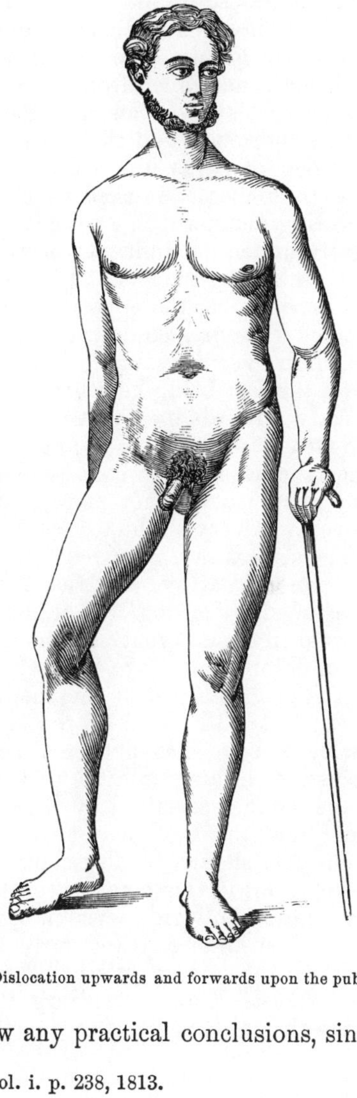

Dislocation upwards and forwards upon the pubes.

The differential diagnosis between a fracture of the neck of the femur and this dislocation may be thus briefly stated. In the fracture there is crepitus, mobility, slight eversion easily overcome, moderate or no shortening, no abduction, the trochanter major rotates on a short radius, the head of the bone cannot be felt. In this dislocation there is no crepitus, the limb is immobile, the eversion is extreme and not easily overcome, there is generally more shortening, the thigh is abducted, the trochanter major rotates upon a longer radius, and the head of the bone can generally be distinctly felt in its unnatural position.

Prognosis.—Sir Astley Cooper remarks that although this accident is easy of detection, he has known three instances in which it was overlooked, and he cannot but regard such errors as evidence of great carelessness on the part of the surgeon who is employed.

The reduction has generally been accomplished, in recent cases, with no great difficulty; and when not reduced the patients have occasionally recovered with very useful limbs.

Treatment.—From the several reported examples of dislocation upon the pubes reduced by manipulation, it would be difficult to draw any practical conclusions, since

[1] Dorsey's Surgery, vol. i. p. 238, 1813.

the methods have differed so widely from each other. I shall mention only three, which may be found in our own journals. One of these has already been mentioned in connection with the history of this process, as a case of compound dislocation, reduced by Dr. Ingalls, of Chelsea, Mass., and the two remaining examples were both reported by E. J. Fountain, of Davenport, Iowa. Dr. Ingalls succeeded by carrying the limb into its greatest state of abduction and rotating the thigh inwards; the replacement of the bone being aided also by pressing upon its head with his fingers thrust into the wound; while Dr. Fountain succeeded equally in both of his cases, by an almost opposite mode of procedure, namely, by adducting the limb forcibly, rotating the thigh inwards and then flexing the thigh upon the body. The first of Dr. Fountain's cases occurred in June, 1854. The patient, an adult male, had fallen from the second story of a house to the ground, fracturing his lower jaw, and dislocating his left hip. The limb was a trifle shortened, and the foot strongly everted. The prominence of the trochanter was lessened, and the head of the bone could be felt upon the pubes. Assisted by Dr. Arnold, he reduced the limb in the following manner: The patient was laid on the floor, and placed completely under the influence of chloroform. The dislocated limb was then "seized by the foot and knee and rotated outwards, the leg flexed and carried over the opposite knee and thigh, the heel kept well up, and the knee pressed down. This motion was continued by carrying the thigh over the sound one as high as the upper part of the middle third, the foot being kept firmly elevated. Then the limb was carried directly upwards by elevating the knee, while the foot was held firm and steady, at the same time making gentle oscillations by the knee, when the head of the bone suddenly dropped into its socket."[1] The time occupied was not more than thirty seconds, and the force employed was very slight.

The second case occurred on the 31st of Oct., 1855, in the person of John McCarthy, an Irish laborer; the dislocation having been occasioned by falling with a horse, while riding. The reduction was effected in about twenty seconds by the same process, and without the aid of chloroform.

It is probable that no one method will succeed equally well in all cases; but if the head of the bone, as in the case dissected by Sir Astley Cooper, has not only actually surmounted the pubes, but pushed itself fairly into the pelvis, then the limb ought to be abducted in the manner practiced by Ingalls, and forcibly rotated outwards, in order that the head may be thus lifted over the pubes; and subsequently it should be flexed upon the body, adducted and brought down. But in this manœuvre we ought to be careful not to continue the rotation outwards after the head of the femur has risen above the pubes, lest the head and neck should grasp, as it were, the psoas magnus and iliacus internus muscles, underneath which they have been thrust. On the contrary, it will be necessary at this point to rotate the thigh again gently inwards, which, by compelling the head

[1] Fountain, New York Journ. Med., Jan. 1856, p. 69 et seq.

to hug the front of the pubes, will enable it, while the flexion is being made, to slide downwards under these muscles toward the socket. If, however, the head of the bone has never risen upon the summit of the pubes, and is not actually engaged under the muscles which pass over it at this point, then the rotation outwards will not be necessary in any part of the procedure.

Baron Larrey has reported a case of dislocation "before the horizontal portion of the pubes," which he reduced "by suddenly raising with his shoulder the lower extremity of the femur, while with both hands he depressed the head of the bone."[1] This is the same of which we have already spoken as being attended with the unusual phenomenon of the thigh placed at a right angle with the body.

If reduction is attempted by extension, the patient ought to be laid on his back upon a table, with the dislocated limb falling off slightly from its side. The extending band, made fast above the knee, should then be secured to a staple in the line of the axis of the dislocated thigh, and of course, below the table; while the counter-extending band, crossing under the perineum, should be made fast in the same line, above the level of the table, and beyond the head of the patient.

When extension is commenced, and the head of the femur has begun to move, the reduction may sometimes be facilitated by lifting

Fig. 272.

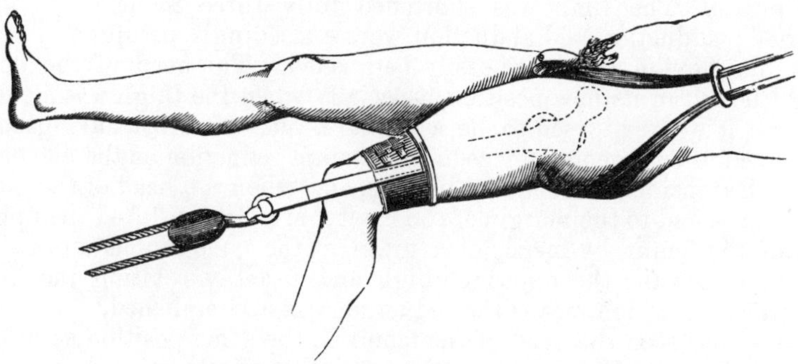

Reduction of dislocation upon the pubes, by extension.

the upper part of the thigh with a jack towel or a band passed under the thigh and over the neck of the surgeon, as we have recommended in both of the backward dislocations.

[1] Larrey, Lond. Med.-Chir. Rev., Dec. 1820, p. 500; vol. i. first ser., from Bullet. de la Fac. de Méd., No. 1.

§ 5. Anomalous Dislocations, or Dislocations which do not properly belong to either of the Four Principal Divisions before described.[1]

1. *Dislocations directly Upwards.*

Syn.—"Sus-Cotyloïdiennes;" Malgaigne. "Sixth dislocation;" Mütter.

Malgaigne affirms that the head, in this dislocation, is situated external to the anterior inferior spinous process, and about one inch below the anterior superior spinous process. But this position is not uniform. It may be found in front of the inferior process or above as well as behind, or external to it.

The symptoms which characterize this accident, are shortening of the limb, slight abduction and extension, with extreme eversion or rotation outwards. The eversion of the toes, together with the slight amount of shortening which has in general been observed, has led several times to the supposition that it was a fracture of the neck of the femur; but the rigidity, and the position of the trochanter and head will usually render the diagnosis clear.

Cummins reports a case which occurred in the practice of Gibson, of New Lanark, where the head of the bone was believed to be situated just below the anterior superior spinous process, and inwards toward the pubes. The limb was shortened fully three inches; the toes everted; adduction and abduction were exceedingly painful and difficult, but flexion was more easily performed. The head of the bone could be felt in its new position, especially when the thigh was moved. At first it was supposed to be a fracture, but this error having been corrected, the surgeons proceeded to attempt reduction on the eleventh day. Extension was made by pulleys, and when the head of the bone had descended to the margin of the cavity, Mr. Gibson lifted the upper end of the femur by means of a towel, at the same moment pressing the knee toward the opposite thigh and forcibly rotating the limb inwards; by which means the reduction was accomplished.[2]

Lente has seen the head of the femur in the same position as in the case reported by Cummins, not as a primitive dislocation, but consequent upon an attempt to reduce a dislocation into the ischiatic notch. The shortening was about two inches; the limb very much rotated outwards; the rotundity of the affected hip greater than that of the other, and the trochanter major one inch further removed from the

[1] Malgaigne, Traité des Frac. et des Lux., tom. ii. p. 869 et seq. Samuel Cooper, First Lines, vol. ii. p. 391. Pirrie's Surg., Amer. ed., 1852, p. 275. Skey's Surg., Amer. ed., 1851, p. 110 et seq. Gibson's Surg., sixth Amer. ed., vol. i. p. 386. Guy's Hospital Reports, vol. i. 1836, pp. 79 and 97; vol. iii. 1838, p. 163. London Lancet, Lond. ed., vol. i., 1848, p. 184; vol. ii., 1840, p. 281; vol. i., 1845, p. 412; vol. ii. p. 159. London Med. Gaz., vol. xix. pp. 657 and 659; vol. x. p. 19; vol. xxxiii. p. 404. Med.-Chir. Trans., vol. xx. p. 112. Lente's paper on "Anomalous Dislocations of the Hip-Joint," in New York Journ. Med. for Nov. 1850, p. 314 et seq. Philadelphia Med. Examiner, No. 51. Amer. Journ. Med. Sci., vol. xvi. p. 14. New York Med. and Phys. Journ., 1826, vol. v. p. 597.

[2] Cummins, Guy's Hospital Reports, vol. iii. p. 163, 1838.

anterior superior spinous process. The head of the bone could be felt distinctly in its new position.

The reduction was effected finally with pulleys, by the aid of chloroform, and by rotation of the limb in various directions.[1]

Morgan also reports a case in which the head of the femur was above the acetabulum, and a little to the outside of the ilio-pectineal eminence.[2]

In a majority of cases these dislocations have been reduced by manipulation alone, or by manipulation aided by pressure. The limb should be seized in the usual manner, at the knee and ankle, carried up toward the face, abducted, then rotated inwards, gently adducted, and finally brought down again to the bed. At the moment when the rotation and adduction commence, the head of the bone should be pressed toward the socket by the hands, and, if necessary, lifted a little over the margin of the acetabulum, by moderate extension at a right angle with the body.

2. *Dislocations Downwards and Backwards upon the Posterior Part of the Body of the Ischium, between its Tuberosity and its Spine.*

James C——, æt. 35, was admitted to the Pennsylvania Hospital on the 23d of January, 1835, under the care of Dr. Hewson. The patient, a muscular man, had been crushed under a falling roof, and, as he thought, with his right thigh separated from his body. When received into the hospital, one hour after the accident, the right thigh was flexed upon the pelvis, and rested upon the left; the right leg was also flexed upon the thigh; the knee was below its fellow, the toes turned inwards, and the whole limb shortened at least one inch. The head of the bone could be felt distinctly resting upon that portion of the ischium which lies between the acetabulum, the tuberosity of the ischium, and the spine.

On the following day, the muscles of the patient having been sufficiently relaxed by suitable means, the pulleys were applied; but, after a second attempt, some of the bands having given way suddenly, the pulleys were removed, when it was found that the reduction had been accomplished, although neither the patient nor his attendants had noticed the return of the bone to its socket. For several days there was entire loss of sensibility and motion in the leg, owing probably to the pressure which had been made upon the sciatic nerve; but these symptoms gradually disappeared, and at the time when the case was reported, about two months after the accident, he was walking with crutches.

Dr. Kirkbride, who has reported this unusual case of dislocation, doubts whether the extension was necessary to the reduction, as the head of the bone was brought very near the margin of the acetabulum

[1] Lente, New York Journ. of Med., Nov. 1850, p. 314.

[2] Pirrie's Surgery, p. 276. See also Phil. Med. Exam., No. 51, Mütter's paper.

by lifting the thigh with a towel, and it probably afterwards entered the socket so soon as the extension was relaxed.[1]

Malgaigne has referred to several similar examples.

3. *Dislocations Downwards and Backwards into the lesser or lower Ischiatic Notch.*

Syn.—"Behind tuber ischii;" Gibson, S. Cooper. "Fifth dislocation;" Gibson.

September 7, 1821, Charles Lowell, of Lubec, Mass., was riding a spirited horse, when the animal, being restive, suddenly reared and fell back on his rider, in such a manner as that the weight of the horse was received on the inside of the left thigh; Mr. Lowell having fallen on his back, a little inclined to the left side. The surgeon, who was immediately called, recognized it as a dislocation, and thought he had succeeded in reducing it; but a day or two later it was seen by a second surgeon, who declared that it was still out of place, and repeated the attempt at reduction, but without success, as the result proved.

In December of the same year Mr. Lowell called upon John C. Warren, of Boston, who was now able to determine, easily, as he affirms, the precise character of the accident. The limb was elongated, contracted, and the head could be felt in its unnatural position. By advice of Dr. Warren, he was taken to the Massachusetts General Hospital, and a persevering attempt was there made to reduce the bone, but with no better success than had attended the efforts previously made.[2]

Mr. Keate has reported a case produced in a very similar way by a horse having fallen backwards with the rider into a deep and narrow ditch; but the position of the limb was somewhat extraordinary, considering that it was a dislocation backwards, the whole limb being very much abducted and the toes being turned outwards, as if the head of the bone was in front of the tuber ischii, rather than behind it. The thigh and leg were much flexed, and the whole limb was shortened from three to three inches and a half. The head of the femur could be distinctly felt "inferior to the ischiatic notch, and on a level with the tuberosity of the ischium." In the first attempt at reduction the head of the bone was thrown into the foramen ovale, from which it was, however, after one or two more attempts by extension, and by lifting with a jack-towel, restored to the socket. Mr. Keate believes that the dislocation was originally into the foramen ovale, but that in the struggles made by the patient to extricate himself, it was thrown backwards into the position in which he found it.[3]

Mr. Wormald has reported a primitive accident of the same kind, occasioned by jumping from a third story window. The patient died soon after, and at the autopsy the head of the femur was found under

[1] Kirkbride, Amer. Journ. of Med. Sci., vol. xvi. p. 13.

[2] New York Med. and Phys. Journ., vol. v. p. 597; 1826. Letter to the Hon. Isaac Parker, &c., by John C. Warren; 1826. North Amer. Med. Journ., vol. iii. p. 169.

[3] Amer. Journ. Med. Sci., vol. xvi. p. 226, 1835. From Lond. Med. Gaz., vol. x. p. 19.

the outer edge of the glutæus maximus, projecting through the torn capsule opposite the upper part of the tuber ischii. The shaft of the femur lay across the pubes, and the limb was considerably shortened and turned inwards.[1]

4. *Dislocations directly Downwards.*

Syn.—"Sous-cotyloïdiennes;" Malgaigne.

The following is one of several similar examples now upon record:—

A man, æt. 50, was admitted into the London Hospital under the care of Mr. Luke. A dislocation of the left femur was easily diagnosticated, but the symptoms were peculiar, inasmuch as the limb was lengthened one inch, without either inversion or eversion; yet the head of the bone could be easily felt, and was thought to be in the ischiatic notch. By manipular movements reduction was easily effected about an hour after the accident. The man subsequently died from the effects of broken ribs. At the autopsy, Mr. Forbes, the house-surgeon, before dissecting the parts, again dislocated the bone. This was done with ease, and it was clear that the original form of dislocation had been reproduced, as the bone could not be made to assume any other position. The head of the bone proved to be displaced neither into the ischiatic notch nor the thyroid hole, but midway between the two, immediately beneath the lower border of the acetabulum. The gemellus inferior and the quadratus femoris had been torn, the ligamentum teres had been wholly detached, and there was a laceration in the lower part of the capsular ligament.[2]

Dr. Blackman, of Cincinnati, informs me that in Jan. 1859, he reduced a sub-cotyloid, incomplete dislocation, in a man æt. 70, by manipulation, Dr. Judkins lifting the thigh upwards and outwards by means of a towel, while Dr. Blackman first flexed and then abducted the limb.

5. *Dislocations Forwards into the Perineum.*

Syn.—"Périnéales;" Malgaigne. "Luxation sur la branche ascendante de l'ischion." D'Amblard. "Inwards on the ramus of the os pubis;" Skey.

D'Amblard published an example of this accident in 1821; occasioned by a violent muscular exertion made by the patient in an effort to spring into his carriage, the symptoms attending which did not differ materially from those which were found to be present in the two following examples, except that while in Parker's patient the toes were turned slightly inwards, in D'Amblard's patient they were a little turned outwards.[3]

Mr. E——, æt. 35, a calker by occupation. The injury was received while at work under the bottom of a canal boat, July 20, 1831, the boat being raised upon props three and a half feet long. The patient was standing very much bent forwards, with his feet far apart,

[1] Wormald, Lond. Med. Gaz., 1836.

[2] Luke, Med. News and Library, vol. xvi. p. 34, March, 1858; from Med. Times and Gaz., Jan. 2, 1858.

[3] Malgaigne, op. cit., tom. ii. p. 876.

between which lay a piece of round timber one foot in diameter, when the props gave way, letting the whole weight of the boat upon himself and his companions. One of the workmen was killed outright. On extricating Mr. E. from his situation, the left leg and thigh were found extended at a right angle with the body, the toes turned slightly inwards, the natural form of the nates was lost, and the head of the femur could be felt distinctly moving, when the limb was rotated, in the perineum, behind the scrotum, and near the bulb of the urethra.

For the purpose of reduction, the patient was laid on his back upon a table, and the pelvis made fast by a muslin band. Extension, accompanied with moderate rotation, was then made in a direction outwards and downwards, bringing the head of the bone over the ascending ramus of the ischium, beyond which it was lying, into the foramen thyroideum; and from this position the bone was replaced in the acetabulum, by carrying the dislocated limb forcibly across the opposite one. The patient soon recovered the use of the joint.[1]

J. B., an Irishman, æt. 40, on entering the St. Louis Hospital, gave the following account of his accident, which had occurred six hours previously. He was engaged in excavating earth, and having undermined a bank, it unexpectedly fell upon his back while he was standing in a bent position, with his thighs stretched widely apart. The weight crushed him to the earth, breaking both bones of his right leg, the radius of the same side and dislocating the left hip into the perineum. The thigh presented a peculiar appearance, being placed quite at a right angle with the body, but somewhat inclined forwards. The part of the hip naturally occupied by the trochanter major presented a depression deep enough to receive the clenched fist; while the head of the bone could be both seen and felt projecting beneath the skin of the raphe in the perineum. Rotation of the limb, which was difficult and excessively painful, rendered the position of the head still more manifest. The patient had also retention of urine, occasioned probably by the pressure of the femur upon the urethra. Having dressed the fractures, Dr. Pope placed the patient under the full influence of chloroform, and then proceeded to reduce the dislocated thigh; for which purpose "two loops were applied, interlocking each other in the groin, and using the leg as a lever, extension, by means of the pulleys, was made transversely to the axis of the body. A steady force was kept up for a short time, and the thigh-bone glided into its socket with a snap that was heard by every attendant and patient in the large ward."[2]

§ 6. Ancient Dislocations of the Femur.

Says Sir Astley Cooper: "I am of opinion that three months after the accident, for the shoulder, and eight weeks for the hip, may be fixed as the period at which it would be imprudent to attempt to make

[1] W. Parker, New York Med. Gaz., 1841; N. Y. Journ. Med., March, 1852, p. 188.

[2] Pope, St. Louis Med. and Surg. Journ., July, 1850; N. Y. Journ. Med., March, 1852, p. 198.

the reduction, except in persons of extremely relaxed fibre, or of advanced age. At the same time, I am fully aware that dislocations have been reduced at a more distant period than that which I have mentioned; but in many instances the reduction has been attended with the evil results which I have just been deprecating." A remark which later surgeons do not seem always to have correctly understood, or which, if they have understood, they have not correctly represented; since it has many times been affirmed of this distinguished surgeon, that he regarded reduction of the hip as impossible after eight weeks, and they have proceeded to cite examples which would prove that he was in error. But long before Sir Astley's day, Gockel mentioned a case of reduction of the femur after six months, and Guillaume de Salicet declared that he had reduced a similar dislocation after one year,[1] and Sir Astley says, that he is "fully aware" of the existence of such facts; yet with a knowledge of what has so frequently followed these attempts, he would not recommend the trial after eight weeks, except under the circumstances by him stated; and notwithstanding the number of these reported successes has been considerably increased in our day, we suspect that Sir Astley's rule will continue to govern experienced and discreet surgeons. Two examples which have recently been published of successful reduction after six months by manipulation, would encourage a hope that the period might be greatly extended, were it not that manipulation also has already failed many times in the case of ancient luxations, and that the attempt has sometimes been followed with disastrous results, even in recent cases.

The following are the two examples of reduction by manipulation after the lapse of six months:—

On the 21st of March, 1856, a man presented himself at the Commercial Hospital, Cincinnati, with a dislocation of the femur upon the dorsum ilii, of six months' standing. The limb was shortened two inches. Dr. Blackman, under whose care he was admitted, administered chloroform, and by manipulating after the method described by Dr. Reid, the reduction was accomplished.[2]

In a letter addressed to me by Dr. Blackman, and dated April 21st, 1859, he informs me that this patient presented himself again before the class about six months since, and the restoration of the functions of the limb was found to be complete.

The second example occurred in the practice of Martial Dupierris, of Havana, Cuba. A Chinese boy named A-sin, aged about sixteen years, arrived at Havana on the fourth of June, 1856, suffering under a severe illness, which confined him for a month or more to his bed, and the existence of the dislocation was not discovered until he had sufficiently recovered to rise upon his feet. It was then ascertained that he had a dislocation of the left femur upon the dorsum ilii. Upon inquiry, Dr. Dupierris learned that the accident had occurred before leaving China, a period of more than six months. The boy was

[1] Malgaigne, op. cit., tom. ii. p. 185; from Gallicinium Medico-practicum, Ulm, 1700, p. 288.

[2] Blackman, Ohio Med. and Surg. Journ., vol. viii. p. 522.

still feeble, the limb somewhat emaciated, and instead of being rigid from muscular contraction, all the muscles "were in a flaccid condition, except the great gluteal, which was painful to the touch." Deeming the use of anæsthetics improper, on account of the boy's feeble condition, these agents were not employed. Dr. Dupierris describes the method of reduction as follows: "The body being held by two assistants by means of two bands, one of which passed beneath the perineum, and the other under the axillæ, traction was made upon the limb by two strong and intelligent assistants. The movement of the head of the bone, resulting from this manœuvre, was very limited, even when the force was much increased; and the excruciating pain, which the patient referred to the iliac region, compelled us for the moment to desist.

"The following day, the patient having obtained a tolerable night's rest by means of a narcotic potion, I concluded to attempt the reduction by flexion, believing that I could thus better prevent any accident which the necessary force might produce; the operator, in adopting this method, having it in his power to follow the head of the bone by pressure upon it with the hand, aiding its movement in the proper direction, or correcting any deviation that may occur. The emaciated condition of the boy was eminently favorable for such a procedure.

"The patient being placed upon his back, and the trunk of the body made steady by assistants, with the left hand I grasped the upper part of the leg, placed the right hand upon the head of the bone in the iliac fossa, and then proceeded to flex the leg upon the thigh, and the thigh upon the pelvis. By this movement the great gluteal muscle was relaxed, and the head of the bone advanced, while with the right hand I directed the latter toward the cotyloid cavity. As soon as I judged the head to be immediately above the centre of the socket, I extended the leg, the thigh remaining flexed at a right angle; and then using the limb as a lever, I rotated it from within outwards, and at the same time extended it by making a movement of circumduction in a similar direction. When by these procedures the limb was brought near to its opposite fellow, a snap audible to the assistants, and of a deeper character than is ordinarily observed in the reduction of recent dislocations, indicated the return of the head of the bone to its natural position; a fact which was further substantiated by the establishment of the original length and form of the member and the subsidence of the pain.

"The after-treatment consisted in placing a pad between the knees, and another between the internal malleoli, and confining the limbs together by two bands, one above the knees, and the other around the lower part of the legs. But in spite of these precautions to prevent re-displacement, the next morning I found that the dislocation had been reproduced. It was again reduced, but for three successive days there was a re-displacement. After this, however, the head of the bone kept its place; passive motion was daily employed, and all suffering ceased. After twenty days of rest, and a liberal use of the lactate of iron, the patient was allowed to get up; and, being provided with a pair of crutches, upon which he exercised himself daily, improved very rapidly. The muscles gradually recovered their bulk and vigor; and at the end of forty-eight days he was enabled to walk without crutches, although with some fear of falling. About the middle of August, he was put to work in a cigar manufactory, and has continued well ever since."

§ 7. Partial Dislocations of the Femur.

Malgaigne declares that certain experiments made upon the cadaver led him, at one time, to the conclusion that all primitive luxations of the femur were incomplete, and that the old complete luxations found in autopsies, had become so consecutively. Later observations have taught him to correct this error, yet he still finds "incomplete backward luxations quite common, and incomplete dislocations in all the other directions much more common."

I have more than once found occasion to call in question the accuracy of Malgaigne's views in relation to partial dislocations, the relative frequency of which he seems constantly disposed to greatly exaggerate. We cannot see the propriety of calling those cases partial dislocations, in which the head of the bone has fairly left the cotyloid cavity, and mounted upon its margin; even if it remains in this position without tearing the capsule; since the articular surfaces are now as completely separated as if the capsule had given way, and the head of the bone had escaped through the laceration. It is in fact a complete luxation. But I doubt very much whether the head of the bone ever rests upon the margin of the acetabulum without tearing the capsule, unless it has previously undergone certain pathological changes, such as I have already described; at least I cannot hesitate to reject all those examples in which the head of the femur is supposed to rest upon the upper or outer margin of the acetabulum; and if I permit myself to speak of incomplete dislocations at all in this connection, I shall reserve the term for those rare cases in which the head of the femur becomes engaged in the cotyloid notch, after breaking down the fibrous band which, in the natural state, is continuous with the rim of the acetabulum.

Of this form of dislocation, I think I have met with two examples; one of which was in the person of the boy Lower, already mentioned, whose thigh was reduced accidentally by his father; and the other occurred in a boy fifteen years of age, residing at that time in Rutland, Vermont. He was brought to me on the 28th of May, 1842, by Dr. Haynes, of Rutland, at which time the dislocation had existed five years. His account of himself was that in walking upon a slippery floor, his left leg slid outwards and backwards in such a manner as that when he fell it was fairly doubled under his back. On the tenth day following the accident, he began to walk with some help, and he has continued to walk ever since, but with a manifest halt. Three months after the injury was received, it was first seen by several surgeons, who pronounced it a dislocation, and attempted reduction without mechanical aid, but were unsuccessful.

When the young man was brought to me, the limb was neither lengthened nor shortened, but the thigh was forcibly abducted and rotated outwards. It could not be flexed nor greatly extended. The head of the femur could be distinctly felt, as it lay anterior to the socket, but not sufficiently far forwards to rest upon the foramen ovale.

J. C. Warren, of Boston, has reported a similar example in a child six years old, who was brought April 21, 1841, to the Massachusetts General Hospital. Dr. Hale, who saw the lad at the end of two weeks, thought it a dislocation, but it had been treated by another surgeon as a case of hip-disease. The dislocation had now existed eight or ten weeks. The limb was a little lengthened, abducted, turned outwards, and advanced in front of the body, with very slight motion of either flexion or extension, and almost no tenderness about the joint. Dr. Warren, also, was able to feel indistinctly the head of the bone "immediately external to, and in contact with, the insertion of the triceps and gracilis muscles."

An attempt was made by manual extension and manipulation to accomplish the reduction, but without success.[1]

It is probable that both the above cases which I have described at length, were examples of partial dislocation; yet I cannot conceal from others a doubt which I actually entertain whether they were not, after all, only examples of hip-joint disease, arrested after having wrought certain slight pathological changes in the joint and the tissues adjacent. If, however, they were not examples of incomplete dislocations of the hip-joint, then I question whether any such cases have ever occurred.

§ 8. Coxo-femoral Dislocations, Complicated with Fracture of the Femur.

Such complications are exceedingly rare, but it will not do to deny their possibility; although in some of the cases reported, the testimony is not so clear as not to leave a doubt whether the surgeons have not erred in their diagnosis.

James Douglas has reported a case of dislocation upon the pubes, complicated with a fracture of the neck of the femur, the actual condition of which was verified by an autopsy; the patient having died twelve years after the injury was received. The head of the femur still remained above the pubes, and was in no way connected with its neck or shaft. The upper end of the femur projected in the groin, lying upon the inside of the femoral artery and vein. Many other curious pathological changes had also occurred.[2]

The well-authenticated examples of reduction of the dislocation, where the femur was broken also, are still more rare; and several of

[1] Warren, Bost. Med. and Surg. Journ., vol. xxiv. p 220.

[2] Amer. Journ. Med. Sci., vol. xxxiii. p. 455, from Lond. and Edin. Month. Journ. of Med. Sci., Dec. 1843.

the recorded examples which my researches have discovered, need additional confirmation.

John Bloxham, of Newport, in the Isle of Wight, claims to have reduced a dislocation of the femur on the pubes, which was accompanied with a fracture of the thigh a little above its middle. The following is the account of this interesting case which we find in the *London Medico-Chirurgical Review*, copied from the *Medical Gazette* of Aug. 24th, 1833. We regret that we are unable to see the account as published in the *Gazette*, which might supply some circumstances important to a full appreciation of the case:—

On the seventh or eighth day after the accident, "the patient was laid upon his back on the bed and kept in that position by means of a sheet passed across the pelvis, and fastened to the bedstead; another sheet was also passed over the left groin, and secured in a similar manner. The dislocated and fractured limb was then inclosed in splints, one of which extended up the back of the thigh as far as the tuberosity of the ischium. Pulleys, which were secured to a staple in the ceiling, placed at the distance of a foot to the right of a point vertical to the patient's navel, were then attached to a bandage fastened round the splints, as high up as possible.

"The foot was raised with the knee extended, so as to bring the limb nearly to a right angle with the line of the tackle, when, by drawing gradually on the cord, in the course of about ten or fifteen minutes, the head of the bone was rendered movable, and was brought considerably more forward. I then began to press on the head of the bone, so as to push it downwards, whilst the pulleys held it partially disengaged from the pelvis. In a few minutes the head of the bone passed over the ridge of the os pubis, and I then directed the foot to be raised a little higher, which, by putting the gluteii muscles more upon the stretch, was calculated to render them more efficient in drawing the bone into its proper place. By this manœuvre, the head of the bone was drawn backwards, and on the foot being more elevated and the cord slackened, it continued to recede from my fingers till the trochanter major made its appearance in the natural situation, and the reduction was found to be perfectly complete.

"Lest the head of the bone should slip backwards on the dorsum ilii, I directed an assistant to apply firm pressure during the latter part of the process, above and behind the acetabulum.

"The apparatus was then removed, the thigh bound up in short splints, and the patient laid upon a double inclined plane. No symptoms of inflammation appeared afterwards about the joint. Passive motion was employed at the end of a week, and occasionally repeated during the whole reparatory process."[1]

Without intending to question the accuracy of the statements in this case, which, in the main, seem to bear the marks of credibility, we must express our surprise that so little difficulty was experienced in the reduction, if the femur was actually broken, no more, indeed, than is usually experienced when the bone is not broken; and that Mr.

[1] Lond. Med.-Chir. Rev., vol. xix. p. 4[illegible]0, Oct. 1833.

Bloxham was able to employ safely passive motion at the end of a week.

Charles Thornhill relates, in the *London Medical Gazette* for July, 1836, a case of fracture of the femur through its upper third, in a man æt. 40, with dislocation into the ischiatic notch; which dislocation, he assures us, was reduced at the end of six weeks. But it is much more probable that, instead of reducing a dislocation, he refractured the bone. During more than one hour and a half, aided by pulleys, tractions and manipulations were made in almost every direction. The upper part of the thigh was lifted with all the strength of one man by means of a jack towel; it was violently rotated, adducted, and abducted. Both the perineal and the knee band gave way, from the excess of the force employed; and, finally, the head of the femur resumed its place with an audible *crash*. After which the "limb was of nearly equal length with the other;" but there remained an "immense deposit" around the acetabulum.[1]

Malgaigne says that M. Etéve found a poor fellow with a dislocation of his left thigh backwards, a fracture near its middle, a penetrating wound of the knee, and a fracture of the fibula in the same leg. Without delay he proceeded to reduce the dislocation by directing two assistants to support the body, three to support the leg, and two more to make extension from a towel tied not very tightly around the thigh above the fracture. The leg was then extended upon the thigh and the thigh flexed upon the pelvis until it was at a right angle with the body; and after a gradual extension had been made in this direction, M. Etéve pushed with all his strength the head of the bone into its socket. Of which case, Malgaigne justly remarks, that the "extension" practiced by the surgeon was only imaginary.[2] If the reduction was accomplished at all, it was by manipulation and pressure.

Finally, Markoe relates in the paper to which we have already several times made allusion, the case of a boy æt. 8, who was admitted into the New York City Hospital on the 29th of June, 1853, with a compound fracture of the right thigh, a simple fracture of the left, and a dislocation of the head of the right femur upwards and backwards upon the dorsum ilii.

When placed upon the bed, the right limb lay obliquely across the abdomen of the boy, with the foot resting against the axilla of the left side. "The house-surgeon, to whose care the case fell on admission, took the injured limb in his hands and very carefully carried it over the abdomen to the right side, and then adducted it and brought it down toward the straight position," during which procedure the head of the bone is supposed to have resumed its place in the socket.[3]

Such is the account furnished of the symptoms and treatment of this extraordinary case; too meagre certainly to entitle it to much confidence, or to permit us to draw from it any practical inferences. We are not even informed what was the name of the young man who

[1] Amer. Journ. Med. Sci., vol. xxv. p. 218.
[2] Malgaigne, op. cit., tom. ii. p. 206; from Gazette Méd., 1838, p. 751.
[3] New York Journ. Med., Jan. 1855, p. 30.

alone saw and treated the case, nor what was his responsibility as a surgeon.

I have been unable to find any other examples of fracture of the femur complicated with dislocation; and, rejecting at least Mr. Thornhill's case as altogether incredible, the proper conclusion would be, that reduction is sometimes possible in recent cases, if the surgeon will resort promptly, before swelling and muscular contraction have taken place, to manipulation combined with pressure upon the head of the bone. Indeed, it is probable that pressure alone is the means upon which the success will finally depend. Richet says that he has several times dislocated the femur in the cadaver; and then having sawn off the head so as to represent a fracture, he has always been able to push the head of the bone easily into its socket.[1] By seizing the moment then when the patient is laboring under the shock, or by placing him completely under the influence of an anæsthetic, no resistance will be offered by the muscles any more than in the cadaver, and the reduction may, perhaps, be as easily effected.

I have no confidence that anything can be accomplished by extension; nor do I think it will be best to wait until the femur has united, since such delay will probably render the reduction impossible.

CHAPTER XVII.

DISLOCATIONS OF THE PATELLA.

§ 1. Dislocations of the Patella Outwards.

Causes.—In the majority of cases it has been occasioned by muscular action; and especially is this liable to occur in persons who are knock-kneed, or whose external condyles have not the usual prominence anteriorly. It may be caused by suddenly twisting the thigh inwards while the weight of the body rests upon the foot, and the leg is thus kept turned outwards; or by falling with the knee turned inwards and the foot outwards. Occasionally it is the result of a blow received upon the inside, or upon the front and inner margin of the patella. In some persons there seems to exist a preternatural laxity of the ligamentum patellæ or of the tendon of the quadriceps extensor which exposes the subject to this accident from very trifling causes. Fergusson says he has known it to be occasioned by a child's stepping upon the knee of a person lying in bed: and Skey says he has seen two cases which occurred spontaneously during sleep. B. Cooper

[1] New York Journ. Med., March, 1854, p. 293; from Bullet. de Thér.

has seen a young lady who frequently dislocated her patella outwards by merely striking her toe against the carpet, or in dancing. Boyer, Sir Astley Cooper, and others, mention similar examples.

Pathological Anatomy.—Most frequently the dislocation is only partial, the inner half of the patella resting upon the articular surface of the outer condyle; and in consequence of the peculiar obliquity of these surfaces, together with the action of the vasti and rectus femoris, the outer margin of the patella becomes tilted forwards.

If the dislocation is more complete, this margin begins to fall over backwards, as in the accompanying drawing; and in more extreme cases the patella lies flat upon the outer side of the condyle, with its inner margin directed forwards.

Fig. 273.

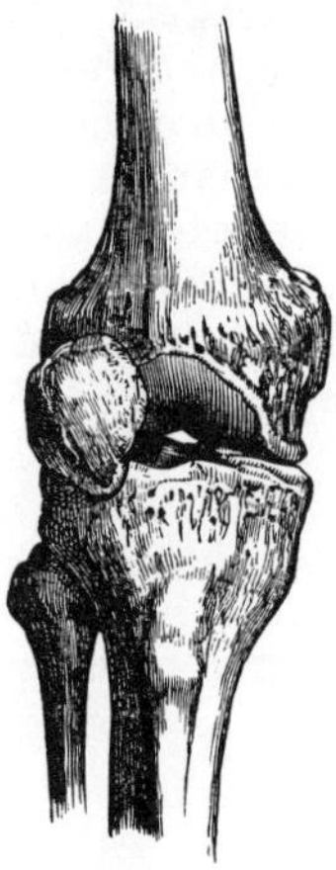

Dislocation of the patella outwards.

When the dislocation is partial, it is probable that neither the capsule nor the ligamentum patellæ usually suffers much laceration; but in complete dislocations, the capsule at least must have given way more or less. Norris, of Philadelphia, reports a case of partial luxation in which the complications were more serious. John Scanlin, æt. 32, was admitted to the Pennsylvania Hospital, on the 27th of August, 1839, in consequence of injuries received a short time previous by having become entangled in machinery. In addition to several fractures in other limbs, he was found to have a subluxation of his left patella outwards, its outer edge being much raised and resting on the side of the external condyle of the femur, while its inner edge was depressed, and firmly fixed in the hollow between the condyles. The internal lateral ligament of the knee was ruptured, allowing the head of the tibia to be moved considerably outwards. A depression existed, also, between the tubercle of the tibia and the lower end of the patella, at the middle and inner side of the knee, evidently produced by a rupture of the ligamentum patellæ in nearly its whole extent. There was almost no swelling, and the limb was moderately flexed. By firm pressure the patella could be restored to position, but as soon as the hand was removed it returned to its original position. At the end of two months "a good degree of motion existed at the knee-joint, which was in no way inflamed or painful."[1]

Symptoms.—The limb is slightly bent, but immovable; the breadth of the knee is considerably increased; the inner condyle projects unnaturally, and the patella is distinctly felt upon the outer side. If the dislocation is partial, the outer margin of the patella forms an irregular sharp ridge in front of the external condyle. If it is complete, the inner margin presents itself in front of the external condyle, and the outer margin looks backwards. Usually the patient suffers great pain so long as the dislocation remains unreduced.

Watson, of New York, saw a case of complete dislocation of the

[1] Norris, Amer. Journ. Med. Sci., vol. xxv., Feb. 1840, p. 276.

patella outwards in a fat young lady, with lax fibre, and occasioned by dancing. He says the knee was slightly but firmly flexed. It was reduced by a very slight pressure with the fingers, and although some inflammation with effusion into the joint ensued, the use of the limb was completely restored in a week or ten days.[1]

Prognosis.—Reduction is in general easily accomplished, but a reluxation is very prone to occur. In the few examples reported of a permanent luxation, the patients have eventually recovered the use of the limb in a great measure. Boyer saw four cases of this kind, in three of which it existed in the left leg and had remained from infancy. The patellæ were easily replaced, but unless confined they soon became displaced again; not one of them found it necessary to apply for surgical aid, as "they suffered no great inconvenience from the luxation, and it exempted them from military service."

After reduction, very little or no inflammation usually follows. Mr. Key has, however, narrated a case in *Guy's Hospital Reports*, of death from suppuration in the knee-joint, following upon the reduction of an *inward* subluxation. The dislocation was produced by a fall while carrying a pail, and was reduced by very gentle pressure; but the patient, a girl, æt. 20, although apparently in good health, was believed to be somewhat strumous.[2]

Treatment.—In order to relax completely the quadriceps extensor, by whose action chiefly the patella is held in its unnatural position, the body should be bent forwards, while at the same moment the leg is extended upon the thigh and the thigh flexed upon the body. The surgeon will accomplish these indications in the most simple manner, by placing the patient in a chair, and then lifting the foot upon his own shoulder, as he kneels or sits before him. Sometimes the patella will resume its position at once when this manœuvre is adopted; but if it does not, slight lateral pressure, made with the fingers, will generally be found sufficient to accomplish the reduction.

In some instances, where other means have failed, the reduction has been effected by violent flexion and extension of the knee, aided by lateral pressure.

I have already mentioned, when speaking of dislocations into the foramen thyroideum, the case of N. Smith, in whose person I found at the same moment a dislocation of the thigh, a subluxation outwards of the tibia, and a complete outward luxation of the corresponding patella. This was occasioned by a fall from a height upon the inside of the knee. I reduced the tibia first, and then easily replaced the patella by lifting the leg and pushing with my fingers against its outer margin.

In many cases the patients themselves have reduced the dislocation immediately, and the surgeon is only consulted in relation to the after treatment. Liston says that this is so constantly the fact or else such dislocations are really so rare that it has never happened to him to have an opportunity of reducing any form of dislocation of the patella.

Not long since a young gentleman æt. 25, residing in Somerset, N. Y.,

[1] Watson, New York Journ. Med., vol. i. p. 306. [2] Op. cit., vol. i. p. 260.

called upon me in consequence of having discovered a floating cartilage in his knee-joint. His account of the matter was that on the first of February, 1858, he was kicked by a cow upon the outside of the right leg about six inches below the knee, and that he immediately found the patella dislocated outwards. After several efforts he finally succeeded in reducing it himself. His knee soon became greatly swollen, so that for five weeks he was unable to walk, and he has been more or less lame to this time. Six months after the accident he discovered a floating cartilage on the inside of the patella about one inch in diameter, which occasionally slips between the joint surfaces, and suddenly trips him up.

§ 2. Dislocations of the Patella Inwards.

Causes.—Less frequent than dislocations outwards, they are occasioned generally by direct blows received upon the outer margin of the patella.

Fig. 274.

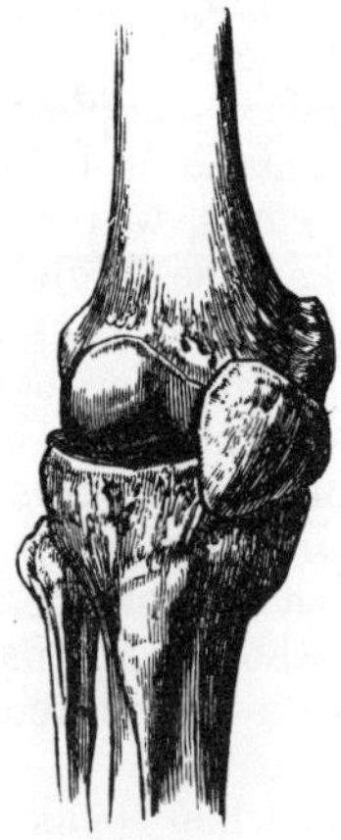

Dislocation of the patella inwards.

The symptoms, pathological anatomy, and treatment will be the same as in dislocations outwards, except so far as these must necessarily vary from the opposite position of the patella.

§ 3. Dislocations of the Patella upon its Axis.

Syn.—"Semi-rotation;" Miller.

These accidents, of which up to the present moment not more than fifteen examples have been recorded, seem to be the result of the same causes which produce lateral luxations; and indeed they may be regarded as only exaggerated forms of incomplete lateral dislocations. In these latter accidents, as we have already noticed, the external or the internal margin of the patella, according as the subluxation is to the outer or inner side, is thrown more or less obliquely forwards; a position into which it is carried partly by the peculiar form of the articulating surfaces; and partly by the action of the vasti and rectus femoris muscles. If now these muscles were to contract suddenly and violently, and the return of the patella to its normal position was prevented by the lodgment of one of its margins in the inter-condyloidean fossa, the other or free margin would be compelled to rise until it became perpendicular to the limb, or it might perhaps even become completely reversed in its socket. The signs of this accident are such as to render an error in the diagnosis almost impossible. The limb is generally found forcibly extended, occasionally it is in a position of moderate flexion, but the projection of the sharp border of the patella directly forwards under the skin, is itself sufficient to determine the true nature of the injury.

Reduction may be effected by the same manœuvres which we have recommended in lateral luxations; but if these measures do not succeed, we may direct the patient to make a violent effort himself to flex and extend the limb, or the surgeon may force the limb into flexion and extension alternately, or he may rotate the tibia upon the femur, and then flex. Finally, he ought to make use of lateral pressure also, upon both margins of the upright patella, but in opposite directions.

Watson, of New York, has related the following example of rotation of the patella upon its inner margin ("Luxation Verticale Externe," *Malg.*).

Henry Burton, aged about thirty-five years, of rather slender frame, while riding on horseback in a crowd, received a blow upon his knee from a horse ridden by another person. When seen by Dr. Watson, soon after the accident, the leg was perfectly straight, but could be flexed to about an angle of 140° without causing pain. "The patella appeared to be slightly drawn up, and it was twisted upon its axis, presenting its outer edge, in a prominent hard line, in front of the knee; its inner edge was resting either in the groove between the condyles of the femur, upon which its posterior face should naturally play, or in the small depression on the anterior face of the femur, immediately above this groove. The anterior surface of the patella was turned inwards, its posterior surface outwards, and it rested nearly at right angles with its natural position. Its upper and lower attachments were both preserved, and could be distinctly felt; and a sort of band appeared to pass from its under, or, as it now lay, its outer face, inwards to the deeper portion of the knee-joint. This band, as I conceived, was caused either by the tension of the capsular ligament, or by the rupture of its edge, as it passes from the outer side of the patella. The position of the bone was so well marked that no one at all acquainted with the anatomy of the part could mistake the nature of the accident.

"With the leg extended, and the anterior muscles of the thigh forced downwards as much as possible, pressure was made upon the patella with the expectation of forcing down its prominent edge. The effort was followed only by an increase of pain, the bone remaining permanently fixed. Another attempt was made to cant its posterior edge inwards, and to bring its anterior edge outwards, without pressing it against the condyles of the femur, by forcing the head of a key against the posterior, now the outer face of the patella (using this as a fulcrum), and pressing the prominent edge of the bone toward the outer condyle. This manœuvre gave him no pain, but was as fruitless in its result as the other. At length the knee was forcibly bent and immediately straightened again; and then by canting the patella as before, and pushing it slightly downwards and inwards, it sprung with a sudden snap into its proper position."[1]

Dr. Joseph P. Gazzam, of Pittsburg, Pa., has met with a similar case. On the 10th of Sept., 1842, James Porter was thrown while wrestling, and immediately found himself unable to rise. Dr. Gazzam saw him about an hour after the accident, and found the patella of the right leg dislocated on its axis, and resting on its inner edge in the groove between the condyles of the femur. Dr. G. proceeded to attempt reduction, but failed, after having made repeated trials by lifting the limb toward the body and by pressure in opposite directions. In consultation with Dr. Addison, it was now determined to divide the ligamentum patellæ, which was done by introducing beneath the skin a narrow-bladed knife, and cutting close to the tubercle of the tibia. Again the attempts at reduction were renewed, but without success. The patella could be moved on its edge more freely than before the cutting, but resisted every effort to replace it. The patient was now bled in the erect posture and until the approach of syncope, but to no purpose. On the following morning, it was determined to adopt, with some modification, the mode practiced so successfully by Dr. Watson. "The thigh was strongly flexed," says Dr. Gazzam, "on the pelvis, and the heel elevated. Then the leg was flexed steadily and forcibly on the thigh, and suddenly straightened. At the moment of straightening the leg, I pressed very strongly against the lower edge of the patella from without, with the head of a door key well wrapped, while Dr. Addison pressed with both thumbs against the upper edge of the bone toward the external condyle. On the fourth trial this manœuvre succeeded, the bone springing into its place with a snap." Recovery was uninterrupted, and two or three months after, the patient had the complete use of his limb.[2]

In a case of the same kind, published originally in *Rust's Magazine*, and which is copied at length by Mr. B. Cooper in his edition of Sir Astley's great work, the reduction was found impossible, notwithstanding the surgeon finally had the temerity to sever completely the tendon of the quadriceps extensor, and the ligamentum patellæ. Extensive suppuration followed, under which the poor fellow finally sank and died.

It is scarcely necessary to say that, rather than expose the patient to such hazards, it would be better to leave the bone unreduced.

[1] Watson, New York Journ. Med., Oct. 1839, p. 302.
[2] Gazzam, Amer. Journ. Med. Sci., vol. xxxi. April, 1843, p. 363.

§ 4. Dislocations of the Patella Upwards.

Occasionally the ligamentum patellæ has been found so much elongated and relaxed, as to permit the patella to glide upwards upon the front of the femur. Heister and Ravaton have each seen an example in which a displacement from this cause existed to the extent of three inches. It is much more common, however, to meet with this dislocation as a result of a rupture of the ligamentum patellæ, as the following example will illustrate.

On the 18th of Dec. 1850, Dennis Mullards, æt. 50, was admitted to the surgical wards of the Buffalo Hospital of the Sisters of Charity. While at work on this same day, he had slipped and fallen, with his knee forcibly flexed under his body. I found the ligament of the patella torn asunder and the patella drawn up two or three inches upon the front of the thigh. We applied at once the dressings used by me for a broken patella, and were able to bring the bone down completely to its place. Three weeks from the time of the receipt of the injury, the dressings were removed, and the patella was found to be nearly but not quite in its original place. From this time we commenced to move the joint: in about ten days more he left the hospital, and I lost sight of him, so that I am unable to speak more definitely of the result.

CHAPTER XVIII.

DISLOCATIONS OF THE HEAD OF THE TIBIA.

Syn.—"Tibia upon the femur:" "dislocations of the leg."

In consequence of the great size and irregularity of the articular surfaces between the tibia and femur, together with the remarkable number and strength of the ligaments which bind the two bones together, dislocations at this joint are exceedingly rare. They are known to take place, however, in four principal directions, namely, backwards, forwards, inwards, and outwards. A dislocation may also occur in either of the diagonals between these points, that is, antero-laterally, or postero-laterally. They may be either complete or incomplete. Velpeau has found upon record thirteen examples of complete dislocations forwards, and eight backwards, but not one of a complete lateral luxation. Velpeau thought also that the antero-posterior luxations were always complete, but Malgaigne has shown that this opinion is erroneous.

Simple flexion and extension, however extreme, are generally insufficient to produce either of these dislocations. They may be produced by a violent blow upon the lower end of the femur, or upon the upper end of the tibia, or by twisting the tibia upon the femur, as when the foot is made fast in a hole, and the body swings around upon the knee.

§ 1. Dislocations of the Head of the Tibia Backwards.

Symptoms.—The head of the tibia is felt in the popliteal space; and, if the dislocation is complete, the pressure upon the popliteal nerve becomes excessively painful.

Fig. 275.

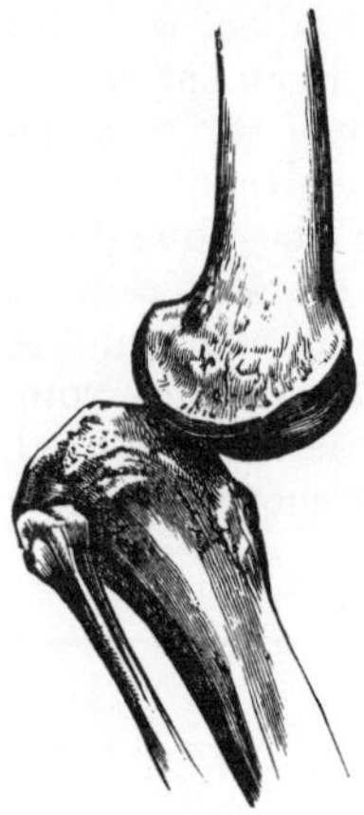

Dislocation of the head of the tibia backwards.

A marked depression exists in front, immediately below the patella, and especially upon the sides of the ligamentum patellæ; the condyles of the femur project strongly in front; the leg may be not at all, or only slightly shortened, or the shortening may amount to one inch or more, and usually it is in a position of extreme extension, or thrown forwards from the line of the axis of the femur; but its position has been found to vary greatly in different cases, the limb being sometimes very much flexed, and in others very slightly flexed, or perfectly straight.

Pathological Anatomy.—The posterior ligament of the joint is torn; the muscles of the ham are put upon the stretch; the popliteal nerves and vessels compressed; and the head of the tibia either rests partly upon the posterior half of the lower articulating surface of the femur, or it passes up and rests only against its posterior articulating surface, which in this direction extends an inch or more upwards. If the dislocation is complete, the crucial ligaments are also torn, and all the parts about the joint suffer extensive injury from stretching, laceration, or compression.

Prognosis.—Malgaigne has seen three examples of incomplete backward luxations which were not reduced, and neither of the persons were very greatly maimed in consequence. One walked with crutches after three or four days, and with a cane after about five weeks. Another did not leave his bed under one month, and it was nearly one year before he could lay aside his crutches; but both of them were finally able to walk at least twelve leagues per day. Malgaigne informs us, however, that in a similar case seen by Lassus, the patient was confined to his bed two years, although he finally recovered a tolerable use of his limb.

If the reduction is promptly effected, the limb kept perfectly quiet a sufficient length of time, and in other respects properly managed, not much inflammation need generally to be anticipated, and the limb may suffer in the end very little, if any maiming.

Treatment.—It will be proper, at first, to attempt the reduction by simple manipulation, as this is often found to succeed when the dislocation is recent and incomplete, and especially when the system is greatly depressed by the shock of the injury. If the dislocation is complete, however, we can hardly anticipate success without the application of some extending force.

In the employment of manipulation we ought to be governed at first by the same rule which we have found so generally applicable in dislocations of the femur, namely, to carry the limb in those directions in which it will move easily, or without much force. If this fails, we may at once resort to forced flexion alternating with extension, rotating or rocking the limb also occasionally from one side to the other, while at the same moment strong pressure is made upon the projecting bones at the knee-joint in opposite directions or in the direction of the articulation.

Finally, it may be necessary to resort to extension, made by means of a lacq, or by the hands of strong assistants, above the ankle, always at first in the direction of the axis of the tibia; the counter-extending band being applied to the perineum, if the leg is straight, but to the lower and under part of the thigh, if the leg is flexed.

A very convenient mode of making extension where we wish to apply more than usual force, is to lay the whole limb over a firm double inclined plane, or fracture splint, securing the thigh to the thigh-piece with a roller, and making the extension with the screw attached to the foot-board. This method, however, while it enables us to use great force in the extension, prevents the surgeon from employing, at the same time, those flexions, extensions, and other manipulations, upon which success so often depends.

Mr. Rose has related in the *Provincial Medical Journal* of June 11th, 1842, a characteristic example of this accident, except that the patella had also suffered a lateral displacement, presenting the usual favorable termination.

A woman was standing upon a low ladder, when a carriage driven furiously came in contact with it, and precipitated her to the ground. Dr. Rose, who saw her almost immediately, found the tibia completely dislocated at the knee, the head being driven behind the condyles of the femur into the ham, with the patella thrown to the outside of the external condyle, and the leg in a state of fixed extension. Immediately, and without difficulty, the bones were restored by applying one hand to the patella, the other to the back of the upper portion of the tibia, and simultaneously pulling and pushing those bones toward their natural positions. The patient was then removed to a bed, and by the diligent use of antiphlogistic remedies inflammation was kept in check, and the case reached a favorable termination without one untoward symptom. After the lapse of only a few weeks, she had completely recovered the use of the knee joint.[1]

Dr. Walsham communicated a case to Sir Astley Cooper, in which the dislocation was not only complete, but the tendon of the quadriceps extensor was ruptured. The leg was bent forwards. The reduction was accomplished very easily by extension made with the hands by four men, in the line of the axis of the limb. In about one month

[1] Rose, Amer. Journ. Med. Sci., vol. xxxi. p. 216.

this man began to walk with crutches, but he was not perfectly recovered until after five months; at which time the crutches were finally laid aside.[1]

§ 2. Dislocations of the Head of the Tibia Forwards.

The signs of this accident are the reverse of those which belong to dislocations backwards. The patella, tibia, and fibula, are prominent in front, while the condyles of the femur may be felt behind, pressing strongly upon the muscles, nerves, and bloodvessels which occupy the popliteal space. In case the dislocation is complete, a shortening may exist to the extent of one or even three inches. Dr. O'Beirne, of Dublin, has mentioned a case to Mr. B. Cooper, in which the shortening was three inches and a half, and Mr. Mayo has seen one example in which the dislocated limb was "fully four inches" shorter than the other.[2] It is quite probable, however, that these latter statements are somewhat exaggerated.

Fig. 276.

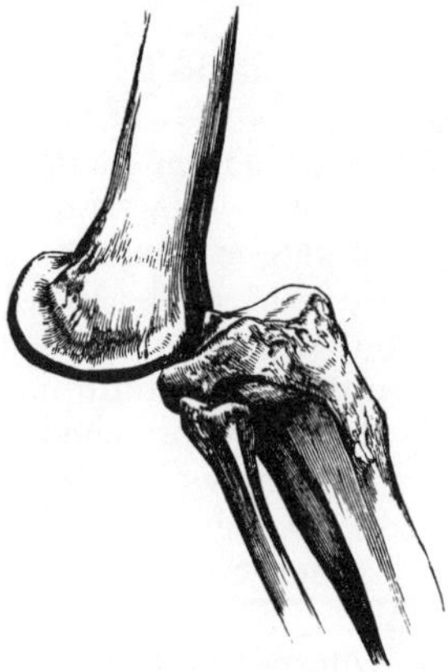

Dislocation of the head of the tibia forwards.

In consequence of the pressure upon the popliteal artery, the pulsations in the branches below are frequently interrupted, and in one instance this pressure was sufficient to produce finally a dry gangrene.

Dr. Gorde relates a case in the *Bulletin de Thérapeutique*, occurring in a woman nearly sixty years old. This woman was returning home at night with a heavy burden, and in a state of intoxication, when she stepped into a ditch as deep as up to the middle of her thighs. The body was thrown forwards by the fall, while the feet stuck at the bottom of the ditch; the whole force of the impulse being sustained by the thighs. The lower end of the femur was found driven downwards and backwards, and lodged under the muscles of the calf of the leg; the limb being shortened three inches. Reduction was promptly effected, and without inflicting any pain of which the patient complained. In six weeks the patient was cured.

Mr. Toogood has reported also, in the *Provincial Medical Journal* of June 18th, 1842, an example of complete dislocation in this direction, in which the appearance was so dreadful, that Mr. Toogood at first despaired of being able to reduce it; but by directing two men to make counter-extension while he made extension, the reduction was immediately effected. At the end of one month the patient was able to leave his bed; and sixteen years after, Dr. Toogood saw him walking

[1] Walsham, Sir A. Cooper on Disloc., 2d Lond. ed., p. 188.

[2] B. Cooper's ed. of Sir Astley Cooper on Disloc., &c., pp. 214—215.

[3] Gorde, Amer. Journ. Med. Sci., vol. xvi. p. 225, May, 1835.

"with very little lameness."[1] Parker, of Liverpool, has reported another example in the *London and Edinburgh Monthly Journal* for December, 1842, which was occasioned by the fall of a heavy spar upon a man's back, and the consequent violent bending of the knee under his body. In this case the limb was slightly flexed, and the patella was loose and floating. The reduction was effected without much difficulty by extension and counter-extension made by two men, while the operator, placing his knee in the ham of the patient, attempted to bring the leg to a right angle with the thigh.[2]

B. Cooper and Malgaigne have each recorded several other examples of this accident.

Dr. White, of this city, politely invited me to see with him a young lad, æt. 10, whose tibia was partially dislocated forwards eight weeks before, by a boy's having hit the top of his knee with his head, while they were at play. His father, who is himself a physician residing near town, reduced the limb very easily, by extension made with his own hands, and by pressing upon the projecting bones. Violent inflammation ensued, but at the time when I saw him, the knee was free from soreness or swelling, and the motions of the joint were nearly restored.

§ 3. Dislocations of the Head of the Tibia Outwards.

Occasionally, owing to a violent wrench of the knee-joint, the lateral ligaments upon one side or the other are ruptured, and consequently the joint surfaces separate somewhat from each, or when the limb is moved, the head of the tibia may slide a little forwards or backwards, or to either side. These are not properly examples of subluxation, nor should we consider as belonging to this class the accident originally described by Mr. Hey, as an "internal derangement of the knee-joint," but which also by some writers has been termed a "subluxation of the knee." Of this latter accident, I will take occasion hereafter to speak a little more particularly.

In subluxation, properly so called, if the direction of the dislocation is outwards, the outer condyle of the femur rests upon the inner articulating surface of the tibia, and if the direction of the dislocation is inwards, the inner condyle of the femur rests upon the outer articulating surface of the tibia.

The signs which characterize this accident are such as cannot easily be mistaken. The limb is not shortened, nor is there anything especially diagnostic in its position, since it has been found to be sometimes flexed, and at other times straight; but the strong lateral projections made by the inner condyle of the femur on the one hand, and by the heads of the tibia and fibula on the other, cannot fail to inform us as to the true nature of the accident.

The treatment will not differ essentially from that which has already been recommended in dislocations of the tibia backwards or

[1] Toogood, Amer. Journ. Med. Sci., vol. xxxi. p. 465. [2] E. Parker, ibid.

forwards. If any other expedients can prove useful, they must be left to the judgment of the surgeon whenever the exigencies of the case shall demand them.

Fig. 277.

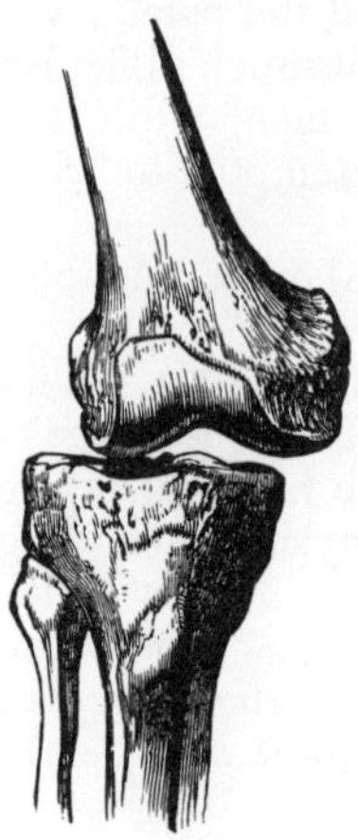

Subluxation of the head of the tibia outwards.

I have already mentioned the case of N. Smith, who, in consequence of a fall from a window, had a dislocation of the right femur, tibia, and patella. The tibia was subluxated outwards, and the leg was partially flexed upon the thigh, with the toes everted. By moderate extension, made with my own hands, united with alternate flexion and extension, the bone was easily and promptly restored to its place. Having reduced the femur also, the limb was laid over a gently inclined plane made of pillows; and cloths moistened with cool water were kept constantly applied to the knee for many days. Very little swelling followed the accident, and his recovery was rapid and complete.

A man was received into the North London Hospital, with a partial dislocation of the tibia outwards, and, although the knee was much swollen, the nature of the injury was easily determined. The knee was immovable, and the toes turned outwards. Mr. Hallam, the house surgeon, reduced it by extension and counter-extension made by his own hands.[1]

Mr. Pitt records a similar case in a young lady, produced by a fall down a flight of stairs. It was reduced easily by extension and counter-extension. Inflammation followed, but it was finally controlled, and she regained the use of her limb.[2]

In one case of subluxation, mentioned by Sir Astley Cooper, and in a second recorded by Bransby Cooper, the recovery of the functions of the joint did not seem to have been so rapid; the joint remaining unstable and tender for a long time afterwards.[3]

§ 4. Dislocations of the Head of the Tibia Inwards.

There is nothing peculiar in either the signs, condition, or treatment of this accident, as distinguished from a dislocation outwards, to demand of us a special consideration.

Sir Astley Cooper has mentioned two cases of subluxation inwards, and Mr. B. Cooper has added to these a third. Sir Astley remarks that in the first accident, the only one indeed which he had himself ever seen, he was struck with three circumstances: first, the great deformity of the knee from the projection of the tibia; second, the ease with which the bone was reduced by direct extension; and third, by the little inflammation which followed. The second case of which

[1] Hallam, Amer. Journ. Med. Sci., vol. xix. p. 251.
[2] Pitt, ibid., vol. xxxi. p. 465.
[3] B. Cooper's ed. of Sir Ast., op. cit., pp. 211–13.

Sir Astley speaks was communicated to him by a Mr. Richards. In this case the fibula was also broken, and the reduction was accomplished only after extension had been made by several persons for half an hour. The limb became excessively swollen, and remained so for many weeks. Eighteen months after the accident the knee continued somewhat stiff, and there was an unnatural lateral motion in the joint, from the injury which the ligaments had sustained. The patient referred to by Bransby Cooper had met with the accident by a fall upon the foot with his leg bent under him; and a fellow workman had reduced the bones by extension and pressure. Mr. Cooper thinks that not only the internal lateral ligament was torn, but also some fibres of the vastus externus and the crucial ligaments. Violent inflammation ensued, which did not permit him to leave the hospital until after about two weeks.[1] Fergusson has seen two examples of unreduced subluxation inwards, in both of which the patients had regained useful limbs.[2]

Fig. 278.

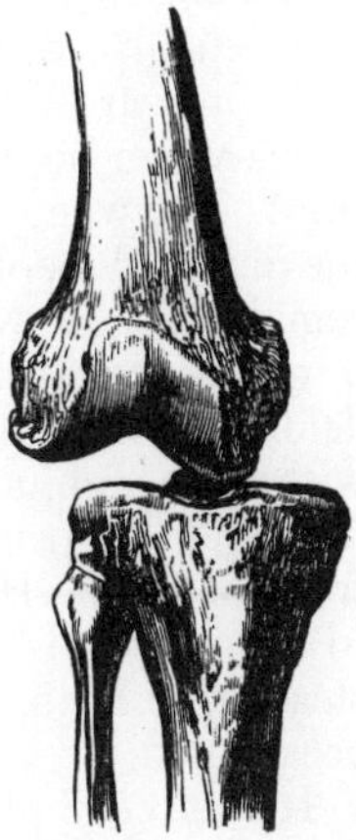

Subluxation of the head of the tibia inwards.

Malgaigne mentions that Boyer, Costallat, and Key, had each seen one similar example; and he also enumerates two additional cases of complete luxation attended with a protrusion of the bone through an external wound; in both of which the reduction was easily effected and the patients recovered.[3]

§ 5. Dislocations of the Head of the Tibia Backwards and Outwards.

In June, 1853, Henry J., of Dansville, N. Y., æt. 24, was thrown by an enraged bull, and his left leg being caught under the knee by the horns, was twisted violently. Dr. Prior, of Dansville, and Batton, of Burns, were called, and found the left knee completely dislocated; the tibia being displaced backwards beyond the condyles of the femur, and also a little outwards. The foot and leg were inclined outwards. With the assistance of four men, extension and counter-extension were made in the line of the axis of the limb, and the reduction was easily accomplished. Pasteboard splints, bandages, &c., were applied to maintain the bones in place; but the swelling came on rapidly, and in the evening these dressings were removed. The limb was now laid over a double inclined plane carefully padded, in order to press the upper end of the tibia forwards, as it manifested a constant inclination to become displaced backwards. This apparatus was employed six weeks, with the exception of two or three days, during which the limb was laid upon pillows, but as the pillows did not sufficiently

[1] B. Cooper, ed. of Sir Ast., op. cit., pp. 211–13. [2] Fergusson, op. cit., p. 284.
[3] Malgaigne, op. cit., tom. ii. p. 956.

support the back of the tibia, the double inclined plane was resumed. After the removal of the plane, during seven weeks longer, an angular splint was kept closely applied to the back of the limb.

Seven months after the accident, on the 23d of January, 1854, Dr. Robinson, of Hornellsville, brought the gentleman to me. I found the bones displaced backwards about three-quarters of an inch, and half an inch outwards, or to the fibular side. This was the position of the bones when he was sitting with his leg bent at a right angle with the thigh, but when he stood erect and bore some weight upon his foot, the outward displacement ceased, and the backward displacement only remained. It was very easy, however, in whatever position the leg might be, to push the bones forwards by the hands until nearly all deformity had disappeared. He could flex the leg to a right angle with the thigh, and straighten it completely, but he could not lift the foot and leg from the floor while sitting with his limb extended in front of him. He was unable to bear sufficient weight upon the foot to use it at all in progression, on account of the inability to fix and steady the limb, but not on account of any pain or soreness which it occasioned.

It was very plain that the surgeons were not in fault for this unfortunate condition; indeed they seem to have exercised throughout great ingenuity and skill in its management.

I directed the young man to Mr. John C. Seiffert, our very ingenious instrument maker, who has since succeeded, I learn, in adapting to his knee a mechanical contrivance which enables him to walk quite well.

Thomas Wells, of Columbia, South Carolina, has described a similar accident, the tibia being dislocated outwards and backwards, which terminated fatally on the fourth day, in consequence mainly of exposure, intemperance, and neglect to apply for surgical aid. The bones were never reduced, and the autopsy disclosed also a fracture of the internal condyle of the femur.[1]

§ 6. Slipping of the Semilunar Fibro-Cartilages.

Syn.—"Internal derangement of the knee-joint;" Hey. "Partial dislocation of the thigh-bone from the semilunar cartilages;" Sir Astley Cooper. "Subluxation of the semilunar cartilages;" Malgaigne. "Subluxation of the knee;" Erichsen. To these we think it proper to add, as giving rise to the same class of symptoms, "Floating cartilages in the knee-joint."

We have already expressed our opinion that this accident is in no proper sense a subluxation of the knee; and we should not, therefore, think it worth while to make any farther allusion to it, were it not necessary in order to enable the student of surgery to distinguish between the phenomena which belong to it and those which belong strictly to subluxations of this joint.

Symptoms.—The patient is suddenly thrown to the ground while walking, as if by an instantaneous loss of power in the affected limb,

[1] Wells, Amer. Journ. Med. Sci. vol. x. p. 25, May, 1832.

this loss of control over the limb being accompanied usually with sharp pain, referred to the region of the knee-joint; or he trips his toe against something in his path, and the toes becoming everted, the leg suddenly gives way under him; in some cases it has happened when the patient was turning in bed, the weight of the bedclothes hanging upon the toes so as to occasion a strain and rotation outwards at the knee-joint, or it follows upon a subluxation of the joint, as in one example which I shall presently relate.

If the patient is walking when the accident takes place, and he falls to the ground, he finds himself unable to move the limb, or to stand upon it; but by manipulation, the difficulty is as easily overcome as it occurred, when immediately the motions of the joint become free, and he walks off as if nothing had happened.

When the accident has once taken place, it is afterwards exceedingly liable to occur from very slight causes, and eventually the knee-joint becomes tender and the capsule fills with synovia, indicating the existence of subacute synovitis.

A single example will illustrate the usual history of these cases.

A young man, from Colesville, N.Y., æt. 23, consulted me on the 27th of Oct. 1858, in relation to the condition of his knee-joint. He stated that, on the 13th of Aug. 1858, while standing with the whole weight of his body resting upon the left leg, a mate struck him on the inside of the lower end of the left femur. The blow was made with the palm of the hand, but with sufficient force to throw him down. It was immediately noticed that the tibia was partially dislocated inwards at the knee-joint. The whole lower part of the limb was inclined outwards. A person present in the room seized upon the foot and by extension easily brought it back to place; the bone resuming its position with an audible snap. After this he continued to walk about until night. Two days after, the knee had become so much inflamed that he was obliged to take to his bed, on which he was confined three weeks. Gradually the swelling subsided, and in about five weeks after the accident he began to walk on crutches. On the 23d of Sept., he was walking in the store without crutches, when he suddenly felt a sensation of slipping in the joint, and he fell to the floor as if he had been tripped up. At the time when he called upon me, this had happened many times, but it has never been attended with pain. The joint was filled with synovia, and tender, yet I could distinctly feel a hard body just to the inside of the ligamentum patellæ, and which moved freely under the finger.

Pathological Anatomy.—The same class of symptoms, with only very slight modifications, belongs probably to several varieties of "internal derangement of the knee-joint;" and first, it will be remembered that the semilunar cartilages upon which the margins of the condyles of the femur rest, are attached to the tibia by several ligaments; but when, from relaxation or a violent strain, any one of these ligaments becomes elongated or gives way, the portion of cartilage which it restrains is permitted to become partially displaced, and by interposing its thick margin between the deeper articulating surfaces the bones are separated and the muscles lose their control over the joint; second, these ligaments may not only yield, but a fragment of one of the cartilages may become actually broken off from the main portion; third, the femur may perhaps escape behind some portion of an interarticular cartilage and thus, instead of the cartilage placing itself between the joint surfaces, the femur itself may have thrust it into this position; fourth, a cartilage or some portion of a cartilage may become hypertrophied, and thus give rise to the symptoms described; fifth, in other cases still, a bony, cartilaginous, fibrinous, or calcareous growth or concretion forming within the joint, and if originally attached, becoming separated from the capsule, may move about more or less freely, and give rise to the same class of symptoms which we have described.

This last variety has generally been described under the name of "floating cartilages;" but since these bodies are not always cartilaginous, and especially since they do not always by any means move so freely as to be properly designated as "floating," the term is less appropriate than that originally given by Hey, and which we have chosen to adopt.

Treatment.—For the purpose of obtaining immediate relief it is generally sufficient to flex the leg completely and then suddenly extend it, or to combine this motion with a slight twisting or rocking of the knee-joint. Sometimes this experiment has to be repeated several times before it is completely successful, and in a few instances it has failed altogether. I think I must have met with ten or twelve examples in the course of my practice, and in no instance has the sudden flexion and extension of the limb failed to overcome the difficulty.

As to the question of subsequent treatment, especially as to whether it is proper to attempt their extirpation when they are found to be loose, or to make any other surgical interference, I prefer to leave its consideration to those general treatises upon surgery where it more properly belongs.

CHAPTER XIX.

DISLOCATIONS OF THE LOWER END OF THE TIBIA.

Syn.—"Tibio-tarsal luxations;" Malgaigne. "Dislocations of the ankle-joint;" Chelius and others.

THE tibia may be dislocated at its lower end in four directions; namely, inwards, outwards, forwards, and backwards. Most of these dislocations complicate themselves with fractures of the fibula, or of the tibia, or with fractures of both bones.

Dupuytren, Malgaigne, and a few other surgeons have reported examples also of dislocations forwards and inwards.

Boyer, with a majority of the French writers, and several English and German surgeons, speak of these dislocations as belonging to the foot; consequently the outward dislocation of Boyer is the inward dislocation of Sir Astley Cooper, Malgaigne, myself and others, who prefer to regard the tibia as the bone dislocated.

§ 1. Dislocations of the Lower End of the Tibia Inwards.

Syn.—"Inward tibio-tarsal luxations;" Malgaigne. "Dislocations of the foot outwards;" Boyer and others.

Causes.—This dislocation is occasioned generally by a fall from a height, upon the bottom of the foot, the foot receiving at the same moment a sufficient inclination outwards to determine the main force of the impulse toward the inner side of the ankle. It may be produced also by a blow received directly upon the outside of the leg just above the ankle, or by a violent twist or wrench of the foot outwards.

Pathological Anatomy.—I have already, in the chapter on fractures of the fibula, stated my opinion that a large majority of those accidents which have been called inward and outward dislocations of the tibia, were merely examples of lateral rotation of the astragalus within the half ginglimoid and half orbicular socket formed by the lower extremities of the tibia and fibula; and that true dislocations, either partial or complete, are at this joint and in these directions very rare occurrences. We shall continue, however, in accordance with the general practice of writers, to call them all dislocations, whether the astragalus simply rotates on its axis, or is displaced laterally and horizontally from the tibia.

Fig. 279.

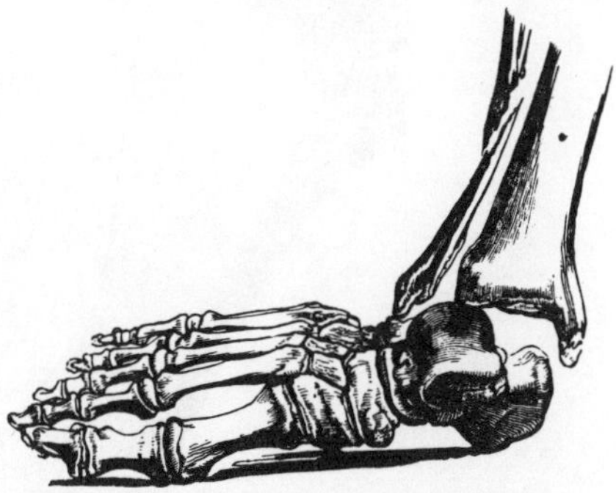

Dislocation of the lower end of the tibia inwards.

In the most common form of the accident, then, when the foot is violently twisted outwards, the astragalus becomes tilted upon its outer and upper margin in such a way as that this margin slides inwards and places itself underneath the middle portion of the lower articulating surface of the tibia; its upper and inner margin descends toward the extremity of the malleolus internus, and the outer face of the astragalus presents obliquely upwards and outwards, instead of directly outwards as it would do in its natural position. This cannot occur without a rupture of the internal tibio-tarsal ligaments, or a fracture of the malleolus internus, or both; indeed, a fracture of the internal malleolus is a very common circumstance in connection with this form of dislocation. Much more frequently, however, the fibula itself gives way at a point within from two to five inches of its lower extremity; or sometimes the fracture in the fibula occurs through that portion which forms the malleolus externus. For more particular information as to the causes and relative frequency of these fractures, I refer the reader to the chapter on fractures of the fibula.

Rarely it happens that instead of this lateral rotation of the astragalus, there occurs a true lateral displacement of the tibia inwards upon the astragalus, and the outer portion of the lower articulating surface of the tibia comes to rest upon the inner portion of the upper articulating surface of the astragalus; or it may slide completely off in the same direction; a result which is usually attended with a laceration of the muscles and integuments, converting the accident into a compound dislocation. In some cases this extreme displacement occürs without such lacerations.

In this form of the accident, the true lateral luxation, the fibula may remain unbroken and undisturbed, the tibia merely having become displaced inwards; or the fibula may give way also above the articulation, while the malleolus internus, and the internal lateral ligaments are equally liable to rupture as in the other form of the accident.

Sometimes in addition to these complications, the lower end of the tibia is found to be broken obliquely upwards and outwards from the articulating surface, leaving that fragment attached to the fibula which corresponds to the inferior peroneo-tibial articulation.

Symptoms.—The foot is more or less violently abducted, the sole of

Fig. 280.

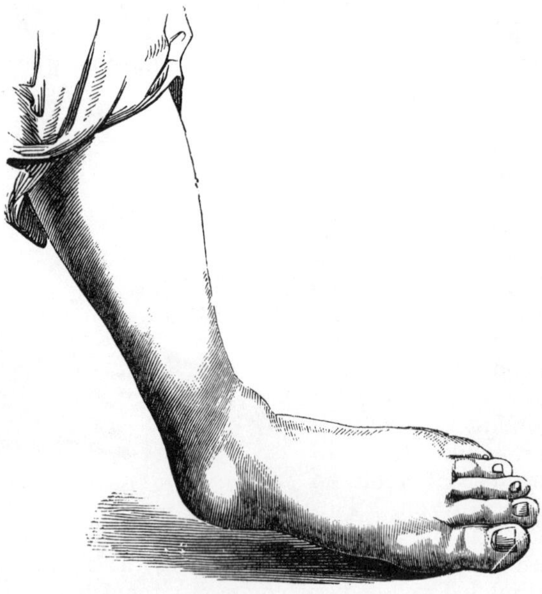

Dislocation of the lower end of the tibia inwards.

the foot presenting downwards and outwards instead of directly downwards; the malleolus internus projects strongly at the inner side of the joint; and at the outer side there is a corresponding depression, generally most marked a little above the articulation near the point of fracture in the fibula. The pain is very great, and the foot is immovably fixed, so far as the volition of the patient can determine motion, but the surgeon can generally move it pretty freely, yet not without causing a great increase of the pain. When the dislocation is complete, and the fibula also is broken, the limb becomes slightly shortened.

Treatment.—When the accident is of the nature of a simple rotation of the astragalus upon its axis, the reduction is often accomplished with the greatest ease by seizing upon the foot, and forcibly adducting it. Not unfrequently the patient himself, or some other person who is present, has effected the reduction before the surgeon is called. In other cases, and especially when it partakes of the nature of a true dislocation, much difficulty is sometimes experienced in the reduction. The surgeon ought then to flex the leg upon the thigh, in order to relax the gastrocnemii muscles, and holding the foot midway between flexion and extension, he should pull steadily upon it with his own hands, while an assistant makes counter-extension, and supports the limb with his hands, grasping the thigh above the knee. At the same moment lateral pressure should be made upon the projecting bone in the direction of the articulation. It is of some use, also, to occasionally flex and extend the limb moderately, and to give to the foot a gentle rocking motion. If more force is needed, it may be applied by placing the limb over a firm double inclined fracture splint, and making the extension by the aid of a screw attached to the footboard, as we have suggested in certain cases of dislocation at the knee. Or we may employ the pulleys after the manner represented in the accompanying drawing.

Fig. 281.

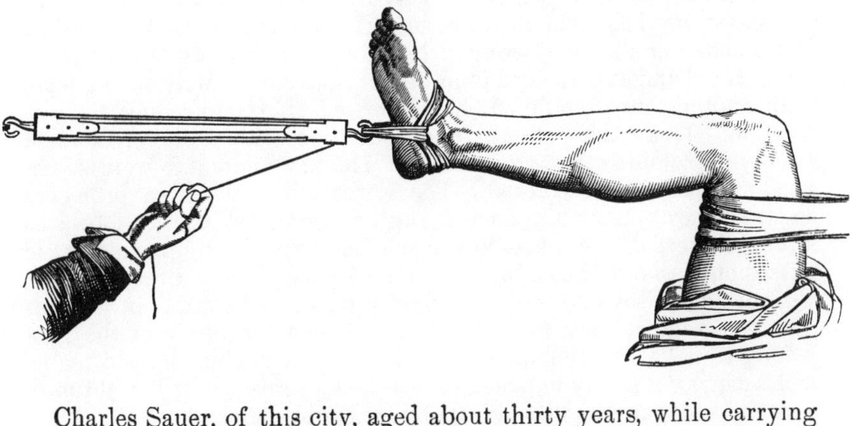

Charles Sauer, of this city, aged about thirty years, while carrying a weight upon his shoulders, on the 6th of May, 1854, slipped upon the side walk and fell, dislocating the left tibia inwards and fracturing the fibula four inches from its lower end. I was in attendance soon after the accident occurred, and found the tibia projecting inwards, with the other symptoms usually accompanying a simple rotation of the astragalus upon its axis. Seizing the foot with my hands, and flexing the leg, while an assistant held up the thigh and made counter-extension, I had scarcely begun to pull upon the foot before the reduction was effected. Dupuytren's splint was at once applied, and the subsequent inflammation was so trivial as scarcely to deserve notice. In six weeks the limb was sound, and free from all anchylosis.

In my report on dislocations, made to the New York State Medical Society for the year 1855, I have mentioned twelve similar examples, in addition to some examples of compound dislocations, all of which were easily reduced, but the results were not always so favorable.

If, as rarely happens, the tibia is broken obliquely into the joint, the complete reduction of the dislocated tibia may be found impossible, owing to the obstacle presented by the displaced fragment.

The following I am disposed to regard as examples of dislocation accompanied with fracture of the tibia within the articulation.

Brockway, of Cortland, N. Y., aged about twenty-seven years, consulted me at my office a few years since in relation to the condition of his foot. I found the tibia dislocated inwards and projecting more than an inch beyond the astragalus; the foot was turned outwards, compelling him to walk upon the inside of his foot; the fibula was bent inwards against the tibia, at a point about four inches above the ankle, which seemed to have been the seat of fracture of this bone. He stated to me that immediately after the receipt of the injury, which was occasioned by a fall from a height upon the bottom of his foot, he had consulted a surgeon, Dr. A. B. Shipman, of Cortland, and that although Dr. Shipman made repeated and violent efforts to effect the reduction, he had been unable to do so. Indeed the bone had never been removed from the position in which it was at first placed.

J. Borland, of Erie Co., N. Y., æt. 31, fell under a rolling log and dislocated his left tibia inwards, breaking off the internal malleolus, and fracturing the fibula four inches from its lower end. Dr. Sweetland, an old and experienced practitioner, was immediately called, who, with another surgeon, failed, after repeated efforts, to reduce the dislocation. I saw the patient, in consultation with these gentlemen, twenty-four hours after the accident. The foot and ankle were somewhat swollen, and discolored. The lower end of the tibia projected so far inwards as to threaten a rupture of the skin; the foot was strongly everted. We first flexed the leg upon the thigh, and made extension with our hands, in the manner I have already directed. This we continued several minutes; finally moving the limb in various directions, and adding forcible pressure upon the inside of the projecting tibia. We then placed the leg over a double-inclined plane, and, securing it firmly in place, we attached a screw to the foot through a sandal and gaiter, and while the leg was well flexed upon the thigh, we renewed the extension and lateral pressure. This was continued with the application of more or less power, during half an hour meanwhile changing the position of the limb occasionally by varying the angle of the splint. Our efforts were prolonged in all more than one hour, when, as we had made no impression upon the bone, and the patient had repeatedly implored us to desist, the attempt was given over. The end of the tibia seemed to rest partly upon the astragalus, and the extension was plainly all that was demanded, but the obstacle was beyond doubt within the articulation, or rather between the tibia and fibula.

Four weeks after the accident, Mr. Borland walked on crutches, and during a year he was compelled to use a cane, but since that time, a period of twelve years, he has walked without any artificial support. For a year or two he felt a yielding in his ankle, as the weight of his body settled upon his limb; but this gradually ceased, and for some years past he has walked without any halt, and seems to step as firmly as before the accident. The foot still inclines outwards; the tibia projects inwards one inch, and the broken ends of the fibula can be felt resting against the tibia, where they are united.

Not long since I had occasion to amputate a limb for a compound dislocation inwards at the ankle-joint, and the possibility of this fracture was confirmed by the dissection. About one-third of the outer portion of the articular surface was broken off obliquely, and the fragment was lying so displaced that a reduction would have been rendered impossible.

Dr. Townsend, of Boston, has reported a case of compound dislocation, in which also amputation became necessary; and, with other injuries, the dissection showed a fragment from the outer margin of the tibia, one inch and a half long, and one inch thick at its widest part, with a very sharp point, displaced and lying almost transversely over the astragalus.[1]

For a more full account of the prognosis and the general management of these cases subsequent to the reduction, I beg again to refer the reader to the chapter on fractures of the fibula; and for my views in relation to the treatment of compound dislocations of the ankle-joint I will refer also to the chapter on compound dislocations of the long bones.

§ 2. Dislocations of the Lower End of the Tibia Outwards.

Syn.—"Outward tibio-tarsal luxations;" Malgaigne. "Dislocations of the foot inwards," of others.

The causes are the same or similar to those which are known generally to produce dislocations inwards; only that the force of the concussion or the direction of the rotation must have been reversed.

The external lateral ligaments, peroneo-tarsal, are either ruptured or the lower portion of the fibula gives way, or both of these circumstances may have happened; while the internal malleolus may also yield to the shock and to the weight of the body now resting upon it.

[1] Townsend, Mass. Hosp. Reports, Bost. Med. and Surg. Journ., vol. xxxiii. p. 277.

The nature of the accident may vary also in respect to the relative position of the articular surfaces; the astragalus may simply rotate on its inner and upper margin, or the tibia, with the fibula of course, may actually slide outwards until the lower end of the tibia more or less completely abandons the upper surface of the astragalus.

The modes of reduction and the general principles of treatment subsequently, will not differ from those which we have mentioned as suitable for dislocations in the opposite direction. The examples which have fallen under my observation are not numerous, but the reduction has always been easily effected. Thus a man, æt. 21, fell from a scaffolding, alighting upon his feet. He says that his left foot struck the ground obliquely and upon its outer margin. I found the fibula projecting very strongly outwards, evidently carrying with it the tibia; the malleolus internus was broken off, and the foot forcibly turned inwards. Without either flexing the leg upon the thigh or calling to my aid any degree of counter-extension except what was made by the weight of the body, I grasped the foot and drew upon it gently while at the same moment I rotated the foot outwards. Immediately the bones resumed their places.

Fig. 282.

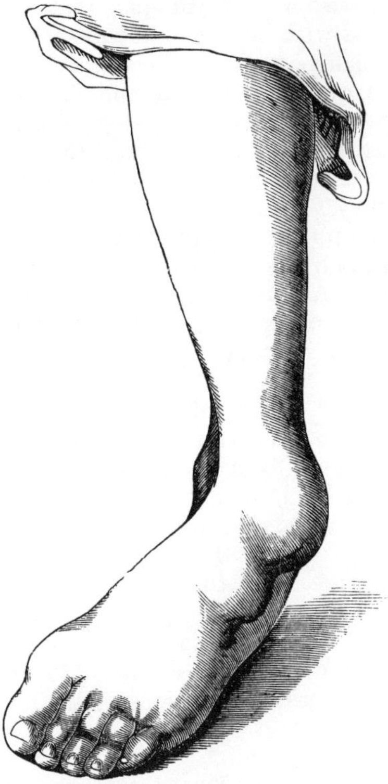

Dislocation of the lower end of the tibia outwards.

In June of 1846, Henry Wilson, æt. 38, consulted me in relation to his foot, which he said had been dislocated four weeks before. He had fallen upon the outside of his foot and turned it suddenly inwards, so that when he looked at it he found the sole presenting toward the opposite side. Seizing upon it with both hands, he pressed it forcibly outwards, and the reduction immediately took place with a snap. Very little soreness followed, nor was he confined to his house a single day. He had continued to walk about with only a slight halt in his gait, nor would he have thought it necessary to consult me at all except that the tenderness had not yet disappeared. He was not aware that the fibula had been broken also until I called his attention to the fact. The fracture had taken place two inches above the ankle; and, although it was already united, the depression occasioned by its having fallen in somewhat toward the tibia was very plainly felt and recognized.

§ 3. Dislocations of the Lower End of the Tibia Forwards.

Syn.—"Forward tibio-tarsal luxations;" Malgaigne. "Dislocations of the foot backwards," of others.

Causes.—This dislocation may be produced by a violent extension of the foot upon the leg; as, for example, when, the foot being engaged under a piece of timber, the body falls backwards to the ground; or when, the leg remaining fixed, a heavy weight descends upon the front of the foot; or it may be caused by a fall upon the bottom of the foot, the foot resting upon an inclined plane; by a blow upon the back of the tibia, or possibly, even by the toes being brought violently in contact with some firm body.

Pathological Anatomy.—The displacement may be very slight, so that the end of the tibia is only a little advanced upon the astragalus; or it may be such that the tibia rests one-half upon the naviculare and one-half upon the astragalus, or it may even desert the astragalus entirely. In these latter examples, the lateral ligaments suffer more or less complete laceration. The fibula is generally broken on a level with the articulation, the malleolus internus also in some cases, and still more rarely a fracture occurs through the posterior margin of the articular surface of the tibia.

Fig. 283.

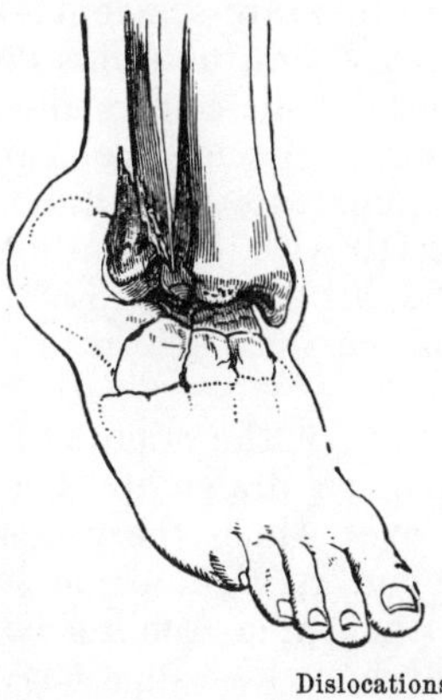

Fig. 284.

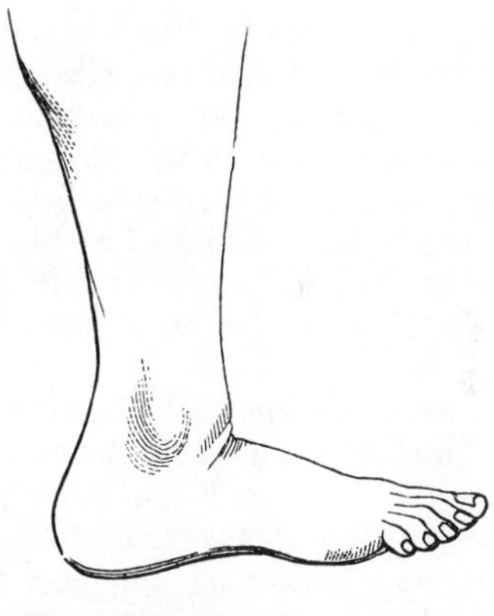

Dislocations of the lower end of the tibia forwards.

Symptoms.—The length of the foot in front of the tibia is diminished, while the projection of the heel is correspondingly increased; the toes are turned downwards, and the heel drawn upwards, and fixed in this position; the end of the tibia may generally be distinctly felt in front of the astragalus; the extensor tendons of the toes are sharply defined, while the tendo-Achillis is curved forwards, and tense.

Treatment.—The reduction is to be attempted by flexing the leg upon the thigh, and making extension from the foot, while, at the same moment, pressure is made upon the front of the tibia and against the heel. When the bone begins to slide into place, the foot should be forcibly flexed upon the leg. A slight lateral motion or rotation in either direction may assist in restoring the bones to place.

In general, the dislocation has been easily reduced, but in a majority of the examples recorded great difficulty has been experienced in maintaining the reduction; and in a few cases it has been found impossible to do so.

In order to maintain the reduction, the leg, flexed upon the thigh, should be laid on its back in a box; and the foot supported firmly against a foot-piece placed at a right angle with the box. In this position, the weight of the leg will tend somewhat to overcome the action of the muscles which are disposed to displace the foot backwards. Generally it will be found necessary to make additional pressure directly upon the front of the leg above the ankle; which, in order that it may not prove mischievous, must be effected with some soft material, and must be applied over a broad surface. Perhaps nothing will better answer these indications than to pass a cotton band, six or eight inches in width, through slits or mortices in the sides of the box; these slits being of a width equal to the width of the band, and placed at a point sufficiently below the level of the spine of the tibia, so that when the band is made fast underneath the box it shall press the leg firmly backwards. To prevent the heel from suffering in consequence of this pressure, it also should be supported, or suspended by another band passing underneath the heel and fastened above to the top of the foot-board.

Dupuytren relates the following example of this rare accident:—

Pierre Froment, æt. 33, was carrying a heavy weight upon his back, and had his right foot in advance, when by accident he came suddenly in contact with a beam placed across his path. Under the fear of being precipitated forwards, he made a sudden effort to throw his body backwards, by which he lost his balance, and fell with the point of the left foot inclined inwards and forwards, and his whole weight was thrown first on the outer side, and then on the front of the ankle-joint.

On examination the leg seemed to be planted upon the middle of the foot; the toes were directed downwards and the heel drawn up. On the instep there was a large bony prominence, over which the extensor tendons of the toes were stretched like tense cords. Behind the joint was a deep hollow, at the bottom of which the tendo-Achillis could be felt, forming a tense, resisting, semicircular cord, with its concavity directed backwards. The fibula was also broken; the lower end of the lower fragment remaining attached to the foot, while the upper end of the same fragment was carried forwards by the displacement of the tibia, so that it lay nearly horizontally, with its broken extremity directed forwards.

Dupuytren directed one assistant to fix the leg, and a second to make extension from the foot, while Dupuytren himself, standing on the outer side of the limb, forced the heel forwards and the tibia backwards. The first attempt succeeded partially, and the second completed the reduction. The limb was then placed in the apparatus employed by this surgeon for a fractured fibula, which we have before described, and laid on its outer side in a semiflexed position. The patient recovered rapidly, and in little more than a month he was able to walk.[1]

But such fortunate results have not usually been observed; indeed Dupuytren encountered much more serious difficulties in two other cases which came under his own notice, one of which he has himself recorded. This was in the person of a woman æt. 48, who was brought to the Hôtel Dieu in 1815, the accident having just happened from a slip in going down stairs. The fibula was broken, and also a fragment was broken from the tibia. The house surgeon reduced the bones and placed the limb in the ordinary apparatus for broken legs, but on the following day Dupuytren found them reluxated, and laid the limb on his own splint, but the pressure requisite to keep the tibia in place soon induced sloughing, ulceration, and abscesses, and after four months' treatment, during which time the tibia had been repeatedly displaced, she left the hospital able to use her limb, but with a certain amount of incurable deformity.[2]

Malgaigne mentions the third example as having been seen by himself in Dupuytren's service in 1832, in which case the attempt to maintain the reduction by a tourniquet resulted in gangrene and finally the death of the patient.[3] Earle lost a patient after amputation made on the eighth day. The tibia could not be kept in place, and the amputation became necessary on account of the final protrusion of the bone through the integuments, which had sloughed.[4]

§ 4. Dislocations of the Lower End of the Tibia Backwards.

Syn.—"Backward tibio-tarsal luxations;" Malgaigne. "Dislocations of the foot forwards," of others.

More rare even than the dislocations forwards, Malgaigne has nevertheless succeeded in collecting five examples.

They appear to have been produced generally by a cause the reverse of that which we have seen to produce so often the preceding dislocation. Thus while the dislocation forwards is produced most frequently when the foot is in violent extension, this dislocation has occurred in at least two or three cases, when the foot was forcibly flexed upon the leg.

The symptoms are strongly marked and characteristic. The length of the foot from the tibia to the ends of the toes is increased one inch or more; the heel being correspondingly shortened, or rather wholly obliterated; a portion of the articulating surface of the astragalus may be distinctly felt in front of the tibia; the posterior surface of the tibia touches the tendo-Achillis; the leg is shortened and the malleoli approach the sole of the foot.

In most cases one or both of the malleoli have been broken; and

[1] Dupuytren, Injuries and Dis. of Bones. London ed., p. 278.
[2] Op. cit., p. 276. [3] Malgaigne, op. cit., p. 1044. [4] Ibid., p. 1044.

R. W. Smith, who has reported one of the examples alluded to, believes that the dislocation is never complete.

Fig. 285.

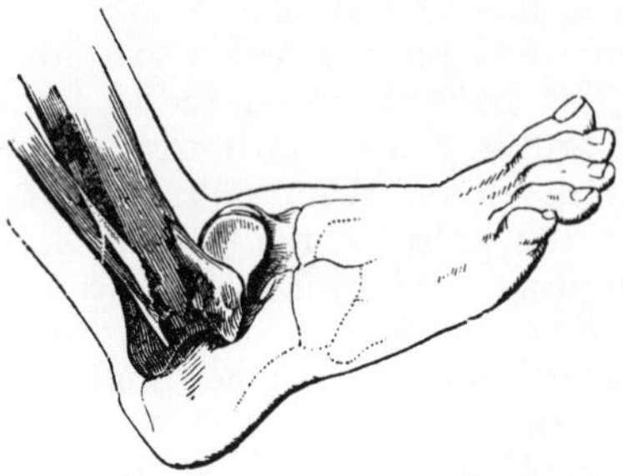

Fig. 286.

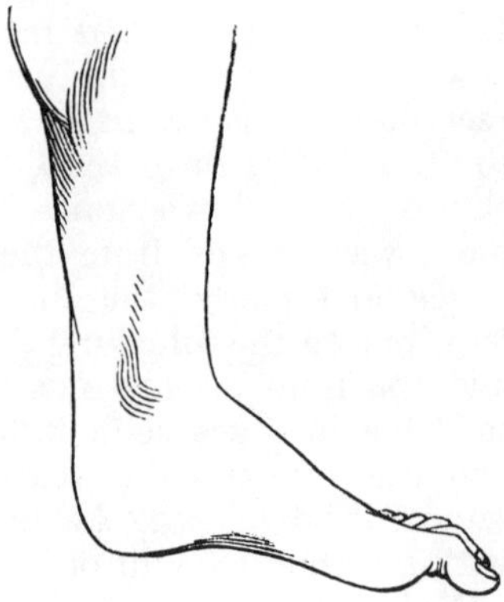

Dislocations of the lower end of tibia backwards.

Reduction should be attempted by a method similar to that which has been recommended in all the other dislocations of the ankle; only with such modifications as the peculiarities of the case must necessarily suggest.

CHAPTER XX.

DISLOCATIONS OF THE UPPER END OF THE FIBULA.

Syn.—"Luxations of the superior peroneo-tibial articulation;" Malgaigne.

SURGEONS have frequently described a condition of the peroneo-tibial articulation, in which the ligaments have become relaxed, giving a preternatural mobility to the head of the bone. It is also not unfrequently displaced upwards, in consequence of an oblique fracture of the tibia. I have myself seen several examples of both these accidents; but simple traumatic dislocations, which can only occur forwards or backwards, are very rare.

§ 1. DISLOCATIONS OF THE UPPER END OF THE FIBULA FORWARDS.

Malgaigne has collected three examples of this luxation, uncomplicated with any other accident, and not apparently due to any abnormal condition of the ligaments, two of which at least seemed to have been produced by the violent action of the muscles which are attached to the anterior face of the fibula. The third example, reported by Thompson, in the *London Lancet*,[1] permits a doubt as to whether the displacement was occasioned by muscular action, or by a direct blow upon the part.

The signs which characterize the anterior luxation are the absence of the head of the fibula in its natural position, and its presence in front, near the ligamentum patellæ; the altered direction of the biceps flexor cruris muscle; and, in one case, considerable deformity in the shape and position of the leg has been observed.

Thompson and Jobard were unable to accomplish the reduction while the leg was extended upon the thigh, but succeeded readily after having flexed the leg. On the other hand, Savournin succeeded with the leg extended, but with the foot flexed upon the leg. Malgaigne, to whom I am indebted for these observations, thinks that flexion of the leg, combined with flexion of the foot, would render the reduction more easy.

In whatever position the limb is placed, the surgeon must rely chiefly upon forcible pressure made with the fingers against the front and upper portion of the displaced bone.

J. E. Hawley, of Ithaca, N. Y., a distinguished practitioner, and late Prof. of Surgery in the Geneva Medical College, has furnished me with a brief account of a case which came under his own observation.

On the 29th of March, 1854, Bambak, while vaulting upon the parallel bars in a gymnasium, unintentionally made a complete somerset, and fell with his right foot upon the edge of a plank. Dr. Hawley, who was immediately called, found his right leg demi-flexed and immovably fixed. The head of the fibula was plainly felt in front of its natural position, near the ligamentum patellæ. The patient was suffering the most intense pain. Extension and counter-extension were made, and while the doctor was pressing with both of his thumbs upon the head of the fibula, it went into its place with an audible snap. The relief was instantaneous. Complete rest was observed for a few days, while cooling lotions were constantly applied, and within a week he was able to attend to his usual duties.

§ 2. Dislocations of the Upper End of the Fibula Backwards.

Sanson has recorded one example, in which the passage of the wheel of a carriage across the upper part of the leg, precisely on a level with the peroneo-tibial articulation, ruptured the ligaments which bind the fibula to the tibia, and caused a displacement which, however, seems to have been spontaneously overcome. Nevertheless there remained a preternatural mobility, permitting the fibula to be pushed easily backwards or forwards upon the tibia.

The only example of a permanent backward displacement is related

[1] Op. cit., 1850, vol. i. p. 385.

by Dubreuil. A man, æt. 32, in order to save himself from falling, sprang suddenly, with his right leg in a position of extreme abduction, and at the same moment he experienced a severe pain in the region of the peroneo-tibial articulation. The head of the fibula was found to be thrown backwards, and formed under the skin a marked prominence; the foot was drawn outwards, and the whole outside of the limb became cold and numb. Dubreuil flexed the leg moderately, and, pressing the head of the fibula from behind forwards, the reduction was easily effected. On the following day, the limb having been straightened, the dislocation was found to be reproduced. It was again replaced, and the knee covered with a leather cap, secured moderately tight. After twelve days of complete rest, the knee was moved gently, and on the seventeenth day the patient walked with the help of a cane. For some time the leg had a tendency to incline outwards; but in about three months the cure was perfectly established.[1]

It is probable that in this case the dislocation resulted from the violent action of the biceps flexor cruris. Such at least is the opinion of both Dubreuil and Malgaigne, and I see no reason to question the correctness of their theory.

CHAPTER XXI.

DISLOCATIONS OF THE INFERIOR PERONEO-TIBIAL ARTICULATION.

NÉLATON relates the only example of a simple luxation of this articulation of which we have any information. The patient who was the subject of this accident, presented himself at the hospital under the care of M. Gerdy on the thirty-ninth day after the accident, which had been occasioned by the passage of the wheel of a carriage obliquely across the leg in such a manner as to push the malleolus externus directly backwards. The lower end of the fibula was in almost direct contact with the outer margin of the tendo-Achillis; the outer face of the astragalus, abandoned by the fibula, could be distinctly felt in nearly its whole extent; the foot preserved its natural position; and he could walk pretty well, only that he was obliged to step with some care. M. Gerdy believed that the bone was too firmly fixed in its new position to be moved, and therefore made no attempt at reduction.

[1] Malgaigne, op. cit., tom. ii. p. 386.

CHAPTER XXII.

TARSAL LUXATIONS.

§ 1. Dislocations of the Astragalus.

Malgaigne, who speaks also of luxations "sub-astragaloid," has thought proper to call the dislocations which we now propose to consider "double dislocations of the astragalus." In the variety first named, the astragalus retains its connections with the tibia, but separates from the scaphoid bone, while its relations to the calcaneum are only slightly disturbed. This we prefer to regard as one of the many varieties of tarsal luxations, and shall appropriate to it no specific appellation, except to designate it as astragalo-scaphoid, or astragalo-calcaneo-scaphoid, according as more or less of the several articulations are disturbed.

In the second named variety, called by Malgaigne a "double" luxation, and which constitutes the subject of this chapter, the astragalus abandons all the articular surfaces against which it is naturally applied, and thrusts itself out from between the tibia, fibula, calcaneum, and scaphoides; so that it may be said to have suffered a triple or quadruple rather than a "double" dislocation, as is implied by the nomenclature adopted by Malgaigne. This we choose to regard as the only true dislocation of the astragalus, and as such we propose to designate it by the simple term "dislocation of the astragalus."

The astragalus may be dislocated forwards, outwards, inwards, backwards; or it may be dislocated obliquely in either of the diagonals between these lines; it may be simply rotated upon its lateral axis without much, if any, lateral displacement; and, finally, it has been occasionally driven between the tibia and fibula, tearing away the intermediate ligaments, and generally fracturing one or both bones of the leg.

Fig. 287.

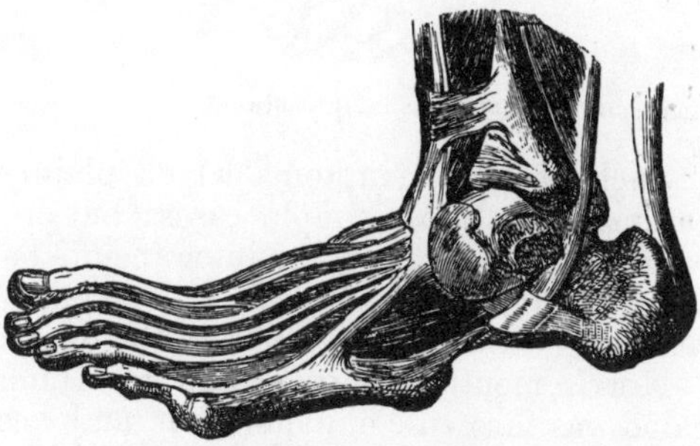

Dislocation of astragalus outwards. Anatomical relations.

Causes.—The causes which have been found chiefly operative in the production of this dislocation are very much the same as those which produce, under other circumstances, a dislocation of the lower end of the tibia. Thus, a fall from a height upon the bottom of the foot, accompanied with a violent abduction, adduction, flexion, or extension, may determine a dislocation of the astragalus inwards, outwards, backwards, or forwards. Sometimes it is accomplished by a mere wrenching and twisting of the foot in machinery, or in the wheel of a carriage, or by being caught between two irregular bodies. It may be produced also by a direct blow.

Symptoms.—The great prominence occasioned by the displacement of the bone in either of these several directions, accompanied generally with more or less lateral deviation of the foot, is alone sufficient to indicate the true nature of the accident. In some cases, also, the foot is forcibly flexed or extended; the leg is shortened in consequence of the tibia having fallen down upon the calcaneum; the superincumbent skin and tendons are rendered tense; blood is effused, and swelling speedily occurs. In the backward dislocation, the position of the foot is not much changed, but the tibia being slightly carried forwards, the length of the dorsal aspect of the foot is proportionably diminished.

Fig. 288.

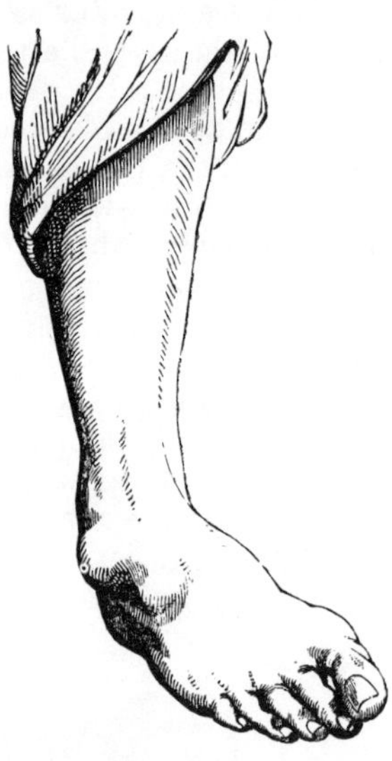

Simple dislocation of the astragalus outwards.

Fig. 289.

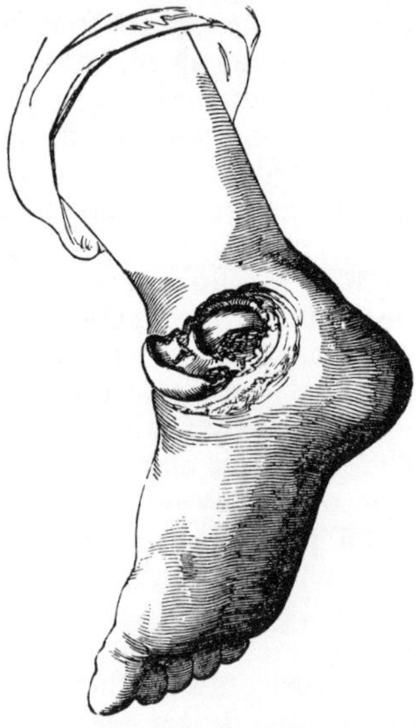

Compound dislocation of the astragalus inwards.

Such are the symptoms which plainly enough indicate the dislocation in the most simple cases; but in a majority of the examples which have been seen, the integuments have been more or less extensively torn, exposing to the eye at once the naked bone, and thus removing all chance of error in the diagnosis.

Norris mentions a case, seen by Hammersley, in which the astragalus was thrown completely out, and was subsequently found in the earth where the patient had received his injury. Inflammation, gangrene and tetanus supervened, and the patient died on the seventh day.[1]

[1] Norris, Amer. Journ. Med. Sci., Aug. 1837, p. 383.

Prognosis.—It will be readily understood that nothing short of very great violence could disturb and completely break up the connections of a bone so compactly and firmly seated as is the astragalus, and that aside of any unusual complications, under the most favorable circumstances, intense inflammation must naturally be anticipated; and with few exceptions this has actually taken place. Even when reduction has been promptly and easily effected, inflammation, gangrene, and death have sometimes speedily ensued. But more often the reduction has been found to be exceedingly difficult or impossible, and complete removal of the bone or amputation has been immediately demanded.

In a limited number of cases, on the other hand, the bone has been easily reduced, and recovery has taken place with a tolerably useful limb; or resection has been practiced with an equally favorable result; in still other cases the bone has been left protruding, and the patient has finally recovered so far as to be able to walk again, but in such a crippled condition as to render the achievement a very doubtful triumph of conservative surgery.

Norris, of Philadelphia, relates the following case, illustrating the imminent danger to which even the life of the patient may be exposed in those examples which are apparently the most simple.

William Summerill, æt. 30, was admitted to the Pennsylvania Hospital on the twenty-sixth of September, 1831. An hour previous, while descending a ladder, he slipped and fell in such a manner as to throw the entire weight of his body upon the outer part of his left foot. The foot was turned inwards, and nearly immovable; a slight depression existed immediately below the lower end of the tibia, and there was a hard rounded projection on the outer part of the foot a little below and in front of the extremity of the fibula; the skin over this projection was not broken or excoriated, but reddened; there was no fracture of either bone of the leg.

The symptoms rendered it plain that the astragalus was dislocated forwards and outwards. Dr. Barton, under whose care the patient was received, proceeded soon after to make attempts at reduction. The muscles of the leg were relaxed as much as possible, and extension made from the foot by seizing the heel and front part of the foot while an assistant made counter-extension at the knee. The bone was also pushed inwards toward the joint by the surgeon. These efforts were continued for a considerable time, but had no effect in changing the position of the bone.

Six hours afterwards, Drs. Harris and Hewson being in consultation, the attempt was again made to accomplish the reduction, but without success; and the surgeons immediately proceeded to excise the bone.

An incision was made parallel with the tendons, commencing a short distance above the projection and extending down far enough to expose fairly the astragalus and its torn ligaments. The bone was then seized with the forceps and easily removed after the division of a few ligamentous fibres that continued to connect it with the adjoining parts. Very little bleeding occurred, only two small arteries requiring the ligature.

After removal, it was discovered that about one-half of the surface which plays in the lower end of the tibia had been fractured, and that it remained firmly attached to the extremity of that bone. No attempt was made to remove this fragment; but the joint being carefully sponged out, the sides of the wound were brought together and closed by sutures, adhesive straps and a roller; after which the foot, placed in its natural position, was laid in a fracture-box.

On the fifth day a slough began to form upon the outside of the foot, which was followed by suppuration at other points, and on the thirteenth day an opening was made to evacuate the pus near the malleolus internus. At the end of about eight weeks the fragment of the astragalus which had been suffered to remain, was found to be carious, and it was removed; the heel also had ulcerated from pressure, and several other bones of the tarsus were discovered to be carious. Fifteen months later, this poor fellow was still in the hospital suffering from hectic, with extensive disease in the bones of the tarsus and ankle-joint. Finally, amputation of the leg was practiced by Dr. Barton, a few days after which he died.[1]

Norris mentions also two examples of simple dislocation of the astragalus at the Pennsylvania Hospital which came under the observation of Dr. Barton, in both of which the bone was left unreduced. In one case inflammation and sloughing soon effected a complete exposure of the protruding bone, but after a time the skin cicatrized. At the end of five months the patient walked and had good use of the joint, though great deformity of the foot existed, and he continued to be subject to ulceration of the newly-formed skin on its outer part. In the other case gangrene supervened soon after the accident, and the patient died.

Norris adds that "the late Professor Wistar removed the astragalus in a case of compound dislocation, and the patient was cured with some motion at the joint."

Dr. Alexander Stevens, of New York, made the same operation in a case of compound dislocation, and after several months, he affirms that the patient "has recovered with very trifling deformity of the foot, and with a flexible joint. He walks with very slight lameness."[2]

The dislocations backwards, of which seven examples only have been recorded, have all with but one exception been left unreduced; yet in at least four instances the patients have recovered with pretty useful limbs. Such was the fact with Liston's and Lizars' patients, and also with Mr. Phillips' two cases, to all of which I shall again refer. It must be noticed, however, that in each of the cases mentioned as followed by a successful termination without reduction, the dislocations were simple.

Turner, of Manchester, has reported one example of compound luxation outwards and backwards, which, finding himself unable to reduce, he removed the astragalus with a tolerably successful result.[3] Finally

[1] Norris, Amer. Journ. Med. Sci., Aug. 1837, p. 378.

[2] Stevens, North Amer. Med. and Surg. Journ., Jan. 1827, p. 200.

[3] Turner, Trans. Provin. Med. and Surg. Journ., vol. ix. Essay on Disloc. of Astrag. with nearly fifty cases.

a case was presented in one of the London hospitals in 1839, of a dislocation inwards and backwards, which was reduced in about ten minutes, by extension accompanied with lateral pressure.[1]

Treatment.—Various attempts have been made by surgical writers to determine the line of treatment which should be adopted in these unfortunate cases, but with very unsatisfactory results, since they are far from having arrived at similar conclusions, nor have they been able always to settle the question definitely for themselves. The difficulty consists in the multiplicity, and lack of uniformity in the complications which attend these accidents, rendering it impossible to establish a classification upon which an uniform treatment may be safely based. There are certain principles, however, which seem to be sufficiently settled to allow of an authoritative announcement; these may be briefly stated as follows: If the dislocation is simple, reduce the astragalus immediately, provided this is possible. If the luxation is complete, and it cannot be reduced, even partially, proceed at once to resection or to amputation. In compound dislocations, resection or amputation affords the only safe resource. In all cases the inflammation is likely to be intense, in order to prevent which complication the surgeon must be unremitting in his use of the appropriate remedies.

Out of eighteen cases of complete excision of the astragalus, collected by Turner, fourteen made good recoveries, and in only one of these fourteen was there anchylosis.

These several points we shall proceed to illustrate a little more fully.

In a recent simple luxation of the astragalus forwards, the leg should be flexed to a right angle with the thigh, and for the purpose of making extension, one assistant should take hold of the foot with both hands in the same manner that a servant draws a boot, that is, with the right hand grasping the heel, and the left placed upon the dorsum of the foot near the toes. A second assistant should seize the lower part of the thigh in order to make counter-extension, while the surgeon presses with the ball of his hand against the head of the astragalus, upwards and backwards. If these simple measures fail, the pulleys ought to be employed as a substitute for the hands in making extension. In applying the extension, the toes must be kept well down, and occasionally the foot should be moved gently from one side to the other.

An oblique dislocation must be reduced, if possible, to an anterior luxation, before an attempt is made to carry the head of the bone back to its place, as by this mode the reduction will be greatly facilitated.

Lateral luxations may be reduced by the same means; but if the astragalus is dislocated outwards the foot must be held forcibly adducted during the extension, and if it is dislocated inwards, the foot must be held strongly in the opposite direction.

Lizars says that he has seen one case of backward luxation, and that all attempts at reduction were unavailing. The limb was, how-

[1] London Lancet, vol. ii. p. 559.

ever, preserved and proved to be useful.[1] Liston was equally unsuccessful in a case which came under his notice.[2] Phillips has reported two cases, in neither of which was the reduction accomplished.[3] Nélaton has seen a compound dislocation which he could not reduce.[4] Mr. Erichsen, however, who admits that when dislocated backwards it has not hitherto been reduced, declares that the surgeons at University Hospital have succeeded in one case recently, in which both the tibia and fibula were broken also.[5] Mr. Erichsen suggests also that in case of a failure by the ordinary means, we should resort to a subcutaneous section of the tendo-Achillis. Mr. Williams, of Dublin, in a similar case, which had been left unreduced, was obliged finally to extract the bone, in consequence of the integuments having sloughed.[6]

Compound dislocations, and such as are otherwise complicated, demand of the surgeon immediate amputation, or exsection, the latter of which ought to be preferred whenever the condition of the limb encourages a reasonable hope that the foot may be saved.

When exsection is practiced, and the bone is found to be broken, as it often is, all the fragments should be carefully removed, since they are certain to become necrosed if left in place. Nor ought the surgeon to hesitate to lay open freely the tissues in every direction, in order that he may accomplish this purpose; even the tendons lying over the protruding bone may be sacrificed unhesitatingly, since after having been so severely bruised, stretched, and lacerated, they are pretty certain to slough. Indeed the more freely the tissues are divided over the bone, the less will be the danger of inflammation, and the safer will be the life and limb of the patient.

In addition to the examples already cited of compound dislocation in which the astragalus was removed, the following, reported by Dr. W. A. Gillespie, of Ellisville, Va., will also illustrate the occasional value of exsection in these severe accidents.

Mrs. A., aged about fifty years, fell from a horse on the 23d of May, 1833, dislocating both ankles. The luxation of the right foot was accompanied with a luxation of the astragalus outwards, which projected through a very large wound in the integuments, and its trochlea was placed at an angle of about 45° with its natural position. Early on the following day it was removed by severing its few remaining connections, and the wound was immediately closed by stitches, adhesive plasters, and light dressings. From the moment of the receipt of the injury, and for several days afterwards, she suffered excruciating pain in the limb, and on the third day tetanus was apprehended, but its full accession was prevented by the free use of opiates. The limb was suspended in N. R. Smith's fracture apparatus; and as gangrene with hectic fever soon threatened the life of the patient, fermenting

[1] Lizars, System of Practical Surg., Edinburgh ed., 1847, p. 161.
[2] Liston, Elements of Surgery, vol. iii. p. 348.
[3] Phillips, Lond. Med. Gaz., vol. xiv. p. 596.
[4] Nélaton, Pathologie Chirurg., t. ii. p. 482.
[5] Erichsen, Science and Art of Surg., Amer. ed., 1859, p. 270.
[6] Williams, Erichsen, op. cit., p. 271.

poultices were diligently applied, and the patient was sustained by wine, bark, and other tonics. Two months after the injury was received, the date at which the report is given, the wound had entirely healed, and her complete recovery was regarded as certain.[1] Many other similar examples have been reported by foreign surgeons.

One word more with regard to the treatment of the wound after excision. A considerable experience in accidents and wounds of this class, that is, wounds accompanied with great contusion and laceration, has convinced me that the practice of closing the surface with sutures, adhesive plasters, bandages, &c., is eminently pernicious. The effusions, which must necessarily occur, and which indeed we think ought to occur, are thus imprisoned beneath the skin, giving rise to swelling, pain, inflammation, and finally suppuration or sloughing. It is far better, in our opinion, to have the wound open, covering it only with cloths constantly kept moist with cool water. For this latter purpose some mode of irrigation is preferable, as being more constant and uniform. To those who have never adopted this treatment of contused wounds, or of wounds generally, we would recommend an early trial, feeling confident that they will never have occasion to regret the experiment.

§ 2. Astragalo-Calcaneo-Scaphoid Dislocations.

It is perhaps quite as common for the astragalus to be dislocated from the scaphoid bone and calcaneum, while it retains its connections with the tibia, as to be luxated from all these bones at the same time. This astragalo-calcaneo-scaphoid dislocation is that which Malgaigne has termed "sub-astragaloid." Produced by the same causes which determine true dislocations of the astragalus, it may occur in the same directions, and is liable to the same complications; nor will either the prognosis or treatment differ essentially from that which is recognized and established in the other accident.

As in dislocations proper of the astragalus, so also in this accident, opposite results have occasionally followed from similar modes of treatment. Thus, Dr. Detmold, of New York, stated in 1856 to the New York Academy of Medicine, that he had recently met with a dislocation of the astragalus, in which the bone retained its proper relations with the tibia, but not with the bones of the tarsus. The patient had fallen from a wagon and caught his foot in the wheel. Dr. Detmold made extension with pulleys, but could not effect the reduction. Subsequently he was obliged to remove the astragalus on account of the suppuration which followed and the consequent exposure of the bone. The wound did not heal kindly, and at length amputation of the leg became necessary.

Dr. Detmold concludes, from this example and others which have come to his knowledge, that if a similar case were to present itself to him again, he would amputate at once.[2]

[1] Gillespie, Amer. Journ. Med. Sci., Aug., 1833, p. 552.
[2] Detmold, New York Journ. Med., May, 1856, p. 383.

The following case, reported by Dr. Thomas Wells, of Columbia, S. C., is of unusul interest, as illustrating the danger of leaving the bone displaced, and also the benefit which may, even under the most unfavorable circumstances, result from its final removal.

Doctor S., æt. 30, was riding in an open carriage, some time during the year of 1819, when his horses became frightened and ran, and in leaping from his vehicle he struck upon his left foot, dislocating the astragalus from its junction with the scaphoid bone, upwards and slightly outwards. Several medical gentlemen made violent efforts to reduce the bone, but without effect. Inflammation and suppuration, accompanied by a high fever, soon followed, and the head of the astragalus becoming carious, protruded through the skin. On the 18th of August, about seven months after the injury was received, he was still suffering from a copious discharge, pain, swelling, and general irritative fever, and it was determined to excise the bone; which was accordingly done by enlarging the wound and detaching its loose connections with the adjacent tissues. The astragalus extracted left a frightful wound, the foot seeming to be nearly separated from the leg. A hollow splint was adjusted to the inside of the foot and leg, so as to preserve the limb perfectly steady and in a proper direction; simple dressings were applied, and an anodyne administered internally. No accidents followed, and at the end of September the wound was healed, and the swelling of the parts had entirely subsided. One year after the operation, he walked without the least difficulty; the ankle being then "perfectly sound." The leg was shortened about one inch, and this deficiency was supplied by a thick heel upon his shoe.[1]

Examples might be cited illustrative of the value of early exsection where reduction could not be accomplished; but after what has already been said upon the subject of dislocations of the astragalus, we shall not regard any farther references as either necessary or useful. If other principles of treatment are to govern the surgeon than those which we have already laid down, they cannot here be stated. They are among those unwritten rules whose existence we cannot always recognize until the case arises upon which they may apply. Yet in the exigency supposed they are as clearly defined, and as imperative, in the mind of the clever surgeon, as any of those laws which have been made the subjects of special record.

§ 3. Dislocations of the Calcaneum.

The calcaneum may, as a consequence of a fall upon the heel, or of a direct blow, be dislocated outwards from the astragalus alone, or upwards and outwards from the cuboid bone at the same time. It has been found also at the same moment dislocated outwards from the astragalus, and inwards upon the cuboid bone.

Chelius says he has seen an old dislocation of the calcaneum, produced in early life by pulling off a boot; from which there finally

[1] Wells, Amer. Journ. Med. Sci., May, 1832, p. 21.

resulted a degeneration like elephantiasis of the leg, rendering amputation necessary.[1]

Mr. South remarks in his notes to Chelius, that the two cases of dislocation outwards of this bone, mentioned by Sir Astley Cooper, were from his (South's) notes (cases 199 and 200). In the first case, that of Martin Bentley, occasioned by the falling of a heavy stone upon his foot, the integuments were not broken, and the position of the foot resembled a varus. "The dislocation was easily reduced, having bent the thigh and knee on the body and fixed the leg, by laying hold of the metatarsus and of the tuberosity of the heel-bone, and drawing the foot gently and directly from the leg, during which extension Cline put his knee against the outside of the joint, and the foot being pressed against it, the heel and the navicular bone readily slipped into their place, and the deformity disappeared." He was discharged from the hospital in five weeks, "having the complete use of his foot."

In the second case, the dislocation, produced also by the fall of a stone upon the foot, was compound, and the patient, Thomas Gilmore, having been brought into St. Thomas's Hospital, the reduction was effected by extending the foot, and rotating it outwards. Six months after, when he left the hospital, he was able to walk pretty well with a stick.

§ 4. Middle Tarsal Dislocations.

The scaphoid and cuboid bones may be dislocated from the astragalus and calcaneum, constituting what is termed, by Malgaigne, a middle tarsal dislocation. It is probable that to some extent the same thing has occurred in many of those cases which are reported as simple dislocations of the astragalus, or as dislocations at the astragalo-scaphoid articulation; but it occurs also occasionally in a degree so perfect and complete as to leave no doubt as to the true nature of the disjunction, and to entitle it to a separate consideration.

Mr. Liston mentions the case of a boy, æt. 14, who fell from a height of forty feet, striking, apparently, upon the extremity of the foot. The scaphoid and cuboid bones were found to be displaced upwards and forwards, so that the foot was shortened about half an inch, and had a clubbed appearance. No attempt was made to reduce the bones, and he left the hospital in three weeks, able to stand on the foot.[2] Sir Astley Cooper has recorded in more detail a similar example. A man, working at the Southwark bridge, London, received upon the top of his foot a stone of great weight. He was immediately carried to Guy's Hospital, and his condition is described as follows: "The os calcis and the astragalus remained in their natural situations, but the fore part of the foot was turned inwards upon the bones. When examined by the students, the appearance was so precisely like that of a club-foot, that they could not at first believe but that it was a natural defect of that kind," but upon the assurance of the man, that previously to the

[1] Chelius, System of Surg., Amer. ed., vol. ii. p. 354.
[2] Practical Surg., also London Lancet, vol. xxxvii. p. 133.

accident his foot was not distorted, extension was made, and the reduction was effected. He was discharged from the hospital in five weeks, having the complete use of his foot.[1]

§ 5. Dislocations of the Os Cuboides.

According to Piédagnel, quoted by Chelius, the cuboid bone may be dislocated upwards, inwards, and downwards, but Malgaigne affirms that he has found no case recorded in which the dislocation has occurred alone, or unaccompanied with a dislocation of one or more of the other tarsal bones.

§ 6. Dislocations of the Os Scaphoides.

Burnett has seen a luxation of the scaphoid bone in which its connections with the astragalus were undisturbed, while at the same time it was completely separated from the cuneiform bones. By strong pressure exercised during several minutes, the os scaphoides was made to fall into its place. The dislocation was compound, yet the wound healed rapidly, and in a short time the recovery was almost complete.[2]

Several examples are recorded of a true luxation of the os scaphoides, in which the bone had abandoned both the astragalus on the one hand, and the cuneiform bones on the other.

Piédagnel mentions a case in which the scaphoid bone was broken longitudinally, and its internal fragment, constituting the largest portion, was displaced inwards through a tegumentary wound. He was unable to effect reduction, and was compelled to amputate the foot.[3]

Walker has reported the first example of luxation forwards, occasioned by jumping upon the ball of the foot. The bone formed a marked projection upon the top of the foot, and a corresponding depression existed below. An attempt was first made to accomplish the reduction by simple pressure with the thumbs; but this having failed, the surgeon bent the extremity of the foot forcibly downwards, and by continuing to press upon the os scaphoides, it fell into its position easily and with a distinct click. In about three weeks the patient was able to walk with only a slight halt, and no deformity remained.[4]

§ 7. Dislocations of the Cuneiform Bones.

The cuneiform bones may be luxated partially, and without having separated from each other, of which two or three examples are recorded; or, which is more common, the cuneiforme internum may be luxated alone. Says Sir Astley Cooper: "I have twice seen this

[1] Sir A. Cooper on Disloc., &c., London ed., 1823, p. 376.
[2] Burnett, Lond. Med. Gazette, 1837, vol. xix. p. 221.
[3] Piédagnel, Journ. Univ. et Heb., tom. ii. p. 208.
[4] Walker, The Medical Examiner, 1851, p. 203.

bone dislocated; once in a gentleman who called upon me some weeks after the accident, and a second time in a case which occurred in Guy's Hospital very lately. In both instances the same appearances presented themselves. There was a great projection of the bone inwards, and some degree of elevation, from its being drawn up by the action of the tibialis anticus muscle; and it no longer remained in a direct line with the metatarsal bone of the great toe. In neither case was the bone reduced; the subject of the first of these accidents walked with but little halting, and I believe would in time recover the use of the foot, so as not to appear lame. The cause of the accident was a fall from a considerable height, by which the ligament was ruptured which connects this bone with the os cuneiforme, and with the os naviculare. The second case, which was in Guy's Hospital, my apprentice, Mr. Babington informs me, happened by the fall of a horse, and the foot was caught between the horse and the curb-stone."[1]

In a case of compound luxation seen by Mr. Key, reduction was effected and in two months the cure was so far completed that the patient walked with only a slight lameness.[2] Nélaton, in a similar case of compound luxation, unable to reduce the bone, removed it completely, and the patient recovered.[3]

Robert Smith has called attention to a species of dislocation of the internal cuneiform bone not before very accurately described; but of which he has presented two examples. It consists in a simultaneous dislocation of the metatarsus and internal cuneiform; that is to say, the first metatarsal bone together with the internal cuneiform is dislocated upwards and backwards upon the tarsus, carrying with it also the four remaining metatarsal bones. In both of the examples seen and recorded by him, the dislocations were ancient, and no account could be obtained of the precise manner in which the accidents had been produced. The feet were foreshortened to the extent of an inch or more, in consequence of the overlapping of the bones, yet the heel in each case preserved its natural relations to the tibia, not being proportionately lengthened as is the case in dislocations of the tibia forwards. The plantar surface of the foot was turned inwards, and instead of being concave it was convex, both in its antero-posterior and transverse diameters. A transverse ridge on the top of the foot also indicated the line of the projecting bones. Both of these cases were verified by a careful dissection.[4]

Dupuytren has reported in his *Treatise on Injuries of the Bones*, a similar case, occurring in a woman æt. 30, who was brought immediately to Hôtel Dieu. She stated that in descending from the bridge of St. Michael with a burden of two hundred pounds, she fell in such a way that the whole weight of the body was received on the right foot, and that at the moment she made an effort to check herself in falling, she experienced extremely severe pain in this part, and heard a very distinct snap; she was unable to raise herself from the ground.

[1] Sir Ast. Cooper, op. cit., p. 383. [2] Key, Guy's Hosp. Rep., 1836, vol. i. p. 544.
[3] Nélaton, Malgaigne, op. cit., p. 1076.
[4] Robert Smith, Treatise on Fractures, &c., Dublin ed., 1854, p. 224 et seq.

On the following morning Dupuytren reduced the bones with very little difficulty by extension, combined with pressure against the dislocated ends. The bones went into place with a loud snap, and in two or three months she left the hospital with only a little lameness.[1]

Mr. Smith, without intending to question the possibility of a simple luxation of the metatarsal bones, of which, indeed, Malgaigne has collected a number of well authenticated examples, is inclined to believe that, when a luxation of the bones of the metatarsus is the consequence of a fall from a height, the individual alighting upon the anterior part of the foot, it is, in general, that variety which has now been described. And this aptness on the part of the cuneiform bone to maintain its connection with the first metatarsal bone, he would ascribe mainly to the fact that both the peroneus longus and tibialis anticus have attachments to each of the bones in question.

CHAPTER XXIII.

DISLOCATIONS OF THE METATARSAL BONES.

LUXATIONS of one or more of the metatarsal bones, at the points of their articulations with the tarsus, have been known to occur in almost every direction. They may be occasioned by crushing accidents, by machinery, or more often perhaps they have been caused by a fall backwards or forwards, when the anterior extremity of the foot was wedged under some solid body and immovably fixed. They may be produced also, probably, by simply striking upon the ball of the foot in falling from a height. We have noticed, however, that Mr. Smith inclines to the opinion that this will, in general, only produce the species of dislocation which he has particularly described.

The symptoms which characterize the dislocation of the whole range of metatarsal bones upwards and backwards will, when the dislocation is complete, resemble very much those which belong to the dislocation described by Smith. The dorsum of the foot will be shortened antero-posteriorly, the two arches of the foot will be lost upon the plantar surface, or even actually reversed, a ridge will traverse the back of the foot and a corresponding depression will exist underneath.

In some cases, however, the dislocation is not complete, the articulations being only sprung, and then there can exist no foreshortening of the foot, and all the other signs will be less striking.

If only a single bone is luxated the diagnosis is generally very

[1] Dupuytren, op. cit., p. 326.

easily made out, unless indeed considerable swelling has already occurred.

Mr. South says that in 1835, a case was admitted to St. Thomas's Hospital, under Mr. Green's care, of dislocation of the last two metatarsal bones, occasioned by the falling of a heavy chest upon the inside of the foot. Upon the top of the foot was a large swelling below and in front of the outer ankle, and behind it a cavity in which two fingers could be easily buried, in consequence of the bases of the metatarsal bones having been thrown upwards and backwards upon the top of the cuboid bone. The reduction was accomplished with much difficulty by continued extension, and as the bones resumed their place a distinct crackling was heard.[1]

Liston reduced a dislocation upwards of the first metatarsal bone; Malgaigne mistook a dislocation of the fourth bone for a fracture, and did not attempt the reduction until the seventh day, when, after five successive trials, the head entered with a noise into its cavity. In a dislocation of the second, third, and fourth metatarsal bones, he also failed to detect the true nature of the accident until the tenth day, when he proceeded to attempt reduction, but failed. Inflammation, suppuration, and delirium followed, and the patient died on the forty-first day. Tufnell failed in a similar case, although his patient finally recovered with a not very useful limb. Malgaigne failed to reduce the bones also in a recent case of luxation of the first four bones, although he used chloroform, and diligently tried various means. The same writer has seen one example of ancient dislocation, which was not recognized by the surgeon. Finally, Monteggia reports a case of dislocation of the last two metatarsal bones, which was not at the time recognized. On the tenth day swelling commenced, and soon after the patient died in convulsions.[2]

These references, drawn chiefly from Malgaigne, sufficiently illustrate the difficulty which surgeons have experienced in the reduction of these bones, when a portion only is displaced. A difficulty which is probably due to the fact that it is almost impossible to make extension upon a single metatarsal bone; indeed, it is probable that by pressure only upon the displaced head can we expect to accomplish much in these accidents, and even this cannot be made to act very effectively, owing to the small amount of surface presented against which the force can be properly applied.

If, on the other hand, all the bones are dislocated at once, the reduction is generally accomplished with ease by simple extension, combined with properly directed pressure. Bouchard and Meynier succeeded without difficulty in two cases of backward dislocation; Smyly was equally successful on the sixth day, in a case of dislocation downwards. Laugier reduced an outward dislocation of all the bones by pressure and extension easily; and Kirk succeeded as well, in an example of the opposite character, all the bones being carried inwards.[3]

[1] South, Note to Chelius's Surg., vol. ii. p. 256.
[2] Malgaigne, op. cit., p. 1077 et seq.
[3] Ibid., p. 1081.

Mr. Sandwith has given us an account of a case which occurred in his own person, from the fall of his horse upon his foot. "I was instantly sensible," says Mr. Sandwith, "of the nature of the injury, and as soon as I was upon my feet, the metatarsus was found to be drawn upwards, and obliquely outwards upon the tarsus, by the action of the flexor muscles. On the removal of the boot, which was cut away, these were the appearances: the foot considerably shortened, the toes turned a little outwards, and a hard swelling, bigger than an egg, upon the tarsus, with tumefaction of the integuments. The pain, which was great at first, was kept under by a warm fomentation.

"The reduction was easily effected by my friends, Messrs. Williams and Brereton, and leeches and bread and water poultices prevented inflammation. For several nights the foot was violently shaken by spasmodic action of the muscles, but the parts preserved their relative situation; and, although it was nearly a year before all lameness ceased, yet at the end of six weeks I was enabled to lay aside my crutches. For the ability to use the foot in so short a time, I was indebted to a contrivance which rendered the foot and ankle inflexible.

"Instead of an elastic sole to the shoe part of the apparatus, one of wood was procured, around the heel of which was nailed a piece of firm unbending leather; this reached as high as the calf of the leg; three small straps with buckles held the leg in situ, and a broader one across the instep secured the foot. The comfort I experienced from this simple apparatus is my reason for describing it so particularly; it has since been found useful in various injuries of the foot and ankle."[1]

In one extraordinary case, however, Dupuytren was not so successful. Paul Eudes, æt. 24, fell, while drunk, into a ditch six feet deep, and alighted on the soles of his feet. This accident was followed by great swelling, and he did not suspect the nature of the injury, or present himself at the hospital until three weeks after. Dupuytren then ascertained that he had dislocated the metatarsal bones of both feet. Several fruitless attempts were made to accomplish the reduction, but to no purpose, and in about two weeks he left the hospital.[2]

CHAPTER XXIV.

DISLOCATIONS OF THE PHALANGES OF THE TOES.

DISLOCATIONS of the toes are less common than those of the fingers, yet a considerable number of cases have been recorded by different surgeons. They are occasioned by blows received directly upon the

[1] Sandwith, Amer. Journ. Med. Sci., Nov. 1828, p. 216, from Lond. Med. Gaz., vol. i.

[2] Dupuytren, op. cit., p. 329.

ends of the toes, by the weight of the body brought to bear suddenly upon their plantar surfaces, as when a horseman springs in his stirrup, or by a fall, in consequence of which the rider hangs in his stirrup, by leaping, &c.

They may be partial or complete; and in the latter case, a slight overlapping is generally observed. In a great majority of cases the direction of the displacement is backwards, or with only a slight lateral deviation. Occasionally, several bones are displaced at the same time, but usually only one suffers displacement. It is more common here to find compound and complicated dislocations than in the case of the fingers.

The position of the toes is not always the same in the same form of dislocations. Thus, in the dislocation backwards, the toe is sometimes reversed upon the foot to nearly a right angle, and at other times it is found lying in the same axis as the metatarsal bone, or the phalanx, from which it is luxated. About one year since, I reduced a backward dislocation of the first phalanx of the second toe in the person of Lewis Brittin, æt. 60, who had fallen from a four story window, striking upon his feet, and breaking both thighs. I did not discover the dislocation of the toe until sixteen hours after the accident. It was then lying parallel with the axis of the metatarsal bone, upon which it was slightly overlapped. The reduction was effected easily by pulling upon the last phalanx with my fingers, while, at the same moment, I pushed the head of the bone toward the socket. No swelling followed, nor has it troubled him at all since his recovery.

With regard to the treatment, surgeons have experienced the same difficulty in certain cases of dislocation of the great toe as we have seen experienced in similar dislocations of the thumb. Occasionally, indeed, the reduction has been found to be impossible. The same doubts have existed also in relation to the causes of this difficulty, and in reference to the means by which it was to be overcome. We shall therefore refer the reader to the chapter on Dislocations of the First Phalanges of the Thumb and Fingers for a more full consideration of this matter.

In case the smaller toes are luxated, the reduction is generally effected with ease, by simple extension, or by extension combined with pressure; sometimes, also, the bone will be more easily put in place by reversing the phalanx more completely, as we have advised in certain cases of dislocation of the fingers.

If the skin is penetrated, it will often be found necessary either to amputate or to practice resection upon the exposed phalanx.

Sir Astley Cooper relates a case of luxation of "all the smaller toes," from the metatarsus, which had not been reduced, and the subject of which was, in consequence, so much maimed that he was unable to labor. It had been occasioned by a fall, from a considerable height, upon the extremities of the toes. A projection existed at the roots of all the smaller toes, the extremity of each metatarsal bone being placed under the first phalanx of its corresponding toe. The swelling, which immediately followed the receipt of the injury, had concealed its nature, and now, several months having elapsed, reduction could not be effected. The only relief which could be afforded him, therefore, was in wearing a piece of hollow cork at the bottom of the inner part of the shoe, to prevent the pressure of the metatarsal bones upon the nerves and bloodvessels.[1]

CHAPTER XXV.

COMPOUND DISLOCATIONS OF THE LONG BONES.

Frequency of Compound as compared with Simple Dislocations.—Compound dislocations, as compared with simple, are of rare occurrence. Of ninety-four dislocations reported by Norris as having been received into the Pennsylvania Hospital for the ten years ending in 1840, only two were compound;[2] and of one hundred and sixty-six dislocations recorded in my observations, only eight were compound.[3]

Relative Frequency in the Different Joints.—In my own recorded cases, four were dislocations of the tibia inwards at the ankle-joint, one was a partial (pathological) luxation forwards at the same joint, one was a luxation of the astragalus, one a luxation of the head of the humerus into the axilla, and one a forward luxation of the radius and ulna at the wrist-joint. Both of the cases reported by Norris were dislocations of the thumb.

Sir Astley Cooper, speaking upon this point, says that the elbow, wrist, ankle, and finger-joints are most subject to these accidents; and that he has seen but two in the shoulder-joint, and one in the knee-joint. He had never seen a compound dislocation at the hip-joint, and he believed that it was "scarcely ever" so dislocated. Mr. Bransby Cooper has, however, reported in detail a very interesting case of this accident, communicated to him by Dr. Walker, of Charlestown, Mass., in which reduction was accomplished by *manipulation* alone, by Dr. Ingalls, on the second day. The patient died at the end of about three weeks.[4] So far as I know, this is the only case upon record. Malgaigne says that a compound dislocation at the hip-joint has probably never occurred.

Among the cases of compound dislocation recorded by Sir Astley and Bransby Cooper, most of which were communicated to these gentlemen by other surgeons, 45 were dislocations of the ankle, 10 of the astragalus, 4 of the ulna at the wrist-joint, 4 of the thumb, 2 of the

[1] Sir Ast. Cooper, op. cit., p. 385.

[2] Norris, Amer. Journ. Med. Sci., April, 1841, p. 335.

[3] For the most of these cases, see Transactions of the New York State Med. Soc. for 1855; article entitled "Report on Dislocations, with especial reference to their Results." By F. H. Hamilton.

[4] A. Cooper, on Dislocations, &c., by B. Cooper, p. 59.

knee, 1 of the shoulder, 1 of the elbow, 1 of the radius and ulna at the wrist, 1 of the scaphoid bone, and 1 of the metatarsal bone of the great toe. Other writers have occasionally described compound dislocations of the clavicle, but I know of no record of a compound dislocation of the lower jaw.

Prognosis, as determined by the Mode of Treatment adopted by most of the Ancient and many of the Modern Surgeons.—By most of the early writers these accidents, whenever they occurred in the larger joints, were regarded as nearly beyond the reach of art. Says Hippocrates: "In cases of complete dislocation at the ankle-joint, complicated with an external wound, whether the displacement be inwards or outwards, you are not to reduce the parts, but let any other physician reduce them if he choose. For this you should know for certain, that the patient will die if the parts are allowed to remain reduced, and that he will not survive more than a few days, for few of them pass the seventh day, being cut off by convulsions, and sometimes the leg and foot are seized with gangrene." Hippocrates adds: "But if not reduced, nor any attempts at first made to reduce them, most of such cases recover."[1]

The same remarks are applied by Hippocrates to compound dislocations of the head of the tibia, of the lower end of the femur, of the wrist, elbow, and shoulder-joints; death occurring in all cases, as he believes, more or less speedily whenever the bones are reduced and retained in place a sufficient length of time, and "were it not that the physician would be exposed to censure," he would not reduce even the bones of the fingers, since it must be expected, he thinks, that their articular extremities will exfoliate even when the reduction is most successful.

I shall presently show, however, that even Hippocrates advised and probably practiced resection in certain cases of these accidents.

Both Celsus and Galen adopt almost without qualification the line of practice laid down by Hippocrates, and affirm equally the danger and almost certain death, consequent upon the reduction of compound dislocations in large joints.[2] Celsus recommends resection in some cases.

Paulus Ægineta, however, and after him Albucasis, Haly Abbas, and Rhazes, do not regard the rules established by Hippocrates, in relation to the non-reduction of the bones, as so imperative, nor the results of the opposite practice as so uniformly fatal.

"Hippocrates remarks," says Paulus Ægineta, "in the case of dislocations with a wound, the utmost discretion is required. For these, if reduced, occasion the most imminent danger, and sometimes death, the surrounding nerves and muscles being inflamed by the extension, so that strong pains, spasms, and acute fevers, are produced more particularly in the case of the elbows, knees, and joints above, for the nearer they are to the vital parts the greater is the danger they induce. Wherefore, Hippocrates, by all means, forbids us to apply reduction and strong bandaging to them, and directs us to use only anti-inflam-

[1] Works of Hippocrates, Sydenham ed., London, vol. ii. p. 634.
[2] Paulus Ægineta, Syd. ed., vol. ii. p. 510.

matory and soothing applications to them at the commencement, for that by this treatment life may sometimes be preserved. But what he recommends for the fingers alone, we would attempt to do for all the other joints; at first, and while the parts remain free from inflammation, we would reduce the dislocated joint by moderate extension, and if we succeed in our object, we may persist in using the anti-inflammatory treatment only. But if inflammation, spasm, or any of the afore-mentioned symptoms come on, we must dislocate it again if it can be done without violence. If, however, we are apprehensive of this danger (for perhaps if inflammation should come on it will not yield), it will be better to defer the reduction of the greater joints at the commencement; and when the inflammation subsides, which happens about the seventh or ninth day, then, having foretold the danger from reduction, and explained how, if not reduced, they will be mutilated for life, we may try to make the attempt without violence, using also the lever to facilitate the process."[1]

In the following quotations from three of the most celebrated writers of the last two centuries, we find but little, if any evidence that the opinions of the fathers upon this subject were not still held in general respect: "If the joint be dislocated, so that it is either uncovered, or a little thrust forth without the skin, the accident is mortal, and of more danger to be reduced than if it be not reduced. For if it be not reduced, inflammation will come upon it, convulsion, and sometimes death. 2. There will be a filthiness of the part itself. 3. An incurable ulcer, and if perhaps it be brought to cicatrize at all, it will easily be dissolved by reason of the softness of it: but if it be reduced, it brings extreme danger of convulsion, gangrene, and death."[2]

"Si vero in magnis articulis tam valida fuit facta luxatio, ut ligamentis ruptis os articuli multum sit protrusum per integumenta, hæc pars ossis vasis privata moritur, citius autem si reponatur, quam si non reponitur; quare sola amputatio restat ad conservationem vitæ."[3]

Heister, who makes no allusion to this subject in the first edition of his great work, published at Amsterdam in 1739, adds the following remarks in his last edition, translated and published in London in 1768: "Dislocations attended with a wound, especially of the shoulder or thigh-bone, are of very bad consequence, and often endanger the life of the patient; in Celsus's opinion (Book VIII. Chap. XXV.), whether the bones be replaced or not, there is generally great danger; and so much the more the nearer the wound is to the joint. Hippocrates has declared that no bones can be reduced with security, beside those of the hands and feet. (*Vectiar.* 19, 5.) See more on this subject in that passage of Celsus just now quoted, though I by no means recommend the following him implicitly."[4]

[1] Paulus Ægineta, Syd. ed., vol. ii. p. 509.

[2] "Chirurgeon's Storehouse." By Johannes Scultetus, of Ulme, in Suevia. London ed., 1674, p. 31.

[3] Johannes de Gorter. Chirurgia repurgata. Lugduni Batavorem, 1742, t. 86.

[4] General System of Surgery, by Dr. Laurence Heister. 8th ed. London, 1768. Vol. i. p. 164.

Such were the extreme views as to the fatality of these accidents, and of the feebleness of our resources entertained by the ancient, and even by the more modern writers almost down to our own day; with only rare exceptions these limbs were condemned either to great and inevitable deformity, or to amputation. Nor, if we speak only of their fatality, have surgeons ceased to regard these accidents as among the most grave with which they have to deal.

Pathology, and Appreciation of the Sources of Danger as compared especially with Compound Fractures.—The danger, according to Sir Astley Cooper, consists in the rapid inflammation of the synovial membranes, which is speedily followed by suppuration and ulceration, whereby the ends of the bones become exposed; and for the repair of which lesions, great general as well as local efforts are required, and a high degree of constitutional irritation results. In addition to which circumstances, "the violence inflicted on the neighboring parts, the injury of the muscles and tendons, and the laceration of bloodvessels, necessarily lead to more important and dangerous consequences than those which follow simple dislocations."

The sources of danger enumerated by Sir Astley Cooper have been regarded as sufficient to account for their extraordinary fatality by the majority of those modern surgical writers who have alluded to the subject; but I must confess that to me they do not appear so. In compound fractures the mortality is far less; yet one might naturally suppose, that when the sharp and irregular fragments are pressing into the flesh, among nerves and bloodvessels, the irritation and inflammation would be equal, if not more than equal to the irritation and consequent inflammation produced by exposing a joint surface to the air; indeed, modern experience has sufficiently shown that these surfaces are much more tolerant of atmospheric exposure, and of the action of many other irritants, than surgeons formerly supposed. A clean incision into a large joint, which exposes the synovial membranes to the air, and which permits the products of inflammation to escape freely, is attended with much less danger than a small puncture which does not at all permit the air to enter, nor the increased synovia and the pus to escape. Very grave results sometimes follow from large wounds into large joints, but under judicious treatment such results are the exception and not the rule.[1] But Sir Astley evidently attributes more of the bad consequences to the exhausting effects of the efforts at repair, than to the immediate inflammation resulting from the exposure of the joint. It is pretty certain, however, that a majority of these patients die at a period too early to render this cause in any considerable degree operative.

As to the bruising of the "muscles and tendons, and laceration of bloodvessels," it cannot be denied that it must usually be greater than in "simple dislocations;" and I will not say that it is not in a given number of instances greater than in the same number of instances of

[1] Upon this point see the very able article entitled "Amputations and Compound Fractures," by John O. Stone, in the New York Journal of Medicine, vol. iii. of 2d series, p. 316, Nov. 1849.

compound fractures. The tissues have often been thrust rudely through by a large and smooth bone, and the tendons have been stretched violently or torn completely asunder; while occasionally large arteries, which are prone to hug the bones about the joints, are lacerated and left to bleed. That the importance of these complications, however, may not be over-estimated, we must state that Sir Astley Cooper himself has remarked how seldom, in compound dislocations of the ankle-joint, the large arteries are injured; that a tearing of the ligaments and of the tendons is almost as likely to occur in simple dislocations as in compound; and, indeed, that in neither case are the tendons usually ruptured, but only thrust aside. Moreover, the skin is often made to give way not so much from the pressure of the round head within, as from the equal pressure of some sharp angular body from without. In all these respects, there are many examples of compound fractures which possess not a whit of advantage; in which cases, nevertheless the surgeon feels very little doubt as to the ultimate cure.

In short, the causes which, according to Sir Astley Cooper, determine the extraordinary fatality of these accidents, do not sufficiently differ from those which operate in compound fractures to occasion so great a difference in results, and the fatality of compound dislocations remains unexplained; or if surgical writers have here and there intimated the true cause, they have failed to give it its proper place and value.

I think the cause of the greater fatality of compound dislocations over compound fractures is to be found in the simple fact that dislocations are generally reduced, and by splints or other apparatus successfully maintained in place, while compound fractures, as my statistical report of cases has proven, are not generally reduced completely, nor can they by any means yet devised, except in a few cases, be maintained in place if reduced. Broken limbs, whether simple or compound in their character, will in a great majority of cases shorten upon themselves in spite of the most assiduous and skilful attempts to prevent it.[1]

In adults most bones break obliquely, and cannot be made to support each other, and even in transverse fractures the broken ends are generally small compared with the articular ends of the same bones, and afford a very uncertain and inadequate support for themselves; not to speak of the difficulty of once bringing their ends into exact apposition where the muscles are powerful, or where they lie embedded in a large mass of flesh so that they cannot be felt. While, on the other hand, dislocated bones, whether simple or compound, are capable when restored to place of supporting themselves; or with only slight assistance, their reduction may be maintained; it is also ordinarily a work of no great difficulty to reduce them.

Herein, then, consists the most important difference between these two classes of accidents, which are in other respects so similar. In the one, the very nature of the injury prevents the complete reduc-

[1] "Report on Deformities after Fractures." Trans. Am. Med. Assoc., vol. viii. ix. and x.

tion, and the consequent violent strain of the muscles, tendons, and other soft tissues; while in the other, the nature of the accident leaves it in the power of the surgeon to reduce the bones, and modern surgery has in a great measure sanctioned the practice of maintaining them in place, in defiance of the efforts of the muscles, and sometimes, no doubt, at the imminent hazard of the life of the patient.

Is it not fair to presume that tissues which have been stretched and lacerated, require rest in order that they may recover from the effects of their injuries? And if the soft parts are really more injured in dislocations than in fractures, does not the indication for rest become, for this very reason, more imperative?

General Inferences.—We have come, then, to regard the shortening of limbs after fractures, within certain limits and in certain cases, as a conservative circumstance rather than as a circumstance which the surgeon should in all cases seek to prevent.

There is abundant evidence that the ancients had some knowledge of the value of rest to the muscles, tendons, &c., in the prevention of inflammation after compound dislocations, since they constantly urge the greater danger of reducing these dislocations, than of leaving them unreduced; and they do not hesitate to recommend, that in case violent inflammation supervenes upon the reduction, the bone shall immediately be again dislocated. Galen speaks very explicitly on this subject, and says that "the danger in reduction consists partly in the additional violence inflicted on the muscles, and partly in their being then put into a stretched state, whereby spasms or convulsions are brought on, and gangrene as the result of the intense inflammation which ensues;" and Paulus Ægineta remarks: "For these, if reduced, occasion the most imminent danger, and sometimes death; the surrounding nerves and muscles being inflamed by the extension," &c.

I have already quoted from Sir Astley Cooper the causes or reasons which he has assigned for the fatality of compound dislocations; and the same reasons have generally been assigned by those who have written since his day; but he has elsewhere, when speaking of exsection, given place to the very idea for which we claim so much prominence, the danger arising from a stretching of the muscles. Mr. Liston, also, and Mr. Miller, when speaking especially of dislocations of the tibia at the ankle-joint, refer to the same source of danger.

Treatment.—Let us see now the alternatives which surgery presents for the treatment of these intractable accidents.

1. Reduction of the bone.
2. Non-reduction.
3. Amputation.
4. Tenotomy.
5. Resection and reduction.

The questions for us to consider are, first, by which of these several methods is the life of the patient rendered most secure? and second, where of two or more methods all are equally safe, by which will he suffer the least maiming or mutilation?

By Reduction.—We have seen already how the old surgeons regarded the practice of reducing compound dislocations of the larger joints.

It is not difficult, however, to find in the records of surgery numerous examples of successful terminations under this practice.

Dr. White, of Hudson, N. Y., has reported a case of this kind in which the dislocation was at the ankle-joint.[1] Pott says he has seen this practice occasionally succeed,[2] and Mr. Scott communicated to the *Lancet* in March, 1837, a case of compound dislocation of the humerus successfully treated by reduction. Sir Astley Cooper also records several cases of compound dislocations at the lower end of the tibia and fibula, successfully treated by reduction.

A careful examination, however, of those cases reported by Sir Astley as having been reduced without resection, and which resulted in cures, does not, in my opinion, leave much substantial evidence in favor of the practice; or perhaps we ought rather to say that it leaves only a qualified evidence of its propriety in certain cases. He has mentioned about sixteen of these examples, comprising dislocations of the lower end of the tibia, or of the tibia and fibula, outwards, also inwards and forwards, all of which, save one quoted from Mr. Liston, have been reported to him by other surgeons, and not one of which had he ever seen himself. Many of the cases are reported very loosely, evidently in reply to circular letters, and from memory, without recorded notes, and by unknown, and in some sense irresponsible surgeons. It is not always said whether the wounds in the soft parts were made by the protrusion of the bones, or by some external violence; yet this is certainly a very material point in determining whether reduction is to be followed by inflammation or not. The results, sometimes only attained after exposure to great hazards, are, after all, often sufficiently unfavorable.

It will be noticed, also, that in Cases 152 and 153, the astragalus was comminuted and removed, either at first or at a later day; and in Cases 154, 155, 156, and 160, the tibia, and also probably the fibula, was broken, and it does not appear but that in consequence of this complication the limb became shortened, and the muscles were thus put at rest, very much as if the bones had been retracted; and in one of the cases enumerated under 161, the lower end of the tibia spontaneously exfoliated. That a comminution, or that any fracture of the astragalus or of the tibia and fibula, should be regarded in these cases as rendering the accident less grave, can only be comprehended by a full appreciation of the value of relaxation of the muscles.

The few cases which remain after this exclusion do indeed illustrate how nature and skill may triumph over great difficulties, but nothing more.

It is possible, also, that some of these examples of recovery after reduction may admit of an explanation entirely consistent with our own views of the true source of the danger in these accidents, if indeed they do not tend actually to confirm our doctrines. I have myself seen one example of complete recovery after the reduction of a compound dislocation at the ankle-joint, although resection was

[1] White, Amer. Journ. Med. Sci., Nov. 1828, p. 109.
[2] Pott, Chirurg. Works, vol. ii. p. 243.

not practiced; but in this case, all the tissues, or nearly all which suffered any injury, were completely torn asunder, and therefore wholly removed from the danger of which we have spoken. The example to which we allude is the following: On the 30th of Oct., 1858, John Bourquard, æt. 30, was caught in the tow-line of a canal boat, causing a compound dislocation of the right ankle-joint. I found the foot, immediately after the accident, thrown completely back against the lower part of the leg, the integuments in front of the joint, as well as all of the tendons and ligaments on this side, being completely torn asunder, while the tendo-Achillis, and the tendons behind both of the malleoli, with the corresponding integuments, were uninjured. This immunity of the tissues behind the malleoli was due to the direction in which the foot was drawn, namely, directly backwards. Everything which had suffered a strain being thoroughly severed, I did not hesitate to attempt to save the limb without resection. The reduction was accomplished very easily. The leg and foot were placed in a box filled with bran, and cool water dressings were applied to the portion which was exposed. On the 22d of November, the limb was removed from the bran to a pillow, the union being sufficient not to demand so much lateral support. About the first of March he left the hospital, the wound having closed, but the ankle remaining swollen and stiff.

I have also during the last year seen two cases in which the foot has been nearly severed from the leg through the ankle-joint, by means of a "reaper." In each case the patient was standing with his back to the machine, and one of the blades cut horizontally from side to side, severing everything except about three inches of integument in front, and the extensor tendons of the toes. In the first instance, having seen the patient, a gentleman nearly sixty years of age, within three or four hours of the time of the receipt of the injury, I found him exceedingly exhausted by the hemorrhage. Both malleoli were cut off smoothly, the knife having severed the limb so exactly through the joint, as to have touched the cartilage at but one or two points. Having secured the bloodvessels, I replaced the foot, and after a few days of attendance I left him in the charge of an excellant young surgeon, Dr. Robertson, of Lancaster, N. Y., to whose diligence and skill the patient is no doubt mainly indebted for his recovery. After the lapse of nearly one year he is able, by the assistance of a shoe furnished with lateral supports, to walk very well. In the second case, which was only brought to my notice some months after the accident occurred, in consequence of a troublesome fistula near the ankle-joint, the recovery had been complete except that a small fragment of one of the malleoli was necrosed and required removal.

Dr. Eli Hurd, of Niagara Co., N. Y., was equally fortunate in a case of compound dislocation of the shoulder-joint. This was in the person of G. T., æt. 30, who was caught in the gearing of a thrashing machine on the 18th of Feb. 1852, which having drawn him in with great force dislocated the head of the left humerus downwards through the integuments into the axilla. Reduction was accomplished according to the method recommended by Nathan Smith, by pulling from each wrist at right angles with the body, while the operator himself seized the naked head of the humerus with his left hand, his right resting upon the top of the shoulder, and pushed it into place. The time occupied in the reduction was about thirty seconds. The forearm was then suspended in a sling, and the venous hemorrhage, occasioned by a rupture of the subclavian vein, was arrested by compression. The tegumentary wound, between three and four inches in length, was subsequently closed by sutures and cool water-dressings were applied. On the fourth day the wound had united by first intention, and the man was walking about his room. In less than a month he was dismissed cured, and in the following harvest he was able to cut his own hay and grain, and to use his arm as before the accident.[1]

Miller and Hoffman reduced successfully a compound dislocation of the knee,[2] and Galli has communicated a similar case to Malgaigne.[3]

Whether either of the three last mentioned examples admit of the same explanation as the preceding three, I am unable to say, but whether they do or do not, they are too exceptional in their character to prejudice the argument materially which we shall hereafter make in favor of resection.

Non-Reduction.—On the other hand, it will be very difficult to find an equal number of cases of compound dislocations, unreduced, which have terminated favorably. The fact is no doubt that at the present day very few surgeons would feel themselves justified in leaving a bone out of place unless they proceeded to amputate. In the *Transactions* of the New York State Medical Society for 1855, I have reported (Case 16 of Tibia and Fibula, p. 87), a compound dislocation at the ankle-joint, which, being unreduced, terminated fatally on the twenty-eighth day. This is the only example of a compound dislocation of a long bone, left unreduced, which has fallen under my observation; excepting, of course, those cases in which amputation was immediately practised.

The united testimony, however, of the old surgeons, who generally neither amputated nor adopted the method of resection, but who recommended and practiced non-reduction, is, that it is much more safe to leave these bones unreduced, than to reduce them without resection; and I see no reason to doubt the correctness of their opinions in this matter. But whether it would be more safe to leave such limbs unreduced, or having practiced resection to restore them, is another question, in which the advantage and comparative safety of the latter practice is too obvious to require explanation or defence.

Amputation.—Says Pott: "When this accident (dislocation of the ankle) is accompanied, as it sometimes is, with a wound of the integuments of the inner ankle, and that made by the protrusion of the bone, it not unfrequently ends in a fatal gangrene, unless prevented by timely amputation, though I have several times seen it do very well without." And Sir Astley Cooper, speaking of compound disloca-

[1] Hurd, Buffalo Med. Journ., vol. ix. p. 119.
[2] Miller and Hoffman, London Med. Repos., vol. xxiv. p. 346.
[3] Galli, Malgaigne, op. cit., t. ii. p. 958.

tions of the ankle-joint, remarks: "Thirty years ago it was the practice to amputate limbs for this accident, and the operation was then thought absolutely necessary for the preservation of life, by some of our best surgeons." Nor is it difficult to see by what reasoning surgeons of "thirty years ago" had fallen back upon this desperate remedy. Both reduction and non-reduction having proven eminently hazardous, in the absence of perhaps both knowledge and experience in resection, they finally adopted the alternative of amputation, as that which after all must give to the patient the best chance for life; and were no other alternatives to be presented, this would be our choice in a large proportion of cases.

It must not be understood, however, that amputation is an expedient wholly free from danger; or, indeed, that the chances of the patient are in the average very greatly increased by this practice. Of thirteen amputations made for compound dislocations at the ankle-joint, in the Royal Infirmary at Edinburgh, only two resulted in the recovery of the patients.[1] Alluding to which, Mr. Fergusson remarks: "An amount of mortality which may well incline the surgeon to act upon the doctrine inculcated by Sir Astley Cooper." (To attempt to save the limb by reduction.) But Mr. Fergusson has added a sentiment which accords very closely with my own experience and opinions. "I fear, however, that in the attempts which have been made to save the foot (by reduction) the results in all the cases have not met with the same publicity; that the instances where amputation has been afterwards necessary, or where death has been the consequence, have not always been recorded; and, from what I have myself seen, I would caution the inexperienced practitioner from being over-sanguine in anticipating a happy result in every example."

By Tenotomy.—As a means of overcoming the resistance of the muscles, and for the purpose especially of facilitating the reduction, tenotomy has been proposed. First by Dieffenbach in cases of ancient unreduced luxations; but Wm. Hey, Jr., was the first to make a practical application of this suggestion in a case of compound dislocation. After cutting the tendo-Achillis, the ankle being dislocated, the reduction was easily effected, but a strong tendency to displacement backwards remained, and he was obliged afterwards to cut the tendons of the tibialis posticus and flexor longus digitorum.[2]

This method, based in some degree upon a very correct notion of the principal sources of difficulty, I regard as totally impracticable, at least to any useful or adequate extent. In order to be efficient, all the tendons passing the articulations must be cut, or nearly all of them; and I doubt whether the judgment of any discreet surgeon will ever sanction such an extreme, I might almost say, such an absurd measure. Nor do I think that in the point of view in which we are now considering this subject, having reference only to the question of danger, if the cutting of the tendons was sufficiently extensive to have any real effect in facilitating the reduction, the practice would be found

[1] Edinb. Med. Monthly, Aug. 1844.

[2] Hey, Trans. of Provinc. Med. and Surg. Assoc., vol. xii. p. 171, 1844.

to have any advantage over other methods known to be eminently dangerous.

By Resection.—Finally, resection presents itself for our consideration as the only remaining surgical expedient.

We have seen that most of the early writers understood the effects of a constant strain upon the muscles in increasing the danger of spasms, inflammation, and death; but in general they have suggested no remedy but non-reduction or amputation. Hippocrates, however, uses the following language, after speaking of resection of protruding bones in accidental amputations, or in fractures of the fingers: "Complete resections of bones at the joints, whether the foot, the hand, the leg, the ankle, the forearm, the wrist, for the most part, are not attended with danger, unless one be cut off at once by deliquium animi, or if continual fever supervene on the fourth day." To which passage the translator adds the following note: "This paragraph on resection of the bones in compound dislocations and fractures contains almost all the information on the subject which is to be found in the works of ancient medicine." Celsus notices the practice of resection in compound dislocations very briefly, as follows: "Si nudum os eminet, impedimentum semper futurum est; ideo quod excedit, abscindendum est."

Mr. Hey, of Leeds, was the first of modern surgeons who called especial attention to the value of resection in compound dislocations.

Subsequently, Mr. Parks, of Liverpool, in an "Account of a new method of treating Diseases of the Joints of the Knee and Elbow," advocates the practice of resection in certain cases of diseases of these joints, but especially in "affections of the joints produced by external violence."

Mr. Levéille, in France also, following, as he affirms, the guidance of Hippocrates, has advocated a similar practice.

Velpeau, Syme, Fergusson, Erichsen, Miller, Liston, Chelius, Lizars, Gibson, Norris, under certain circumstances, and especially where the bones cannot otherwise be reduced, and where the dislocations occur in certain joints, and especially the elbow and ankle-joints, recommend resection. To which names we may add that of Sir Astley Cooper, who has considered the subject, as applied to the ankle-joint, quite at length, and who says: "I have known no case of death when the extremities of the bone" (tibia, at the ankle) "have been sawed off, although I shall have occasion to mention some cases which terminated fatally when this was not done."

Why resection should diminish the danger to life, by placing at rest the injured muscles, has been already sufficiently considered; but it seems not improbable that, if synovial membranes are actually more susceptible of violent and dangerous inflammations than the other tissues about the joints, then would this source of danger be removed just in proportion as the synovial membranes themselves are removed. Such, indeed, was the argument used by Sir Astley; and Mr. South, in a note to Chelius, when referring to this fact, has made the following statement:—

"In compound dislocations of the ankle-joint, with protrusion of the shin-bone through the wound, most English surgeons saw off the joint end, not merely to render reduction more easy, but also, according to Sir Astley Cooper's opinions, to lessen the suppurative process, by diminishing the synovial surface. This mode of practice is certainly not commonly followed in reference to other joints, and the younger Cline was always opposed to its being resorted to in dislocated ankle."

The following case, having occurred under my own eye, will serve to illustrate the value of the principle which I have been endeavoring to establish:—

Samuel Adamson, of Buffalo, æt. 24, was caught by the cable of a vessel, June 17, 1855, dislocating the left tibia at its lower end inwards, and breaking the fibula two inches above the ankle. I was immediately called, and found the tibia protruding through the skin about three inches. The periosteum was torn up, and the cartilaginous surface of the end of the bone was roughened. His thigh was also severely bruised and lacerated, but the bone was not broken.

Dr. Boardman assisting me, we attempted to reduce the bones, but with our hands we found it impossible to do so. I proceeded immediately to remove about one inch and a half of the lower end of the tibia with the saw. The remaining portion was then brought easily into place, and the wound dressed with sutures, adhesive straps, bandages, and light splints. On the same day he became an inmate of the marine wards at the Hospital of the Sisters of Charity, and was placed under the care of Dr. Wilcox, through whose politeness I was permitted to see him frequently.

The wound in the leg healed kindly, with only a slight amount of inflammation and suppuration. Violent inflammation, however, occurred in the thigh, followed by extensive suppuration and sloughing. This, in fact, proved to be by far the most serious injury, and that which most endangered his life and delayed his recovery.

After about two months, the ankle was in such a condition as to require little or no further attention. The fragments of the fibula had shortened upon each other and were united, so that the tibia rested upon the astragalus. It was nearly two months, however, before he began to walk, owing to the condition of his thigh.

Aug. 24, 1856, fourteen months after the accident, Adamson called at my office. He was then employed again as a sailor on board the schooner Sebastopol, and performed all the duties of an ordinary deck hand. His leg is shortened one inch and a quarter; from which, it seems, that there has been some deposit upon the end of the bone, which has compensated for one-quarter of an inch of that which I removed. The ankle is perfect in its form, being neither turned to the right nor to the left, and he treads square and firm upon the sole of his foot. There is considerable freedom of motion, especially in flexion and extension. Occasionally it becomes a little swollen and painful.

In a case of compound dislocation of the upper end of the humerus, occurring also under my own observation, and recorded in the *Transactions of the New York State Medical Society for* 1855 (p. 27, Case 14), in which reduction was followed by death, I have now much reason to believe that if I had practiced resection before the reduction, my patient's chances for recovery would have been greatly increased; perhaps also the case of compound dislocation at the wrist-joint recorded in the same vol. (p. 68), in which, having reduced the bones, I was subsequently compelled to amputate, may equally illustrate the hazard to which the practice of reduction without resection must often expose the patient.

The same remarks I will venture to apply to the case of compound dislocation of the hip, of which I have already spoken as having occurred in the practice of Dr. Walker, of Charlestown, Mass. Had the head of the femur been resected before its reduction, I cannot doubt but that the unfortunate man's chances for recovery would have been very greatly improved.

Thus, if we consider the question of the life of the patient only, the argument and the testimony seem to favor resection in a great majority of cases of compound dislocations occurring in large joints, and in a considerable number of cases of similar accidents in the smaller joints. It is certainly more safe than non-reduction or reduction without resection, and it is probably quite as safe as amputation or tenotomy.

But there is another question, which is, in our estimation, secondary to the one now considered, but which is often in the estimation of the patient himself, of the first importance—namely, by which method will he suffer the least maiming or mutilation?

This question I do not find it difficult to answer. Certainly it is not by non-reduction or by amputation; and, putting tenotomy aside, it is now a question only between reduction without resection, and reduction with resection. These two methods, one of which experience has shown to be fraught with danger, and the other of which experience has shown to be relatively safe, are now to be compared in a point of view in which their antagonisms are perhaps less conspicuous, yet sufficiently marked.

First. In either case the inflammation consequent upon the injury may be violent, and the recovery slow and tedious. The same arguments, however, which we have applied to the question of the comparative danger of the two modes, must apply with nearly equal force to this question of maiming; since the amount of maiming must often be governed by the intensity and duration of the inflammation, and upon this point the testimony has been shown to be in favor of resection.

It will be observed that not only is the danger of maiming rendered more considerable by reduction without resection, because the inflammation is so much more likely to extend to the tendons and muscles, causing them to adhere to each other, and to become subsequently atrophied, a condition from which they often never completely recover, but also because the ligaments and capsules of the joints, with the synovial surfaces, are in consequence encroached upon, and the freedom of motion is ever afterwards greatly restricted, if not completely lost. This marked impairment of the functions of the joint does not always happen, but it cannot be denied that it does generally. Indeed it is by no means uncommon for these accidents to be followed, after ulcerations of the cartilage, by copious bony deposits in and around the joints.

How is it, on the other hand, with these joints after resection? I have thus far heard of no cases in which complete anchylosis resulted; but in all considerable freedom of motion has returned, and in some the restoration in this respect has been nearly or quite as complete as before the accident.

Says Dr. Kerr, of Northampton: "Several cases of compound dislocation of the ankle have fallen under my care, and it has been uniformly my practice to take off the lower extremity of the tibia, and to lay the limb in a state of semiflexion upon splints; by this means a great deal of painful extension, and the consequent high degree of inflammation, are avoided. The splints I used are excavated wood, and much wider than those in common use, with thick movable pads stuffed with wool. I keep the parts constantly wetted with a solution of liquor ammoniæ acetatis, without removing the bandage. In my very early life, upwards of sixty years ago, I saw many attempts to reduce compound dislocations without removing any part of the tibia; but, to the best of my recollection, they all ended unfavorably, or, at least in amputation. By the method which I have pursued, as above mentioned, I have generally succeeded in saving the foot, and in preserving a tolerable articulation."

Sir Astley Cooper has made a valuable experiment to determine the condition of the new joint under these circumstances; and the vast number of cases in which resection has now been practiced in cases of caries of the articulating surfaces, and their results, add still more substantial proofs as to the usefulness of the joints after such operations.

"I made an incision upon the lower extremity of the tibia, at the inner ankle of a dog, and cutting the inner portion of the ligament of the ankle-joint, I produced a compound dislocation of the bone inwards. I then sawed off the whole cartilaginous extremity of the tibia, returned the bone upon the astragalus, closed the integuments by suture, and bandaged the limb to preserve the bone in this situation. Considerable inflammation and suppuration followed; and in a week the bandage was removed. When the wound had been for several weeks perfectly healed, I dissected the limb. The ligament of the joint was still defective at the part at which it had been cut. From the sawn surface of the tibia there grew a ligamento-cartilaginous substance, which proceeded to the surface of the cartilage of the astragalus to which it adhered. The cartilage of the astragalus appeared to be absorbed only in one small part; there was no cavity between the end of the tibia and the cartilaginous surface of the astragalus. A free motion existed between the tibia and astragalus which was permitted by the length and flexibility of the ligamentous substance above described, so as to give the advantage of a joint where no synovial articulation or cavity was to be found. This experiment not only shows the manner in which the parts are restored, but also the advantage of passive motion; for if the part be frequently moved, the intervening substance becomes entirely ligamentous; but if it be left perfectly at rest for a length of time, ossific action proceeds from the extremity of the tibia into the ligamentous substance, and thus produces an ossific anchylosis."

Second. Is it not probable, moreover, since the limb can be retained in place so much more easily after resection, that it will actually, in a majority of cases, be found to have been retained in place more perfectly? Even after simple dislocations, especially in those occurring at the ankle-joint, great deformity and much maiming are the not unfrequent results, and that too when all diligence and care have been employed. It has been impossible always to maintain a perfect apposition in the articulating surfaces. How much greater must be this difficulty in cases of compound dislocations!

Third. The only argument which remains in favor of reduction without resection is the necessary shortening of the limb after resection. But this need seldom perhaps to exceed three-quarters of an inch, and often not more than half an inch; an amount of shortening which, as I have had occasion to prove when treating of fractures, does not necessarily produce a halt, and which indeed is often not known to exist by the patient himself.

Finally. It must not be inferred that the author intends to recommend resection as a universal practice in cases of compound dislocations of the long bones. He has only sought to determine in a general manner its relative value as compared with other modes of procedure; and especially has it been his intention to bring more prominently into view the importance of rest and relaxation to the muscles, as an element in the treatment most essential to success. To declare its special application to cases would demand a treatise more elaborate than it was proposed to write. If, however, one were to speak of the individual bones only, there seems sufficient authority in the facts and arguments already presented to conclude that resection is applicable to certain compound dislocations of the clavicle, humerus, radius and ulna, fingers, femur, tibia and fibula, and toes; in short to all of these accidents occurring in the long bones of the extremities.

If an attempt is made to save the limb without resection, it is scarcely necessary to say that the success will depend, in a great measure, upon the care, attention, and skill bestowed upon the treatment. Cool or tepid water-dressings, according as the indications or the sensations of the patient seem to demand, are among the most valuable remedial agents. The limb must be maintained in a position of rest, combined with moderate elevation; and the bran-dressings, recommended in compound fractures, will be found occasionally useful.

CHAPTER XXVI.

CONGENITAL DISLOCATIONS.

§ 1. General Observations and History.

We have omitted, until this moment, to speak of Congenital Dislocations, because, whatever theory of causation we adopt, dissections have shown that they are generally, in some sense, pathologic, or are accompanied with such essential modifications of the anatomical structures as to separate them entirely from ordinary traumatic luxations, which alone constitute the proper subjects of consideration in the present treatise. In relation to congenital dislocations, we shall find it necessary to establish systems of etiology, symptomatology, prognosis, and treatment, having very few points in common with traumatic dislocations. Exceptions to this rule will occur, in examples of intra-uterine traumatic luxations, existing at birth without either original or accidental malformations of the articulations, or of the adjacent muscular, tendinous, or ligamentous structures; yet only in sufficient numbers to warrant the intrusion of the subject in this place.

It is probable that congenital displacements may occur in all the articulations of the skeleton; and in most of them their existence has been already established by dissections. Until within a few years, however, the attention of surgeons has been almost entirely directed to congenital dislocations of the shoulder and hip.

Hippocrates, in his treatise "De Articulis," speaks expressly of dislocations of the hip occurring in the mother's womb, comprising them under the same order with the different varieties of club-foot.

Avicenna and Ambrose Paré have each mentioned original dislocations of the hip; but the first to record an example with any degree of accuracy was Kerkring; in which case, death having occurred during infancy, he was able to verify his opinion by an autopsy. Chaussier has reported, in the *Bulletin de la Faculté et de la Société de Médecine*, An. 1811 and 1812, the case of an infant, upon which he discovered, at birth, two dislocations, one at the scapulo-humeral articulation, and the other at the coxo-femoral. In 1788, Paletta, of Milan, published, under the title of *Adversaria Chirurgica*, a collection of observations, in which, among other things, he has described certain congenital malformations of the hip-joint; and in 1820, he published another work, entitled *Exercitationes Pathologicæ*, where he enters into a more complete exposition of the nature and causes of these deformities

In 1826, Dupuytren read, before the Academy of Sciences, a memoir upon the lameness produced by the original displacement of the femurs; and in the *Leçons Orales*, published in the collections of the

Sydenham Society, may be found a full record of the views and observations of this distinguished surgeon.

The writings of Dupuytren seem, more than anything previously written, to have directed the attention of surgeons and pathologists to this interesting subject, and to have given a new impulse to investigation.

From this time, various treatises have been written by eminent surgeons, many of which are characterized by profound thought, careful investigation, and practical experiment.

Among those who have furnished us lately with elaborate treatises, or with more precise practical information upon this subject, the following names deserve especially to be mentioned: Breschet,[1] Caillard-Billionière,[2] Lehoux,[3] Sandiforte,[4] Duval and Lafond, Humbert and Jacquier, Bouvier,[5] Sédillot,[6] Gerdy, Poliniére, Wrolik,[7] Guérin,[8] Parise,[9] Pravaz,[10] Carnochan,[11] and Robert Smith.[12]

§ 2. Etiology.

Hippocrates says that the bones of the extremities may be disarticulated during intra-uterine life by falls or blows, or by injuries of any kind, inflicted directly upon the abdomen of the mother.

Ambrose Paré, while admitting the efficiency of the several causes named by Hippocrates, believed also that the contractions of the womb, and violence employed by the accoucheur were occasionally adequate to the production of the same results. He taught, moreover, that the position of the fœtus itself might favor the displacement; and that, in some instances, an articular abscess, insufficient depth of the socket with a laxity of the ligaments, were competent to determine the expulsion of the head of the femur from its natural position.

Sédillot regards a softening and relaxation of the ligaments as the most frequent cause.

Parise and Malgaigne are disposed to attribute a majority of these cases to hydrarthrosis, or water in the joints. Says Malgaigne: "For myself, after having long meditated upon this subject, I have come to think that inflammation of the joints enjoys a grand rôle, both in coxo-femoral dislocations and in many others, and even also in various

1 Breschet, Répertoire d'Anatomie et de Physiologie.

2 Caillard-Billionière, Thèse Inaugurale, 1828.

3 Lehoux, Thèse Inaugurale, 1834, Paris.

4 Sandiforte, Thesis, Sustained before the Faculty of Med. of Leyden.

5 Duval and Lafond, Humbert and Jacquier, Bouvier. See Pravaz.

6 Sédillot, Journ. de Connais. Med.-Chirurg., 1838.

7 Gerdy, Poliniére, Wrolik. See Pravaz.

8 Guérin, Recherches sur les Luxations Congénitales; par Jules Guérin, Paris, 1841.

9 Parise, Archiv. Gén. de Méd., 1842.

10 Pravaz, Traité Théorique et Pratique des Luxations Congénitales du Femur, suivi d'un Appendice sur la Prophylaxie des Luxations Spontanées; par Ch. G. Pravaz, Lyon, 1847.

11 Carnochan, A Treatise on the Etiology, Pathology, and Treatment of Congenital Dislocations of the Head of the Femur; by John Murray Carnochan, New York, 1850.

12 R. Smith, A Treatise on Fractures in the Vicinity of Joints, and on Certain Accidental and Congenital Dislocations, Dublin, 1854.

congenital malformations generally ascribed to arrest of development." This writer admits, however, that it will not do to generalize too much in this matter, and that the etiology of congenital luxations is probably as complex as that of luxations after birth.

Chaussier seems to have regarded muscular contraction, or the occurrence of an intra-uterine convulsion, as the cause of the example of congenital dislocation of both humerus and femur seen and recorded by him. Since whom Guérin has greatly extended the application of this doctrine, having embraced in the same etiologic formula all or nearly all congenital dislocations. Guérin ascribes to muscular contraction in one form or another, and to corresponding muscular paralysis, not only dislocations of the femur and other long bones, but also club-foot, torticollis, and various other deviations of the spine. He affirms, moreover, that he has established incontestably the dependence of this abnormal state of the muscular system upon the absence or disappearance more or less complete of corresponding portions of the central nervous systems.

Breschet and Delpech maintained similar views, especially in relation to the dependence of the several varieties of club-foot upon some morbid condition of the cerebro-spinal axis. While Carnochan remarks as follows: "It appears most in accordance with science to refer the muscular spasmodic retraction, upon which congenital dislocations of the head of the femur from the cotyloid cavity depend, to a perverted condition of the excito-motor apparatus of the medulla spinalis, and more especially of that portion of it which is in direct relation with the reflex-motor nervous fibres, distributed to the pelvi-femoral muscles surrounding, and in connection with, the ilio-femoral articulation."

Palletta ascribes these deformities solely to an original defect of the germ; and Dupuytren also declares that, in the case of a congenital dislocation of the hip, the causes are coeval with the earliest organization of the parts, and that the displacement is due rather to a defect in the depth or completeness of the acetabulum, than to accident or disease.

Breschet and Delpech, both of whom, as we have already stated, refer them to some morbid condition of the cerebro-spinal axis, imagine that in consequence of this morbid condition of the nervous centres there exists an arrest of development in the bones, muscles, ligaments, sockets, and, in short, through all the apparatus of the joint which is the seat of the deformity.

If we proceed to analyze these various opinions, we shall find that they are so far susceptible of classification, as that they may be arranged under the three following divisions.

First, the physiological doctrines; according to which congenital dislocations are due to an original defect in the germ, or to an arrest of development.

Second, the pathologic doctrines; which refer them to some supposed lesion of the nervous centres, to contraction or paralysis of the muscles, to a laxity of the ligaments, to hydrarthrosis, or to some other diseased condition of the articulating apparatus.

Third, the mechanical doctrines; which recognize no intra-uterine dislocations except those which are strictly traumatic. The causes being understood to be the peculiar position of the fœtus in utero, violent contractions or the constant pressure of the walls of the uterus, falls and blows upon the abdomen, and unskilful manipulation of the child in delivery.

After a full and careful consideration of this subject, we are prepared to admit the occasional agency of all the causes enumerated, and the probable concurrence of two or more in many instances; nor do we see the propriety of rejecting, as Malgaigne has done, all that large class of malformations which seem to depend upon an arrest of development, or those which appear to be due mainly or solely to intra-uterine paralysis, of both of which many examples have been reported.

§ 3. Congenital Dislocations of the Inferior Maxilla.

Malgaigue affirms that "we know of no congenital dislocation of the jaw," and that we are "not to take seriously the pretended luxation observed by Guérin upon a dérencéphalous infant." The example recorded by Robert Smith he rejects also, declaring that he does "not comprehend how one can see in it a luxation."

For myself, I know of no reason why we should not take "seriously" the case mentioned by Guérin, since, so far as appears in his very brief report of the same, it might have been a true luxation. The specimen was before the academy, and if Malgaigne, from a personal examination, has become satisfied that a dislocation did not exist, he ought to have so informed us. But since he does not speak of having made it the subject of especial examination, we shall feel compelled to accept of it as reported by Guérin.

As to the objections offered to Mr. Smith's case, namely, that "aside of the complete absence of its history, the subject did not present the characteristic signs of a luxation; and the dissection discovered neither maxillary condyle, nor glenoid cavity," we must reply, the dissection seems to us to have furnished such evidence that the deformity was congenital as to render its history unnecessary; the signs were characteristic, not indeed of a traumatic luxation, but of a congenital dislocation, such as may be supposed to have been the result of an arrest of development, or of an original aberration of the germ.

The following is a summary of the very complete account of this case given by Robert Smith.

On the fifth of May, 1840, Edward Lacy, æt. 38, an idiot from infancy, died at the Hardwick Hospital, in consequence of gangrene of the lungs. While making the autopsy, a singular deformity of the face was discovered. The right and left sides seemed as though they did not belong to the same individual, the left being in every respect more fully developed. Upon removing the integuments, the muscles of the right side were found to be much smaller than those of the left, and especially the masseter. These latter having been removed also, the condition of the right temporo-maxillary articulation was carefully studied.

When the mouth was closed, the external lateral ligament, instead of being directed backwards, was seen descending obliquely forwards, to be attached to a very imperfectly developed condyle situated at least one-quarter of an inch in front of its natural position. There was neither an inter-articular cartilage nor cartilage of incrustation, the joint surfaces being invested by a thick periosteum alone; nor was there any distinct capsular ligament.

Nearly the whole of the right side of the inferior maxilla was smaller than the left. The condyle was short and curved, being directed nearly horizontally inwards, and resembling much more the coracoid process than the condyle of the inferior maxilla. The coronoid process was very small and thin, and the sigmoid notch could scarcely be said to exist.

The articular eminence of the temporal bone was absent, there being in its place merely a flat surface destitute of cartilage; which surface presented upon its inner side a shallow and semicircular sulcus where the hook-like condyle of the lower jaw had played.

The malar, superior maxillary, and sphenoid bones of the right side had also suffered corresponding changes of form and relative size.

The motions permitted in the lower jaw were more extensive than those which it enjoys in its normal condition, that is, upon the right side the ramus could be moved very freely forwards and backwards, while upon the left, the condyle underwent a species of rotation upon its axis. During life the patient was observed to be constantly performing this motion, and the right side of the face was continually affected with spasmodic twitches. When the mouth was closed, the front teeth of the upper jaw projected beyond those of the lower, and when opened the deformity was in all respects greatly increased.[1]

Mr. Smith takes this occasion also to express his dissent from the views maintained by Ribes, namely, that the formation of the glenoid cavity is consequent upon the growth of the condyle, and that, were this process not formed, there would not exist either a glenoid cavity or an articular eminence. It is true that neither the glenoid cavity nor the articular eminence is found in the fœtus. Until the seventh month of intra-uterine life, there exists at this point of the temporal bone only a plane surface, and the glenoid cavity with its corresponding eminence is developed in proportion to the growth and development of the condyle. But Mr. Smith justly observes that although the development of the condyle does precede that of the glenoid cavity, "it by no means follows that the formation of the latter is due to the pressure of the former." The cavity, or rather the transverse eminence in front of the plane surface, does not exist in fœtal life, because, owing to the peculiar form of the inferior maxilla at this period, its existence is not necessary. The vertical portion of the jaw (vertical only in the adult) is in the fœtus nearly in the same line with the axis

[1] Robert Smith, op. cit., p. 283.

of the shaft, and consequently when the mouth is opened by the action of the muscles, the condyles are pressed upwards and backwards instead of upwards and forwards, as in the adult. A displacement forwards cannot therefore very well occur; and the protection of the articular eminences is not required. As age advances the angles of the jaw increase, the portions upon which the condyles rest become more vertical, and finally a displacement forwards would occur whenever the mouth was well opened if the articular eminences were not present to afford a sufficient protection in front.

In the case of Lacy the fœtal condition of the bones upon one side remained during life, there being neither cavity nor eminence, and the condyle itself being only imperfectly developed; but the angle of the jaw had assumed the form which belongs to the adult, and the ascending ramus was vertical, consequently the condyle became somewhat displaced forwards.

Chronic rheumatic arthritis is occasionally found in the temporo-maxillary articulation of old persons; and it may be important to distinguish it from congenital luxation, with which, owing to the absorption of the articular eminence, and the consequent displacement of the condyle, it might possibly be confounded.

Says Mr. Smith: "In a majority of instances, this remarkable disease attacks those of advanced age, and is symmetrical; but occasionally it occurs during the period of adult life. In the latter case it is generally more rapid in its progress, is accompanied by greater pain, and is more liable to implicate the neck of the condyle, and the ramus of the jaw."

When the condyle is implicated it becomes enlarged, and can be felt beneath the zygoma, in front of the meatus externus. The lymphatic glands of this region are sometimes enlarged, and the progress of the malady is attended with a constant but not generally severe pain.

The deformity of the face varies according as one or both articulations are affected. When the malady is confined to one joint, the chin is thrown slightly forwards, but chiefly to the opposite side; and when both are implicated the chin is simply advanced so that the teeth project beyond those of the upper jaw.

As the disease progresses, the glenoid cavity enlarges by absorption, and at length a considerable portion or the whole of the articular eminence disappears, and the jaw becomes gradually displaced through the action of the external pterygoids. The disease does not extend in the temporal bone beyond the articulating surface of the glenoid cavity. The condyle assumes a variety of forms, sometimes being greatly enlarged in all its diameters, while its upper surface may be flattened, or conical. The inter-articular cartilage disappears; but Mr. Smith has never yet found any foreign bodies in the joint, and in only one instance have the surfaces been polished or eburnated as we often see in examples of chronic rheumatic arthritis occurring in the hip, knee, and other joints.

The following is an excellent summary of the diagnostic marks between congenital, accidental, and rheumatic dislocations, given by this writer:—

"1. In the congenital luxation, the mouth can be freely opened and closed; in chronic rheumatism these motions can be performed, but not without uneasiness to the patient, an uneasiness which sometimes amounts to severe pain; in luxations from accident, the mouth cannot be closed.

"2. An involuntary flow of saliva accompanies the accidental luxation alone, although in some cases of chronic rheumatism there is an increased secretion of that fluid.

"3. In congenital luxation, the teeth of the upper jaw project beyond those of the lower; the reverse is observed in accidental luxation and in chronic rheumatism.

"4. In congenital luxation there is no fulness in the cheek, such as the coronoid process produces in cases of accidental luxation, and the enlarged condyle in some instances of chronic rheumatic arthritis."[1]

§ 4. Congenital Dislocations of the Spine.

Says Guérin, of the subluxation occipito-atloidean there are two varieties: "First. Backwards, consisting in an exaggerated flexion of the head, upon the front of the neck and chest, with a commencement of sliding backwards of the occipital condyles upon the articular facets of the atlas. Here are two examples in fœtal enencéphalous monsters. Second. Forwards. Those who follow my consultations can recollect having seen last year an infant, about two or three months old, who offered a remarkable example. The head was exactly applied against the posterior part of the neck, and upper part of the back. There was probably a sliding of the condyles forwards, with elongation of the anterior ligaments."[2]

The existence of the first of these varieties has since been denied by Guérin himself;[3] and it will be noticed that he only speaks of the second as a *probable* subluxation forwards. Neither of them can therefore be regarded as established.

Guérin farther remarks that he has observed subluxations in the other regions of the spinal column many times; and he showed to the Academy a fœtus in which the spine presented, besides the occipito-altoidean displacement, a series of angular flexions in the antero-posterior direction, with sliding of the articular surfaces.

In attempting to appreciate the value of Guérin's observations upon this point, it must be remembered that he regards all cases of congenital torticollis, and other deviations of the spine, as examples of subluxation; and, in some sense, we think the theory of this distinguished surgeon may be regarded as correct. The amount of articular displacement between each of the adjacent vertebræ may be very inconsiderable in any such case, yet, however trivial, if it exceeds the limits

1 R. Smith, op. cit., p. 292.
2 Guerin, op. cit., 1841, p. 29.
3 Guérin, Gaz. Méd., 1851, p. 227.

of natural motion, it may properly enough be regarded as the commencement of a luxation.

§ 5. Congenital Dislocations of the Pelvic Bones.

Bassius speaks of a diastasis or separation of the sacro-iliac symphysis, observed by him in newly-born children, and in infants; but, according to Malgaigne, his account of these cases is not such as to warrant any conclusions as to the true nature of the displacements.

Congenital extrophy of the bladder is accompanied always with a deficiency of the central and upper portions of the pubic bones, the result manifestly of an arrest of development; but these cases, of which I have seen two examples, are not properly examples of congenital dislocations, but only of diastases, the separated portions remaining in their normal positions with reference to each other, except that they are not prolonged sufficiently to meet in the median line.

Guérin declares, however, that he has seen congenital displacement, or overriding of the iliac bone upon the sacrum, accompanied with coxo-femoral dislocation and curvature of the spine. The same writer mentions an example, in a fœtal monster, of diastasis of the pubic bones, and of the sacro-iliac symphysis, accompanied with a turning out of the pubis upon the external face of the ischium.[1]

§ 6. Congenital Dislocations of the Sternum.

Seger alone has reported one example of luxation of the xiphoid cartilage from the sternum.

A woman, in her fifth month of pregnancy, fell and dislocated her shoulder. Just four months after this, she was brought to bed with an infant, well formed, except that, soon after it was born, the ensiform cartilage was observed to be remarkably movable, especially when the child hiccoughed, to which it was very subject. The cartilage was separated from the sternum by the breadth of the little finger. No treatment was employed; the cartilage gradually became restored to its place, and in about one year it was firmly united to the sternum.[2]

§ 7. Congenital Dislocations of the Clavicle.

Malgaigne says that a congenital dislocation at the sterno-clavicular articulation has never been observed; but Guérin declares that he has established the existence of three varieties, namely:—

1. A luxation of the sternal end of the clavicle inwards and forwards; this extremity of the clavicle lying in front of the sternal fourchette. In illustration of which he presented to the Academy a

[1] Guérin, op. cit., p. 32.
[2] Seger, Ephem. Nat. Curios., 1677, from Malg., op. cit., p. 410.

plaster cast of a girl eight years old, in whom the displacement existed upon both sides.

2. Inwards and upwards. Observed by him in a girl eight years old; but which displacement took place only when the arm was moved, and through the contraction of the sterno-cleido-mastoideus muscle.

3. Backwards. Of which he presented two examples in the corresponding sides of a fœtal monster.

I believe I have already referred to Fergusson's case of dislocation of the sternal end of the clavicle forwards, which occurred during birth. The end rested in front of the sternum, and could be pushed into its place with great ease; but when left alone it immediately slipped out again. Nothing was done, a new joint formed, and the child afterwards possessed as much power in the one arm as in the other.[1]

Guérin says that he has seen a dislocation upwards and outwards at the acromial end of the clavicle in a fœtus of three months.

In regard to the treatment of either of these displacements of the clavicle, we need only remark that a reduction ought to be attempted: and, if practicable, without much confinement of the little patient, it should be maintained until the bones have become fixed in their natural positions. It is quite probable that this can never be accomplished, at least perfectly; but it will nevertheless be proper always to make the attempt.

§ 8. Congenital Dislocations of the Shoulder. (*Upper End of the Humerus.*)

Guérin affirms that he has established the existence of three varieties of scapulo-humeral dislocations, namely:—

1. Dislocation of the head of the humerus downwards; of which variety he presented to the Academy a plaster cast taken from a boy ten years old. The displacement existed in both arms, but much more pronounced in the right than in the left arm. It was due wholly to paralysis of the muscles about the joint, and to elongation of the capsule.

2. Downwards and inwards; complete upon one side and incomplete upon the other, in the same person. The head of each humerus was applied against the ribs, and the arms maintained in an abduction almost horizontal, under the influence of the retraction of the deltoid muscles. "The same case," Guérin remarks, "has been confirmed by Roux."

3. Subluxation upwards and outwards: seen on both sides in a fœtal monster, which was offered to the Academy for examination; and in one arm of a young man fifteen years old, of which Guérin presented a plaster cast. "It is characterized by a sliding of the head of the humerus in the direction indicated; this sliding being favored by a corresponding displacement of the coracoid and acromion processes."[2]

[1] Fergusson, System of Surg., 4th Amer. ed., 1853, p. 203.
[2] Guérin, op. cit., p. 30.

Malgaigne, who regards "all luxations in consequence of paralysis as essentially posterior to birth," will not admit the first example mentioned by Guérin; but, as we stated before, the objections made by Malgaigne have failed to convince us of the propriety of rejecting all of this class of reported examples. Of the second case, mentioned by Guérin as having been confirmed by Roux, Malgaigne declares that he has consulted Roux upon this matter, and that he affirms that "he has never seen a congenital luxation of the shoulder."

Robert Smith has met with but two of the forms of congenital luxation of the humerus described by Guérin, namely, that in which the head of the humerus is displaced forwards, and that in which it is displaced backwards. Of the first variety he has seen several examples.

The first was in the person of Alexander Steele, æt. 29, who presented both a dislocation of the head of the humerus under the coracoid process of the left scapula, and pes equinus in the foot of the left leg. The muscles of the arm and shoulder upon that side were feeble and greatly atrophied. The humerus was shortened; its head being of the natural size and form, but when the arm hung by the side it dropped so far from its socket as to permit the thumb to be placed between the head and the acromion process. By pressing the humerus forwards the finger could be placed in the outer part of the glenoid cavity; and, although the head could be moved about thus freely, it seemed naturally to occupy only the anterior half of the glenoid fossa.

Robert Smith's second example of subcoracoid congenital luxation was presented in the person of Mr. H., æt. 20, the condition of whose left shoulder resembled almost precisely that of Mr. Steele. "The deformity had existed from his birth, but became much more obvious and striking as he increased in age and stature."

In the third example the child had attained nearly the age of one year before the condition of the limb attracted attention, which was then excited, not by the deformity of the shoulder but by the atrophied condition of the muscles of the arm. The child had never complained of pain about the joint, nor had he ever met with any accident. No doubt this also was an example of paralysis, and it is not improbable that it was congenital, but the evidence upon this point is not very conclusive. When seen by Mr. Smith, he was nine years old, the shoulder and arm presenting the same appearance as in the other cases mentioned.

The fourth was also subcoracoid and symmetrical, the same deformity existing in both shoulders. This was in the person of a female, æt. 29, who had been for many years a patient in a lunatic asylum, and who died of chronic inflammation of the meninges of the brain.

Mr. Smith, who himself made the autopsy, first noticed the condition of the left shoulder. The muscles were atrophied; the head of the humerus could be felt lying under the coracoid process; the elbow projected from the side, but could be readily brought into contact with it. The right shoulder presented the same appearance, but the deformity was somewhat less, and the head of the humerus was not so directly underneath the coracoid process.

From the external appearances presented by the two shoulders, Mr. Smith did not doubt that these deviations from the natural state of the parts were not the result of violence.

Proceeding to remove the soft parts upon the left side, scarcely any trace was found of a glenoid cavity in its natural situation, but immediately underneath the coracoid process, upon the costal surface of the scapula, was formed an oblong socket completely surrounded by a capsular ligament, which ligament included also that small portion of the original socket which remained. The head of the humerus was changed in form, being oval, and fitted, in some measure, to both the old and new sockets upon which it seemed to rest alternately.

Upon the right side, although the condition of the bones was somewhat different, the characteristic features of the deformity were similar.

Malgaigne, who quotes Mr. Smith as saying that these dislocations must have been congenital, and for no other reason than because they were symmetrical, has scarcely done this author justice. Says Mr. Smith: "The position of the glenoid cavity, the remarkable form of the head of the humerus, the presence of a perfect glenoid ligament, the absence of any trace of disease, and the existence of the deformity upon each side, *all* indicate the original nature of the malformation."

The only example of backward luxation seen by Smith was also symmetrical, and seems to be equally well authenticated. This was in the person of a woman named Doyle, æt. 42, a lunatic also, who died Feb. 8, 1839, in Dublin. She had been a patient in the lunatic asylum fifteen years, and was subject to severe epileptic convulsions, which ultimately proved fatal.

Mr. Smith made the autopsy on the day following her death. The convolutions of the brain were small and atrophied, as is frequently observed in idiots.

The two shoulders resembled each other so perfectly, both in external appearance and in their anatomy, that Mr. Smith has only found it necessary to describe particularly the condition of one.

The coracoid process was remarkably prominent, but the acromion was not so prominent as in accidental dislocations of the shoulder. The head of the humerus could be seen and felt distinctly moving with the shaft, upon the dorsal surface of the scapula. On removing the integuments, muscles, &c., no trace of a glenoid cavity was found in its natural situation; but upon the external surface of the neck of the scapula was a well-formed socket, which received the head of the humerus. This socket was covered with cartilage of incrustation, and surrounded by a perfect capsule. The tendon of the biceps arose from the top and internal margin of the socket. The form of the acromion process was changed; the scapula smaller than natural; the head of the humerus irregularly oval, its anterior half alone being in contact with the glenoid cavity; the great tubercle natural, but the lesser was elongated and curved, forming a process of an inch in length, around the base of which the tendon of the biceps muscle played.[1]

Gaillard relates the case of a female child, upon whom the left arm was discovered to be deformed a few days after birth, and the elbow separated from the side. Later, the arm was found to be nearly immovable, and only at the end of four years was the dislocation recognized; but no attempt at reduction was then made. When sixteen years old, she was seen by Gaillard, who found the head of the humerus in the infra-spinous fossa. The scapula, clavicle, and arm were preternaturally small; the forearm, although well developed, could not be completely extended nor supinated.

Despite these unfavorable circumstances, Gaillard determined to make an attempt to accomplish the reduction. Four times in the space of eight days he submitted the arms to extension made at right angles with the body, by means of sixteen pound weights, the extension being continued from twenty to twenty-five minutes, and occasionally his own exertions being added to the weights. On the fourth attempt, the head of the bone was drawn gradually forwards, and by a rotatory motion it was finally made to slip into its socket; but it became immediately displaced. The next day Gaillard reduced it anew, and retained it in place one hour. Six days later it was again reduced, and, by the aid of bandages, permanently retained in place. The slight pain and swelling which followed soon disappeared; and, by the aid of careful exercise, at the end of two years the arm had increased in length, and the patient could use the arm and hand so much better than before, as to encourage a hope that the recovery would be complete.[2]

Aristide Rodrigue, of Hollidaysburg, Penn., in a letter to the editor of the *American Journal of Medical Sciences*, gives the following brief account of a case of intra-uterine dislocation of the shoulder, complicated with a fracture of the forearm.

"The woman when about four months gone with child, fell on her left side, striking a board, and felt herself much hurt at the time: at the full period she was delivered of a full-grown large boy with the following deformity: dislocation of the humerus into the axilla; fracture of both bones of forearm of left side, lower third. Dislocation could not be reduced; union of the bones of the forearm by ossific matter complete; bones passing each other, and hand at an angle of about 40°; the child did well otherwise; now, four years old, strong and healthy; humerus has grown nearly apace with the other; forearm has not, and remains short and deformed as at birth; the hand is of the same size with that of the sound side."[3]

[1] Robert Smith, op. cit.

[2] Gaillard, Mém. de l'Acad. de Méd., 1841, from Malg., p. 569.

[3] Rodrigue, loc. cit., Jan. 1854, p. 272.

§ 9. Congenital Dislocations of the Radius and Ulna Backwards.

It is not uncommon to meet with examples of a slight subluxation backwards of these bones in feeble and newly-born infants; which condition is probably due to a relaxation and elongation of the capsule. It is characterized by a preternatural mobility of the joint, and especially by the circumstance that the limb is capable of abnormal extension, or flexion backwards, as it is sometimes called. Guérin has seen this condition more advanced, the bones of the forearm having actually overlapped somewhat upon the lower end of the humerus, so that the articular surface of this latter, presented itself in the fold of the elbow. This was especially observed in a girl of fourteen and a boy of thirteen years, and also in the two arms of a fœtal monster.[1]

Chaussier relates that a young woman at the commencement of the ninth month of pregnancy, perceived suddenly movements of the fœtus so violent that she almost lost her consciousness. These movements were repeated three times in the space of six minutes, after which everything returned to its natural order, and the accouchement took place naturally and at the usual term. The infant was pale and feeble, and presented a complete backward luxation of the radius and ulna.[2]

§ 10. Congenital Dislocations of the Head of the Radius.

Examples of this luxation have been reported by Dupuytren, Cruveilhier, Sandifort, Adams, Dubois, Verneuil, Deville, Robert Smith, and Guérin, most of which were in the direction backwards, some outwards, but only one of them forwards; some were double, the same deformity being presented in both arms, and others were single. In a few examples the dislocations were complicated with a consolidation of the radius to the ulna, and in others with a deficiency of the ulna or with some deformity indicating its congenital origin.

Of the symmetrical or double dislocation backwards Dupuytren furnishes the following example, presented to him in 1830, by M. Loir: "The abnormal position which the head of either radius had assumed was at the back part of the lower extremity of the humerus, beyond which it extended for the space of at least an inch. This disposition of parts was absolutely identical on the two sides, and had all the characters of a congenital affection."[3]

In the example of outward luxation, mentioned by Deville, there was an almost complete absence of the ulna, the head of the radius mounting upwards more than three *centimetres* above the level of the articulation.[4]

Guérin, who has described the only example of a forward luxation, says it was observed by him in a girl of seven years, and that it was

[1] Guérin, op. cit., p. 31. [2] Chaussier, from Malgaigne, op. cit., t. ii. p. 268.
[3] Dupuytren, Injuries and Dis. of Bones, p. 117.
[4] Deville, Bulletins de la Soc. Anat., 1849, p. 153.

symmetrical. The two radii lay in front of the humeri near the coronary fossettes.[1]

§ 11. Congenital Dislocations of the Wrist.

Guérin thinks he has seen three forms of congenital luxation of the wrist. First, a dislocation forwards characterized by a sliding of the wrist before the bones of the forearm, and by the projection posteriorly of the lower ends of the radius and ulna; seen in an infant of six months, and in two adults. Second, backwards and upwards; seen in a child of six years, and accompanied with an incomplete paralysis of all the muscles of the forearm and hand. Third, backwards and outwards; in a girl of fourteen years, accompanied with incomplete paralysis.[2]

Guérin has also seen three examples of dislocation outwards in fœtal monsters, and one of dislocation inwards, as the result of arrest of development.

Robert Smith believes that the case of simple dislocation of the wrist or of the carpus forwards, mentioned by Cruveilhier in his *Anatomie Pathologique*, was an example of congenital luxation; and he relates two other cases equally remarkable which came under his own observation. One was in the person of Deborah O'Neil, a lunatic and epileptic, who died when thirty-six years old. Both upper extremities were deformed from birth; the right presenting an example of dislocation of the carpus forwards, and the left of dislocation of the carpus backwards. The dissection showed that there had been an arrest of development, especially in the bones of the forearm and carpus. The second was in the person of a young woman who died of phthisis in the Richmond Hospital; the right wrist presenting an example of congenital dislocation of the carpus forwards from arrest of development also.[3]

Marrigues describes a very singular congenital displacement which he found upon a newly-born infant. The radius and ulna were widely separated below, and in the interspace was lodged the whole of the first range of the carpal bones; the hand being strongly turned inwards.[4]

§ 12. Congenital Dislocations of the Fingers.

Chaussier found in a fœtus the last three fingers of the left hand dislocated at the metacarpo-phalangeal articulation. The thighs, knees, and feet were also dislocated.[5]

A. Bérard speaks of an incurvation backwards of the last two phalanges of the fingers as having been occasionally seen in newly-born children of the female sex; and Malgaigne adds that he has himself

[1] Guérin, op. cit., p. 31. [2] Ibid., p. 717.
[3] R. Smith, op. cit., pp. 238, 251.
[4] Marrigues, Malgaigne, from Journ. de Méd., 1775, t. ii. p. 31.
[5] Chaussier, Malgaigne, op. cit., t. ii. p. 751.

seen a woman who had, from birth, all the *phalangettes* carried backwards to an angle of 135°, leaving the heads of the phalanges projecting forwards under the skin.[1]

Robert has seen, in a girl six years old, a congenital lateral luxation of the *phalangette* of the index finger, which was inclined outwards at an obtuse angle. The external condyle of the lower extremity of the proximal phalanx was slightly atrophied, and the internal presented a corresponding projection. Robert cut the internal lateral ligament by a subcutaneous incision, but without any favorable result.[2]

§ 13. Congenital Dislocations of the Hip.

Dupuytren thought that double dislocations of the hip-joint, as congenital accidents, were more common than single dislocations, but in the experience of Pravaz the rule has been reversed, he having met with but four double dislocations in a total of nineteen.

Congenital dislocations of the femur have been noticed much oftener in females than in males. Of forty-five examples mentioned by Dupuytren and Pravaz, only seven or eight were males.

They may be complete or incomplete. Of the complete luxations, four varieties have been noticed.

Upwards and backwards, upon the dorsum ilii. This variety is by far the most common.

Upwards and forwards; the head of the femur resting upon the eminentia ilio-pectinea.

Downwards and forwards into the foramen thyroideum; of which variety Chaussier alone mentions one example; but Delpech found in an infant, born paralytic, the head of the femur lodged habitually *near* the foramen thyroideum.

Directly upwards; seen by Guérin, Pravaz, and others; the head of the femur being placed immediately without the anterior inferior spinous process of the ilium.

Guérin has observed, moreover, a single variety of subluxation; characterized by the incomplete displacement of the head of the femur in the direction upwards and backwards, so that it rested upon the edge of the cotyloid cavity: "Observed often in newly-born children, and with those in whom the muscular dislocations are effected spontaneously after birth."

Both Delpech and Guérin have called attention to two varieties of what the latter terms, pseudo-luxations; of which the first simulates a dislocation upwards and backwards, and the second a dislocation downwards and forwards. In these examples, the extreme adduction or abduction of the thighs might lead to a belief that the bones were dislocated, when in fact the abnormal position of the limbs are due only to muscular contraction, without actual articular displacement.

In the remarks which follow, we shall have special reference to that form of congenital dislocation of the femur in which the head of the

[1] Bérard, Malgaigne, op. cit., p. 773.

[2] Robert, from Malg., op. cit., p. 773.

bone rests upon the dorsum ilii, as being that which will be presented in a vast majority of cases, and which, characterized by the same general phenomena, may be regarded as typical of all the others.

Symptomatology.—First. When the dislocation is double.

In these examples the deformity is often found to be symmetrical; the opposite limbs being of precisely the same length, and in the same relative positions; a circumstance which, when it exists, may render the diagnosis more difficult, or may cause it to be for a long time entirely overlooked. It is in such cases especially, that the deformity is not usually discovered until the child begins to walk.

The first circumstance which would naturally arrest our attention, if the person who is the subject of this double dislocation is stripped and placed erect before us, is the great apparent length of the arms and of the body in comparison with the lower extremities. We may next observe that the great trochanters are carried upwards and backwards, so as to make a remarkable projection in this direction; the lumbar portion of the spinal column is thrown very much forwards, and the dorsal portion backwards. The thighs incline inwards, so as almost to cross each other; the whole of the lower extremities are imperfectly developed and feeble, the toes are generally pointed directly forwards, or they may be noticed to turn inwards.

When the person stands, and his limbs are not in motion, the heel is usually brought down fairly to the floor; but in walking, and especially in the attempt to run, he touches only the balls and toes of his feet. "When they are about to walk," says Pravaz, "we see them lift themselves upon the points of the feet, to incline the superior part of the trunk toward the member which is about to support the weight of the body, and to lift the other from the ground with an effort, in order to carry it forwards. At this moment one of the trochanters, that which corresponds to the column of sustentation, appears to approach the iliac crest more nearly than when the patient is standing upon his two feet." In consequence of which mobility of the thigh-bones, the patient assumes a peculiar waddling gait, which is not only ungraceful but exceedingly fatiguing.

The difficulty of progression is, however, very variable in different persons. Sometimes the patient requires no aid whatever, and at other times he cannot walk without assistance. Generally it increases with age. It is especially deserving of notice that in rapid progression the mobility of the heads of the femurs is appreciably less than in slow progression, which is explained by the more constant and vigorous contraction of the muscles about the joint, when the motions of the limb are rapid.

In the recumbent posture, the thighs may be drawn down easily to almost their natural positions. The only exception to this rule, according to Carnochan, "is when the head of the femur has escaped from the natural capsule in which it was originally inclosed, and a new socket has been formed upon the dorsum of the ilium."

Abduction is performed with difficulty; adduction and rotation, especially inwards, being less restricted.

Second. When the dislocation is only upon one side.

In these cases the symptoms are essentially the same as in the double dislocation; with only such slight differences and peculiarities as would naturally suggest themselves to the surgeon, and which will not, therefore, demand from us a special consideration.

Pathology.—The head of the femur is sometimes merely changed in form and consistence, the neck also undergoing corresponding alterations in its size, form, direction, &c.; at other times the head is absent altogether, and with it a considerable portion, or the whole of the neck has disappeared.

The pelvic bones are usually more or less deformed. The acetabulum may be entirely deficient, or it may present itself as an irregular bony protuberance, without cartilage, fibro-cartilage, or ligaments. Sometimes it exists as an oval or triangular cavity, which is expanded at its superior and posterior margin into a distinct fossa, where the head of the femur, descending from the dorsum ilii, occasionally rests A new cavity is formed usually upon the side of the pelvis, which is shallow and without an elevated margin, or it may be deeper, and more complete in its construction, by the addition of an osseous border. In either case, the new socket is often lined with a true periosteum and synovial membrane; but not unfrequently it is unprotected by any soft tissue, the surface being hard and polished like ivory.

The head of the femur, having escaped from its original capsule, through a button-like opening, rests in this socket constantly. In still other examples the head of the femur remains within its capsule, and may be observed to play backwards and forwards between the two sockets; or the head and neck being absorbed, and the capsule remaining entire, the latter is converted into a long narrow sac, somewhat contracted in its centre, or finally into a firm ligamentous cord, which, being attached to the stunted upper extremity of the femur, limits its motions in the direction of the crest of the ilium. In this case no new socket is formed.

A portion of the pelvi-femoral muscles are contracted, in consequence of an approximation of their points of origin and insertion, and remaining in a state of comparative, if not absolute, inertia, they become atrophied, or pass into a condition of fatty degeneration, while other muscles, in consequence of the increased labor which they have to perform, become hypertrophied, or degenerate into a fibrous tissue.

Treatment.—Says Dupuytren: "Of what possible utility can it be to practice extension of the lower extremities in these cases, even supposing the limbs could be thus brought to their natural length? Is it not evident that the head of the femur, finding no cavity fitted to receive and hold it, would, when abandoned to itself, resume its former abnormal position? There is something more rational and feasible in adopting a palliative course of treatment. When we call to mind the natural proneness which the heads of thigh-bones have to ascend to the external iliac fossæ, and that this tendency is partly due to the superincumbent weight of the body, and in part to muscular action, a just conception may be formed of the indications on which the employment of palliative remedies should be founded. The object should be to relieve the lower limbs of the superincumbent weight, on the one hand, and on the other to moderate the muscular action. Both of these indications are in part fulfilled by repose; and the attitude most conducive to this effect is the sitting posture, in which the weight of the upper part of the body is not transmitted to the lower extremities, but is centred in the tuberosities of the ischia. Therefore, laboring persons afflicted with this infirmity should be recommended to adopt a sedentary occupation, as a calling which requires much standing and walking about would dangerously aggravate their deformity. Yet one would scarcely be willing to condemn such individuals to perpetual repose; and to avoid this it is necessary to discover some means for diminishing the inconveniences which attend the upright posture, the act of walking, and other exercises. Experience has taught me hitherto but two methods of obtaining this important object: the first consists in the daily employment of a perfectly cold bath, in which all the body should be immersed for the space of three or four minutes, the head being protected by an oiled-silk cap; the water may be fresh or salt; and the only precautions necessary to take are to avoid bathing when the body is in a state of perspiration, or when the catamenial discharge is present. These baths have a local, as well as general, tonic effect. The second method consists in the constant use, at least during the day, of a belt, which embraces the pelvis, fitting closely over the great trochanters, and keeping them at a constant height, so as to bind the parts together, and prevent that continual unsteadiness of the body which results from the loose connections of the heads of the thigh-bones. For the proper fulfilment of these indications, certain precautions are necessary in the construction of this cincture; in the first place, it should occupy the narrow interval between the crest of the ilium and great trochanters, completely filling this space, and therefore being about three or four fingers' breadth, according to the age and size of the patient. It should further be well padded with wool or cotton, and covered with doe-skin, so that it may not abrade the parts to which it is applied; and there should be a piece let in on either side, so as to receive and support the trochanters without entirely covering them; it should be buckled behind, and padded straps be carried under the thigh, and across the tuberosity of the ischium, on either side, to prevent the zone from slipping up. I do not mean to assert that I have ever succeeded in completely getting rid of the inconveniences of congenital dislocations of the thigh-bones, but I have prevented their increasing, and have rendered supportable what I could not cure. The testimony of some patients to the value of this treatment has been of a most unequivocal character; for, being worried by the pressure of the belt, they have laid it aside, but have speedily restored it again, as they found that without it they had neither a sense of firmness in the hip, nor confidence in walking."

In relation to which opinions the same excellent writer subsequently made the following candid admissions: "I at first thought that no benefit would be derived in these cases from the employment of continual traction on the lower extremities, for reasons already stated; but the experiments of MM. Lafond and Duval tend to throw some doubt on the correctness of this conclusion. These distinguished practitioners tested the influence of extension, in their orthopædic institution, on a child eight or nine years of age, who was the subject of double congenital dislocation of the hip; after the uninterrupted employment of this treatment for some weeks, I satisfied myself that the limbs had resumed their natural length and direction; but I was not a little astonished to find that, after extension had been persisted in for three or four months continuously, the greater part of the beneficial results remained for several weeks undiminished. It would be idle, it is true, to generalize on this single case; but as an isolated example of the utility of extension it is interesting, and it may be the forerunner of more important results."[1]

Since which time Humbert and Jacquier, who, as well as Duval and Lafond, confined themselves to the treatment of deformities, claim to have met with equal success in the management of these cases by extension alone; and, still more lately, Guérin, of Paris, and Pravas, of Lyons, by the adoption of the same general principle more or less modified, have added new triumphs, and greatly enlarged its application.

The means recommended and practiced by Guérin, are: first, preparatory extension destined to elongate the muscles as much as possible; second, subcutaneous section of the muscles which mechanical extension has not sufficiently elongated; third, extension of the ligaments, and even, if extension does not suffice, their subcutaneous section; fourth, manœuvres destined to effect reduction; fifth, treatment designed to consolidate the reduction, and consisting in the application of the apparatus proper to maintain the extension and separation of the divided tissues, and to retain the head of the femur in its place; finally, in the gradual execution of movements proper to complete the coaptation of the surfaces, and to establish little by little the physiological movements of the joint.

Other surgeons have confined their efforts to the reduction of the dislocation, and they have, consequently abandoned all those cases in which, owing to the complete absence of the natural socket, or to the want of sufficient mobility in the limb, the reduction was deemed impossible; but Guérin has gone a step farther, and has sought to establish a new socket upon some point of the pelvic bones as near as possible to its natural articular fossa. "The means which I adopt," says Guérin, "are based upon a recognition of the processes which nature employs for the attainment of the same purpose, and of which mine are but an imitation. I have shown that the essential condition of the formation of artificial cavities is perforation of the articular capsule, and the placing in contact of the luxated extremity with an osseous surface, and that the condition of the maintenance of this abnormal rapport is the intimate adherence of the borders of the rent with the circumference of the new cavity. Now it appeared to me that art could realize, in all points, the conditions which preside at the spontaneous formation of artificial joints. To this end I commence by practicing under the skin, and at the point corresponding to that where

[1] Dupuytren, op. cit., pp. 176–8.

it is most convenient to fix the luxated extremity, scarifications of the capsule, down to the bone to which it is attached. By this means the dislocated extremity is placed in immediate contact with the bony surface upon which it reposes. It makes upon this point a beginning of the work of organization resulting from the adhesion and fusion of the scarified points with the corresponding points of this surface. Then, in order to circumscribe and imprison the luxated extremity, in this place of election, I practice all about deep scarifications, which tend to excite the same work of organization and to establish fibro-cellular adhesions between the incised borders of the capsule and the contiguous bony surfaces.

"Finally, when the fibro-cellular adhesions are supposed to be sufficiently solid to resist the movements of the new articulation, I provoke, little by little, the development of the cavity destined to embrace the luxated extremity by the means which nature herself employs in analogous circumstances; that is to say, by circumscribed and frequent movements of this articulation."[1]

The treatment ought to be commenced as early as possible, no examples of success having been recorded in persons over fifteen years of age; while the youngest child whose treatment is reported as successful was three years of age.

For the purpose of making the requisite extension, and of maintaining the bone in place, Pravaz (who does not, however, adopt Guérin's practice of establishing for the head of the bone a new socket, but only seeks to reduce and maintain it in its old socket) has invented several forms of apparatus adapted to the different stages of progress in the treatment. Heine, of Cannstadt, Guérin, and others have also suggested special contrivances for the same purpose; but no surgeon who understands fully the principle upon which the cure is supposed to be accomplished, will be at a loss for apparatus suitable for making the necessary extension, or for maintaining the reduction when once it has been effected.

The length of time required for the completion of a cure, where a cure is possible, must vary according to the age and health of the patient, and according to the pathological condition of the joint, and may be found to extend from a few months to one or more years. It is unnecessary to say that where the accomplishment of the cure demands a period of several years, the treatment must be intermittent and greatly varied, so as to suit all the changing circumstances in the condition of the patient.

Finally, if after a fair trial we fail to accomplish a cure, or if the condition of the child will not warrant even the attempt, we ought as far as possible to seek to prevent an increase of the deformity, by such means as our ingenuity may suggest, or by such judicious appliances and general management as we have seen recommended by Dupuytren.

South says that he has seen one case of double dislocation in which the walking was at first extremely difficult, but from the fifteenth

[1] Guérin, op. cit., pp. 81–3.

year and onwards the patient so improved, that at the twentieth year scarcely any trace of the peculiar gait could be discovered.[1]

§ 14. Congenital Dislocations of the Patella.

Palletta found a dislocation of the patella in the cadaver of a young man, which he supposed to be congenital.[2] Michaëlis has reported two cases; one in a young man of seventeen years, and the other in a girl of fourteen, each of whom affirmed that it had existed from birth.[3] Both of these examples presented themselves at the hospital on account of hydrarthrosis of the knee-joints, and Malgaigne, who had himself seen a similar case, is disposed to regard them all as examples of pathological rather than congenital luxations. Périat reports a case in which the dislocation was only produced by walking, and in relation to the authenticity or pertinence of which Malgaigne seems also to entertain a doubt.[4]

South says that he has seen a congenital dislocation on both legs, in an aged man. The patella rested entirely upon the outer faces of the external condyles, leaving the front of the knee-joint completely uncovered. When the limbs were extended the patellæ could be easily made to resume their natural positions, but on the patient's making the slightest movement they were again displaced. The knees were very much inclined inwards, the feet outwards, and his gait was difficult and unsteady.[5]

§ 15. Congenital Dislocations of the Knee.

The head of the tibia has been found, at birth, dislocated forwards, backwards, inwards, outwards, inwards and backwards, outwards and backwards, and simply rotated inwards.

Most of these luxations were incomplete; and of them all, the dislocation forwards has been observed much the most often.

A subluxation forwards of the head of the tibia has been seen by Guérin in a fœtal monster, accompanied with extreme retraction of the extensor muscles of the leg.[6] Cruveilhier has dissected a fœtus affected with a similar subluxation.[7]

In these examples the displacement forwards at the articular surface was but slight, and the anterior flexion of the limb inconsiderable; but when the dislocation is complete, or nearly so, the deformity is in all respects very much increased; as the following examples will illustrate:—

Dr. D. H. Bard, of Troy, Vermont, has reported an example of

[1] South, Note to Chelius, op. cit., vol. ii. p. 245.
[2] Palletta, Exercitationes Pathologicæ, p. 91.
[3] Michaëlis, Rev. Méd. Chirurg., tom. xv. p. 56.
[4] Périat, Malgaigne, op. cit., tom. ii. p. 932.
[5] South, Note to Chelius, op. cit., vol ii. p. 247. [6] Guérin, op. cit., p. 33.
[7] Cruveilhier, Atlas de l'Anat. Patholog., 2e livr., pl. 2.

complete anterior luxation of the tibia, seen by himself, in a new-born infant. The leg was found drawn forwards upon the thigh at an acute angle, so that the toes pointed toward the face of the child, and the bottom of the foot was directed forwards. By the application of moderate force, the limb could be straightened and even flexed completely. These motions inflicted no pain. It was especially noticed that in bringing down the leg from its position of extreme anterior flexion (extension) more force was required in the first part of the manœuvre than in the last; and that if, having brought the leg down, it was left to itself, it immediately resumed the abnormal position, moving at first slowly, but after a time much more rapidly.

The limb was confined by bandages for a short time, and it did not afterwards show any disposition to return to its unnatural position. The child did well, and when it began to use its legs, no difference could be discovered between them.[1]

Chatelain was consulted in relation to a similar case, in which the restoration of the limb to its natural position was also easily effected, and by means of three metallic splints, applied during about fifteen days, the cure was consummated. Chatelain directed, however, that the leg should be kept flexed upon the thigh eight days longer.[2]

Kleeberg found a child with the leg so much flexed forwards (extended) upon the thigh that the popliteal region became the lowest point of the limb; in front and above the articular extremity of the tibia could be felt, and the condyles of the femur made a corresponding projection behind into the popliteal space. This was plainly an example of complete luxation; and, contrary to what was observed in Bard's case, flexion of the limb backwards was difficult and painful.

The treatment was commenced by securing the limb in a straight position by means of a splint and roller; subsequently, Kleeberg carried the limb back to an obtuse angle, and finally, it was kept eight days in a position of extreme flexion. A complete cure was said to have been accomplished in about two weeks.[3]

Guérin has seen a subluxation backwards, accompanied with a slight rotation of the head of the tibia outwards, in a girl fourteen years old; and which, he affirms, was congenital, characterized by a permanent flexion (backwards) of the leg upon the thigh, and a sliding of the condyles of the tibia backwards.

This girl was under Guérin's treatment, but with what result is not stated.[4]

Chaussier found both tibiæ displaced backwards in an infant otherwise deformed.[5]

Robert speaks of an example of lateral subluxation in a man, which had existed from birth. The right knee was thrown inwards, and the left outwards.[6]

Guérin "operated" publicly upon a child, two years old, who had a

[1] Bard, Amer. Journ. Med. Sci., Feb. 1835, p. 555, from Bost. Med. and Surg. Journ., Nov. 26, 1834.

[2] Chatelain, Bibliothèque Méd., tom. lxxv. p. 85.

[3] Kleeberg, Malgaigne, op. cit., p. 983.

[4] Guérin, sur les Lux. Congén., p. 33.

[5] Chaussier, Malgaigne, op. cit., p. 984.

[6] Robert, Malg., op. cit., p. 985.

congenital dislocation of the head of the tibia backwards and inwards, accompanied with a slight rotation of the leg inwards.[1] In what manner he operated, and with what result, he does not inform us.

The same writer speaks of a subluxation backwards and outwards, with rotation in the same direction, a deformity which, he affirms, is very frequent, and which appears especially after birth, although the causes which produce it have given their first impulse during intra-uterine life.

The case quoted from Robert, by Malgaigne, as an example of dislocation inwards, seems to have been rather a case of semi-rotation of the articular surfaces, the inner condyle being thrown back into the popliteal space, while the outer condyle still retained its natural position.

§ 16. Congenital Dislocations of the Tarsal Bones.

Under this general term may be included all those varieties of subluxation of the several bones which compose the tarsus, and which are known as examples of talipes or club-foot; such as tibio-astragaloid luxations, astragalo-scaphoid, calcaneo-astragaloid, calcaneo-cuboid, &c.

Although these deformities may properly enough claim a place in a chapter on congenital dislocations, they have so long been the subjects of special treatises as to justify their exclusion from the present volume.

§ 17. Congenital Dislocations of the Toes.

Observed occasionally at the metatarso-phalangeal articulations; the articular facets of the first phalanges suffering a subluxation upwards, or laterally upon the corresponding metatarsal bones.

Guérin has noticed especially a congenital, lateral subluxation of the great toe.[2]

[1] Guérin, sur les Lux. Congén., p. 33.

[2] Guérin, op. cit., p. 34.

INDEX.

PART I.—FRACTURES.

PART II.—DISLOCATIONS.

THE END.

ERRATA.

Page 86, line 20, *for* "one hundred and four fractures," *read* "twelve partial fractures."
" " " 31, *for* "Symes," *read* "Syme."
" 269, 270, 272, and 273, *for* "proned" and "supined," *read* "pronated" and "supinated."

NORMAN PUBLISHING ®

Collaborators on the production of *A Practical Treatise on Fractures and Dislocations*:

Jill Lustig, Project Manager
Seventeenth Street Studios, Designer
Martha Nicholson Steele, Editor
Technical Publications, Electronic Page Composition
Thomson-Shore, Printer and Binder

The display and text type for the new Introduction is Bodoni, a Postscript font from Adobe Systems.

The edition is limited to 750 copies.

79.95 limited edition
(THIS 1991 REPRINT EDITION
(@ 95.00)
20863